A Lange Medical Book

INTERNAL MEDICINE ON CALL

Third Edition

P9-CES-259

Edited by

Steven A. Haist, MD, MS, FACP
Professor of Medicine
Division of General Internal Medicine
Department of Internal Medicine
University of Kentucky Medical Center
Lexington, Kentucky

John B. Robbins, MD
General Internist
Private Practice
Internal Medicine Associates
Bozeman, Montana

Series Editor
Leonard G. Gomella, MD
The Bernard W. Godwin, Jr. Associate Professor of Prostate Cancer
Department of Urology
Jefferson Medical College
Thomas Jefferson University Medical Center
Philadelphia, Pennsylvania

Lange Medical Books/McGraw-Hill
Medical Publishing Division

New York Chicago San Francisco Lisbon London
Madrid Mexico City Milan New Delhi San Juan
Seoul Singapore Sydney Toronto

McGraw-Hill
A Division of The McGraw-Hill Companies

Internal Medicine On Call, Third Edition

Copyright © 2002 by the **McGraw-Hill Companies, Inc.** All rights reserved. Printed in the United States of America. Except as permitted under the United States Copyright Act of 1976, no part of this publication may be reproduced or distributed in any form or by any means, or stored in a data base or retrieval system, without the prior written permission of the publisher.

Previous editions copyright © 1997 and 1991 by Appleton & Lange

1234567890 DOC/DOC 98765432
ISSN:1052-6854
ISBN: 0-8385-4278-6

Notice

Medicine is an ever-changing science. As new research and clinical experience broaden our knowledge, changes in treatment and drug therapy are required. The authors and the publisher of this work have checked with sources believed to be reliable in their efforts to provide information that is complete and generally in accord with the standards accepted at the time of publication. However, in view of the possibility of human error or changes in medical sciences, neither the authors nor the publisher nor any other party who has been involved in the preparation or publication of this work warrants that the information contained herein is in every respect accurate or complete, and they disclaim all responsibility for any errors or omissions or for the results obtained from use of the information contained in this work. Readers are encouraged to confirm the information contained herein with other sources. For example and in particular, readers are advised to check the product information sheet included in the package of each drug they plan to administer to be certain that the information contained in this work is accurate and that changes have not been made in the recommended dose or in the contraindications for administration. This recommendation is of particular importance in connection with new or infrequently used drugs.

The book was set in Helvetica by Pine Tree Composition, Inc.
The editors were Janet Foltin, Harriet Lebowitz, and Regina Y. Brown.
The production supervisor was Richard Ruzycka.
The index was prepared by Katherine Pitcoff.
The art manager was Charissa Baker.

R.R. Donnelley & Sons Company was the printer and binder.

This book was printed on acid-free paper.

INTERNATIONAL EDITION ISBN 0–07–121235–3
Copyright © 2002. Exclusive rights by the McGraw-Hill Companies, Inc., for manufacture and export. This book cannot be re-exported from the country to which it is consigned by McGraw-Hill. The international Edition is not available in North America.

Contents

GALANTI

Associate Editors viii
Contributors x
Preface xix

I. On-Call Problems 1
1. Abdominal Pain 1
2. Acidosis 9
3. Alkalosis 18
4. Anaphylactic Reaction 24
5. Anemia 27
6. Arterial Line Problems 34
7. Aspiration 36
8. Bradycardia 39
9. Cardiopulmonary Arrest 44
10. Central Venous Line Problems 53
11. Chest Pain 57
12. Coagulopathy 66
13. Coma, Acute Mental Status Changes 72
14. Constipation 82
15. Cough 86
16. Delirium Tremens (DTs): Major Alcohol Withdrawal 90
17. Diarrhea 97
18. Dizziness 104
19. Dyspnea 111
20. Dysuria 117
21. Falls 122
22. Fever 127
23. Fever in the HIV-Positive Patient 135
24. Foley Catheter Problems 141
25. Headache 143
26. Heart Murmur 151
27. Hematemesis, Melena 158
28. Hematochezia 162
29. Hematuria 166
30. Hemoptysis 170
31. Hypercalcemia 175
32. Hyperglycemia 180

33. Hyperkalemia 186
34. Hypernatremia 190
35. Hypertension 194
36. Hypocalcemia 198
37. Hypoglycemia 202
38. Hypokalemia 206
39. Hypomagnesemia 210
40. Hyponatremia 214
41. Hypophosphatemia 220
42. Hypotension (Shock) 224
43. Hypothermia 229
44. Insomnia 234
45. Irregular Pulse 238
46. Jaundice 242
47. Joint Swelling 245
48. Leukocytosis 251
49. Leukopenia 255
50. Nausea & Vomiting 261
51. Oliguria/Anuria 266
52. Overdoses 274
53. Pacemaker Troubleshooting 283
54. Pain Management 287
55. Polycythemia 291
56. Pruritus 296
57. Pulmonary Artery Catheter Problems 303
58. Seizures 308
59. Syncope 315
60. Tachycardia 323
61. Thrombocytopenia 333
62. Transfusion Reaction 338
63. Wheezing 341

II. Laboratory Diagnosis 345
III. Procedures 390

1. Arterial Line Placement 390
2. Arterial Puncture 391
3. Arthrocentesis (Diagnostic & Therapeutic) 392
4. Bladder Catheterization 394
5. Bone Marrow Aspiration & Biopsy 397
6. Central Venous Catheterization 399
7. Endotracheal Intubation 407
8. Gastrointestinal Tubes 410
9. Intravenous Techniques 411
10. Lumbar Puncture 412

11. Paracentesis 418
12. Pulmonary Artery Catheterization 421
13. Skin Biopsy 430
14. Thoracentesis 431
IV. Fluids & Electrolytes 435
V. Blood Component Therapy 437
VI. Ventilator Management 442
1. Indications & Setup 442
2. Routine Modification of Settings 447
3. Troubleshooting 448
A. Agitation 448
B. Hypoxemia 450
C. Hypercarbia 454
D. High Peak Pressures 456
4. Weaning 458
VII. Therapeutics 461
1. Classes of Generic Drugs, Minerals, Natural Products, & Vitamins 462
2. Generic Drugs: Indications, Actions, Dosage, Supplied, & Notes 470
3. Minerals: Indications/Effects, RDA/Dosage, Signs/Symptoms of Deficiency and Toxicity, and Other 589
4. Natural Products: Uses, Dose, Cautions, Adverse Effects, and Drug Interactions 590
5. Vitamins: Indications/Effects, RDA/Dosage, Signs/Symptoms of Deficiency and Toxicity, and Other 594
6. Tables 597

Appendix 618
Table A–1. Fahrenheit/centigrade temperature conversion 618
Table A–2. Pounds/kilograms weight conversion 619
Table A–3. Glasgow Coma Scale 619
Figure A–1. Calculating body surface area 620
Table A–4. Endocarditis prophylaxis 621
Table A–5. Specimen tubes for venipuncture 622

Index 623

Commonly Used Resuscitation Drugs and Techniques ..... Inside front and back covers

Associate Editors

Aimee G. Adams, PharmD
Ambulatory Care Specialist
Assistant Professor
College of Pharmacy
University of Kentucky
Lexington, Kentucky

James A. Barker, MD
Scott & White Clinic
Associate Professor
Pulmonary & Critical Care Medicine
Texas A & M College of Medicine
Temple, Texas

David P. Haynie, MD
Cardiovascular Specialist, PA
Private Practice
Lewisville, Texas

William J. John, MD
Senior Clinical Research Physician
US Affiliate, Oncology
Eli Lilly Company
Lexington, Kentucky

Rita K. Munn, MD
Associate Professor
Division of Hematology and Oncology
Department of Internal Medicine
University of Kentucky Medical Center
Lexington, Kentucky

Kelly M. Smith, PharmD
Drug Information Specialist
Clinical Associate Professor
College of Pharmacy
University of Kentucky
Lexington, Kentucky

Benjamin J. Stahr, MD, FCAP
Pathologist
Greensboro Pathology Associates
Moses H. Cone Memorial Hospital
Greensboro, North Carolina

Contributors

Aimee G. Adams, PharmD
Ambulatory Care Specialist
Assistant Professor
College of Pharmacy
University of Kentucky
Lexington, Kentucky

David A. Adkins, MD
Fellow
Division of Pulmonary and Critical Care Medicine
Department of Internal Medicine
University of Kentucky Medical Center
Lexington, Kentucky

Jerri L. Alley, MD
Dermatologist
Private Practice
Harrisonburg Dermatology
Harrisonburg, Virginia

James A. Barker, MD
Scott & White Clinic
Associate Professor
Pulmonary & Critical Care Medicine
Texas A & M College of Medicine
Temple, Texas

Donald R. Barnett, MD
Primary Care
Veterans Administration Medical Center
Topeka, Kansas

P. Ricky Bass, MD
Assistant Professor
Departments of Internal Medicine and Pediatrics
University of Louisville
Louisville, Kentucky

David J. Bensema, MD
General Internist
Private Practice
Lexington, Kentucky

Rolando Berger, MD
Professor of Medicine
Division of Pulmonary and Critical Care Medicine
Department of Internal Medicine
University of Kentucky Medical Center
Lexington, Kentucky

Larry T. Breeding, MD
Cardiologist
Private Practice
Cardiology Associates of East Tennessee
Knoxville, Tennessee

Eric W. Byrd, MD
General Internist
Private Practice
Hendersonville Internists, Inc.
Hendersonville, North Carolina

Robert T. Davis, MD
Associate Professor of Medicine
Division of General Internal Medicine
Department of Internal Medicine
University of Kentucky Medical Center
Lexington, Kentucky

David W. Dozer, MD
Gastroenterologist
Private Practice
Milwaukee Digestive Diseases Consultants, SP
Milwaukee, Wisconsin

Rita M. Egan, MD, PhD
Rheumatologist
Private Practice
Bluegrass Rheumatology Associates
Lexington, Kentucky

G. Paul Eleazer, MD
Professor of Medicine
Department of Internal Medicine
University of South Carolina
Columbia, South Carolina

Kim R. Emmett, MD
Assistant Professor
Division of General Medicine
Section Chief of Geriatrics
Department of Medicine
University of Tennessee Graduate School of Medicine
Knoxville, Tennessee

Joan B. Fowler, PharmD, BCPP, CGP
Creative Educational Concepts, Inc.
Lexington, Kentucky

David K. Goebel, MD
Hematologist/Oncologist
Private Practice
Tri-State Regional Cancer Center
Ashland, Kentucky

John J. Gohmann, MD
Medical Oncologist
Private Practice
Central Baptist Hospital
Lexington, Kentucky

Leonard G. Gomella, MD
The Bernard W. Godwin, Jr. Associate Professor of Prostate Cancer
Department of Urology
Jefferson Medical College
Thomas Jefferson University Medical Center
Philadelphia, Pennsylvania

Tricia L. Gomella, MD
Assistant Professor, Part-time
Division of Neonatology
Department of Pediatrics
Johns Hopkins University
Baltimore, Maryland

Steven A. Haist, MD, MS, FACP
Professor of Medicine
Division of General Internal Medicine
Department of Internal Medicine
University of Kentucky Medical Center
Lexington, Kentucky

David P. Haynie, MD
Cardiovascular Specialist PA
Private Practice
Lewisville, Texas

David M. Hiestand, MD
Medicine/Pediatrics Resident
Department of Internal Medicine and
Department of Pediatrics
University of Kentucky Medical Center
Lexington, Kentucky

William J. John, MD
Senior Clinical Research Physician
US Affiliate, Oncology
Eli Lilly Company
Lexington, Kentucky

Alan T. Lefor, MD
Director, Surgical Education and Academic Affairs
Director, Division of Surgical Oncology
Cedars-Sinai Medical Center
Professor of Clinical Surgery
Department of Surgery
University of California, Los Angeles
Los Angeles, California

Jerry J. Lierl, MD
Associate Professor
Division of Cardiology
Department of Internal Medicine
University of Cincinnati
Cincinnati, Ohio

Shantae L. Lucas, MD
Hematologist/Oncologist
Private Practice
Cancer Care of Western North Carolina
Asheville, North Carolina

Ralph A. Manchester, MD
Medical Chief
University Health Service
Associate Professor of Medicine
General Medicine Unit
Department of Medicine
University of Rochester School of Medicine and Dentistry
Rochester, New York

Andrew D. Massey, MD
Associate Professor of Medicine
Department of Internal Medicine
University of Kansas School of Medicine–Wichita
Wichita, Kansas

Rick R. McClure, MD, FACC
Cardiologist
Cardiovascular Consultants, PSC
Private Practice
Lexington, Kentucky

Thomas B. Montgomery, MD
Associate Professor
Division of General Internal Medicine
Department of Internal Medicine
University of Kentucky Medical Center
Lexington, Kentucky

William C. Moore, MD
General Internist
Private Practice
Ferrell Duncan Clinic, Inc.
Springfield, Missouri

Rita K. Munn, MD
Associate Professor
Division of Hematology and Oncology
Department of Internal Medicine
University of Kentucky Medical Center
Lexington, Kentucky

John C. Parker, MD
Fellow
Division of Endocrinology, Nutrition and Metabolism
Department of Medicine
Duke University
Durham, North Carolina

Carol B. Peddicord, MD
General Internist
Private Practice
Albany, Kentucky

Holly G. Pursley, MD
Instructor
Division of General Internal Medicine
Department of Internal Medicine
University of Kentucky Medical Center
Lexington, Kentucky

Michael S. Pursley, MD
Fellow
Division of Cardiovascular Medicine
Department of Internal Medicine
University of Kentucky Medical Center
Lexington, Kentucky

John B. Robbins, MD
General Internist
Private Practice
Internal Medicine Associates
Bozeman, Montana

David W. Rudy, MD
Assistant Professor of Medicine
Division of General Internal Medicine
Department of Internal Medicine
University of Kentucky Medical Center
Lexington, Kentucky

Steven I. Shedlofsky, MD
Professor of Medicine
Division of Digestive Diseases and Nutrition
Department of Internal Medicine
University of Kentucky Medical Center
and Veteran's Administration Hospital
Lexington, Kentucky

Kelly M. Smith, PharmD
Drug Information Specialist
Clinical Associate Professor
College of Pharmacy
University of Kentucky
Lexington, Kentucky

Benjamin J. Stahr, MD, FCAP
Pathologist
Greensboro Pathology Associates
Moses H. Cone Memorial Hospital
Greensboro, North Carolina

R. Douglas Strickland, MD
Gastroenterologist
Private Practice
Holston Valley Hospital
Gastroenterology Associates
Kingsport, Tennessee

Gregg M. Talente, MD
Assistant Professor
Division of General Internal Medicine
Brody School of Medicine
East Carolina University
Greenville, North Carolina

Timothy A. Winchester, MD
General Internist
Private Practice
Lexington, Kentucky

Preface

The third edition of *Internal Medicine On Call* is a user-friendly reference that will assist in the initial evaluation and treatment of the most frequently encountered problems in internal medicine. It will serve as an aid to house officers and medical students when they are called about medical problems, whether common or potentially life-threatening. *Internal Medicine On Call* provides a concise and practical approach to these problems and serves to bridge the gap between textbooks and patient care. Unlike many books or manuals, *Internal Medicine On Call* is organized by the presenting problem or complaint rather than the diagnosis. We have not attempted to provide a comprehensive discussion, but rather the essential elements in the initial assessment and management of each problem. This will aid the house officer or student when called to evaluate a patient with a specific problem.

Each on-call problem is introduced with a case scenario. This is followed by the questions the clinician should initially ask. A differential diagnosis is given with key points to help one arrive at the final diagnosis. A database section includes key points on the physical examination, laboratory tests, and other tests that are important in making the diagnosis. A plan for the treatment of specific diagnoses is also included. Recommendations for treatment are specific with regard to dosage and dosing intervals, but it is emphasized that hepatic and renal disease as well as other factors (eg, age) can greatly affect the metabolism of drugs. In addition, variations in institutional practices exist. For these reasons, treatment may need to be individualized from patient to patient or from institution to institution.

House officers and medical students often have questions regarding frequently used medications, laboratory tests, and procedures including step-by-step instruction, as well as indications and contraindications. These areas, as well as ventilator management and transfusion therapy, have been included to provide house officers and medical students a manual to answer many of the questions that arise in the day-to-day management of their patients.

The third edition of *Internal Medicine On Call* includes significant changes from the second edition. Each problem has been updated to include the latest diagnostic tests and treatment. Three new problems, *Dizziness, Overdoses,* and *Pruritus,* have been added, as well as new laboratory tests such as troponin, which have become widely used since the printing of the second edition. Section VII, Therapeutics (formerly called Commonly Used Medications), includes sections on minerals, natural products (herbals), and vitamins, as well as over 100 new medications.

We are grateful to Tricia Gomella, MD, for providing the "on-call" concept originally used in her book *Neonatology: Basic Management, On Call Problems, Diseases, and Drugs,* first published in 1988. We thank McGraw-Hill for providing us the forum to present a unique approach for medical student and house officer education. In particular, we want to thank our copy editor,

Linda Conheady, whose diligence and keen eye for detail has helped us improve the quality of the third edition of *Internal Medicine On Call.* We also want to thank Janet Foltin, our editor at McGraw-Hill, whose support and guidance has been invaluable.

Finally, we want to thank Sonni Webb and Mary Robbins, RN, for their efforts in the completion of this book. Without their assistance and support, the completion of this manual would not have been possible.

We sincerely hope that this manual will enhance your training and help you to provide the best care for your patients.

Steven A. Haist, MD, MS, FACP
Lexington, Kentucky

John B. Robbins, MD
Bozeman, Montana

April 2002

I. On-Call Problems

1. ABDOMINAL PAIN

I. Problem. A 34-year-old woman admitted for control of her diabetes develops acute abdominal pain that increases in severity over several hours.

II. Immediate Questions

A. What are the patient's vital signs? Acute abdominal pain may signify a condition as benign as gastroenteritis or as catastrophic as an infarcted bowel or perforated viscus. The significant morbidity and mortality of the acute surgical abdomen can be obviated by early diagnosis. *Tachycardia* and *hypotension* would suggest circulatory or septic shock from perforation, hemorrhage, or fluid loss into the intestinal lumen or peritoneal cavity. Orthostatic blood pressure and pulse changes would also be helpful in ascertaining the presence of volume loss. *Fever* occurs in inflammatory conditions such as cholecystitis and appendicitis. When the temperature exceeds 102°F, gangrene or perforation of a viscus should be suspected. Fever may not be present in elderly patients, patients on corticosteroids, or patients who are immunocompromised.

B. Where is the pain located? Abdominal pain is produced by three mechanisms: (1) *tension* within the walls of the alimentary tract (biliary or intestinal obstruction); (2) *ischemia* (strangulated bowel, mesenteric vascular occlusion); and (3) *peritoneal irritation.* The first two causes result in visceral pain, a dull pain perceived in the midline and *poorly localized.* Generally, *pain arising from the GI tract* is perceived in the midline because of the symmetric and bilateral innervation of these organs. *Unilateral pain* is likely caused by organs with unilateral innervation such as the kidney, ureter, or ovary. Generally, *midepigastric pain* is caused by disorders of the stomach, duodenum, pancreas, liver, and biliary tract. Disease of the small intestine, appendix, upper ureters, testes, and ovaries results in *periumbilical pain. Lower abdominal pain* is caused by processes in the colon, bladder, lower ureters, and uterus. Inflammation of the parietal peritoneum results in more severe pain that is *well localized* to the area of inflammation. It is also important to realize that *referred pain* (pain originating from a site more central than where it is perceived) occurs because the cutaneous dermatomes and visceral organs share the same spinal cord level.

C. Does the pain radiate? Pain that becomes rapidly generalized implies perforation and leakage of fluid into the peritoneal cavity. Biliary pain can radiate from the right upper quadrant to the right inferior scapula. Pancreatic and abdominal aneurysmal pain may radiate to the back. Ureteral colic classically is referred to the groin and thigh.

D. **When did the pain begin?** Sudden onset suggests perforated ulcer, mesenteric occlusion, ruptured aneurysm, or ruptured ectopic pregnancy. A more gradual onset (> 1 hour) implies an inflammatory condition such as appendicitis, cholecystitis, diverticulitis, or an obstructed viscus such as bowel obstruction.

E. **What is the quality of the pain?** Intestinal colic occurs as cramping abdominal pain interspersed with pain-free intervals. Biliary colic is not a true colicky pain in that it usually presents as sustained persistent pain. Unfortunately, the terms *sharp, dull, burning,* and *tearing,* although used by patients to describe pain, seldom assist in determining the etiology.

F. **What relieves the pain or makes it worse?** Pain with deep inspiration is associated with diaphragmatic irritation, such as with pleurisy or upper abdominal inflammation. Patients with intestinal or ureteral colic tend to be restless and active, whereas patients with peritonitis attempt to avoid all motion. Coughing frequently exacerbates abdominal pain from peritonitis.

G. **Are there any associated symptoms?** *Vomiting* may result from intestinal obstruction or may result from a visceral reflex caused by pain. In conditions causing an acute surgical abdomen, the vomiting usually follows rather than precedes the onset of pain. *Hematemesis* suggests gastritis or peptic ulcer disease. *Diarrhea* may result from gastroenteritis, but may also result from ischemic colitis or inflammatory bowel disease. *Obstipation* (absence of passage of stool or flatus) suggests mechanical bowel obstruction. *Hematuria* points to genitourinary disease such as nephrolithiasis. *Cough* and *sputum production* might occur if lower lobe pneumonia is present.

H. **For women, what is the patient's menstrual history?** A missed period in a sexually active woman would suggest ectopic pregnancy. A foul vaginal discharge might indicate pelvic inflammatory disease.

I. **What is the patient's past medical history?** Is there a history of peptic ulcer disease, gallstones, diverticulosis, alcohol abuse, abdominal operations suggesting adhesions, or an abdominal aortic aneurysm? Is there any known history of cardiac arrhythmias or other cardiac disease that could result in embolization to a mesenteric artery?

III. **Differential Diagnosis.** There are several potential causes of acute abdominal pain, some of which are listed in Table 1–1. Many of these diseases can be managed medically; others require urgent surgery. Abdominal pain can result from extra-abdominal processes as well as intra-abdominal disease.

A. **Intra-abdominal disease**

1. **Hollow viscera.** Perforation of a hollow viscus represents a surgical emergency.

TABLE I–1. COMMON CAUSES OF ACUTE ABDOMEN: CONDITIONS IN ITALIC TYPE OFTEN REQUIRE SURGERY.

- **Gastrointestinal tract disorders**
  Nonspecific abdominal pain
  Appendicitis
  Small and large bowel obstruction
  Incarcerated hernia
  Perforated peptic ulcer
  Bowel perforation
  Meckel's diverticulitis
  Boerhaave's syndrome
  Diverticulitis
  Inflammatory bowel disorders
  Mallory-Weiss syndrome
  Gastroenteritis
  Acute gastritis
  Mesenteric adenitis
- **Liver, spleen, and biliary tract disorders**
  Acute cholecystitis
  Acute cholangitis
  Hepatic abscess
  Ruptured hepatic tumor
  Spontaneous rupture of the spleen
  Splenic infarct
  Biliary colic
  Acute hepatits
- **Pancreatic disorders**
  Acute pancreatitis
- **Urinary tract disorders**
  Ureteral or renal colic
  Acute pyelonephritis
  Acute cystitis
  Renal infarct
- **Gynecologic disorders**
  Ruptured ectopic pregnancy
  Twisted ovarian tumor
  Ruptured ovarian follicle cyst
  Acute salpingitis
  Dysmenorrhea
  Endometriosis
- **Vascular disorders**
  Ruptured aortic and visceral aneurysms
  Acute ischemic colitis
  Mesenteric thrombosis
- **Peritoneal disorders**
  Intra-abdominal abscesses
  Primary peritonitis
  Tuberculous peritonitis
- **Retroperitoneal disorders**
  Retroperitoneal hemorrhage

Boey JH: Acute abdomen. In Way LW, ed. Current Surgical Diagnosis and Treatment *10th ed. Appleton & Lange; 1994.*

   a. **Upper abdomen:** Esophagitis, gastritis, peptic ulcer disease, cholecystitis, cholelithiasis, and biliary colic.
   b. **Midgut:** Small bowel obstruction or infarction.
   c. **Lower abdomen:** Inflammatory bowel disease, appendicitis, large bowel obstruction, diverticulitis.

2. **Solid organ**
   a. **Hepatitis**
   b. **Pancreatitis**
   c. **Splenic infarction or abscess**
   d. **Pyelonephritis/Urolithiasis**
3. **Pelvis**
   a. **Pelvic inflammatory disease**
   b. **Ruptured ectopic pregnancy**
4. **Vascular system**
   a. **Ruptured aneurysm**
   b. **Dissecting aneurysm**
   c. **Mesenteric thrombosis or embolism**

B. **Extra-abdominal disease.** To prevent unnecessary surgery, these causes of acute abdominal pain should be considered.
   1. **Diabetic ketoacidosis**
   2. **Acute adrenal insufficiency**
   3. **Acute porphyria**
   4. **Pneumonia involving lower lobes**
   5. **Pulmonary embolism involving lower lobes**
   6. **Pneumothorax**
   7. **Sickle cell crisis**

C. **Special populations.** In these patients, pain is secondary to unusual causes or unusual presentation of common problems.
   1. **Elderly patients.** Pain is often present without signs and symptoms commonly seen in younger patients.
   2. **Patients with HIV.** See Section I, Chapter 23, Fever in the HIV-Positive Patient, p 135.
   3. **Patients with hemophilia. Hematoma of bowel wall.**

D. **Rare causes**
   1. **Celiac axis compression syndrome**
   2. **Painful rib syndrome**
   3. **Wandering spleen syndrome**
   4. **Abdominal migraine**
   5. **Fitz-Hugh–Curtis syndrome.** Perihepatitis secondary to gonococcal or chlamydia salpingitis.

IV. Database

A. **Physical examination key points.** See Table 1–2.
   1. **Vital signs and general appearance.** See Section II.A. Does the patient appear uncomfortable? Is the patient jaundiced? and Is there a position that provides some relief of the pain? Patients with peritonitis resist movement, whereas patients with colic writhe in pain.
   2. **Lungs.** Percuss for dullness at the bases, suggests a pleural effusion or consolidation. In addition to dullness, the presence of crackles or bronchial breath sounds suggests a pneumonia, infarction, or atelectasis associated with decreased inspiratory effort because of pain.
   3. **Heart.** Look for jugular venous distension, S_3 gallop, or a displaced apical impulse indicative of congestive heart failure that might predispose to passive congestion of the liver or mesenteric ischemia. An irregular pulse could indicate atrial fibrillation, which might result in mesenteric artery embolism.
   4. **Abdomen**
      a. **Inspection.** Examine for the presence of distension (obstruction, ileus, ascites), ecchymoses (hemorrhagic pancreatitis), caput medusae (portal hypertension), and surgical scars (adhesions).

TABLE I–2. PHYSICAL FINDINGS WITH VARIOUS CAUSES OF ACUTE ABDOMEN.[1]

Condition	Signs
Perforated viscus	Scaphoid, tense abdomen; diminished bowel sounds (late); loss of liver dullness; guarding or rigidity
Peritonitis	Motionless, absent bowel sounds (late); cough and rebound tenderness; guarding or rigidity
Inflamed mass or abscess	Tender mass (abdominal, rectal, or pelvic); punch tenderness; special signs (Murphy's, psoas, or obturator)
Intestinal obstruction	Distension; visible peristalsis (late); hyperperistalsis (early) or quiet abdomen (late); diffuse pain without rebound tenderness; hernia or rectal mass (some)
Paralytic ileus	Distension; minimal bowel sounds; no localized tenderness
Ischemic or strangulated bowel	Not distended (until late); bowel sounds variable; severe pain but little tenderness; rectal bleeding (some)
Bleeding	Pallor, shock; distension; pulsatile (aneurysm) or tender (eg, ectopic pregnancy) mass; rectal bleeding (some)

[1] *Reproduced with permission from Boey JH: Acute abdomen. In Way LW, ed.* Current Surgical Diagnosis and Treatment. *10th ed. Appleton & Lange; 1994.*

b. **Auscultation.** Listen for bowel sounds (absent or an occasional tinkle with ileus, hyperperistaltic with gastroenteritis, high-pitched rushes with small bowel obstruction).

c. **Percussion.** Tympany is associated with distended loops of bowel. Shifting dullness and a fluid wave suggest ascites with peritonitis.

d. **Other signs.** Pain with active hip flexion or with extension of the patient's right thigh while lying on the left side (*psoas sign*) could result from an inflamed appendix. *Obturator sign* (pain on internal rotation of the flexed thigh) can occur with appendicitis.

5. **Rectum.** Evaluation of acute abdominal pain is not complete until a rectal exam has been performed. A mass suggests the presence of rectal carcinoma. Lateral rectal tenderness occurs with appendicitis, a condition in which examination of the abdomen may not reveal localized findings. If stool is present, evaluate for occult blood.

6. **Female genitalia.** Examine for pain with cervical motion and cervical discharge that may suggest pelvic inflammatory disease. Also palpate for adnexal masses that would indicate an ectopic pregnancy, ovarian abscess, cyst, or neoplasm.

B. **Laboratory data.** The decision to operate is seldom made solely on the basis of laboratory data. This information serves mainly as an adjunct in (1) cases in which the etiology of the pain is unclear, or (2) to assist preoperative assessment in individuals for whom the diagnosis is certain and the decision to operate has already been made.

1. **Hematology.** An increased hematocrit suggests hemoconcentration from volume loss (pancreatitis). A low hematocrit may suggest a process that has resulted in chronic blood loss, or possibly acute intra-abdominal hemorrhage or an acute gastrointestinal (GI) hemorrhage. With acute blood loss, however, the hematocrit may not decrease for several hours. An elevated white blood cell count (WBC) suggests an inflammatory process such as appendicitis or cholecystitis.
2. **Electrolytes, blood urea nitrogen (BUN), creatinine.** Bowel obstruction with vomiting can result in hypokalemia, azotemia, and volume contraction alkalosis. A strangulated bowel or sepsis may result in a metabolic gap acidosis. An elevated BUN/creatinine ratio is seen with volume depletion and GI bleeding.
3. **Liver function tests including bilirubin, transaminases, and alkaline phosphatase.** Results are elevated in acute hepatitis, cholecystitis, and other biliary tract disease.
4. **Amylase/lipase.** Markedly elevated levels are associated with pancreatitis. However, in up to 30% of patients with acute pancreatitis, amylase may be initially normal, especially in patients with lipemic serum. Conversely, amylase can also be elevated in conditions other than pancreatitis, such as acute cholecystitis, perforated ulcer, small bowel obstruction with strangulation, and ruptured ectopic pregnancy. Serum lipase will help differentiate pancreatitis from the other causes of hyperamylasemia.
5. **Arterial blood gases (ABG).** Hypoxemia is often an early sign of sepsis and may occur with pancreatitis. As mentioned, metabolic acidosis may result from ischemic bowel or sepsis.
6. **Pregnancy test.** All premenopausal women with acute right or left lower abdominal pain should be tested for human chorionic gonadotropin (HCG) levels to rule out ectopic pregnancy, regardless of whether or not they missed their last period.
7. **Urinalysis.** Hematuria may indicate nephrolithiasis; pyuria and hematuria can be present in urinary tract infections. In addition, pyuria is occasionally present with appendicitis.
8. **Cervical culture.** Obtain a cervical culture for chlamydia and gonorrhea when pelvic inflammatory disease (PID) is suspected.

C. Radiology and other studies

1. **Flat & upright abdominal films.** These films can be readily obtained and may provide important information. Watch for the following indicators: gas pattern; evidence of bowel dilation; air-fluid levels; presence or absence of air in the rectum; pancreatic calcifications; biliary and renal calcifications; aortic calcifications; loss of psoas margin (suggesting retroperitoneal bleeding); and presence or absence of air in the biliary tract.
2. **Chest film.** A CXR may reveal lower lobe pneumonia, pleural effusion, or elevation of a hemidiaphragm indicating a subdiaphrag-

matic inflammatory process. Free air under the diaphragm suggests a perforated viscus and is most often seen on the upright chest film. As many as 15–20% of cases of perforation do not manifest this sign.

3. **Ultrasound (US).** This readily obtainable and noninvasive test is the preferred modality for right upper quadrant pain or gynecologic disease. US may reveal the presence or absence of gallstones, biliary tract dilation, or ectopic pregnancy.
4. **CT.** The most sensitive test when considering many possible diagnoses. CT has a sensitivity of 96% and a specificity of 83–89% for appendicitis.
5. **Electrocardiogram (ECG).** An ECG is needed to rule out an acute myocardial infarction (MI) or pericarditis, which may present with acute upper abdominal pain.
6. **Paracentesis.** See Section III, Chapter 11, Paracentesis, p 418. With known ascites and acute abdominal pain, this test is required to rule out the possibility of spontaneous bacterial peritonitis. If ascites is suspected but has not been documented, an ultrasound should be performed before an attempted paracentesis.
7. **Other studies** may be obtained in a more leisurely fashion to determine the nature of the pain, provided the patient does not appear to have a case of acute abdominal pain requiring surgery. These tests can include the following:
   a. **Intravenous pyelogram (IVP)**
   b. **Abdominal CT scan**
   c. **Hepato-iminodiacetic acid (HIDA) scan,** to rule out acute cholecystitis
   d. **Contrast bowel studies,** such as an upper GI and small bowel series, to look for evidence of occult perforation or mechanical obstruction. A barium enema may be helpful in evaluation for sigmoid or cecal volvulus.
   e. **Endoscopic studies,** such as esophagogastroduodenoscopy (EGD), colonoscopy, or endoscopic retrograde cholangiopancreatography (ERCP).
   f. **Arteriography.** This may be necessary in patients in whom mesenteric artery ischemia is suspected.

V. **Plan.** As mentioned previously, the initial goal in evaluating acute abdominal pain is to determine whether or not surgical treatment is indicated to prevent further morbidity. When pain has been present 6 or more hours and has not improved, there is an increased likelihood that the patient will require surgical exploration to determine the cause. Often the specific etiology of the patient's abdominal pain is not determined until laparotomy. The use of analgesics remains controversial, but many surgeons now favor the use of moderate doses of pain medication to make the patient more comfortable and facilitate further examination (See Section I, Chapter 54, Pain Management,V, p 289).

A. **Observation.** With the exception of conditions requiring urgent surgical exploration (Table 1–3), most cases of abdominal pain can be initially managed with close observation, correction of any fluid or electrolyte disturbances, and judicious use of analgesics.

1. **Surgery consultation.** Any patient developing acute abdominal pain should be evaluated by a general surgeon.
2. **Gastric decompression.** When mechanical obstruction is suspected or vomiting is present, a nasogastric tube should be placed for decompression. (See Section III, Chapter 8, Gastrointestinal Tubes, p 410).
3. **Intravenous fluids.** Septic or circulatory shock should be treated with vigorous intravenous volume replacement. If hypotension persists, vasopressors such as dopamine may be needed (See Section I, Chapter 42, Hypotension, V, p 227).
4. **Serial physical examinations.** Periodic examinations by the same clinician are helpful in determining a change in the patient's condition and establishing a diagnosis or need for surgery.

B. **Surgery.** Indications for an urgent operation without a period of observation or establishment of a specific preoperative diagnosis are outlined in Table 1–3.

TABLE I–3. INDICATIONS FOR URGENT OPERATION IN PATIENTS WITH ACUTE ABDOMEN.[1]

- **Physical findings**
  - Involuntary guarding or rigidity, especially if spreading
  - Increasing or severe localized tenderness
  - Tense or progressive distension
  - Tender abdominal or rectal mass with high fever or hypotension
  - Rectal bleeding with shock or acidosis
  - Equivocal abdominal findings along with
    - Septicemia (high fever, marked or rising leukocytosis, mental changes, or increasing glucose intolerance in a diabetic patient)
    - Bleeding (unexplained shock or acidosis, falling hematocrit)
    - Suspected ischemia (acidosis, fever, tachycardia)
    - Deterioration on conservative treatment
- **Radiologic findings**
  - Pneumoperitoneum
  - Gross or progressive bowel distension
  - Free extravasation of contrast material
  - Space-occupying lesion on CT scan with fever
  - Mesenteric occlusion on angiography
- **Endoscopic findings**
  - Perforated or uncontrollably bleeding lesion
- **Paracentesis findings**
  - Blood, bile, pus, bowel contents, or urine

[1] *Reproduced with permission from Boey JH: Acute abdomen. In Way LW, ed.* Current Surgical Diagnosis and Treatment. *10th ed. Appleton & Lange: 1994.*

REFERENCES

Balthazar EJ, Birnbaum BA, Yee J et al: Acute appendicitis: CT and ultrasound correlation in one hundred patients. Radiology 1997;202:137.

Fishman MB, Aronson MD: Approach to the patient with abdominal pain. In: Fletcher SW, Fletcher RH, Aronson MD, editors-in-chief. UpToDate [CD-ROM]. Version 8.2. Wellesley, MA;2000. www.uptodate.com

Jung PJ, Merrell PC: Acute abdomen. Gastroenterol Clin North Am 1988;17:227.

Ray BS, Neill CL: Abdominal visceral pain in man. Ann Surg 1947;126:709.

Silen W: *Cope's Early Diagnosis of the Acute Abdomen.* 18th ed. Oxford University Press;1991.

Wagner JM, McKinney P, Carpentar JL: Does this patient have appendicitis? JAMA 1996;276:1589.

2. ACIDOSIS

I. **Problem.** A 30-year-old male is brought into the emergency room unconscious. A friend found him at home. No other history is available. Physical examination is unremarkable except for rapid, shallow breathing. An arterial blood gas (ABG) reveals a pH of 7.10.

II. **Immediate Questions**

A. **Is the acidemia from a metabolic, respiratory, or mixed acidosis?** A quick look at the pCO_2 on the ABG slip will reveal whether the disturbance is a primary metabolic or respiratory acidosis. If the pCO_2 is less than 40 mm Hg, then the primary disturbance is a metabolic acidosis. If the pCO_2 is greater than 40 mm Hg, the disturbance may be a primary respiratory acidosis or may be a mixed disturbance. Many ABG slips list the base excess (BE). The BE may help determine the etiology of the acidosis. If the BE is positive, the acidosis is respiratory; if the BE is negative, the acidosis is at least partially metabolic. Remember, the BE is calculated from the pH; the calculation assumes that both the pH and pCO_2 are correct.

B. **What are the patient's vital signs?** Metabolic acidosis is often the result of lactic acid production from hypoperfusion and hypoxia. If there is hypotension or if the patient is orthostatic, immediate fluid resuscitation is indicated. Vasopressor agents may also be needed. (See Section I, Chapter 42, Hypotension, p 224). Bradypnea may suggest a narcotics overdose. Tachypnea may arise from hyperventilation as respiratory compensation for a metabolic acidosis; or from increased respiratory effort with hypoventilation (eg, pulmonary edema), resulting in a respiratory acidosis.

C. **Are there any arrhythmias or ectopy?** With a profound acidemia from any cause, there may be disturbances of cardiac rhythm or ventricular ectopy. Obtain an ECG and monitor the patient.

D. **What is the serum bicarbonate?** To fully understand an acid–base problem, it is imperative to obtain the serum bicarbonate from an electrolyte panel. A high serum bicarbonate is evidence for a primary respiratory acidosis. A low serum bicarbonate is evidence for either a primary metabolic acidosis or a mixed metabolic and respiratory acidosis.

E. **Do the values for serum bicarbonate, pH, and pCO_2 fit?** Once you have the serum bicarbonate, you should make sure the pH, pCO_2, and HCO_3^- fit:

$$pH = pK_a + \log \frac{HCO_3^-}{H_2CO_3}$$

which can be simplified to:

$$H^+ = 24 \times \frac{pCO_2}{HCO_3^-}$$

In this patient with a pH of 7.10, if the pCO_2 is 20 mm Hg and the serum bicarbonate is 6 mmol/L, then:

$$H^+ = 24 \times \frac{20}{6}$$

$$H^+ = 80$$

Does a pH of 7.10 equal a $[H^+]$ of 80 nmol/L? There are some simple rules to help convert pH to $[H^+]$. At a pH of 7.40, the $[H^+]$ = 40 nmol/L. pH is a log scale, and for every 0.3 change in pH, the $[H^+]$ doubles or is halved. For instance, if pH = 7.70, $[H^+]$ = 20 nmol/L, and at pH = 8.00, $[H^+]$ = 10 nmol/L. In this patient, if pH = 7.10, then $[H^+]$ = 80 nmol/L. Also, around a pH of 7.40 (7.25–7.48), the $[H^+]$ changes 1 nmol/L for every 0.01 change in pH. Lastly, on the back of many ABG slips, there may be a scale showing the relationship between pH and $[H^+]$. If the numbers do not fit reasonably well (± 10%) into the equation

$$[H^+] = 24 \times \frac{pCO_2}{HCO_3^-}$$

then it is difficult to determine the acid–base disturbance, and the blood gas and serum bicarbonate should be repeated. For instance, if pH = 7.30, pCO_2 = 45 mm Hg, and HCO_3^- = 30 mmol/L, a superficial interpretation might be respiratory acidosis; however, closer scrutiny is necessary.

A pH of 7.30 corresponds to a H^+ of 50 nmol / L

$$50 = 24 \times \frac{45}{30}$$

$$50 \neq 36$$

The pH, the pCO_2, or the HCO_3^- is in error. For instance, if there had been too much heparin in the syringe, the pH would be falsely low.

F. Is the compensation appropriate? Checking to see whether the compensation is appropriate may unmask mixed disturbances.

1. For **respiratory acidosis,** immediate compensation is through buffers. In the short term, one expects the HCO_3^- to increase by 1 mmol/L for every 10 mm Hg increase in pCO_2 over normal (40 mm Hg). Renal compensation is not present for up to 24 hours. For chronic respiratory acidosis, expect an increase in the HCO_3^- of 3.5–4.0 mmol/L for every 10 mm Hg increase in pCO_2. It will take several days (3–5 days) for maximal renal compensation for a respiratory acidosis. For instance, in a 25-year-old with an acute episode of asthma, the ABG revealed a pCO_2 of 90. One would expect the bicarbonate to increase by 5 mmol/L from the calculation 1 mmol/L × (90 mm Hg – 40 mm Hg)/10 mm Hg. One would also expect the HCO_3^- to be 31 mmol/L from the calculation 26 mmol/L (normal bicarbonate range 23–29) + 5 mmol/L. If the bicarbonate were 25 mmol/L, then a relative metabolic acidosis would be present along with the primary respiratory acidosis. If the bicarbonate were 36 mmol/L, then a metabolic alkalosis would also be present along with the primary respiratory acidosis.
2. For **metabolic acidosis,** compensation begins immediately through buffers and hyperventilation; however, steady state may not be reached for up to 24 hours. The expected change in $pCO_2 = (1.5 \times HCO_3^-) + 8 \pm 2$. For instance, in a 40-year-old with renal failure, the serum bicarbonate was found to be 14 mmol/L. The expected change in pCO_2 would be $(1.5 \times 14) + 8 \pm 2$, or 29 ± 2. One would expect the pCO_2 to be between 27 and 31 mm Hg. If the actual pCO_2 were 19 mm Hg, then a respiratory alkalosis would also be present along with the primary metabolic acidosis. If the actual pCO_2 were 36 mm Hg, then a relative respiratory acidosis would be present along with the primary metabolic acidosis.

III. Differential Diagnosis. An acidemia is either from a metabolic or respiratory acidosis. There are many causes for both, and sometimes a patient may have more than one cause.

A. Respiratory acidosis. By definition, respiratory acidosis occurs secondary to hypoventilation. Hypoventilation can be caused by lung, chest, or central nervous system (CNS) disorders.

1. **Lungs**
   a. **Asthma.** May progress from a respiratory alkalosis to respiratory acidosis. A normal or elevated pCO_2 indicates impending respiratory failure, and may indicate the need for prompt intubation.
   b. **Pulmonary edema.** Mild pulmonary edema usually causes a respiratory alkalosis. Severe pulmonary edema may cause a respiratory acidosis, and intubation will probably be required.

c. **Pneumonia.** Again, pneumonia usually causes respiratory alkalosis. But if more than one lobe is involved, or if there is underlying chronic obstructive disease, pneumonia may cause a respiratory acidosis.
d. **Upper airway obstruction.** Causes of obstruction may include foreign bodies, tumors, or a laryngospasm.
e. **Pneumothorax.** Usually causes respiratory alkalosis; can cause a respiratory acidosis.
f. **Large pleural effusion.** Usually causes a respiratory alkalosis; can cause a respiratory acidosis.

2. **Chest abnormalities**
   a. **Kyphoscoliosis.** Resulting in a restrictive defect.
   b. **Scleroderma.** Resulting in a restrictive defect.
   c. **Marked obesity (Pickwickian syndrome)**
   d. **Muscular disorders.** These include muscular dystrophy, severe hypophosphatemia, or myasthenia gravis.
   e. **Peripheral neurologic disorders, such as Guillain-Barré syndrome.**
3. **CNS disorders**
   a. **Drugs or toxins.** Causes respiratory drive depression.
      i. **Ethanol intoxication at levels of 400–500 mg%**
      ii. **Barbiturates, especially overdoses**
      iii. **Narcotics**
      iv. **Benzodiazepines.** Especially when taken with alcohol.
   b. **Cerebrovascular accident**
   c. **Brain stem bleed or cervical spinal cord injuries**

B. **Pseudorespiratory alkalosis.** Arterial hypocapnia is present; however, there is an increase in the mixed venous pCO_2. Seen in severe cardiac dysfunction and associated pulmonary hypoperfusion with normal pulmonary function. Total body carbon dioxide is increased, resulting in an increase in H^+ and an acidosis.

C. **Metabolic acidosis.** This can be divided into gap and nongap acidosis. The anion gap can be calculated as follows:

$$\text{Anion gap} = [Na^+] - ([Cl^-] + [HCO_3^-])$$

The normal anion gap is 8–12 mmol/L. An increase in anion gap may result from an increase in an unmeasured anion. Other causes of an elevated anion gap include dehydration; alkalosis; use of penicillin antibiotics that contain large amounts of sodium, such as carbenicillin; and therapy with sodium salts or organic acids such as sodium lactate, acetate, and citrate. Sodium citrate is used in whole blood and packed red cells as an anticoagulant. However, only a metabolic acidosis will cause an appreciable increase in the anion gap.

1. **Normal anion gap (metabolic nongap acidosis)**
   a. **Loss of bicarbonate through the GI tract**

i. **Diarrhea**
ii. **Small bowel fistula**
iii. **Pancreatocutaneous fistula**
iv. **Ureterosigmoidostomy**
v. **Chloride-containing exchange resins,** such as cholestyramine; or with calcium chloride or magnesium chloride

b. **Loss of bicarbonate through the kidneys**
i. **Renal tubular acidosis.** If the history does not reveal an obvious cause such as diarrhea, then you need to consider renal tubular acidosis.
(a.) **Distal renal tubular acidosis.** Causes include hypercalcemia, amphotericin B, and medullary sponge kidney.
(b.) **Proximal renal tubular acidosis.** Proximal tubular reabsorption of HCO_3^- is impaired. Causes include lead, cadmium and mercury toxicity, and amyloidosis.
ii. **Carbonic anhydrase inhibitors**

c. **Other causes not from gastrointestinal or renal loss of HCO_3^-**
i. **Early renal failure**
ii. **Hydrochloric acid**
iii. **Hyperalimentation**
iv. **Dilutional**

2. **Elevated anion gap (metabolic gap acidosis)**

a. **Lactic acidosis.** Results from overproduction or impairment of lactate utilization by the liver, often from tissue hypoperfusion and hypoxia.
i. **Shock. Cardiogenic, hypovolemic, septic shock.**
ii. **Severe anemia**
iii. **Hypoxia**
iv. **Malignancy**
v. **Seizures**
vi. **Ethanol**
vii. **Crush injury**

b. **Renal failure.** Loss of acid secretion, and failure to filter anions.

c. **Ketoacidosis**
i. **Diabetic ketoacidosis**
ii. **Alcoholic ketoacidosis**
iii. **Starvation ketoacidosis**

d. **Toxins**
i. **Salicylates.** These compounds cause an isolated metabolic gap acidosis (10%), an isolated respiratory alkalosis (30%), but most commonly a mixed metabolic gap acidosis and respiratory alkalosis (57%).

ii. **Methanol.** Metabolized to formic acid and formaldehyde. May cause blindness, abdominal pain, and headache.

iii. **Ethylene glycol.** Metabolized to oxalate, glycolaldehyde, and hippurate. Renal failure, neurologic disturbances, hypertension, and cardiovascular collapse may occur.

Note: Isopropyl alcohol ingestion does not cause an acidosis, because isopropyl alcohol is metabolized to acetone. It may therefore cause a positive nitroprusside test for ketones. It may cause gastritis.

iv. **Toluene.** Seen in glue sniffing or huffing. Can cause metabolic gap acidosis (hippurate anion) or metabolic nongap acidosis.

e. The anion gap is also helpful in differentiating a pure metabolic acidosis, a mixed metabolic gap acidosis and metabolic nongap acidosis, and a mixed metabolic gap acidosis and metabolic alkalosis. For instance, if the HCO_3^- were 14 with a gap of 23, this would most likely represent a pure metabolic gap acidosis as calculated by:

23 mmol/L Actual gap
−10 mmol/L Normal gap
13 mmol/L Expected change in HCO_3^- from normal

26 mmol/L Normal HCO_3^- (range 23–29)
−13 mmol/L Expected change in HCO_3^-
13 mmol/L Expected HCO_3^-

Actual HCO_3^- 14 mmol/L = expected gap of 13 mmol/L

An HCO_3^- of 19 with a gap of 25 would most likely represent a *mixed metabolic acidosis and metabolic alkalosis* as calculated by:

25 mmol/L Actual gap
−10 mmol/L Normal gap
15 mmol/L Expected change in HCO_3^- from normal

26 mmol/L Normal HCO_3^- (range 23–29)
−15 mmol/L Expected change in HCO_3^-
11 mmol/L Expected HCO_3^-

The actual HCO_3^-, however, is 19 mmol/L, 8 mmol/L higher than expected. Thus, there must also be a metabolic alkalosis in addition to the metabolic gap acidosis.

An HCO_3^- of 8 mmol/L with a gap of 22 mmol/L would most likely represent a *mixed metabolic gap acidosis and metabolic nongap acidosis* as calculated by:

$$\begin{array}{rl} 22\ \text{mmol/L} & \text{Actual gap} \\ -\underline{10}\ \text{mmol/L} & \text{Normal gap} \\ 12\ \text{mmol/L} & \text{Expected change in } HCO_3^- \end{array}$$

$$\begin{array}{rl} 26\ \text{mmol/L} & \text{Normal } HCO_3^- \text{ (range 23 – 29)} \\ -\underline{12}\ \text{mmol/L} & \text{Expected change in } HCO_3^- \\ 14\ \text{mmol/L} & \text{Expected } HCO_3^- \end{array}$$

The actual HCO_3^-, however, is 8 mmol/L, or 6 mmol/L lower than expected. Thus, there must also be a metabolic nongap acidosis in addition to the metabolic gap acidosis.

IV. Database

A. Physical examination key points

1. **Vital signs.** A low respiratory rate suggests hypoventilation; a high rate points toward respiratory failure or compensation for a metabolic acidosis. Hypotension suggests hypoperfusion.
2. **Skin.** Changes, which characterize scleroderma, indicate a restrictive defect. Cool, clammy, and mottled skin on the extremities suggests shock.
3. **HEENT.** Ketosis or fruity odor on breath suggests diabetic ketoacidosis. Look for tracheal shift from a space-occupying lesion or venous distension (congestive heart failure or tension pneumothorax). Pinpoint pupils are consistent with drug overdose.
4. **Lungs.** Evaluate for absent or decreased breath sounds, stridor in upper airway obstruction, wheezes, and rales.
5. **Abdomen.** Peritoneal signs indicate an acute abdomen; marked distension may inhibit respiration.
6. **Neuromuscular examination.** Generalized weakness or focal neurologic signs, depressed level of consciousness, obtundation, and coma should be noted.

B. Laboratory data

1. **Hemograms.** Anemia may be associated with renal failure. Anemia may cause ischemia resulting in lactic acidosis. Leukocytosis with a left shift may suggest sepsis.
2. **Electrolytes.** Serum chloride is usually elevated in metabolic nongap acidosis. Serum potassium is usually increased with acidosis, but may be low in diabetic ketoacidosis or renal tubular acidosis. The serum potassium may be especially helpful in determining the acid–base status given the serum bicarbonate prior to the ABG analysis. For instance, a serum bicarbonate of 34 mmol/L could indicate a

primary metabolic alkalosis, or compensation for a chronic respiratory acidosis. If the potassium were 5.6 mmol/L, this would argue that the bicarbonate of 34 mmol/L was from compensation for a chronic respiratory acidosis. If the potassium were 3.1 mmol/L, this would argue that the bicarbonate of 34 mmol/L was from a metabolic alkalosis. The potassium, BUN, and creatinine may be elevated with renal failure. The creatinine may be falsely elevated with ketoacidosis.

3. **Metabolic gap acidosis.** The following tests *must be* ordered:
   a. **Glucose.** If elevated, may indicate diabetic ketoacidosis.
   b. **Ketone levels.** May indicate alcoholic, starvation, or diabetic ketoacidosis.
   c. **Lactate.** Lactic acidosis may be seen with alcohol use, severe anemia, sepsis, hypoperfusion (either generalized or local), hypoxemia, end-stage liver disease, and postictally.
   d. **Salicylate level**
   e. **Ethanol**
   f. **Methanol**
   g. **Ethylene glycol**
   h. **Paraldehyde.** Very rare cause of metabolic acidosis.
   i. **BUN and creatinine**
4. **Metabolic nongap acidosis.** If the history does not reveal an obvious cause such as diarrhea, then you need to consider renal tubular acidosis.
   a. **Distal renal tubular acidosis.** Inability to lower urine pH below 5.5 with NH_4Cl (ammonium chloride).
   b. **Proximal renal tubular acidosis.** Urine pH will decrease to < 5.5; however, the excretion of HCO_3^- is increased to $> 15\%$ when serum HCO_3^- is raised to the normal range.
5. **Respiratory acidosis.** Order a serum and urine drug screen. If there is hypoventilation with decreased respirations, you need to rule out a drug overdose. Also, with an intentional salicylate overdose, ingestion of other substances must be ruled out, as intentional overdoses often involve multiple substances.

C. **Radiologic and other studies.** If there is respiratory acidosis, radiologic studies may be needed.
   1. **Chest x-ray (CXR).** Rule out pneumothorax, pulmonary edema, pleural effusion, or infiltrative processes.
   2. **CT scan of head.** Consider with hypoventilation and altered mental status or with focal neurologic exam.
   3. **Electromyography (EMG).** May be helpful in assessment of neuromuscular disorders.

V. **Plan.** In general, for both respiratory and metabolic acidosis, treatment of the underlying cause of the acidemia is the primary goal. In emergent situations, the two methods for short-term reversal of metabolic and respiratory acidosis are: (1) to administer IV sodium bicarbonate; and (2) to hyperventilate the patient. Be sure to check serial pH values to monitor the progress of therapy.

A. Severe acidosis (pH < 7.20). Use continuous cardiac monitoring for potential arrhythmias.

B. Metabolic acidosis. Sodium bicarbonate is the mainstay for therapy. Sodium acetate, citrate, and lactate can be used, but all three must be metabolized to bicarbonate, and if hypoperfusion is a problem, the metabolism of one of the precursors to bicarbonate may be delayed.

1. **Bicarbonate therapy.** Although controversial, the present recommendation is to administer IV bicarbonate if the pH < 7.10. The goal is to raise the HCO_3^- to 10–15 mmol.
   a. Calculate the amount of sodium bicarbonate needed to raise the HCO_3^- to a given level.

   $$NaHCO_3 \text{ needed} = \text{wt (in kg)} \times 0.80^* \times (\text{desired } HCO_3^- - \text{measured } HCO_3^-).$$

   b. Give 50% of this amount over the first 12 hours as a mixture of bicarbonate with D5W. A normal bicarbonate drip is made by adding 3 ampoules of $NaHCO_3$ (50 mEq/ampoule) to 1 L of D5W.
   c. Complications of bicarbonate therapy include:
      i. **Hypernatremia**
      ii. **Volume overload**
      iii. **Hypokalemia. Caused by intracellular shifts of potassium as the pH increases.**
      iv. **Overshoot metabolic alkalosis. From overaggressive therapy.**
2. **THAM (0.3 *N* tromethamine).** Is a commercial carbon dioxide–consuming alkalinizing solution. Not clinically proven to be more beneficial than sodium bicarbonate. Side effects include hyperkalemia, hyperglycemia, and respiratory depression.
3. **Treatment of underlying causes**
   a. **Sepsis and hemorrhagic shock.** Volume resuscitation with normal saline is indicated. Vasopressors may be needed. See Section I, Chapter 42, Hypotension, Section V, p 227.
   b. **Renal failure.** Dialysis as needed.
   c. **Diabetic ketoacidosis.** Normal saline and insulin for diabetic ketoacidosis. See Section I, Chapter 32, Hyperglycemia, Section V, p 183.
   d. **Alcoholic ketoacidosis.** Normal saline and dextrose for alcoholic ketoacidosis, along with replacement of other electrolytes and vitamins such as thiamine and folate as needed.
   e. **Starvation ketosis.** Normal saline and dextrose.
   f. **Salicylate intoxication.** Treated with alkalinization of urine. Intravenous fluids containing $NaHCO_3$ (3 ampoules 50 mEq in 1 L of D5W or 2 ampoules $NaHCO_3$ in 1 L D5 1/4NS) are ad-

ministered at 100–250 mL/hr. Check urine pH every 1–2 hours. Urine pH should be maintained at or above 7.5–8.0. ABG and serum bicarbonate should be followed closely, and severe alkalemia (pH > 7.55) avoided. Hemodialysis may be required.

g. **Methanol and ethylene glycol ingestion.** Treated with ethanol infusion (desired serum concentration of ethanol is 100–120 mg/dL), which decreases the accumulation of toxic metabolites. More recently fomepizole (4-methylpyrazole) has been shown to be a safe and effective treatment alternative to ethanol. Hemodialysis may be required.

C. **Respiratory acidosis.** The main goal is to treat the underlying cause.

1. If indicated, intubate the patient and treat with mechanical ventilation. If a patient is already intubated and has a significant respiratory acidosis, then increase alveolar ventilation by increasing tidal volume (up to 8–10 mL/kg), while following peak inspiratory pressures, or by increasing the respiratory rate. See Section I, Chapter 19; Dyspnea, V, p 115; and Section VI, Ventilator Management, Chapter 3C, p 454.
2. In an emergent situation, disconnect the patient from the ventilator and hyperventilate by hand. The importance of good pulmonary toilet (ie, suctioning of secretions) cannot be overemphasized. Sedation is often a necessary adjunct to mechanical ventilation. See Section VI, Ventilator Management, Chapters 3A (p 448) and 3C (p 454).

REFERENCES

Adrogue HJ, Madias NE: Management of life-threatening acid-base disorders. N Engl J Med 1998;338:26.

Brent J, McMartin K, Phillips S, Aaron C, Kulig K: Fomepizole for the treatment of methanol poisoning. N Engl J Med 2001;344:424.

Kaehny WD: Pathogenesis and management of respiratory and mixed acid-base disorders. In: Schrier RW, ed. *Renal and Electrolyte Disorders.* 5th ed. Lippincott-Raven;1997:172.

Narins RG, Emmett A: Simple and mixed acid-base disorders: A practical approach. Medicine 1980;59:161.

Shapiro JI, Kaehny WD: Pathogenesis and management of metabolic acidosis and alkalosis. In: Schrier RW, ed. *Renal and Electrolyte Disorders.* 5th ed. Lippincott-Raven;1997:130.

3. ALKALOSIS

I. **Problem.** You are consulted to see a 60-year-old male with a pH of 7.65, who is 3 days status post cholecystectomy.

II. **Immediate Questions**

A. **Is the alkalemia from a metabolic, respiratory, or mixed alkalosis?** A quick look at the pCO_2 on the arterial blood gas (ABG) slip will reveal whether the disturbance is a primary metabolic or respiratory alkalosis. If the pCO_2 is > 40 mm Hg, the primary disturbance is a metabolic alkalosis with at least partial respiratory compensation. If the pCO_2 is < 40 mm Hg, the disturbance may be a primary respiratory alkalosis or a mixed disturbance. Many arterial blood gas slips list the base excess (BE), which may help determine the etiology of the alkalosis. If the BE is negative, the alkalosis is respiratory; if the BE is positive, the alkalosis is at least partially metabolic. Remember, the BE is calculated from the pH, and assumes that both the pH and pCO_2 are correct.

B. **What are the patient's vital signs?** An elevated respiratory rate, fever, hypotension, or all three may indicate sepsis. Respiratory alkalosis is associated with sepsis. Tachypnea may also indicate anxiety, CNS disease, or pulmonary disease.

C. **What medications is the patient taking?** Diuretics can cause a contraction alkalosis. Acetate in hyperalimentation solutions, antacids, exogenous steroids, or large doses of penicillin or carbenicillin may cause an alkalosis. Salicylate overdose and progesterone can cause a respiratory alkalosis.

D. **Is a nasogastric tube in place? Is the patient vomiting?** Loss of HCl from the stomach is a common cause of metabolic alkalosis.

E. **Is there any history of mental status changes, seizures, paresthesias, or tetany?** Alkalemia may cause the above; and if so, prompt action is indicated.

F. **Is there any ventricular ectopy?** Severe alkalemia may cause ventricular arrhythmias unresponsive to the usual pharmacologic treatments.

Caution: Mortality in critically ill surgical patients is associated with a high serum pH. One study indicated that mortality was 69% in patients with a pH > 7.60, but fell to 44% in patients with a pH between 7.55 and 7.59.

G. **Is there any associated chest pain?** Severe alkalemia causes arteriolar constriction resulting in a decrease in coronary blood flow. The anginal threshold is also reduced.

H. **What is the serum bicarbonate?** To fully understand an acid–base problem, you must obtain the serum bicarbonate from an electrolyte panel. A low serum bicarbonate is evidence of a primary respiratory alkalosis with at least partial metabolic compensation. A high serum bicarbonate is evidence for either a primary metabolic alkalosis or a mixed metabolic and respiratory alkalosis.

I. **Does the serum bicarbonate fit the pH and pCO_2?** See Section I, Chapter 2, Acidosis, Section II.E., p 10.

J. **Is the compensation appropriate?** Checking to see if the compensation is appropriate may unmask mixed disturbances.

1. For respiratory alkalosis, immediate compensation takes place through buffers. The compensation for acute respiratory alkalosis is a decrease of 2 mmol of HCO_3^- (range 1–3 mmol) for each 10 mm Hg decrease in pCO_2. Renal compensation is complete between 2 and 4 days. The compensation for chronic respiratory alkalosis is a decrease of about 5 mmol of HCO_3^- for each 10 mm Hg decrease in pCO_2. For instance, in a 35-year-old woman who is 36 weeks pregnant, the ABG revealed a pCO_2 of 25. One would expect the HCO_3^- to decrease by 7.5 mmol from the calculation 5 mmol/L × (40 mm Hg – 25 mm mg)/10 mm Hg. One would expect the HCO_3^- to be 18.5 or 26 mmol/L (normal HCO_3^-) – 7.5 mmol (expected change in HCO_3^-). If the HCO_3^- were 25 mmol, a relative metabolic alkalosis would be present along with the primary respiratory alkalosis, since the serum bicarbonate is higher than expected. If the HCO_3^- were 13 mmol, there would be a metabolic acidosis along with the primary respiratory alkalosis, since the serum bicarbonate is lower than expected.
2. For metabolic alkalosis, compensation begins immediately through buffers and hypoventilation. Hypoventilation as a means of compensation is limited by resulting hypoxemia. Seldom will the pCO_2 be > 55 mm Hg secondary to compensation. The expected increase in pCO_2 is 0.6 mm Hg (range 0.25–1.0 mm Hg) for each 1-mmol increase in HCO_3^-. For instance, in a 60-year-old status post cholecystectomy, the HCO_3^- was 36 mmol/L. The expected pCO_2 is 46 mm Hg (36 mmol/L – 26 mmol/L) × 0.6 mm Hg per 1 mmol/L change in HCO_3^-. If the pCO_2 were 40 mm Hg, there would be a relative respiratory alkalosis along with the primary metabolic alkalosis. If the pCO_2 were 55 mm Hg, there would be a respiratory acidosis along with a primary metabolic alkalosis.

III. Differential Diagnosis. Alkalemia results either from a metabolic or respiratory alkalosis. There may be many causes for both, and sometimes a patient may have more than one cause.

A. Respiratory alkalosis. By definition, respiratory alkalosis occurs secondary to hyperventilation. Hyperventilation can result from either central or peripheral stimulation of respiration. Common causes include medications, CNS disease, pulmonary disease, anxiety, and systemic disorders.

1. **Medications**
   a. **Salicylate overdose.** Causes an isolated respiratory alkalosis (30%), isolated metabolic gap acidosis (10%), and most commonly a mixed metabolic gap acidosis and respiratory alkalosis (57%).
   b. **Progesterone**
2. **CNS disease.** See Section I, Chapter 13, Coma, Acute Mental Status Changes, p 72.

   a. **Cerebrovascular accident**
   b. **Infection**
   c. **Tumor.** Primary or metastatic.
   d. **Trauma**
3. **Pulmonary disease.** See Section I, Chapter 19, Dyspnea, p 111.
   a. **Interstitial lung disease**
   b. **Pneumonia.** Usually causes respiratory alkalosis; if multiple lobes or underlying lung disease, may cause respiratory acidosis.
   c. **Asthma.** If mild to moderate, will cause a respiratory alkalosis; if severe, respiratory acidosis may result.
   d. **Pulmonary emboli**
   e. **Pneumothorax**
4. **Anxiety**
5. **Pulmonary edema.** If mild, causes a respiratory alkalosis; if severe, may cause a respiratory acidosis.
6. **Pain**
7. **Pregnancy.** Secondary to progesterone.
8. **Liver disease.** Cirrhosis.
9. **Fever**
10. **Early sepsis**
11. **Hyperthyroidism**
12. **Iatrogenic**
13. **Hypoxemia**
14. **Residence at high altitude**

B. **Pseudorespiratory alkalosis.** Arterial hypocapnia is present; however, there is an increase in the mixed venous pCO_2. Seen in severe cardiac dysfunction and associated pulmonary perfusion with normal pulmonary function. Total body carbon dioxide is decreased, resulting in an increase in H^+ and an acidosis.

C. **Metabolic alkalosis.** Can be divided into chloride-responsive and chloride-unresponsive. The urine Cl^- is $<$ 10–20 mmol/L with the chloride-responsive causes, and $>$ 20–30 mmol/L with the chloride-unresponsive causes (provided no diuretic has been given). Severe metabolic alkalosis is usually the chloride-responsive type.

1. **Chloride-responsive causes**
   a. **Gastric losses.** Vomiting or nasogastric tube.
   b. **Diarrhea.** Chloride wasting.
   c. **Diuretics**
   d. **Correction of chronic hypercapnia**
   e. **Sulfates, phosphates, or high-dose penicillins**
   f. **Massive blood transfusion.** Citrate is used as an anticoagulant and is metabolized to HCO_3^-. One unit of whole blood and one unit of packed red cells contain 17 and 5 mEq of citrate, respectively.

2. **Chloride-unresponsive causes**
   a. **Cushing's syndrome.** Elevated glucocorticoids from a variety of causes including pituitary adenoma, adrenal adenoma, and ectopic production. Also causes hypertension, glucose intolerance, fluid retention, and osteoporosis.
   b. **Hyperaldosteronism.** Rare cause of hypertension. Also associated with hypokalemia and hypernatremia.
   c. **Exogenous steroid ingestion**
   d. **Bartter's syndrome.** Also causes hypokalemia. Hyperreninemia and hyperaldosteronemia secondary to hyperplasia of the juxtaglomerular apparatus. Patients are normotensive.
   e. **Potassium or magnesium deficiency**
   f. **Calcium carbonate–containing antacids**
   g. **Milk-alkali syndrome**
   h. **Refeeding with glucose after starvation**

IV. Database

A. Physical examination key points

1. **Vital signs.** Tachypnea may indicate pulmonary disease, pulmonary edema, or CNS respiratory stimulation. An elevated temperature may indicate an infection or sepsis.
2. **Chest.** Examination must be thorough; look for evidence of pneumothorax, pleural effusion, pneumonia, bronchospastic disease, and pulmonary edema.
3. **Abdomen.** Look for evidence of chronic liver disease such as ascites and caput medusae.
4. **Skin.** Check for evidence of chronic liver disease such as palmar erythema, Dupuytren's contractures, and spider angiomas. Also look for changes associated with Cushing's syndrome, such as buffalo hump, purple striae, and easy bruisability.
5. **Neurologic exam.** Check for focal abnormalities as evidence for tumor, cerebrovascular accident, and infection. Tremor and hyperreflexia may suggest hyperthyroidism.

B. Laboratory data

1. **Anion gap.** May unmask a mixed metabolic gap acidosis and metabolic alkalosis. See Section I, Chapter 2, Acidosis, III.B.
2. **Serum electrolytes.** Hypokalemia and hypomagnesemia may cause a metabolic alkalosis. Hypokalemia, hypomagnesemia, hypocalcemia, and hypophosphatemia may result from alkalosis.
3. **Respiratory alkalosis**
   a. **Salicylate level.** If elevated, check serum and urine drug screen for other ingested substances.
   b. **Liver function tests**
   c. **Thyroid function studies**
   d. **Blood cultures**

4. **Metabolic alkalosis.** You will need a spot urine for chloride. A urine chloride below 10–20 mmol/L represents a **chloride-responsive** alkalosis. A urine chloride above 20 mmol/L represents a **chloride-unresponsive** alkalosis.
5. **Chloride-unresponsive metabolic alkalosis.** You may need to rule out Cushing's syndrome and primary aldosteronism.

C. **Radiologic and other studies.** If respiratory alkalosis, consider the following:

1. **Chest x-ray.** To look for pulmonary disease and pulmonary edema.
2. **CT scan of head.** Rule out CNS disease.

V. **Plan.** It is essential to identify the cause of the alkalemia and treat it.

A. **Respiratory alkalosis**

1. **If hypoxic,** give supplemental oxygen.
2. **If anxious,** give sedative. Diazepam 1–5 mg PO or 1–2 mg IV; or lorazepam 1–2 mg PO or 0.5 mg IV.
3. **If nonintubated,** increase $FiCO_2$ (fraction of inspired carbon dioxide). Use a rebreathing mask (or a paper bag). Would consider for pH > 7.55.
4. **If the patient is intubated,** decrease minute ventilation. Decrease the rate or tidal volume. Be sure the tidal volume is set for 8–10 mL/kg. The respirator may need to be changed from assist control to intermittent ventilation. Increasing the amount of dead space would also increase the pCO_2.
5. **Salicylate overdose.** Consider alkalinization of urine. Alkalinization of urine should be done cautiously in a patient who is already alkalotic. Follow serum pH and serum bicarbonate closely. See Section I, Chapter 2, Acidosis, Section V, p 16, for instructions on alkalinization of urine. Hemodialysis may be required.

B. **Metabolic alkalosis**

1. In the presence of severe alkalemia with seizures or ventricular arrhythmias, prompt, immediate action is needed. Treatment includes increasing the pCO_2, or administering an acid such as hydrochloric acid. HCl 0.1–0.2 N solution (100–200 mmol of H^+ per liter) is administered slowly through a central line. The amount of required HCl to be administered can be calculated by taking the desired change in HCO_3^- and multiplying by the weight in kg and by 0.50 (bicarbonate space). For instance, in a 80-kg man with a pH of 7.68, if the actual bicarbonate is 52 mmol/L and the desired is 40 mmol/L, the required amount of HCl would be (52 mmol/L − 40 mmol/L) $\times$ 80 kg $\times$ 0.5 = 480 mmol, or about 2.5 liters of 0.2 N solution.
2. **Ammonium chloride and arginine hydrochloride.** Both are precursors to HCl; however, there is significant risk (an increase in ammonia with ammonium chloride in patients with liver failure and hyperkalemia with arginine hydrochloride with renal failure).

3. **Bicarbonate precursors.** Acetate salts (amino acids) found in hyperalimentation solutions or solutions containing lactate should be eliminated.
4. **If chloride-responsive,** give normal saline.
5. **If chloride-unresponsive,** treat underlying disorder.
   a. If potassium or magnesium deficient, will often need massive replacement.
   b. Evaluation and specific treatment of endogenous mineralocorticoid disorders.

REFERENCES

Adrogue HJ, Madias NE: Management of life-threatening acid-base disorders. N Engl J Med 1998;338:107.

Kaehny WD: Pathogenesis and management of respiratory and mixed acid-base disorders. In: Schrier RW, ed. *Renal and Electrolyte Disorders.* 5th ed. Lippincott-Raven;1997:172.

Narins RG, Emmett A: Simple and mixed acid-base disorders: A practical approach. Medicine 1980;59:161.

Shapiro JI, Kaehny WD: Pathogenesis and management of metabolic acidosis and alkalosis. In: Schrier RW, ed. *Renal and Electrolyte Disorders.* 5th ed. Lippincott-Raven;1997:130.

Wilson RF, Gibson D, Percinel AK et al: Severe alkalosis in critically ill surgical patients. Arch Surg 1972;105:197.

4. ANAPHYLACTIC REACTION

I. **Problem.** Within 10 minutes of receiving an intramuscular injection, a patient develops diffuse pruritus, wheezing, and shortness of breath.

II. **Immediate Questions.** Anaphylaxis can be a life-threatening situation and requires immediate evaluation and treatment.

A. **What are the patient's vital signs?** Tachycardia is a common finding and can result from arrhythmia or as a response to hypoxia, fear, or hypotension. Hypotensive shock, which can occur with or without other symptoms, poses the greatest danger from anaphylaxis and must be recognized and treated promptly.

B. **Can the patient still communicate?** The ability to provide appropriate answers to simple questions implies adequate cerebral oxygenation. Inability to speak, dysphonia, hoarseness, or stridor could indicate upper airway obstruction from laryngospasm or laryngeal edema.

C. **What medication(s) did the patient receive?** Anaphylaxis can result from a variety of agents, including medications, foods (especially shellfish and nuts), latex, blood products, venoms, and pollens. The most common medications causing anaphylaxis are penicillins, cephalosporins, sulfonamides, angiotensin-converting enzyme (ACE) inhibitors, chemotherapeutic agents, and local anesthetics. Nonimmunologically mediated anaphylactoid reactions result from opiates, nonsteroidal anti-inflammatory drugs, and radiocontrast material. Any medicines suspected of causing an anaphylactic reaction must be stopped immediately.

III. Differential Diagnosis. Signs and symptoms of anaphylaxis are produced by the release of biologically active mediators such as histamine from basophils and mast cells. This release can either be mediated immunologically through the interaction of antigen with IgE residing on the basophils and mast cells, or it can occur as the result of a nonimmunologic release of mediators. These mediators affect several organ systems, including the skin, upper and lower airways, cardiovascular system, and gastrointestinal tract. Anaphylaxis may involve only one or all of the preceding organ systems and thus must be distinguished from other disease processes occurring at these sites.

A. Upper airway obstruction. This could result from epiglottitis, aspiration of foreign body, vocal cord dysfunction syndrome, globus hystericus, or with other causes of laryngeal edema such as hereditary angioedema. Angioedema involving the tongue and lips secondary to ACE inhibitor therapy is commonly seen today.

B. Lower airway obstruction. Think of status asthmaticus, bolus aspiration, cardiogenic pulmonary edema, or pulmonary embolism.

C. Syncope. See Section I, Chapter 59, Syncope, p 315.

D. Flushing syndromes. Think about carcinoid syndrome, postmenopausal state, "red neck" syndrome with vancomycin, or autonomic epilepsy. Pheochromocytoma usually causes pallor; however, 10–15% of the cases of pheochromocytoma have flushing.

E. Urticaria. This condition can be produced by a wide variety of causes other than anaphylaxis.

F. Excess histamine states. These are found in systemic mastocytosis, basophilic leukemia, and acute promyelocytic leukemia.

G. Serum sickness. Usually occurs 5–7 days after exposure to agent, compared with anaphylaxis, which occurs in 5–60 minutes. This may be seen with beta-lactams (especially oral cefaclor) and horse serum–based rattlesnake antivenom.

IV. Database. Knowledge of the patient's prior history of allergies and current medications is essential. The temporal relationship between administration of medication and the onset of symptoms is also important, since anaphylaxis usually occurs within 1 hour of administration.

A. Physical examination key points

1. **Vital signs.** Hypotension must be recognized immediately.
2. **HEENT.** Evaluate for swelling of lips, tongue, and oropharynx.
3. **Lungs.** Listen for stridor (suggests upper airway obstruction) and wheezing (suggests bronchospasm).

4. **Skin.** Generalized flushing, urticaria, and angioedema may occur.
5. **Extremities.** Look for cyanosis.
6. **Mental status.** Impaired mentation may indicate significant respiratory compromise or hypotension and would suggest the need for immediate respiratory and/or blood pressure support.

B. **Laboratory data**
1. **Serum tryptase.** A protease specific to mast cells, reaches a peak 1 hour after an anaphylactic reaction occurs and remains elevated for approximately 6 hours. A serum tryptase during this period would help confirm the diagnosis.
2. ***N*-methyl-histamine.** A histamine metabolite, remains elevated in the urine for several hours after an anaphylactic reaction and can be measured by a 24-hour urine sample for *N*-methyl-histamine.

C. **Radiologic and other studies**
1. **Chest x-ray.** Can be obtained after the patient is stabilized to exclude other causes of respiratory distress, such as pneumonia and congestive heart failure.
2. **Electrocardiogram.** Acute myocardial infarction can present with severe dyspnea. Anaphylaxis can also cause myocardial ischemia and arrhythmias (mainly in the elderly population).

V. **Plan.** Treatment should be initiated quickly—without waiting for the results of laboratory testing. Any medicines suspected of causing an anaphylactic reaction must be stopped immediately. Initial therapy consists of epinephrine, oxygen, and nebulized beta$_2$-agonist.
1. **Epinephrine.** Epinephrine 0.3–0.5 mL of 1:1000 dilution subcutaneously or intramuscularly should be given immediately for laryngeal edema, bronchospasm, or urticaria. This may be repeated every 10–15 minutes up to a total of three doses. Patients with hypotension, poor tissue perfusion, and IV access will require intravenous epinephrine given as 0.5–1.0 cc of 1:10,000 dilution in bolus fashion (can be given in intervals of 5–10 minutes). If no improvement is seen, a continuous infusion of epinephrine (1–4 μg/min) titrated to effect may be administered. If IV access cannot be obtained immediately, deliver twice the above IV dose down the endotracheal tube.
2. **Oxygen.** Oxygen by face mask should be instituted if the patient appears dyspneic. Intubation may be required if the patient is severely somnolent or hypoxemic. Tracheostomy may be necessary if upper airway edema precludes intubation. The goal is to maintain $pO_2 > 60$ mm Hg.
3. **Bronchodilators.** Albuterol (0.5 mL of 0.5% solution in 2.5 mL of saline) can be administered by nebulizer for persistent bronchospasm.
4. **Antihistamines.** Diphenhydramine (Benadryl) 25–50 mg IV/IM/PO Q 6 hr and cimetidine 300 mg IV Q 8 hr (or other H_2

blockers) should follow epinephrine to reduce the effects of histamine release. This may alleviate hypotension as well as lessen the symptoms associated with mild urticaria.

5. **Glucocorticoids.** Methylprednisolone 120 mg IV × 1 dose then 60 mg IV Q 6 hr should be given in patients with anaphylactic bronchospasm. This may also help the late-phase response that sometimes occurs 6–12 hours after the initial presentation.
6. **Glucagon.** Patients on beta-blockers may be resistant to treatment with epinephrine and can develop refractory hypotension and bradycardia. Glucagon 1 mg IV/IM/SC bolus × 1 dose is administered for inotropic and chronotropic effects not mediated through beta-receptors.
7. **Blood pressure support.** Hypotension usually responds to epinephrine; however, normal saline may be necessary for patients who fail to respond, as well as glucagon, as noted above. Vasopressor medications like dopamine should be used for persistent hypotension despite aggressive fluid administration.
8. **Monitoring.** Telemetry or intensive care unit admission is mandatory for anaphylaxis requiring epinephrine therapy. Relapse of anaphylaxis (late-phase response) can occur hours after the initial presentation. Close monitoring through the first 24 hours is essential. Even with rapid and appropriate treatment, patients may fail to respond. Always be prepared for the possible need for emergent intubation or tracheostomy.

VI. **Prevention.** Patients who have experienced anaphylaxis should be evaluated by an allergist.

A. **EpiPen.** Patients should be provided with, and instructed regarding the use of, a self-administered epinephrine injection device.

B. **Medic Alert bracelet.** Patients at risk for anaphylaxis should wear a Medic Alert bracelet at all times to expedite diagnosis and appropriate treatment in the event of subsequent anaphylaxis.

REFERENCES

Bochner BS, Lichtenstein LM: Anaphylaxis. N Engl J Med 1991;324:1785.

Freeman TM: Anaphylaxis: Diagnosis and treatment. Primary Care 1998;25:809.

Kemp SF, Lockey RF: Anaphylaxis: A review of 266 cases. Arch Intern Med 1995;155:1749.

Ring J, Behrendt H: Anaphylaxis and anaphylactoid reactions. Clin Rev Allergy Immunol 1999;28:723.

Winbery SL, Lieberman PL: Anaphylaxis. Immunol Allergy Clin North Am 1995;15:447.

5. ANEMIA

I. **Problem.** A 50-year-old man is admitted for pneumonia. Laboratory testing reveals a hemoglobin of 11.2 g/dL (7.0 mmol/L).

II. Immediate Questions

A. **What are the patient's vital signs?** If the patient is not hypotensive or severely tachycardic, transfusion therapy is not emergently indicated.

B. **Is the patient symptomatic?** In the absence of angina, congestive heart failure, syncope, pre-syncope, or hemodynamic compromise, transfusion therapy is not emergently indicated.

C. **Is there evidence of acute or recent blood loss such as hematemesis, melena, or hematochezia?** Gastrointestinal (GI) blood loss can be divided into acute or chronic, upper GI (see Section I, Chapter 27, Hematemesis, Melena, p 158) and lower GI (see Section I, Chapter 28, Hematochezia, p 162). Patients more frequently succumb from acute upper GI blood loss than from lower GI blood loss.

D. **Is there a history of hematuria or menorrhagia?** Long-standing hematuria or menorrhagia can cause iron deficiency anemia.

E. **What medications does the patient take?** Aspirin and nonsteroidal anti-inflammatory drugs (NSAIDs) may lead to GI blood loss. Alkylating agents (melphalan, *cis*-platinum), folate antagonists (trimethoprim-sulfamethoxazole, pentamidine), anticonvulsants (phenytoin), and anti-inflammatory drugs (phenylbutazone) may cause marrow suppression or aplasia. Penicillin, sulfonamides, and methyldopa (Aldomet) may cause hemolysis. Alcohol, isoniazid, and trimethoprim may cause maturation defects.

F. **Is there significant organ dysfunction or a current inflammatory disease?** Severe liver, kidney, adrenal, and thyroid dysfunction may lead to anemia. Rheumatoid arthritis, systemic lupus erythematosus (SLE), vasculitides, and chronic osteomyelitis are associated with anemia of chronic disease.

G. **Does the patient have other medical problems associated with excess total body water that may lead to a pseudoanemia, such as congestive heart failure, cirrhosis, and pregnancy?** In the setting of increased plasma volume relative to the red blood cell (RBC) mass, an apparent anemia may be manifest or an existing anemia may be made more apparent.

H. **Does the patient have a personal or family history of anemia, thalassemia, sickle cell anemia, or glucose-6-phosphatase deficiency?** Hereditary disorders of hemoglobin usually present nonacutely, and a family history may be suggestive of an inherited cause of the anemia.

I. **Does the patient have an autoimmune disease?** Pernicious anemia, the most common cause of vitamin B_{12} deficiency, may be associated with other autoimmune endocrinopathies such as Hashimoto's thyroiditis, insulin-dependent diabetes mellitus, and Addison's disease.

III. Differential Diagnosis. There are over 100 causes of anemia. Visualizing the peripheral smear and paying careful attention to the RBC indices are essential when evaluating an anemia. Anemia may result from decreased production of RBCs, blood loss, or increased destruction of RBCs.

A. Pancytopenia. The platelet and white blood cell (WBC) counts are decreased along with the hemoglobin (HGB) and HCT. Pancytopenia is usually caused by marrow invasion, failure, or suppression; most commonly caused by drugs, carcinoma, hematologic malignancies, and inflammatory diseases. It may be idiopathic.

B. Anemia with a low mean corpuscular volume (MCV). Associated with microcytic RBCs on the peripheral smear. Iron deficiency is the most common etiology and is seen in approximately 20% of menstruating females. Hypochromic, microcytic RBCs, target cells, basophilic stippling, marked anisocytosis, and poikilocytosis are seen with thalassemias. Sideroblastic anemia and anemia of chronic disease may also be associated with low MCV. The MCV should never be < 70 if it is due to chronic disease. Microcytic anemias can easily be differentiated by looking at the peripheral smear and various laboratory studies. Serum iron, total iron binding capacity or transferrin, ferritin, and hemoglobin electrophoresis may be helpful (Table 1–4).

C. Normal-MCV anemias. Many anemias are associated with a normal MCV. Anemia of chronic disease is probably the most common normocytic anemia. Chronic infections (tuberculosis, osteomyelitis), collagen vascular diseases, and malignancies may produce an anemia with a normal MCV. Kidney, liver, thyroid, and adrenal dysfunction may also lead to a normal-MCV anemia. Correction of the underlying disorder should correct the anemia. Acute GI blood loss results in a normal-MCV anemia.

D. High-MCV anemias. Many anemias are macrocytic, but only a few are megaloblastic. Folate and vitamin B_{12} deficiencies are the most common megaloblastic anemias. Vitamin B_{12} deficiency can be secondary to pernicious anemia (lack of intrinsic factor), bacterial overgrowth, ileal disease, and rarely, dietary deficiency. Vitamin B_{12} stores last 3–4 years. Folate deficiency is often caused by dietary de-

TABLE I–4. CAUSES OF MICROCYTIC ANEMIA.

	Iron Deficiency	β-Thalassemia	Chronic Disease	Sideroblastic Anemia
Iron	Low	Normal/increased	Low	Increased
TIBC	Increased	Normal	Low	Normal
Ferritin	Low	Normal/increased	Normal/increased	Increased
Hemoglobin A_2[1]	Normal	Increased	Normal	Normal

[1]A type of hemoglobin detected by hemoglobin electrophoresis.

ficiency but may be secondary to increased needs such as with pregnancy or hyperthyroidism. If there is no obvious cause of folate deficiency, then the possibility of malabsorption must be considered. Along with macrocytic RBCs, the peripheral smear of folate or vitamin B_{12} deficiency may demonstrate hypersegmented neutrophils and nucleated RBCs. Other anemias that may be associated with macrocytes are myelodysplasias, aplastic anemias, acquired sideroblastic anemias, anemias induced by chemotherapy (antimetabolites), and anemia associated with hypothyroidism and chronic liver disease. An increased MCV may be seen in the presence of a markedly increased reticulocyte count, because reticulocytes are large cells that increase the mean RBC size.

E. **Anemias with increased reticulocytosis.** Many anemias listed above are associated with an increased reticulocyte count. A *reticulocyte* is a very young RBC ~ 1 day old. Because the RBC life span is 120 days, the normal reticulocyte count is 1/120, or ~ 1%. An increased reticulocyte count indicates that the bone marrow is producing RBCs faster than normal. This is usually due to red cells having a shortened life span or to acute blood loss. The peripheral smear may reveal large polychromatophilic RBCs that are reticulocytes; however, a reticulocyte stain is needed to perform a definitive reticulocyte count. Examples of anemias with an increased reticulocyte count include acquired or autoimmune hemolytic anemias and congenital hemolytic anemias (sickle cell anemia, thalassemias). Correction of a particular deficit such as B_{12} deficiency by the administration of vitamin B_{12} will also lead to a reticulocytosis.

IV. Database

A. Physical examination key points

1. **Vital signs.** Make sure the patient is not hypotensive. The patient may be *orthostatic*. Look for a decrease in systolic blood pressure of 10 mm Hg and/or an increase in heart rate of 20 bpm on movement from a supine to a standing position after 1 minute. Orthostatic changes suggest acute blood loss.
2. **Skin.** Telangiectasia, palmar erythema, and jaundice may indicate liver disease. Isolated jaundice may point toward hemolysis.
3. **Oropharynx.** Glossitis is commonly seen in iron and B_{12} deficiency.
4. **Heart.** Murmurs indicate either hemolysis from valvular disease or a flow murmur resulting from the anemia.
5. **Abdomen.** Check for splenomegaly, which is associated with hemolysis, thalassemias, chronic leukemias, lymphomas, and occasionally acute leukemias. Could also indicate portal hypertension secondary to cirrhosis. Also look for ascites and hepatomegaly.
6. **Rectum.** Test for stool Hemoccult to look for acute or chronic GI blood loss.

7. **Neurologic examination.** Loss of vibration and position sense as well as dementia are associated with B_{12} deficiency but may also represent effects of alcohol.

B. **Laboratory data**

1. **Peripheral smear.** Review of the peripheral smear is essential. Note the size and shape of the RBCs and the presence or absence of platelets. Nucleated RBCs, reticulocytes, schistocytes, sickle cells, and target cells may aid in the diagnosis. Examine WBC morphology for hypersegmented neutrophils.
2. **Reticulocyte count.** The most important laboratory test after reviewing the peripheral smear. An increased reticulocyte count indicates either an appropriate response to anemia or shortened RBC survival through blood loss or hemolysis. A low reticulocyte count indicates that the marrow is responding inappropriately to the anemia either secondary to a nutritional deficiency or marrow failure from fibrosis or replacement (lymphoma, leukemia, carcinoma).
3. **Iron and total iron binding capacity (TIBC) or transferrin.** Occasionally a ferritin should also be obtained if the anemia is microcytic. Will aid in the diagnosis of iron deficiency anemia. Iron deficiency anemia results in a low iron and a normal or elevated TIBC or transferrin; the ferritin is also low. If the patient has a very low MCV (< 70) and a normal iron and TIBC, the likelihood of thalassemia is high. It is important to realize that many acute and chronic illnesses can dramatically affect the iron and TIBC, making their utility in the diagnosis of anemia low. If the question of iron deficiency requires a definite answer, a bone marrow exam with iron stains is indicated.
4. **B_{12} and folate.** Order these tests for any patient suspected of having B_{12} and folate deficiency prior to transfusion. If folate deficiency is secondary to malnutrition, a serum folate may be normal after one or two well-balanced meals. If folate deficiency is suspected and the patient has recently eaten, then consider checking an RBC folate.
5. **Haptoglobin and urine hemosiderin.** A low haptoglobin and a positive urine hemosiderin are indicative of hemolysis.
6. **Direct and indirect Coombs' test.** These tests may indicate that the hemolysis is immunologic. A direct Coombs' measures the presence of antibody and/or complement on the RBC; an indirect Coombs' detects antibody in the plasma that has dissociated from the RBC but is directed at the RBC. The direct Coombs' is the more valuable test in evaluating the possibility of immunohemolytic disease, whereas the indirect Coombs' is primarily of value as a blood banking procedure. Detection of an antibody in the plasma but not on the RBC indicates it is an alloantibody rather than an autoantibody. Most immunohemolytic anemias are due to warm–reacting antibodies, usually IgG. These are manifest

by a direct Coombs' that is positive for IgG with or without complement.

7. **Platelet count.** May be elevated in early iron deficiency. Decreased in folate and vitamin B_{12} deficiency as well as with marrow replacement.

C. **Radiologic and other studies.** Not usually needed unless GI blood loss is suspected; then order as clinically indicated.

V. Plan

A. Anemia with hemodynamic compromise or complications

1. If the patient is hemodynamically unstable or having angina, a transfusion is urgently indicated. In such cases, the source of blood loss is usually obvious. For specific information on transfusion, consult Section V, Blood Component Therapy, p 437.
2. Be sure the patient has adequate intravenous access if there is evidence of acute bleeding.

B. **Anemia without hemodynamic compromise or complications.** If the patient is not hemodynamically compromised, proceed with the workup in an orderly fashion. In many cases, the cause of the anemia is not obvious. Furthermore, laboratory testing is not always diagnostic. If the patient has an unremarkable history and physical, ambivalent laboratory testing, and no obvious underlying infectious, malignant, or inflammatory disease, a bone marrow biopsy is indicated.

C. **Iron deficiency anemia.** The source of blood loss must be found. This usually entails an upper endoscopy of the upper GI tract and a flexible sigmoidoscopy and air-contrast barium enema, or a colonoscopy. Keep in mind that heavy menstrual losses are the most common cause of iron deficiency anemia in young women. Once the source of blood loss is determined, the iron stores need to be repleted. Most patients tolerate oral iron as ferrous sulfate 325 mg PO tid between meals. Treatment must be continued for 3–6 months after normalization of the CBC to ensure adequate repletion of iron stores. Gradually increasing the dose over several days from Q day to bid to tid will improve tolerance to oral iron. Vitamin C 500–1000 units with each dose of iron may improve absorption.

D. **Folate deficiency.** This condition is usually due to dietary insufficiency (pregnancy, chronic alcoholism). In this setting, daily folate supplementation at 1 mg PO is indicated.

E. **Vitamin B_{12} deficiency.** Inadequate dietary intake is a rare cause of B_{12} deficiency. True pernicious anemia can be diagnosed by the use of Schilling's test, which involves giving a loading dose of 1000-mg vitamin B_{12} to saturate receptor sites. This dose is followed by the administration of radiolabeled B_{12} and measurement of the radioactivity in a 24-hour urine sample. If the amount of radioactive B_{12} in the urine is small, oral intrinsic factor can be given along with a second dose of radioactive B_{12} and a 24-hour urine can be recollected. An abnormal first step and a normal second step help differentiate between pernicious anemia and other causes of vitamin B_{12} deficiency (eg, bacterial overgrowth and ileal diseases). The history may also give an obvious etiology for B_{12} deficiency (status post gastrectomy or ileal resection). Vitamin B_{12} is replaced by administration of 30–100 μg IM daily for 2–3 weeks, then 100–200 μg IM every 2–4 weeks for life.

F. Hemolytic anemia. In the face of an elevated reticulocyte count with no obvious source of blood loss, a destructive process must be considered. Immune-mediated processes can be diagnosed by use of the Coombs' test. In the setting of Coombs' negative hemolytic anemia, other disease processes must be considered, such as disseminated intravascular coagulation or microangiopathic hemolytic anemia. A review of the peripheral smear will be helpful. A concomitant low platelet count, low fibrinogen, and elevated prothrombin time, partial thromboplastin time, and fibrin degradation products point toward disseminated intravascular coagulation, (see Section I, Chapter 12, Coagulopathy, V, p 70). The possibility of an inherited disorder such as thalassemia, sickle cell anemia, or an enzymopathy must be ruled out. Hemoglobin electrophoresis and review of the peripheral smear are indicated. If an enzymopathy is considered, specific assays are indicated (glucose-6-phosphate dehydrogenase, pyruvate kinase, etc). The possibility of paroxysmal nocturnal hemoglobinuria must be considered in cases where the etiology is unclear. Ham's test is indicated in this instance. Discussion of specific treatments for hemolytic anemias is beyond the scope of this book.

G. Anemia of chronic disease. This is usually a diagnosis of exclusion. However, if the patient has end-stage renal disease, endogenous erythropoietin levels may be low and the patient may respond to replacement therapy. In other cases, the etiology may be obvious, as with advanced malignancy. There is no specific diagnostic test for this disorder; treatment is of the underlying disease. It is generally manifest by a low reticulocyte count, a low iron and a low TIBC or transferrin, and normal bone marrow morphology. These are not specific findings, however.

REFERENCES

Bolinger A: Anemias. In: Koda-Kimbel MA, Young LY, eds. *Applied Therapeutics: The Clinical Use of Drugs.* 5th ed. Applied Therapeutics, Inc.;1992.

Lux SE: Introduction to anemia. In: Handin RI, Lux SE, Stossel TP, eds. *Blood: Principles and Practice of Hematology.* Lippincott;1995:1383.

Izaks GJ, Westendorp RGJ, Knook DL: The definition of anemia in older persons. JAMA 1999;281:1714.

Toh B-H, van Driel IR, Gleeson PA: Pernicious anemia. N Engl J Med 1997;337:1441.

6. ARTERIAL LINE PROBLEMS

(See also Section III, Chapter 1, Arterial Line Placement, p 390).

I. **Problem.** You are called to the intensive care unit to see a patient in whom a low, dampened arterial line pressure is being obtained.

II. **Immediate Questions**

A. **Does the pressure accurately reflect the patient's status?** Mental status changes (see Section I, Chapter 13, Coma, Acute Mental Status Changes, p 72), tachycardia, and a decreased urine output would be expected with hypotension.

B. **Is the problem with the catheter itself or with the monitoring apparatus (tubing, transducer, electronic equipment)?** If the patient's clinical status does not reflect the low blood pressure obtained by the arterial line, the problem may lie in the equipment.

C. **Is an extremity at risk?** Thrombosis secondary to the arterial line can cause ischemia and tissue loss.

D. **Has the quality of the tracing changed recently?** Find out if the tracing was satisfactory earlier. A good tracing followed by a poor one suggests either deterioration in clinical status or a new problem with the catheter.

III. **Differential Diagnosis.** A low or dampened blood pressure may result from problems with the monitoring equipment, problems with the arterial line catheter, or actual hemodynamic deterioration of the patient.

A. **Patient status.** If the patient's hemodynamic status has deteriorated, the decrease in blood pressure or dampening of the waveform is actually indicative of the patient's status. Often, other clinical indicators of the patient's status such as mental status changes, tachycardia, decreased urine output, and electrocardiographic changes suggest that the patient is genuinely hypotensive.

B. **Monitoring apparatus problems**

1. Air is present in the tubing/transducer.
2. The tubing is kinked.
3. Electrical equipment is faulty.

C. **Catheter problems**

1. There are kinks in the catheter.
2. A thrombus is present in the catheter or in the vessel.
3. The catheter tip is resting against the wall of the artery because of the way the catheter was anchored (by suture or taping).
4. The catheter has punctured the arterial wall, causing bleeding and compression of the catheter.

IV. **Database**

A. **Physical examination key points**

1. **Blood pressure.** If the arterial line pressure is low, perform a brachial artery cuff pressure. If the reading confirms hypotension,

prompt action is indicated. The manual blood pressure is usually within 10–20 mm Hg of the arterial line pressure, unless severe vasoconstriction is present; in which case indirect measurement may underestimate direct measurement by 20–30 mm Hg.

2. **Pulses.** Check at once for distal pulses and for swelling or tenderness in the area of the catheter insertion. Failure to find a pulse or the presence of a decrease in pulse, with significant swelling at the catheter site, represents a potentially serious vascular compromise.
3. **Inspection of the equipment**
   a. Check for air in the lines or the transducer. The search must be thorough and will almost certainly require the assistance of the nursing staff.
   b. Have nursing staff confirm that the electrical equipment is working properly.
   c. Attempt to withdraw blood through the catheter. Inability to do so suggests either that the catheter tip is poorly positioned or that there is a kink or a thrombus in the catheter, at the catheter tip, or in the artery. ***Caution:*** Do not attempt to flush a catheter through which blood cannot be drawn!

V. Plan

A. Maintaining perfusion to the extremity. A limb may be susceptible to ischemic injury as the result of systemic hypotension, a large catheter-to-vessel ratio, bleeding into surrounding tissues, inadequate flushing techniques, or prolonged catheter indwelling time.

1. Failure of the pulse to return will probably necessitate a surgical attempt at thrombus removal or repair of the artery. Consult a vascular surgeon immediately.
2. If bleeding from the artery into the surrounding tissue seems likely, watch carefully for compartmental syndrome (pain, pain with extension of the digits, pallor, hypesthesia, and loss of motor function). Surgical evacuation of the blood may be necessary. Consult a vascular surgeon at once if compartmental syndrome is suspected.
3. Search for evidence of infection. If infection is present, culture and treat appropriately, and remove the catheter.

B. Monitoring apparatus problems

1. Flush the transducer and tubing thoroughly.
2. Retape the tubing to eliminate kinks.
3. Replace faulty electrical equipment.
4. An armboard may prevent the catheter or tubing from extra-arterial kinking.

C. Catheter problems

1. Loosen sutures or tape to reposition the catheter tip away from the wall.
2. If a thrombus or kink in the intra-arterial catheter is suspected, the line will probably have to be removed and relocated.

3. In general, do not attempt to place a new arterial line over a guide wire. Remove the old catheter and replace it with a new one, preferably at a different site. Perforation of the catheter with the guide wire may cause a foreign body embolus, damage to the arterial wall, or dislodgement of a thrombus in or at the tip of the catheter. All these potentially serious complications make the risk of using a catheter guide wire to assess a dampened waveform unwise.

7. ASPIRATION

I. **Problem.** After a generalized seizure, a patient is observed to vomit and subsequently develops acute respiratory distress.

II. **Immediate Questions**

A. **What are the vital signs?** On the basis of the history, it must be assumed that the patient has aspirated gastric contents. This can result in acute respiratory compromise, through lodging of particulate matter in the larynx or trachea, by induction of laryngospasm, or through the rapid onset of pulmonary edema. Both *tachycardia* and *tachypnea* are often present. In severe episodes of respiratory compromise, *respiratory arrest* or *shock* may also occur.

B. **Is the patient able to communicate?** Aphonia may result from lodging of particulate matter in the larynx or trachea; it requires immediate intervention to dislodge the bolus by either the Heimlich maneuver or forceful coughing.

C. **Is the patient cyanotic?** Cyanosis would indicate severe respiratory compromise and probable need for emergent intubation.

D. **Does the patient need to be repositioned?** To prevent further aspiration of gastric contents, the patient should be placed in a lateral decubitus position with the head down.

III. **Differential Diagnosis.** *Aspiration* is defined as the entry of oropharyngeal contents into the larynx below the vocal cords. Three distinct aspiration syndromes are recognized: (1) acidic gastric contents; (2) nonacid and/or particulate material; and (3) oropharyngeal bacterial pathogens. These syndromes should be distinguished from one another as well as from other causes of acute respiratory distress, because the complications and treatment differ for each.

A. **Acid aspiration.** Aspiration of gastric contents with a pH < 2.5 results in immediate alveolar injury and chemical pneumonitis. Noncardiogenic pulmonary edema and shock may occur. Clinically, there is abrupt onset of dyspnea, fever, wheezing, rales, and hypoxemia.

B. **Particulate aspiration.** This can result in mechanical obstruction and bronchospasm. Pneumonia can ensue if particulate material remains lodged in peripheral airways.

C. **Oropharyngeal bacteria.** Saliva contains 10^8 organisms per milliliter. Aspiration of saliva into the lower airway can cause an early pneumonitis followed by necrotizing pneumonia or abscess in 3–14 days.

D. **Asthma.** See Section I, Chapter 63, Wheezing, p 341.

E. **Pneumonia.** Pneumonia can be difficult to distinguish from acute aspiration of gastric contents, since both can result in sputum production, tachycardia, tachypnea, fever, rales, and radiographic infiltrates.

F. **Pulmonary embolism.** This diagnosis must be considered in the differential of any patient developing acute respiratory distress.

G. **Foreign body aspiration.** This occurs mainly in younger children and occasionally in debilitated elderly people who aspirate a food bolus.

H. **Upper airway obstruction.** Acute edema of the vocal cords or glottis may follow aspiration. A high-pitched wheeze is heard over the larynx (*stridor*).

IV. **Database.** Attempt to identify those conditions that predispose to aspiration, including impairment of consciousness, swallowing, and esophageal dysfunction. Disorders resulting in *impairment of consciousness* include anesthesia, alcohol abuse, seizure disorder, acute cerebrovascular accident, cardiopulmonary arrest, and drug overdose. *Esophageal dysfunction* predisposes to aspiration and includes esophageal stricture, hiatal hernia, and nasogastric intubation. *Impaired swallowing* may result from a cerebrovascular accident, polymyositis, myasthenia gravis, Parkinson's disease, an artificial airway, or cancer involving the head and neck. Be aware that deficits in the pharyngeal phase of swallowing may persist for 2–3 days after extubation of a patient with an artificial airway.

A. **Physical examination key points**

1. **Vital signs.** See Section II.A.
2. **HEENT.** Check dentition for loose or missing teeth and evidence of gingivitis.
3. **Neck.** Examine for evidence of tumor involving the oropharynx. Also look for any evidence of prior surgical procedures or radiation of the head and neck.
4. **Lungs.** Wheezing and crackles can occur after aspiration of gastric contents. Wheezing and diminished breath sounds may result from aspiration of particulate material. Listen for stridor (laryngeal wheeze).
5. **Skin.** Examine for presence of cyanosis.
6. **Neurologic examination.** Determine the degree of consciousness and the presence or absence of a gag reflex. Note, however, that even with an intact gag reflex dysphagia and aspiration may still occur.

B. Laboratory data

1. **Arterial blood gases.** Hypoxemia and hypercapnia may occur and, if present, intubation may be required.
2. **Hemogram.** Aspiration of acid contents and pneumonia can cause a leukocytosis and left shift.
3. **Sputum Gram's stain and culture.** If the patient manifests fever, leukocytosis, and sputum production 2–3 days after aspiration, a sputum Gram's stain and culture may be helpful in confirming pneumonia and directing subsequent antibiotic therapy. However, aspiration pneumonia is often anaerobic and may be polymicrobial.

C. Radiologic and other studies

1. **Chest x-ray** may show:
   a. Hyperaeration from air trapping on the side of foreign body aspiration.
   b. Infiltrate in dependent segments of the lungs. Infiltrates may not be seen immediately after aspiration; therefore, if the initial CXR is normal but there is a strong clinical suspicion of aspiration, repeat the CXR in 4–5 hours. Bilateral alveolar infiltrates may occur with acute acid aspiration, resulting in acute respiratory distress syndrome.
   c. A wedge-shaped, pleural-based density suggests pulmonary infarction from pulmonary embolism.
   d. Clear fields and hyperinflation are common in uncomplicated asthma.
   e. Lung abscess formation does not generally occur until 7–14 days following aspiration and will not be observed on initial films.
2. **Other studies.** Ventilation/perfusion ($\dot{V}/\dot{Q}$) scan if a pulmonary embolism is suspected.

V. Plan. Aspiration should be suspected in any patient with a predisposing factor who develops sudden respiratory distress. Early treatment is important because death from respiratory failure can occur if the condition is not recognized early. Ideally, the best treatment is prevention.

A. Prevention

1. For patients being administered tube feedings, gastric emptying should be confirmed and the head of the bed elevated to 45 degrees. Flexible, small-bore feeding tubes are preferable to stiffer large-bore tubes. Duodenal placement of the tube may confer a slight reduction in risk of aspiration compared to gastric feeding.
2. Unconscious patients should be placed in a lateral, slightly head-down position whenever possible.
3. When not being used for enteral feedings, nasogastric tubes should be placed only when continuous suction is required.
4. As many as one-third to one-half of patients presenting with acute cerebrovascular accidents will experience aspiration. Consider or-

dering videofluoroscopy in these patients to determine aspiration risk and appropriate feeding.

B. Oxygenation. Supplemental oxygen should be given in an amount sufficient to ensure oxygen saturation greater than 90%.

C. Intubation and positive pressure breathing. Will be required in the patient for whom supplemental oxygen therapy is not sufficient to maintain adequate oxygenation, or in the patient who is obtunded and unable to protect her or his airway.

D. Medications

1. Bronchodilators such as albuterol 0.5 mL with 3 mL normal saline may relieve bronchospasm.
2. Prophylactic corticosteroids have not been shown to decrease subsequent morbidity and mortality from aspiration and are not indicated.
3. Prophylactic antibiotics likewise have not been shown to diminish morbidity and mortality. Antibiotics should be administered only if the patient continues to manifest fever, leukocytosis, purulent sputum, and infiltrates 2–3 days after the initial aspiration. For patients with in-hospital aspiration, a regimen that provides coverage for gram-negative aerobes, anaerobes, and possibly *Staphylococcus aureus* should be used.

E. Fiberoptic bronchoscopy. Is indicated when lobar or segmental collapse is present, when foreign body aspiration is suspected, or when abscess drainage is required.

REFERENCES

Elpern E: Pulmonary aspiration in hospitalized adults. Nutr Clin Pract 1997;12:5.

Marik PE: Aspiration pneumonitis and aspiration pneumonia. N Engl J Med 2001;344:665.

Marom E, McAdams HP, Erasmus JJ et al: The many faces of pulmonary aspiration. Am J Radiol 1999;172:121.

Teofilo L: Pulmonary aspiration. Comp Ther 1997;23:371.

Tietjen PA, Kaner RD, Quin CE: Aspiration emergencies. Clin Chest Med 1994;15:117.

8. BRADYCARDIA

I. Problem. A nurse on the telemetry unit notifies you that a 66-year-old woman has a heart rate of 40 beats per minute (bpm). She was admitted earlier in the day with syncope.

II. Immediate Questions

A. What are the patient's other vital signs? Heart rate must always be considered in relationship to the blood pressure (BP) and other signs of the patient's condition. A patient with a BP below 90 mm Hg and bradycardia requires more immediate attention than a patient with bradycardia, a normal BP, and no other associated symptoms.

B. **What has the patient's heart rate been since admission?** The range of normal heart rates is wide and is influenced by many factors, such as activity, age, medications, presence of pain or fever, and type of illness. Bradycardia can be seen in both healthy and ill patients.

C. **Does the patient have any symptoms possibly related to the bradycardia?** Such as fatigue, dizziness, syncope, nausea, dyspnea, chest pain, decreased urinary output, or altered mental status.

III. Differential Diagnosis

A. **Sinus bradycardia.** Defined as a sinus node rhythm below 60 bpm. Changes in sinus rate are modulated primarily by parasympathetic nervous system tone. Causes of sinus bradycardia include the following:

1. **Increased parasympathetic tone.** Sinus bradycardia can be precipitated many times by sudden stressful or painful events. An example is a vasovagal syncopal episode related to nervousness, or to fear from venipuncture.
2. **Sinoatrial node dysfunction.** Characterized by the presence of bradycardia at inappropriate times. Sinus node dysfunction can also be manifested by periods of sinoatrial node arrest, or sinoatrial exit block, or by alternating sinus bradycardia and atrial tachyarrhythmias, commonly referred to as *sick sinus syndrome.*
3. **Myocardial infarction.** Sinus bradycardia is seen frequently with inferior wall infarctions, involving the proximal portion of the right coronary artery and its branch to the sinoatrial node. The presence of sinus bradycardia during the early phases of an acute myocardial infarction is, in general, a good prognostic sign. It does not require therapy, as long as left ventricular cardiac output is adequate and hypotension or congestive heart failure (CHF) is absent. In fact, raising the heart rate in this instance may raise cardiac demand and cause further ischemia or infarction.
4. **Cushing's reflex.** Sinus bradycardia in combination with hypertension is associated with an increase in intracranial pressure (hemorrhagic stroke, meningitis, intracranial tumor, or trauma).
5. **Other medical disorders.** Sinus bradycardia can occur in patients with hypothyroidism, hypothermia, obstructive sleep apnea, advancing age, carotid sinus hypersensitivity, and certain infiltrative diseases of the myocardium, such as amyloidosis and sarcoidosis.
6. **Drug effect.** Sinus bradycardia is a common secondary effect of several classes of medications, including beta-blockers, digoxin, calcium channel blockers, clonidine (Catapres), lithium carbonate, and certain antiarrhythmic drugs such as amiodarone (Cordarone) and sotalol (Betapace).

B. **Atrioventricular (AV) node blocks**

1. **Mobitz type I second-degree AV block (Wenckebach).** Characterized by progressive, cyclical prolongation of the PR interval with each cardiac cycle until a ventricular beat is dropped. This results in intermittent AV block in a repeated cycle.
   a. **Acute myocardial infarction.** Most commonly seen early in inferior wall infarctions related to ischemia affecting the atrioventricular nodal branch of the right coronary artery.
   b. **Drug effect.** Excessive serum levels of certain cardiac medications can result in Wenckebach-type second-degree AV block (digoxin, beta-blockers, calcium channel blockers, and amiodarone).
   c. **Infections.** A Wenckebach rhythm is occasionally seen during the acute phases of rheumatic fever and Lyme disease, when the inflammatory process affects the cardiac conduction system.
   d. **Other.** Wenckebach rhythms can occasionally be seen in asymptomatic, otherwise normal adults; they are related to the level of parasympathetic nervous system tone, such as in highly trained aerobic athletes, particularly during sleep.
2. **Mobitz type II second-degree AV block.** Cyclical AV block without the progressive prolongation of the PR interval. The QRS complex of conducted beats may be prolonged because of disease involvement of the bundle of His.
   a. **Acute myocardial infarction.** Large anterior wall infarctions are a more common cause than inferior infarctions.
   b. **Degenerative fibrosing diseases.** Involving the bundle of His.
   c. **Infectious diseases.** Such as viral myocarditis, acute rheumatic fever, and Lyme disease.
3. **Third-degree AV block.** This rhythm is associated with the same conditions as Mobitz type II second-degree heart block. Third-degree AV block occurs when there is no conduction of the P waves from the sinoatrial node through the atrioventricular node to the ventricle. This results in the P waves and QRS complexes being independent of one another. Usually the ventricular rate and rhythm are controlled by a secondary intraventricular pacemaker, which is normally suppressed when AV conduction is intact.
4. **Malfunctioning pacemaker.** See Section I, Chapter 53, Pacemaker Troubleshooting, p 283.

IV. Database

A. **Physical examination key points**

1. **Vital signs.** Obtain the patient's BP during the bradycardic rhythm, and assess the patient's level of consciousness.
2. **Neck veins.** Intermittent cannon "A" waves in the jugular venous pulsations are observed in the presence of complete AV dissocia-

tion. A *cannon "A" wave* is an exaggerated A wave in the jugular venous pulse that results from right atrial contraction on an already closed tricuspid valve, caused by simultaneous atrial and ventricular contraction. This results in backward ejection of right atrial blood into the superior vena cava and jugular veins.

3. **Lungs.** Rales during periods of bradycardia suggest congestive heart failure from inadequate left ventricular cardiac output.
4. **Heart.** Listen for murmurs and gallops. An S_4 gallop may be present during an acute myocardial infarction. A new cardiac murmur may be seen in myocardial infarction, acute rheumatic fever, and myocarditis. See Section I, Chapter 26, Heart Murmur, p 151.
5. **Skin.** Cool, pale extremities suggest an inadequate cardiac output.
6. **Mental status.** Inadequate cerebral perfusion may result in an altered level of consciousness.

B. Laboratory data

1. **Electrolytes.** Exclude hypokalemia if the patient is on digoxin.
2. **Digoxin level.** Bradycardia can be a sign of digitalis intoxication.
3. **Thyroid hormone levels.** Rule out hypothyroidism as a cause.

C. Electrocardiogram and rhythm strip

1. Identify P waves and their timing and relationship to the QRS complexes. Leads I, II, aVR, aVF, and V_1 demonstrate the morphology of the P waves best. The absence of P waves suggests an AV nodal rhythm, or atrial fibrillation with a slow ventricular response, as the cause of the bradycardia.
2. An increasing PR interval with a dropped QRS complex, recurring in a cyclical pattern, indicates Mobitz type I second-degree heart block.
3. P waves that occur intermittently without an associated QRS complex, but with an otherwise constant PR interval, suggest Mobitz type II second-degree heart block. The QRS duration is usually prolonged.
4. Third-degree heart block is present when the P waves and QRS complexes demonstrate no relationship to each other.
5. Look for evidence of myocardial ischemia or infarction. ST segment elevation or depression, T wave inversion, and the presence of new Q waves are common findings.
6. Look for the presence and timing of pacemaker spikes, if appropriate. See Section I, Chapter 53, Pacemaker Troubleshooting, p 283.

V. Plan. Therapy is dictated by the most likely cause of the bradycardia and the presence of symptoms. Some bradycardic rhythms do not require any treatment.

A. Drugs

1. Consider stopping or holding doses of medications associated with bradycardic rhythms. If the patient is asymptomatic, and oth-

erwise fine, discontinuing a medication such as propranolol is all that needs to be done.

2. **Atropine.** 0.5–1.0 mg IV push, up to a total dose of 2.0 mg, is the initial treatment of **symptomatic** sinus bradycardia. Remember, be careful in raising the heart rate of a patient with a recent myocardial infarction, because myocardial demand could increase the likelihood of precipitating further myocardial injury.
3. Since atropine is only a temporary measure, its effects are not likely to last beyond an hour or so. Transcutaneous cardiac pacing (TCP) if available, dopamine 5–20 μg/kg/min, or epinephrine 2–10 μg/min can be used following atropine if the heart rate is not adequate to maintain hemodynamic stability.
4. If digitalis overdose or intoxication is responsible for a potentially life-threatening, hemodynamically unstable arrhythmia, and rapid treatment is necessary, consider giving the patient intravenous digoxin immune Fab fragments (**Digibind**). The dose is based on the amount of digoxin acutely ingested or the serum digoxin concentration and body weight. See dosing charts provided with the drug.

B. Treatment of bradycardia secondary to a CNS event. Initial steps to decrease intracranial pressure include hyperventilation, furosemide, and dexamethasone if there is an increase in intracranial pressure resulting in bradycardia. See Section I, Chapter 13, Coma, Acute Mental Status Changes, V, p 81.

C. Temporary pacemakers. Temporary pacemakers include external and transvenous devices. External pacemakers can be applied quickly in an emergent situation such as cardiac arrest. A transvenous pacemaker should be placed at the bedside using central venous cannulation and fluoroscopy when the patient is more hemodynamically stable.

1. **Indications for temporary pacing**
   - **a.** Mobitz type II second-degree or third-degree AV block associated with an acute myocardial infarction.
   - **b.** Symptomatic AV block associated with drug toxicity that is likely to be prolonged (amiodarone toxicity).
   - **c.** Sinus bradycardia with severe congestive heart failure.
   - **d.** Prolonged sinus pauses (> 3.5 seconds) associated with syncope.
2. **Indications for permanent pacing**
   - **a.** Sick sinus syndrome **with** symptoms as a result of bradycardia or sinus pauses.
   - **b.** Mobitz type II second-degree or third-degree AV block.
   - **c.** Occasionally, patients with cardiomyopathies and class III CHF may benefit from placement of a dual-chambered permanent pacemaker in order to raise heart rate and cardiac output.

REFERENCES

Mangrum JM, DiMarco JP: The evaluation and management of bradycardia. Primary Care 2000;342:703.

Miller JM, Zipes DP: Management of patient with cardiac arrhythmias. In: Braunwald E, Zipes DP, Libby P, eds. *Heart Disease: A Textbook of Cardiovascular Medicine.* 6th ed. Saunders;2001:700.

Wagner GS, ed: *Marriott's Practical Electrocardiography.* 9th ed. Williams & Wilkins;1994.

9. CARDIOPULMONARY ARREST

I. Problem. You are the first member of a code team to arrive at the bedside of a patient found unresponsive by the nurse.

II. Immediate Questions

A. Is the patient unresponsive? Cardiopulmonary resuscitation (CPR) begins with an attempt to arouse the patient. Call the patient by name and gently shake him or her by the shoulders. If the patient is unresponsive, send someone to call a code and begin CPR.

B. Is the patient in optimal position for CPR? The patient must be supine and lying on a firm and flat surface to provide effective external chest compression. The head must be at the same level as the thorax for optimal cerebral perfusion.

C. Is the airway obstructed? In an unconscious patient, the tongue and epiglottis may fall posteriorly and occlude the airway. A head tilt/chin lift maneuver will lift these structures and open the airway. Vomitus or foreign material should be removed from the mouth by either a finger sweep or suction.

D. After establishment of airway patency, is the patient breathing? Respiration can be assessed for no more than 10 seconds by looking for chest movement, listening for air movement, and feeling for breath on the rescuer's face (rescuer's face is turned to face the patient's chest; rescuer's cheek is above the patient's mouth). If breathing is not present, then institute rescue breathing with two full breaths, preferably via either a pocket mask or Ambu bag if available.

E. Is there evidence of adequate circulation? Establish the presence of a carotid pulse. If no pulse is felt after 10 seconds of palpation, begin external chest compressions. After basic and then advanced cardiac life support has been instituted, asking other questions may help elucidate the cause of the patient's arrest.

F. What medications has the patient been taking? Cardiac medications are particularly important. Drugs that prolong the QT interval, such as quinidine and procainamide, amiodarone, and sotalol, may predispose to *torsades de pointes,* characterized by recurrent ventricular tachycardia and ventricular fibrillation. Phenothiazines and tricyclic antidepressants may also cause this condition. Digoxin (Lanoxin) is a frequent cause of a variety of cardiac arrhythmias.

G. **Has the patient received any administered medications that could have resulted in an anaphylactic reaction?** See Section I, Chapter 4, Anaphylactic Reaction, p. 24.

H. **Is there any history of electrolyte disturbance or conditions that could predispose to electrolyte disturbance?** Hypokalemia and hypomagnesemia can predispose to arrhythmias. Hyperkalemia can cause complete heart block and cardiac arrest.

I. **What are the patient's medical problems?** Inquire specifically regarding a prior history of cardiac disease. Is there any recent history to suggest an acute stroke or any conditions that predispose to acute pulmonary embolism, such as recent surgery? The aggressiveness of CPR can be directed by knowing whether the patient has any terminal medical problems such as advanced cancer.

III. **Differential Diagnosis.** Cardiopulmonary arrest can result from either a primary cardiac disturbance or from primary respiratory arrest. There are a wide variety of causes of cardiopulmonary arrest; some of the more common are listed here:

A. **Cardiac**
   1. **Acute myocardial infarction**
   2. **Acute pulmonary edema**
   3. **Ventricular arrhythmias**
   4. **Third-degree heart block**
   5. **Cardiac tamponade**

B. **Pulmonary**
   1. **Pulmonary embolism (usually massive)**
   2. **Acute respiratory failure**
   3. **Aspiration**
   4. **Tension pneumothorax (large)**

C. **Hemorrhagic.** Acute severe hemorrhage such as from a ruptured aortic aneurysm or rapid gastrointestinal bleeding.

D. **Metabolic**
   1. **Electrolyte disturbances.** Hypokalemia, hyperkalemia, and hypomagnesemia can induce arrhythmias.
   2. **Acidosis and alkalosis**
   3. **Hypothermia and rewarming.** During the treatment of acute hypothermia, rewarming may induce ventricular fibrillation or other arrhythmias.

E. **Drug overdoses.** Especially tricyclic antidepressants, digitalis, and beta- and calcium channel blockers.

IV. **Database**

A. **Physical examination key points.** The initial assessment of airway, breathing, and circulation is described in Section II, p. 44. Resuscitation should obviously be initiated before a detailed physical examination is performed. Other signs to watch for are:

1. **Tracheal deviation.** This would indicate the possibility of tension pneumothorax.
2. **Distended neck veins.** May indicate a tension pneumothorax or a hemodynamically significant pericardial effusion.

B. **Laboratory data.** These should be obtained early in resuscitation efforts but should not delay initiation of specific therapy.

1. **Arterial blood gases.** Acidosis could be the cause of an arrhythmia or result from prolonged hypoperfusion. A low pO_2 can result from a variety of causes, including pulmonary edema and pulmonary embolus, or again it may be the result of prolonged hypoperfusion.
2. **Serum electrolytes.** Particularly potassium and magnesium.
3. **Complete blood count.** Keep in mind that with massive hemorrhage the hematocrit may not have had sufficient time to equilibrate and therefore may not be an accurate indicator of the severity of blood loss.

C. **Radiologic and other studies**

1. **Continuous cardiac monitoring.** 3-lead monitoring is acceptable; however, a 12-lead ECG should be obtained as early as possible.
2. **Chest x-ray.** A CXR should be obtained to determine the position of the endotracheal tube or any central venous line. This should obviously be performed after the patient is stabilized.

V. **Plan.** A full description of definitive therapy for each of the causes of cardiopulmonary arrest is beyond the scope of this text. The reader is referred to the excellent reference at the end of this chapter. In general, the best success in performing CPR has been achieved in patients in whom basic life support has been initiated *within 4 minutes* of the time of arrest and advanced cardiac life support *within 8 minutes.* Fairly early recognition of unresponsiveness and initiation of CPR is crucial. Once basic life support has been instituted, the next goal should be to determine the cardiac rhythm. Ventricular fibrillation is treated with immediate defibrillation. The next priority is endotracheal intubation followed by establishment of venous access via an antecubital vein or other large, visible superficial vein. Once a 12-lead ECG has been obtained, the physician may be able to establish a specific cause of the arrest and direct treatment accordingly. Listed here are brief summaries of the management of the major cardiac causes of arrest.

A. **Ventricular fibrillation (see Figure 1–1).** Immediate defibrillation is the most important step in the treatment of ventricular fibrillation. In fact, defibrillation should be attempted prior to attempts to intubate the patient or establish intravenous access. Defibrillation is facilitated by the use of quick-look paddles now available on most defibrillators.

1. The first attempt should be with 200 joules. If the patient remains in ventricular fibrillation, the second attempt should use 200–300 joules, administered immediately. If fibrillation still persists, a third countershock with 360 joules should be delivered.
2. If the patient remains in ventricular fibrillation after three countershocks, CPR should be resumed. The patient should be intubated, intravenous access should be established, and the patient should be connected to a 12-lead ECG. Epinephrine (1 mg of a 1:10,000 solution) should be administered every 3–5 minutes or a one-time dose of vasopressin (40 U IV) given followed by epinephrine every 5 minutes (if needed). Epinephrine is probably the most important pharmacologic agent used during CPR.
3. Within 30–60 seconds, defibrillation should be attempted again with 360 joules. If the patient remains in ventricular fibrillation, a 300-mg bolus of amiodarone should be administered.
4. After administration of amiodarone, defibrillation should again be attempted. If fibrillation persists, a second bolus of 150 mg of amiodarone or a 1.5 mg/kg bolus of lidocaine can be administered, followed by another attempt at defibrillation.
5. Upon return to spontaneous circulation after either step 3 or 4, a constant infusion of 1 mg/min of amiodarone or 2–4 mg/min (15–50 mg/kg/min) of lidocaine should be started.
6. If ventricular fibrillation still persists, procainamide at a rate of 30 mg/min for a total dose of 17 mg/kg can be given followed by defibrillation.

B. **Sustained ventricular tachycardia with no palpable pulse.** This arrhythmia should be managed like ventricular fibrillation.

C. **Ventricular tachycardia with a palpable pulse**

1. **Stable monomorphic ventricular tachycardia (with decreased ejection fraction).**
   a. Amiodarone is the drug of choice, especially in patients with decreased ejection fractions. An initial loading dose of 150 mg over 10 minutes should be given followed by infusion of 1 mg/min. An additional 150-mg bolus over 10 minutes can be used 15 minutes after the first dose if needed. Lidocaine can be used as well with initial 0.5–0.75 mg/kg IV bolus, and this can be administered every 5–10 minutes as necessary until a total loading dose of 3 mg/kg has been given.
   b. If amiodarone or lidocaine fails to convert the patient, synchronized cardioversion with an initial energy level of 100 joules may be attempted, followed by 200 joules, 300 joules, and 360 joules if necessary. Premedicate the patient with a sedative and analgesic whenever possible.
2. **Stable monomorphic ventricular tachycardia (with normal ejection fraction).** Use one agent if possible to avoid adverse side effects (ie, proarrhythmic effects of dual drugs). Procaina-

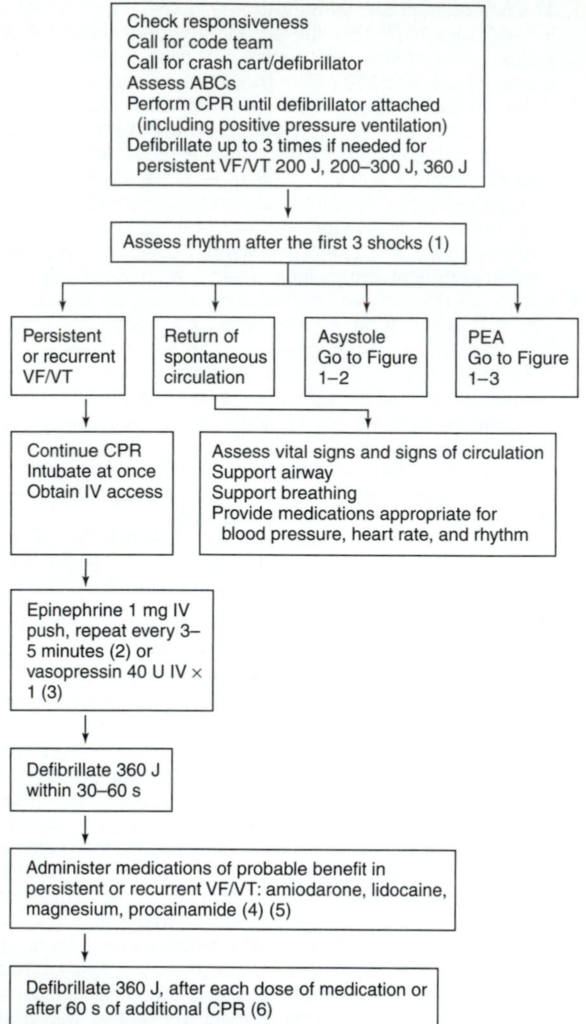

Figure 1–1. Algorithm for ventricular fibrillation and pulseless ventricular tachycardia (VF/VT). (*Reproduced with permission from American Heart Association: Guidelines 2000 for cardiopulmonary resuscitation and emergency cardiovascular care. Circulation 2000 [August 22]:102.*)

Footnotes to Figure I–1

(1) Hypothermic cardiac arrest is treated differently after this point. See Section I, Chapter 43, Hypothermia, p. 229.

(2) The recommended dose of epinepherine is 1 mg IV push every 3–5 min. If this approach fails, consider high-dose epinephrine 0.2 mg/kg IV push, every 3–5 min; however, there is evidence this may be harmful.

(3) No evidence to support use of vasopressin for asystole or PEA or to support using more than one dose. If no response in 5–10 minutes after vasopressin, start or restart epinephrine administration.

(4) Amiodarone 300 mg IV push, consider additional dose of 150 mg IV. No more than 2.2 g should be given in a 24-hr period.
Lidocaine 1.0–1.5 mg/kg IV push. Consider repeat dose in 3–5 min to total loading dose of 3 mg/kg.
Magnesium sulfate 1–2 g IV (if hypomagnesemia present, or polymorphic VT [torsades de pointes])
Procainamide 30 mg/min in refractory VF (maximum total 17 mg/kg)

(5) Sodium bicarbonate (1 mEq/kg IV), for conditions known to provoke cardiac arrest:
If preexisting hyperkalemic,
If preexisting bicarbonate-responsive acidosis,
If overdose with tricyclic antidepressants,
To alkalinize the urine in drug overdoses (aspirin),
If intubated and continued long arrest interval,
Upon return of spontaneous circulation after long arrest interval.
Note: May be harmful in respiratory acidosis.

(6) Follow either CPR-drug-shock-repeat sequence or CPR-drug-shock-shock-repeat sequence.

mide and sotalol are the top choices. Procainamide can be administered IV in 100-mg increments Q 5 min until the arrhythmia is suppressed, the QRS complex widens more than 50%, or a loading dose of 17 mg/kg has been given. Other acceptable drugs are amiodarone and lidocaine dosed as above.

3. **Stable polymorphic ventricular tachycardia.** Identification of ischemia and correction of electrolytes are first priority. If baseline ECG has a normal QT interval, refer to treatment of stable monomorphic ventricular tachycardia with decreased ejection fraction (amiodarone or lidocaine followed by cardioversion). If baseline ECG has a prolonged QT interval, consider torsades de pointes. In this case magnesium, lidocaine, or isoproterenol is effective as well as overdrive pacing.
4. **Unstable ventricular tachycardia**
   - **a.** If the patient has a pulse but is hemodynamically unstable (hypotension, unconsciousness, pulmonary edema), antiarrhythmic therapy should be deferred; instead, immediate *synchronized* cardioversion with 100 joules should be administered.
   - **b.** If an unstable ventricular tachycardia does not convert with 100 joules, administer 200–300 joules; if still unsuccessful, 360 joules.
   - **c.** Following cardioversion, an amiodarone bolus followed by continuous infusion should be administered. Alternatively, a continuous infusion of lidocaine can be administered to prevent recurrence of the arrhythmia.

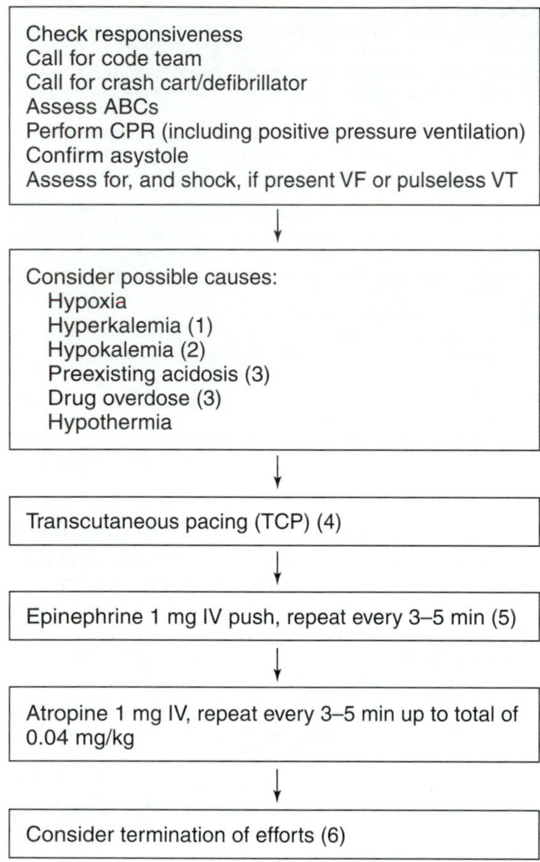

Check responsiveness
Call for code team
Call for crash cart/defibrillator
Assess ABCs
Perform CPR (including positive pressure ventilation)
Confirm asystole
Assess for, and shock, if present VF or pulseless VT
Consider possible causes:
Hypoxia
Hyperkalemia (1)
Hypokalemia (2)
Preexisting acidosis (3)
Drug overdose (3)
Hypothermia
Transcutaneous pacing (TCP) (4)
Epinephrine 1 mg IV push, repeat every 3–5 min (5)
Atropine 1 mg IV, repeat every 3–5 min up to total of 0.04 mg/kg
Consider termination of efforts (6)

Figure 1–2. Asystole treatment algorithm. (*Reproduced with permission from American Heart Association: Guidelines 2000 for cardiopulmonary resuscitation and emergency cardiovascular care. Circulation 2000 [August 22]:102.*)

D. Asystole (see Figure 1–2). This rhythm has an extremely poor prognosis.

1. Epinephrine 1 mg should be administered IV and repeated Q 3–5 min.
2. Because massive parasympathetic discharge can occasionally result in asystole, an initial dose of atropine 1 mg may be adminis-

Footnotes to Figure I–2

(1) Sodium bicarbonate 1 mEq/kg if patient has known preexisting hyperkalemia.
(2) KCl 40–60 mmol/hr IV, if > 40 mmol/hr must be administered through a central line; for rates > 15 mmol/hr cardiac monitoring is mandatory; be sure concomitant hypomagnesemia is not present.
(3) Sodium bicarbonate 1 mEq/kg:
If known preexisting bicarbonate-responsive acidosis,
If intubated and continued long arrest interval,
Upon return of spontaneous circulation after long arrest interval,
Hypoxic lactic acidosis,
If overdose with tricyclic antidepressants,
To alkalinize the urine in drug overdoses (eg, aspirin).
Note: May be harmful in respiratory acidosis.
(4) Evidence does not support TCP for asystole.
(5) The recommended dose of epinephrine is 1 mg IV push every 3–5 min. If this approach fails, consider high-dose epinephrine 0.2 mg/kg push, every 3–5 min. Vasopressin is not recommended for asystole.
(5) Assess effectiveness of ABCs, IV access, and medications. If asystole has continued for > 5–10 min despite resuscitation, then discontinue resuscitation efforts. If the cause is hypothermia, drowning, or reversible drug overdose, consider continuing for longer period of time.

tered if there is no response to the epinephrine. This dose may be repeated after 3–5 minutes if there is no response to a total dose of 0.04 mg/kg.

3. Sodium bicarbonate and calcium chloride are no longer recommended for management of asystole.
4. In general, pacemaker therapy will not be successful if the heart fails to respond to either of the preceding measures.
5. Keep in mind that, occasionally, fine ventricular fibrillation may be mistaken as asystole. This problem can be avoided by evaluating the ECG in several leads.

E. Pulseless electrical activity (PEA) (see Figure 1–3). This condition is characterized by the presence of electrical activity on the ECG but no detectable pulse. It is important to recall that some causes of this condition can be reversed if they are recognized and treated appropriately.

1. PEA is caused by a variety of conditions including hypoxemia, severe acidosis, pericardial tamponade, tension pneumothorax, hypovolemia, and pulmonary embolus. It is therefore important to evaluate for potentially reversible causes such as pericardial tamponade and pneumothorax.
2. If tamponade is suspected, pericardiocentesis should be performed.
3. If tension pneumothorax is suspected, insertion of a catheter-over-needle device in the second intercostal space in the midclavicular line should be attempted.
4. Otherwise, treatment consists of epinephrine 1 mg IV along with CPR. If the heart rate is slow, atropine 1 mg IV should be given with repeated doses after 3–5 minutes to a total dose of 0.04 mg/kg.
5. A fluid challenge should also be administered. Give 500 mL of normal saline over 15 minutes.

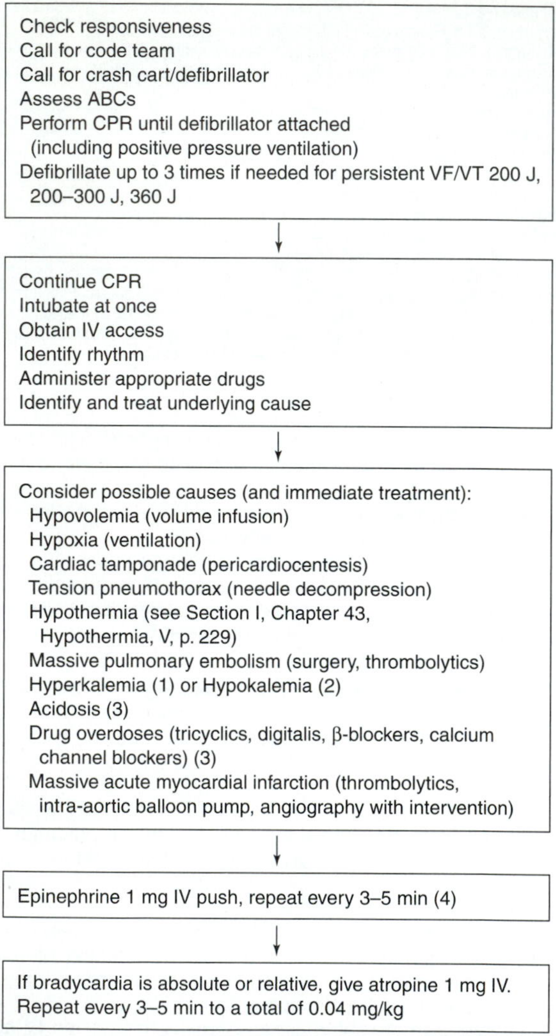

Check responsiveness
Call for code team
Call for crash cart/defibrillator
Assess ABCs
Perform CPR until defibrillator attached (including positive pressure ventilation)
Defibrillate up to 3 times if needed for persistent VF/VT 200 J, 200–300 J, 360 J

↓

Continue CPR
Intubate at once
Obtain IV access
Identify rhythm
Administer appropriate drugs
Identify and treat underlying cause

↓

Consider possible causes (and immediate treatment):
- Hypovolemia (volume infusion)
- Hypoxia (ventilation)
- Cardiac tamponade (pericardiocentesis)
- Tension pneumothorax (needle decompression)
- Hypothermia (see Section I, Chapter 43, Hypothermia, V, p. 229)
- Massive pulmonary embolism (surgery, thrombolytics)
- Hyperkalemia (1) or Hypokalemia (2)
- Acidosis (3)
- Drug overdoses (tricyclics, digitalis, β-blockers, calcium channel blockers) (3)
- Massive acute myocardial infarction (thrombolytics, intra-aortic balloon pump, angiography with intervention)

↓

Epinephrine 1 mg IV push, repeat every 3–5 min (4)

↓

If bradycardia is absolute or relative, give atropine 1 mg IV. Repeat every 3–5 min to a total of 0.04 mg/kg

Figure 1–3. Algorithm for pulseless electrical activity (PEA = rhythm on monitor without detectable pulse). (*Reproduced with permission from American Heart Association: Guidelines 2000 for cardiopulmonary resuscitation and emergency cardiovascular care. Circulation 2000 (August 22):102.*)

Footnotes to Figure I–3

(1) Sodium bicarbonate 1 mEq/kg if patient has known preexisting hyperkalemia.

(2) KCl 40–60 mmol/hr IV, if > 40 mmol/hr must be administered through a central line; for rates > 15 mmol/hr cardiac monitoring is mandatory; be sure concomitant hypomagnesemia is not present.

(3) Sodium bicarbonate 1 mEq/kg:

If known preexisting bicarbonate-responsive acidosis,
If intubated and continued long arrest interval,
Upon return of spontaneous circulation after long arrest interval,
Hypoxic lactic acidosis,
To alkalinize the urine in drug overdose (eg, aspirin),
If overdose with tricyclic antidepressants.
Note: May be harmful in respiratory acidosis.

(4) The recommended dose of epinephrine is 1 mg IV push every 3–5 min. If this approach fails, consider high-dose epinephrine 0.2 mg/kg every 3–5 min. Vasopressin is not recommended for PEA.

6. The administration of calcium chloride for this condition is no longer recommended.
7. Coronary or pulmonary thrombosis should also be considered as possible causes of PEA.

REFERENCES

American Heart Association: Guidelines 2000 for cardiopulmonary resuscitation and emergency cardiovascular care. Circulation 2000;102 (August 22).

10. CENTRAL VENOUS LINE PROBLEMS

(See also Section I, Chapter 57, Pulmonary Artery Catheter Problems, p 303)

I. **Problem.** The nursing staff calls to report that a subclavian line has stopped functioning.

II. **Immediate Questions**

A. **If the central line is used for central venous pressure (CVP) monitoring, what does the waveform look like?** The CVP waveform drops on inspiration, rises with expiration, and should show monophasic to triphasic fluctuations with each cardiac cycle. If there is no waveform, the catheter may not be patent, or there may be a thrombus in the vein or catheter.

B. **Do intravenous fluids flow easily into the catheter, or does fluid leak from the insertion site?** Again, these developments might indicate a thrombosed central vein or a kinked catheter.

C. **Is the patient febrile?** A fever in conjunction with a malfunctioning catheter suggests a central line infection, deep vein thrombosis, or both. If there is any suspicion of associated infection or thrombosis, malfunctioning lines should be removed immediately and cultured.

D. **Are there any arrhythmias?** A central line catheter that extends into the right atrium or right ventricle can cause atrial or ventricular ectopy and arrhythmias.

E. **What is the line's purpose? What is its relative necessity?** If drugs are being administered centrally that should not be given peripherally (vincristine or Adriamycin as a continuous infusion), the situation is different from one in which the central line could be replaced by a peripheral line.

III. Differential Diagnosis

A. **Clotted catheter.** This can occur when central lines are allowed to run dry or are running very slowly. Blood backs up into the catheter lumen and thrombosis occurs.

B. **Misdirected catheter.** Subclavian catheters from either the right or the left side may be inadvertently placed retrograde into the ipsilateral internal jugular vein. This results in a line that cannot be used to measure central venous pressure. Much more rarely, subclavian or internal jugular attempts end up in the long thoracic vein, again failing to function properly. The catheter may also extend into the right atrium or right ventricle rather than the proximal venous circulation.

C. **Kinked catheter.** Catheters can kink at the skin or more deeply. From the right subclavian insertion site, it is not uncommon for catheters within relatively stiff sheaths to kink at the turn from the subclavian vein to the brachiocephalic vein as it joins the superior vena cava. Kinking at this bend is uncommon for single-lumen catheters or triple-lumen catheters not inside a sheath. Internal jugular lines and left subclavian lines are not generally subject to this problem. It should be stressed that any line can be misdirected and kink. The catheters are easily seen fluoroscopically and radiographically; a chest x-ray will usually allow you to diagnose this problem.

D. **Infected catheter.** Central line sepsis will usually not result in any apparent malfunction of the catheter. Fever, sepsis, and positive blood cultures all may result from the spread of skin flora to the intravascular segment of the catheter.

E. **Thrombosis of the vein of insertion.** Any deep vein accessed for central line insertion can thrombose as a result of the trauma associated with the procedure, as well as the presence of a foreign body within the vein. Clinically, these events resemble natural deep vein thrombosis and can result in associated bland or septic pulmonary emboli.

IV. Database

A. Physical examination key points

1. **Vital signs.** An elevated temperature suggests an infection. If the catheter has been in place more than 3 days, you must assume the central venous catheter is the source of the fever.
2. **Extremities.** Look for evidence of deep vein thrombosis. Unilateral edema and venous engorgement suggest deep vein thrombosis.

3. **Skin.** Examine the insertion site for evidence of tissue infiltration, bleeding, catheter kinking, or leakage. Also, erythema around the insertion site may result from a localized infection.

B. Laboratory data

1. **Complete blood count with differential.** An elevated white blood count with an increase in banded neutrophils is often present with catheter-related sepsis.
2. **Prothrombin time (PT), partial thromboplastin time (PTT), platelet count.** Should be obtained if a central line needs to be changed and a coagulopathy is suspected, such as in patients with severe liver disease or malnutrition.
3. **Blood cultures.** Should be obtained as part of routine evaluation of a fever. Remember, if a central venous catheter has been in place for more than 3 days, there is a significant risk of catheter-related sepsis.

C. Radiologic and other studies

1. **Chest x-ray.** Useful in determining whether a catheter is in the correct position or kinked.
2. **Culture of catheter tip.** If catheter-related sepsis or infection is suspected, the catheter must be removed and the tip sent for culture.
3. **Impedance plethysmography and Doppler ultrasound.** Noninvasive tests for suspected extremity venous thrombosis.
4. **Venography.** The gold standard for diagnosing venous thrombosis. If there is a history of allergy to contrast media, venography should be preceded by treatment with corticosteroids and diphenhydramine.
5. **Nuclear venogram.** Can diagnose venous thrombosis and pulmonary embolism simultaneously with lower extremity injection.

V. Plan. For replacement of central venous catheters, see Section III, Chapter 6, Central Venous Catheterization, p 399.

A. Clotted catheter. A line can sometimes be salvaged by aspirating the catheter while it is slowly pulled out. Sterile technique and a small syringe are necessary. Use of a guide wire, manual flushing, or injection of urokinase 5000 U (5000 U/mL) may result in embolization. However, these measures seldom cause any significant problem, probably because of the small volume of the embolus. The only completely safe approach, however, is aspiration. The risk of replacement of the line has to be weighed against the risk of using any of the other techniques besides aspiration. Other factors must be considered, such as the length of time the catheter has been in place, the necessity of a central rather than peripheral placement, and the presence of fever or local evidence of infection.

B. Misdirected catheter. This situation usually requires removal and replacement. With fluoroscopic guidance, a guide wire might be manipulated into the superior vena cava, which then can guide the catheter correctly. If fluoroscopy is not an option, a new puncture may be unavoidable. If the catheter is in the right atrium or right ventricle and does not have to be removed for other reasons, it can be partially withdrawn, using sterile technique, so that it is in the superior or inferior vena cava.

C. **Kinked catheter.** A new line that is kinked at the site of insertion can sometimes be salvaged by repositioning the line with new skin sutures. More proximal kinks can sometimes be fixed by replacing the catheter over a guide wire. If the kink is within a sheath or where the catheter emerges from the sheath, the sheath can sometimes be withdrawn, leaving the catheter in the same place, provided there is enough catheter left onto which the sheath can be withdrawn. The best way to deal with this problem is to prevent it by avoiding the right subclavian approach in patients who have shallow chests in the lateral dimension. In these patients, the lines must negotiate a sharp angle from the subclavian to the superior vena cava.

D. **Infected catheter.** An infected or possibly infected central line *must be removed.* This virtually always requires replacement elsewhere if central venous access is still desired. Intravenous line–associated sepsis is caused in large part by skin contamination. The practice of removing the line over a guide wire and traversing the same insertion site with the replacement line is **not** recommended. A new site is a better idea. It is important to draw two sets of blood cultures from the suspect line as well as two sets from the peripheral veins before the line is removed, and to culture the tip of the catheter after it is removed. The use of antibiotic- or antiseptic-impregnated catheters is associated with reduction in catheter infection. The clinical application of this research is not yet evident in catheters available for routine use.

E. **Thrombosis of the vein of insertion.** This also requires line removal and replacement at a site distant from the thrombosed vein. Heparin 80 U/kg IV bolus followed by 18 U/kg continuous infusion is recommended unless contraindicated for other reasons. The PTT should be checked 6 hours after the infusion is begun; the heparin dose should be adjusted so that the PTT is one and one-half to two times the control. If sepsis is also suspected, antibiotics are necessary, as is a surgical consultation for possible removal of the infected vein. Vancomycin 1000 mg every 12 hours is the preferred antibiotic if normal renal function is present. Vancomycin covers *Staphylococcus epidermidis* as well as *Staphylococcus aureus.* Be sure to decrease the dose if renal insufficiency is present.

REFERENCES

Fares LG, Block PH, Feldman SD: Improved house staff results with subclavian cannulation. Am Surg 1986;52:108.

Gil RT, Kruse JA, Thill-Baharozian MC et al: Triple- vs. single-lumen central venous catheters. Arch Intern Med 1989;149:1139.

Maki DG, Stolz SM, Wheeler S et al: Prevention of central venous catheter-related bloodstream infection by use of an antiseptic-impregnated catheter. Ann Intern Med 1997;127:257.

Mansfield PF, Hohn DC, Fornage BD et al: Complications and failures of subclavian-vein catheterization. N Engl J Med 1994;331:1735.

Raad I, Darouiche R, Dupuis J et al: Central venous catheters coated with minocycline and rifampin for the prevention of catheter-related colonization and bloodstream infections. Ann Intern Med 1997;127:267.

11. CHEST PAIN

I. **Problem.** A 48-year-old man with a history of tobacco abuse is admitted for elective bronchoscopy. On the evening of his admission, he develops substernal chest pain lasting 15 minutes in duration.

II. **Immediate Questions.** Because of potentially serious conditions, patients complaining of chest pain should be evaluated urgently. By far, the most important tool in identifying the cause of chest pain is a meticulous history.

   A. **Does the patient have a prior history of coronary artery disease, and if so, does the current pain resemble previous episodes of angina pectoris?** If the patient has a documented history of coronary artery disease, particularly if the current episode resembles previously known anginal pain, assume the pain represents myocardial ischemia and treat accordingly.

   B. **What is the location, quality, and severity of the pain?** Location (substernal, epigastric); radiation (jaw, arms, back); quality (burning, crushing, tearing, stabbing, sharp); and severity of pain are features that may suggest a particular diagnosis. Because the same spinal cord segments innervate several intrathoracic and extrathoracic structures, the location and quality of different causes of chest pain may overlap.

   C. **Are there any factors that are known to precipitate or relieve the pain?** Sharp pain worsened by coughing or deep inspiration suggests pleuritis, pericarditis, or pneumothorax. Although classical angina is brought on by exertion, acute myocardial infarction (MI) may produce chest pain at rest, especially in the early morning. Movement of the arms or trunk that reproduces pain would indicate a musculoskeletal origin; however, pericarditis can also cause chest pain worsened by movement of the trunk. The pain of esophagitis is frequently exacerbated by recumbency. Relief of chest pain with sublingual nitroglycerin implies myocardial ischemia, although chest pain resulting from esophageal spasm and gallbladder colic may also be relieved. Myocardial ischemia is relieved in 3–5 minutes, whereas esophageal spasm is relieved in 10 minutes by sublingual nitroglycerin.

D. **Has there been any recent trauma, fall, or thoracic procedure?** Fractured ribs, chest wall contusions, or other musculoskeletal conditions such as recent excessive physical activity can result in chest pain.

III. **Differential Diagnosis.** The differential diagnosis includes a variety of conditions, ranging from musculoskeletal chest wall pain to life-threatening conditions such as acute MI and dissecting aneurysm. The clinician's initial goal is to exclude potentially catastrophic conditions, and if such conditions are identified, institute immediate therapy.

A. **Cardiac causes of chest pain**

1. **Acute myocardial infarction.** Pain is characterized as a severe, crushing, retrosternal pain that may radiate into the arms and neck. This pain is generally described as the worst ever experienced, and generally persists 30 minutes or longer. One seldom relieves it with one or two nitroglycerin tablets, and frequently morphine sulfate is required for relief. The pain of MI may begin at rest or even during sleep and is only infrequently preceded by strenuous physical activity. Associated symptoms include nausea, diaphoresis, dyspnea, and palpitations. Because more than 50% of the deaths caused by acute MI occur within the initial 2 hours, the physician must maintain a high index of suspicion for MI when evaluating any patient with acute chest pain.
2. **Angina pectoris.** The pain of angina is similar to that of MI, although it generally lasts less than 20 minutes and is not nearly as severe. Relief can generally be obtained with sublingual nitroglycerin. The pain is generally exacerbated by exertion, but can also occur at rest or with emotional stress. Any recent change in a stable pattern of angina, such as occurrence with rest or increased frequency or severity, should imply an unstable pattern that mandates close monitoring and aggressive medical therapy. Although coronary artery disease is the most common cause of angina pectoris, other potential causes include coronary artery spasm, aortic stenosis, and angina precipitated by thyrotoxicosis, anemia, and a low diastolic blood pressure.
3. **Acute pericarditis.** Pain is usually described as sharp, but may be dull, and is frequently pleuritic. The pain may be worsened by recumbency and relieved by sitting and leaning forward. Rotation of the trunk may precipitate pain. Possible causes include the following:
   a. **Infection.** Most commonly viral, but may also be bacterial, fungal, or tuberculous.
   b. **Myocardial infarction.** Pericarditis may occur in the first 2–3 days after infarction or may not occur until 1–4 weeks after MI (Dressler's syndrome).
   c. **Uremia**

d. **Malignancy.** Most often breast cancer, lung carcinoma, or lymphoma.
e. **Connective tissue diseases.** Including rheumatoid arthritis, scleroderma, systemic lupus erythematosus, or acute rheumatic fever.

B. **Vascular causes of chest pain**

1. **Acute aortic dissection.** Usually described as an excruciatingly severe pain that is tearing in nature and may radiate to the back (especially if the descending aorta is involved). The pain is most severe at its onset. A prior history of hypertension or connective tissue disorders such as Marfan's syndrome is usually present. On presentation, however, the blood pressure may be normal or even low. Aortic dissection is a potentially life-threatening condition that must be recognized and treated early.
2. **Primary pulmonary hypertension.** The pain is frequently similar to angina. It is usually mild, may be associated with syncope or dyspnea, and may occur with exertion.

C. **Pulmonary causes of chest pain**

1. **Pulmonary embolism (PE) with infarction.** Infarction results in inflammation of the overlying pleura and thus causes pleuritic chest pain. Embolism without infarction may cause a more vague, nondescript chest pain. Dyspnea is often present. Hemoptysis may be present if there is underlying pulmonary infarction. Several conditions predispose to deep venous thrombosis or PE; they include pregnancy; postoperative state; prolonged immobilization; malignancy (especially adenocarcinoma); obesity; exogenous estrogen use; paraplegia; cerebral vascular accident with resultant hemiplegia; congestive heart failure; and hypercoagulable states such as protein C, protein S, factor V Leiden, or antithrombin III deficiency; or the presence of a lupus anticoagulant or anticardiolipin antibody. Pulmonary embolism is a potentially fatal condition that is too often underdiagnosed. It should be suspected in any hospitalized patient who develops acute shortness of breath or chest pain, especially with any of the above risk factors.
2. **Pneumothorax.** This is characterized by the acute onset of pleuritic chest pain associated with dyspnea. *Tension pneumothorax* is a potentially life-threatening condition that is characterized by hypotension, tracheal deviation, venous distension, and severe respiratory distress. There are three broad categories of causes of pneumothorax:
   a. **Spontaneous.** This most often occurs in 20- to 30-year-old males and in older patients with bullous emphysema.
   b. **Iatrogenic.** Pneumothorax may be a complication of subclavian vein catheterization or thoracentesis. Barotrauma from mechanical ventilation, especially in patients requiring high inspiratory pressures, may also cause pneumothorax.

c. **Traumatic.** Any patient with a penetrating chest injury, as well as patients with rib fractures, may sustain a pneumothorax.

3. **Pleurodynia.** This is frequently associated with Coxsackie virus.
4. **Pneumonia/pleuritis.** The pain is typically pleuritic and associated with fever, productive cough, and rigors.

D. **Gastrointestinal causes of chest pain**

1. **Gastroesophageal reflux.** This condition is usually described as a burning pain that is made worse with recumbency and relieved by antacids.
2. **Esophageal spasm.** This condition is easily confused with angina pectoris. It may cause substernal chest pain or tightness that is relieved by nitrates. Intermittent dysphagia, if it occurs, suggests esophageal disease; however, it may be difficult by history alone to distinguish esophageal spasm from angina. Remember that both conditions may occur together.
3. **Gastritis.** Alcohol use, stress that is associated with severe burns, trauma, major surgery, or intensive care unit admission, and use of nonsteroidal anti-inflammatory drugs (NSAIDs) all may induce inflammation of the gastric mucosa, resulting in epigastric and lower chest pain.
4. **Peptic ulcer disease (PUD).** This is typically described as an epigastric discomfort that may be burning or gnawing and frequently radiates to the back. Pain may be either relieved or exacerbated by eating. Antacids frequently relieve it.
5. **Biliary colic.** This condition is characterized by postprandial pain that occurs 1–2 hours after eating and may last several hours. In contrast to the term *colic,* the pain is actually constant and intense and may last several hours. The pain is usually located in the right upper quadrant and radiates to the right scapula; however, the pain may also be perceived largely in the epigastrium and lower chest and therefore may be confused with angina.
6. **Pancreatitis.** There is usually a prior history of gallstones or alcohol ingestion. Pain is usually midepigastric with radiation to the back. Similar to pericarditis, it may be exacerbated by recumbency and relieved by sitting upright and leaning forward. Often nausea and vomiting accompany it.

E. **Musculoskeletal chest pain.** Pain is usually reproduced by palpation over the costochondral or sternochondral junctions. Pain is fairly well localized.

1. **Costochondritis.** Point tenderness is elicited over the costochondral junction.
2. **Muscle strain/spasm.** Most typically, there is a preceding history of exercise or overexertion.
3. **Rib fractures after trauma**

IV. Database

A. Physical examination key points

1. **Vital signs**
   a. **Hypotension.** An ominous sign that may result from any one of several potentially catastrophic causes, including massive MI, cardiac tamponade, tension pneumothorax, acute massive PE, rupture of a dissecting aneurysm, or gastritis or peptic ulcer disease with hemorrhage.
   b. **Hypertension.** May result from any painful condition, but must be particularly looked for in the setting of acute MI or aortic dissection where emergent therapy to reduce the pressure is essential.
   c. **Fever.** May result from PE, MI, pneumonia, or pericarditis.
   d. **Tachycardia.** Can be from sinus tachycardia associated with pain, but could also indicate ventricular tachycardia that has developed because of myocardial ischemia. If untreated, ventricular tachycardia may progress into ventricular fibrillation. (See Section I, Chapter 60, Tachycardia, p 323). PE frequently causes sinus tachycardia or acute atrial fibrillation.
   e. **Bradycardia.** A frequent occurrence with inferior MI, this may result from either sinus node dysfunction or atrioventricular heart block (second- or third-degree). (See Section I, Chapter 8, Bradycardia, p. 39)
2. **HEENT.** Evidence of oral thrush, especially in an immunosuppressed patient, could indicate *Candida* esophagitis.
3. **Neck.** Significant venous distension may occur with either an acute tension pneumothorax or cardiac tamponade. Pain with hyperextension of the neck may indicate a cervical nerve or disk problem as a cause of referred shoulder and chest pain. Tracheal deviation suggests tension pneumothorax.
4. **Chest.** Localized chest wall tenderness may result from a contusion, costochondritis, or rib fracture.
5. **Lungs**
   a. Absent breath sounds and hyperresonance to percussion indicate a pneumothorax.
   b. Crackles and signs of pneumonic consolidation such as increased tactile fremitus or egophony may occur with pneumonia.
   c. A pleural friction rub may result from pneumonia, pulmonary infarction, or any process resulting in pleuritis.
   d. Bibasilar crackles and/or wheezes may occur with decompensated congestive heart failure resulting from myocardial ischemia or infarction.
   e. Lung examination may be normal in a patient with acute PE.
6. **Heart**
   a. The point of maximal impulse (PMI) may not be palpable in a patient with a pericardial effusion. Heart sounds may likewise be distant. In a patient with acute pericarditis, a friction rub may be present, but this is an evanescent finding and therefore the patient must be reexamined periodically.

b. Most often, the cardiac exam is normal in a patient with acute MI or angina pectoris. If there is significant associated left ventricular dysfunction, an S_3 gallop may be heard. An S_4 gallop may also be present. A harsh systolic ejection murmur over the aortic outflow area may indicate aortic stenosis, which can cause angina pectoris even in the presence of normal coronary arteries. In the setting of a recent MI, a new holosystolic murmur at the apex suggests papillary muscle dysfunction or rupture. If dissection is suspected, listen for a decrescendo diastolic murmur of aortic regurgitation at the left lower sternal border, which may develop if the dissection spreads to involve the aortic ring.

7. **Abdomen.** For a discussion of abdominal conditions that can also produce epigastric and lower chest pain, see Section I, Chapter 1, Abdominal Pain, p. 1.
8. **Neurologic exam.** A careful and detailed exam is important in any patient in whom aortic dissection is suspected. The dissection may occlude cerebral or spinal arteries and thereby cause a variety of neurologic deficits.
9. **Extremities**
   a. In a patient with suspected PE, examine for evidence of deep venous thrombosis; however, the physical exam is notoriously inaccurate in this condition and may be entirely normal despite the presence of significant venous thrombosis. Be sure to examine the upper extremities.
   b. In patients with suspected dissection, it is important to examine the pulses bilaterally in both upper and lower extremities for symmetry.

B. Laboratory data

1. **Hemogram.** Leukocytosis may result from any form of inflammation such as pulmonary infarction or MI. If there is an increase in banded neutrophils, suspect a bacterial infection such as pneumonia.
2. **Arterial blood gases.** Should be obtained if a pulmonary process is suspected, such as embolism, pneumothorax, and pneumonia. It should also be ordered with decompensated cardiac function resulting in pulmonary edema.
3. **Cardiac enzymes.** Serial measurements of creatine phosphokinase (CK) with isoenzymes every 8–12 hours over the first 24–48 hours may help to confirm or exclude an MI. Note that CK may not become elevated until several hours after the beginning of infarction. Therefore, a single measurement of CK cannot be used to exclude the diagnosis of MI. Troponin I is cardiac specific, is elevated in the first 4–6 hours after an acute MI, and will remain elevated for 5–9 days.

C. **Radiologic and other studies**

1. **Electrocardiogram.** An ECG should be obtained in any patient with a new complaint of chest pain. If available for comparison, an old ECG is helpful. New T wave changes, ST segment depression or elevation, or the presence of new Q waves will be helpful in identifying the cause of the chest pain as myocardial ischemia/infarction. Patients presenting with MI may initially have an entirely normal ECG, and the diagnosis of MI cannot be excluded on the basis of a normal ECG. With a pulmonary embolism, sinus tachycardia, nonspecific ST-T wave changes, right axis deviation, right bundle branch block, P pulmonale, right ventricular hypertrophy, or the classic S_I, Q_{III}, T_{III} (S wave in I and Q wave and inverted T wave in III) may be present.
2. **Chest x-ray.** Request a CXR in any patient in whom the etiology of the chest pain is unclear. It may be helpful in diagnosing pneumothorax, pneumonia, and pleural and pericardial effusions. A widened mediastinum suggests dissection of the thoracic aorta.
3. **Echocardiogram.** This can be performed on an emergent basis if cardiac tamponade is suspected. Also helpful in diagnosing thoracic aortic dissection and assessing regional wall abnormalities in acute MI.
4. **Contrast CT scan.** This should be obtained in any patient in whom aortic dissection is suspected.
5. **Spiral CT of the chest.** Helpful for ruling in pulmonary embolus. A negative test does not rule out the diagnosis.
6. **Ventilation/perfusion ($\dot{V}/\dot{Q}$) lung scan.** A lung scan may be helpful if pulmonary emboli are suspected. Impedance plethysmography and Doppler ultrasound of the lower extremities may also be obtained if there is a strong suspicion for acute deep venous thrombosis.

V. **Plan.** In assessing any patient with acute chest pain, the overriding goal is to exclude the presence of the previously mentioned life-threatening conditions. In the acute setting, it is better to maintain a high index of suspicion for these conditions.

A. **Emergency management (for all patients with chest pain)**

1. **Oxygen.** Administer oxygen therapy with 2–4 L/min by nasal cannula. If the patient has a history of chronic obstructive airway disease, it is preferable to administer 24% O_2 by Venturi face mask initially.
2. **Intravenous access.** Establish at least one intravenous line for administration of medications should the patient's condition deteriorate.
3. **Nitroglycerin.** If chest pain is still present and the systolic blood pressure is above 90, 0.4 mg nitroglycerin may be administered sublingually.
4. **12-lead ECG**

5. **Stat portable CXR and ABG.** If your initial assessment suggests any evidence of a pneumothorax, pneumonia, or heart failure.

B. **Myocardial ischemia.** If your initial assessment suggests the possibility of acute MI, the following are brief guidelines offered for the initial treatment. A full discussion of acute MI is beyond the scope of this section.

1. **Aspirin.** Administer two chewable aspirin (consider ticlopidine [Ticlid] if there is a history of aspirin hypersensitivity).
2. **Nitrates**
   a. Nitroglycerin in a dose of 0.4–0.6 mg may be administered sublingually every 5 minutes, provided that the systolic blood pressure remains above 90. It is preferable to administer the nitroglycerin while the patient is recumbent. This may provide relief for angina pectoris and possibly unstable angina pectoris.
   b. The pain of acute MI is seldom relieved by the administration of nitroglycerin sublingually and requires treatment with either intravenous nitroglycerin or morphine. If the nitroglycerin is effective but pain recurs, begin a nitroglycerin infusion initially at 10 μg/min and increase by 10 μg/min every 10 minutes until relief of pain or to a maximum dose of 200 μg/min. The systolic blood pressure must be maintained above 90 during the administration of nitroglycerin. Hemodynamic monitoring with a pulmonary artery catheter (see Section III, Chapter 12, Pulmonary Artery Catheterization p 421) is often necessary if hypotension persists.
3. **Morphine sulfate.** If pain is not relieved by nitroglycerin sublingually or intravenously, 3–5 mg of morphine IV every 5–10 minutes can be administered for relief. Close monitoring of the patient's blood pressure and respirations is necessary, because hypotension and respiratory suppression may occur. These adverse effects may be reversed with naloxone (Narcan) 0.4 mg IV.
4. **Beta-blockers.** Should strongly be considered. Metoprolol 5 mg every 2–5 minutes for 3 doses intravenously; or atenolol 5 mg every 5 minutes for 2 doses intravenously. Watch for bradycardia and acute heart block (second- or third-degree), especially in a patient with suspected right ventricular infarction.
5. **Heparin.** Unfractionated heparin 70 U/kg bolus, followed by 15 U/kg/hr continuous infusion. Dose is titrated to a PTT 1.5–2 times control value (usually 50–60 seconds); some cardiologists prefer the PTT to be 2–2.5 times the control value. Low molecular weight heparins may also be used. Dalteparin (Fragmin) 120 U/kg SC Q 12 hr, up to a maximum of 10,000 units per dose, or enoxaparin (Lovenox) 1 mg/kg SC Q 12 hr can be used. Treatment is usually continued for 2–8 days after the patient has stabilized.
6. **Transfer to a coronary care unit or intensive care.** This is especially important in the first 24 hours of MI, when arrhythmia monitoring and ready access to a defibrillator are essential.

7. **Platelet glycoprotein IIb/IIIa inhibitors.** Should be considered in the setting of chest pain with ST depression in two contiguous leads or typical chest pain with a history of coronary artery disease. In patients undergoing percutaneous coronary intervention, abciximab (ReoPro) 0.25 mg/kg IV bolus, followed by infusion of 0.125 μg/kg/min (maximum of 10 μg/min) for 18–24 hours. Infusion should be discontinued 1 hour following percutaneous coronary intervention. Eptifibatide (Integrilin) 180 μg/kg IV bolus, followed by infusion of 2 μg/kg/min. Eptifibatide may be administered for up to 96 hours. Tirofiban (Aggrastat) 0.4 μg/kg/min initial infusion for 30 minutes, followed by 0.1 μg/kg/min continuous infusion. Tirofiban may be given for up to 108 hours after presentation. Aspirin and heparin should be used along with the platelet glycoprotein IIb/IIIa inhibitors.
8. **Thrombolytic therapy.** This discussion is beyond the scope of this section, but *should always be considered* in any patient presenting with chest pain that is consistent with a MI; at least 1 mm ST-segment elevation in two contiguous leads and no contraindication to thrombolytics. See the discussions of alteplase, anistreplase, and streptokinase in Section VII, Therapeutics.

C. **Aortic dissection.** The initial treatment goal is to reduce pain and to reduce blood pressure if elevated. Surgical correction is indicated for all ascending thoracic aneurysms.

1. **Transfer to a coronary or intensive care unit.** Make arrangements for immediate transfer where hemodynamic monitoring can be instituted.
2. **Immediate vascular surgical consult**
3. **Intravenous esmolol or labetalol.** Esmolol is given as a 30-mg bolus followed by 3 mg/min and titrated up to 12 mg/min. Labetalol is given as 10 mg over 2 minutes followed by 20- to 80-mg doses every 10–15 minutes up to a total dose of 300 mg, and then a maintenance dose of 2 mg/min, titrating up to 5–20 mg/min. If there is a contraindication to using beta-blockers, then intravenous verapamil or diltiazem can be used.
4. **Relieve pain.** Morphine sulfate 3–5 mg may be administered IV every 10 minutes. Again, close monitoring of the blood pressure and respirations is necessary.

D. **Pulmonary embolism**

1. **Oxygen.** Ensure adequate oxygenation.
2. **Heparin.** After checking a baseline prothrombin time and partial thromboplastin time (PTT), administer a bolus of heparin 80 U/kg IV and follow it with a continuous IV infusion of 18 U/kg/hr. Repeat the PTT in 4–6 hours and adjust the heparin to maintain a PTT approximately 1.5–2.5 times the control value (50–70 seconds).
3. **Surgical or radiological consultation.** For placement of a venocaval filter if systemic anticoagulation is contraindicated.

4. **Thrombolytic therapy or surgical consultation for embolectomy.** Should be considered for massive PE with hypotension. ***Caution:*** Thrombolytics are contraindicated postoperatively.

E. **Acute pneumothorax**
   1. **Decompression.** An acute tension pneumothorax should be treated by immediate placement of a 16-gauge needle into the second intercostal space in the midclavicular line. This potentially life-saving measure can be instituted while the patient awaits placement of a chest tube.
   2. **Oxygen.** A spontaneous pneumothorax occurring in an otherwise healthy person and involving 20% or less of the lung can usually be treated with oxygen and observation. Chest tube insertion or pneumothorax catheter placement with aspiration should be used to treat all other pneumothoraces.

F. **Pericarditis**
   1. **Indomethacin (Indocin) 25–50 mg tid.** Generally effective for pain relief in most cases of pericarditis.
   2. **Emergent echocardiogram.** If tamponade is suspected and confirmed, a cardiology consultation for pericardiocentesis should be requested.

G. **Gastritis/esophagitis**
   1. **Antacids.** Mylanta-II 30 mL every 4–6 hours may provide immediate relief.
   2. **H_2 antagonists.** Cimetidine (Tagamet), ranitidine (Zantac), famotidine (Pepcid), or nizatidine (Axid) may also relieve symptoms. Hydrogen proton pump inhibitors such as omeprazole (Prilosec) are also effective.
   3. **Elevating head of the bed.** Elevation by 6 inches on blocks may help to reduce the reflux that occurs with recumbency.
   4. ***H pylori** antibody.* May be helpful in making a diagnosis of peptic ulcer disease.

H. **Costochondritis.** Treat with NSAIDs such as ibuprofen 800 mg Q 8 hours.

REFERENCES

Raschke RA, Reilly BM, Guidry JR et al: The weight-based heparin dosing nomogram compared with a "standard care" nomogram. Ann Intern Med 1993;119:874.

Silverman ME: *Examination of the Heart: The Clinical History.* 3rd ed. American Heart Association;1990.

12. COAGULOPATHY

I. **Problem.** After cardiac catheterization, a patient has oozing from the femoral arterial puncture site.

II. Immediate Questions

A. What is the patient's blood pressure? Determine immediately if the bleeding is extensive enough to cause hypovolemia and shock (Refer to Section I, Chapter 42, Hypotension, p 224). If central lines need to be placed, determine extent of the coagulopathy before inserting needles into major noncompressible vessels. Hypotension and coagulopathy can also be seen with sepsis.

B. How much external bleeding is there? Look at wounds or needle puncture sites to see if there is active bleeding.

C. Do factors exist that increase the likelihood of generalized bleeding? In critically ill individuals, disseminated intravascular coagulation (DIC) should be considered. In general, when you have a bleeding patient, inquire about liver disease; nutritional status; family history of bleeding disorders; any bleeding with prior surgical procedures (including dental extractions); and use of medications such as aspirin, nonsteroidal anti-inflammatory drugs (NSAIDs), antiplatelet drugs, or anticoagulants.

III. Differential Diagnosis

A. Inadequate hemostasis. This is the most common cause of localized bleeding in the postoperative patient. The bleeding is usually minimal.

B. Platelet disorders

1. **Thrombocytopenia.** See Section I, Chapter 61, Thrombocytopenia, p 333.
   a. **Decreased production.** This is often secondary to chemotherapy, fibrosis, neoplasia, or infection (tuberculosis, histoplasmosis) involving the bone marrow. Ethanol, thiazides, estrogens, and other drugs can impair platelet production. Vitamin B_{12}, folic acid, or iron deficiencies may result in decreased production.
   b. **Sequestration.** Caused by splenic enlargement resulting from portal hypertension, neoplasia, infection, or storage diseases.
   c. **Destruction.** Idiopathic thrombocytopenic purpura (ITP), thrombotic thrombocytopenic purpura (TTP), collagen vascular diseases, and reactions to drugs (penicillins, sulfa drugs, quinidine, thiazides, heparin, and others) can cause platelet destruction.
   d. **Dilution.** May occur with a large volume of blood transfused over a short interval.
2. **Qualitative platelet disorders**
   a. **Inherited disorders**
      i. **von Willebrand's disease (vWD).** Autosomal dominant adhesion defect with many variants; prevalence as high as 1%.

ii. **Bernard-Soulier syndrome.** Inherited adhesion defect characterized by giant platelets and absence/dysfunction of glycoprotein Ib/IX.

iii. **Glanzmann's thrombasthenia.** Inherited aggregation defect with absence/dysfunction of glycoprotein IIb/IIIa.

b. **Acquired disorders**

i. **Drugs.** Aspirin and NSAIDs affect cyclooxygenase metabolism (aspirin for the life of the platelet, NSAIDs in the presence of the drug). Glycoprotein IIb/IIIa inhibitors and other antiplatelet agents affect platelet aggregation only in the presence of the drug.

ii. **Uremia.** Abnormal platelet aggregation caused by an unknown mechanism.

C. **Coagulation defects**

1. **Congenital**

a. **Hemophilia A.** Factor VIII deficiency, X-linked recessive. Incidence of 1/10,000 male births.

b. **Hemophilia B.** Factor IX deficiency, X-linked recessive. Incidence of 1/100,000 male births.

c. **Congenital deficiencies of other coagulation factors.** These are much less common than factor VIII and IX deficiencies.

2. **Acquired**

a. **Disseminated intravascular coagulation (DIC).** DIC is associated with sepsis, trauma, burns, and malignancy; it may be a complication of pregnancy and delivery, liver disease, and heat stroke.

b. **Vitamin K deficiency.** Vitamin K is required for synthesis of factors II, VII, IX, and X. The most frequent setting for deficiency is the malnourished patient receiving antibiotics.

c. **Severe liver disease.** Cirrhosis, hepatitis, hemochromatosis, biliary cirrhosis, or cancer. Coagulopathy is caused by decreased production of coagulation factors, production of abnormal coagulation factors, or a failure to clear activated coagulation factors.

d. **Autoantibodies.** Circulating anticoagulant antibodies occur in postpartum women and in autoimmune diseases such as systemic lupus erythematosus (SLE).

IV. **Database.** The most important factor in diagnosing a coagulopathy is understanding and utilizing appropriate laboratory tests. It is imperative to draw blood for needed tests prior to instituting therapy or transfusions.

A. **History and physical examination key points**

1. **Vital signs.** *Orthostatic hypotension* (a decrease in systolic blood pressure of 10 mm Hg, and/or an increase in heart rate of 20 bpm 1 minute after changing from a supine to a standing position) sig-

nifies a major loss of blood. Also look for resting or supine tachycardia or hypotension. Fever or hypothermia suggests DIC as the cause.

2. **Skin and incisions.** Petechiae, purpura, easy bruising, and oozing from intravenous sites suggest a systemic rather than a local cause. Examine any incision for hematoma or for active bleeding.
3. **Abdomen.** Splenomegaly, hepatomegaly, or ascites provides clues to the diagnosis.
4. **Extremities.** Hemarthrosis may be seen with hemophilia or other causes of coagulopathy.
5. **Neurologic exam.** To assess for CNS bleeding.

B. **Laboratory data**

1. **Complete blood count.** Follow serial hematocrits with ongoing bleeding. An adequate platelet count does not imply adequate function of platelets. Generally, platelet counts of 50,000–100,000 are adequate to maintain hemostasis if function is normal.
2. **Prothrombin time (PT) and partial thromboplastin time (PTT).** The PTT assesses all coagulation proteins except factors VII and XIII. The PT will be elevated if there is a deficiency of factor I, II, V, VII, or X (Table 1–5). Factor VII has the shortest half-life; a deficiency in factor VII is the usual cause in generalized problems such as liver disease. In SLE, there may be a circulating anticoagulant, which usually prolongs the PTT and less frequently the PT. This condition generally does not cause a bleeding diathesis but may predispose to thrombosis.
3. **Peripheral blood smear.** May reveal fragments and helmet cells in DIC and TTP. May suggest other causes of thrombocytopenia such as vitamin B_{12} or folate deficiency. The presence of nucleated red blood cells suggests the presence of marrow infiltrative disorders (eg, prostate cancer) as the cause.
4. **Renal function.** Uremia will inhibit platelet function.

TABLE I–5. COMMON CAUSES OF COAGULOPATHY DIFFERENTIATED BY ALTERATIONS IN PROTHROMBIN TIME, PARTIAL THROMBOPLASTIN TIME, AND PLATELET COUNT

PT	PTT	Platelets	Most Common Causes
↑	–	–	Deficiency or inhibitor of factor VII (early liver disease, vitamin K deficiency, warfarin therapy, dysfibrinogenemia, some cases of DIC
–	↑	–	Deficiency or inhibitor of factors VIII, IX, or XI; vWD; heparin
↑	↑	↓	DIC, liver disease, heparin therapy associated with thrombocytopenia
–	–	↓	Increased platelet destruction, decreased platelet production, hypersplenism, hemodilution
–	–	↑	Myeloproliferative disorders
–	–	–	Mild vWD, acquired qualitative platelet disorders (eg, uremia)

DIC = disseminated intravascular coagulation; vWD = von Willebrand's disease.

5. **Thrombin time (TT).** The TT assays functional fibrinogen; it can also assay for heparin effect and presence of fibrinogen degradation products.
6. **Fibrinogen, fibrin split products, and D-dimer assay.** In DIC, fibrinogen may be decreased and fibrin split products are increased. Fibrinogen is an acute-phase reactant. The absolute fibrinogen level may be normal, but a downward trend is helpful. D-dimer increase may suggest ongoing DIC.
7. **Bleeding time.** This test evaluates platelet function. Uremia, liver disease, and aspirin therapy within the last week may adversely affect function. Thrombocytopenia (platelets < 50,000 per microliter) can increase the bleeding time. Bleeding time is also prolonged by rare disorders of collagen that may impair integrity of the vessel wall. Bleeding time may be prolonged in vWD, but normal bleeding time should not preclude testing.
8. **Blood replacement.** Type and cross-match if needed.
9. **Future studies.** Save one or two tubes of blood prior to transfusion therapy to assay for any coagulation factors or other studies that may be ordered later.

C. Radiologic and other studies

1. **X-ray/CT.** Obtain a CXR if there is indication of intrathoracic bleeding; obtain a CT scan of the head if intracranial bleeding is suspected.
2. **Bone marrow aspiration and biopsy.** Might be performed to assess platelet production in the presence of unexplained thrombocytopenia or if leukemia or another infiltrative marrow disorder is suspected.

V. Plan. Assess the rate of bleeding and differentiate between mechanical bleeding and true coagulopathy. Almost all external bleeding that is mechanical can be controlled by applying direct pressure and elevation. Treatment of coagulopathy requires appropriate laboratory tests to make the diagnosis, and then institution of the correct treatment. In the acute setting, assess the amount of blood loss and the volume status, and treat with IV fluids if hypovolemia is present. For further information regarding transfusion of blood products, refer to Section V, Blood Component Therapy, p 437.

A. Thrombocytopenia

1. Use random donor platelet transfusion, usually 5–10 U at a time, for a platelet count below 20,000 or with higher platelet counts if there is ongoing bleeding. Platelet transfusions are generally not indicated in immune thrombocytopenias unless there is active bleeding. Patients receiving multiple platelet transfusions may develop HLA antibodies and have better incremental increases in the platelet count with HLA-matched single donor platelets. Immunocompromised patients should receive irradiated platelets to avoid a graft-versus-host reaction. Such patients include bone

marrow transplant patients and possibly patients with acute leukemia or lymphoma who are undergoing aggressive therapy.

2. For a drug reaction, discontinue the drug and transfuse platelets if necessary.
3. In the presence of ITP, no treatment is usually needed until the platelet count is below 10,000 unless there is bleeding. For counts below 10,000, IV immunoglobulin (IG) (for Rh-negative patients) or WinRho (for Rh-positive patients) with or without prednisone may be used. Chronic ITP is treated with prednisone, cyclophosphamide, azathioprine, or danazol. The best long-term results are obtained with splenectomy. Platelet transfusions prior to splenectomy are very short-lived in ITP.
4. Document functional defect with bleeding time and treat the underlying condition, such as uremia. Discontinue drugs adversely affecting function.

B. von Willebrand's disease (vWD)

1. Cryoprecipitate or fresh-frozen plasma are plasma products of choice. (See Section V, Blood Component Therapy, p 437).
2. Deamino-8-D-arginine vasopressin (DDAVP), a vasopressin analogue, increases von Willebrand factor (vWF) levels by releasing stores from endothelium. DDAVP can be effective for certain types of vWD with mild bleeding, but is contraindicated in type IIb since it may exacerbate thrombocytopenia.

C. Hemophilia A. Specific recommendations for factor replacement depend on site of bleeding and severity of factor deficiency and are beyond the scope of this book. The reader is referred to a standard hematology text for this information. The half-life of factor VIII is about 8–12 hours. Because many factor VIII concentrates are now available, treatment of choice should be only with genetically engineered products that minimize risk of transmission of viral hepatitis and human immunodeficiency virus (HIV).

D. Hemophilia B. As with hemophilia A, the reader is referred to a standard hematology text for specific recommendations for factor replacement. Factor IX concentrate has a half-life of approximately 24 hours. Several factor IX preparations are available. There is concern about some preparations containing activated coagulation factors that may induce thrombosis or DIC. New preparations probably avoid this risk. Newly diagnosed patients should receive only heat-treated products to avoid transmission of viral hepatitis or HIV.

E. DIC. Treat the underlying cause. Support the bleeding patient with fresh-frozen plasma, platelet transfusions, and blood transfusions. Heparin therapy in chronic DIC decreases the bleeding severity and incidence of thromboembolic events. Results of studies using heparin to treat acute DIC (especially from sepsis) have been less encouraging. The dose of heparin used varies from 5 to 140 U/kg intravenously every 4 hours to 15–20 U/kg/hr by continuous infusion. Lower doses (< 50 U/kg every 4 hours) are recommended if marked thrombocytopenia is present.

F. **Vitamin K deficiency/liver disease.** If immediate treatment is needed, transfuse with 2–4 units of fresh-frozen plasma and follow the PT/PTT. Because factor VII, which has a half-life of 6 hours, is metabolized quickly, repeated infusions may be needed in 6–12 hours. In all cases, begin treatment with vitamin K 10 mg SC every day for 3 consecutive days. Vitamin K may be given intravenously, but because of rare anaphylactic reactions, it must be given slowly—the rate should not exceed 1 mg/min. IV vitamin K has a faster onset and shorter time to maximal effect than SC vitamin K. If the coagulopathy is secondary to vitamin K deficiency, a response to vitamin K should be evident after 24 hours. If there is no response to vitamin K, the coagulopathy is not due to vitamin K deficiency.

REFERENCES

Grosset ABM, Rodgers GM: Acquired coagulation disorders. In: Lee GR, Foerster J, Lukens J et al, eds. *Wintrobe's Clinical Hematology.* 10th ed. Lippincott Williams & Wilkins;1999:1733.

Rodgers GM, Bithell TC: The diagnostic approach to the bleeding disorders. In: Lee GR, Foerster J, Lukens J et al, eds. *Wintrobe's Clinical Hematology.* 10th ed. Lippincott Williams & Wilkins;1999:1557.

13. COMA, ACUTE MENTAL STATUS CHANGES

I. **Problem.** You are called to the emergency room to evaluate a 63-year-old man with confusion and lethargy.

II. **Immediate Questions**

A. **What are the patient's vital signs?** Hypotension from any etiology can decrease cerebral perfusion and lower the level of consciousness. Fever might implicate an infectious process such as pneumonia or urinary tract infection (UTI) as the cause. This is particularly true in the elderly patient. Meningitis should be suspected in any patient presenting with acute mental status changes and fever. Respiratory rate and pattern are also important diagnostic clues.

B. **What is the time course of the mental status alteration?** When possible, it is important to question the patient's family or friends while obtaining the history. If the alteration is long-standing or recurrent, the patient may have dementia or psychiatric illness.

C. **What medications is the patient taking?** Medications, especially in the elderly, may alter mental status. If the patient is hospitalized, review the medication orders and then check the medication administration record to define the actual quantity of analgesic or sedative given.

D. Is there a history of trauma? Recent head trauma may result in a subdural or epidural hematoma. The elderly, alcoholics, and patients receiving oral anticoagulation are particularly susceptible.

E. Is there evidence of central nervous system pathology such as headache, hemiparesis, ataxia, or vomiting? Increased intracranial pressure from tumor, subdural hematoma, or cerebral hemorrhage may lead to delirium, lethargy, or coma.

F. Does the patient drink ethanol or use any recreational medications? Exposure to drugs or toxins is the most common cause of coma. Intoxication with ethanol or other substances, as well as alcohol withdrawal (see Section I, Chapter 16, Delirium Tremens (DTs): Major Alcohol Withdrawal, p 90) can cause alterations in the level of consciousness.

G. What is the pertinent past medical history? Hyperglycemia from diabetes mellitus (see Section I, Chapter 32, Hyperglycemia, p 180) or hypoglycemia (see Section I, Chapter 37, Hypoglycemia, p 202) from its treatment can cause altered mental status. Severe liver disease, renal failure, or hypothyroidism can depress the level of consciousness or cause delirium. Respiratory failure with hypoxemia causes agitation followed by lethargy. Ventilatory failure with hypercapnia causes somnolence. A seizure disorder might present as stupor in the postictal state.

H. Is there a history of psychiatric illness? Patients with depression may present with confusion and disorientation. Patients with catatonic schizophrenia may not be responsive to verbal or other cues.

I. Are there occupational or environmental exposures? Consider carbon monoxide, cyanide, organic solvents, lead, or arsenic as the cause.

J. Is the patient in the perioperative period? Perioperative delirium is common. Potential causes include intraoperative hypotension or anoxia; infection, myocardial ischemia or infarction; and medications such as anticholinergics, sedatives, and narcotics.

K. Is there a history of non–tonic-clonic seizures? Non–tonic-clonic seizures should always be considered in a patient with unexplained mental status changes.

III. Differential Diagnosis

A. Trauma

1. **Subdural hematoma.** The most common intracranial mass lesion resulting from head injury.
2. **Epidural hematoma.** Usually associated with a skull fracture resulting in a lacerated meningeal vessel, particularly the middle meningeal artery.

3. **Concussion.** Cerebral dysfunction that clears within 24 hours, a clinical diagnosis.
4. **Contusion.** Usually associated with neurologic deficits that persist longer than 24 hours. Small hemorrhages are present in the cerebral parenchyma on CT scan.

B. **Metabolic causes**
1. **Exogenous**
   a. **Medications.** The following are a few of the many medications that can alter the content or level of consciousness: narcotics, benzodiazepines, barbiturates, amphetamines, tricyclic antidepressants, H_1 and H_2 antagonists, antiparkinsonian agents, phenytoin (Dilantin), digoxin, corticosteroids, lithium, psychotropics, and salicylates.
   b. **Toxins**
      i. **Environmental/occupational.** These include carbon monoxide, cyanide, organic solvents, and heavy metals such as lead and arsenic.
      ii. **Drugs of abuse.** Intoxication with ethanol, amphetamines, methanol, or ethylene glycol. Withdrawal from ethanol, barbiturates, benzodiazepines, or opiates (see Section I, Chapter 16, Delirium Tremens, Alcohol Withdrawal, p 90).
2. **Endogenous**
   a. **Fluids/electrolytes**
      i. **Sodium.** Hyponatremia (see Section I, Chapter 40, Hyponatremia, p 214) and hypernatremia (see Section I, Chapter 34, Hypernatremia, p 190) may cause confusion. With hyponatremia, the severity of the mental status alteration is related to the level and rate of sodium decrease.
      ii. **Potassium.** Hypokalemia (see Section I, Chapter 38, Hypokalemia, p 206) or hyperkalemia (see Section I, Chapter 33, Hyperkalemia, p 186). Potassium abnormalities infrequently cause mental status changes. Hypokalemia may precipitate hepatic encephalopathy in the cirrhotic patient.
      iii. **Calcium.** Hypocalcemia (see Section I, Chapter 36, Hypocalcemia, p 198) or hypercalcemia (see Section I, Chapter 31, Hypercalcemia, p 175).
      iv. **Magnesium.** Hypomagnesemia (see Section I, Chapter 39, Hypomagnesemia, p 210). Often there is associated hypokalemia and hypocalcemia. The patient may be anxious, delirious, or psychotic. Hypermagnesemia is a rare cause of coma.
      v. **Acidemia or alkalemia.** Mental status changes often result from underlying acidemia or alkalemia. Acute, and to a lesser extent, chronic hypercapnia can cause confusion, hallucinations, and coma. See Section I, Chapter 2, Acidosis, p. 9 and Chapter 3, Alkalosis, p. 18.

vi. **Osmolarity disturbances.** Common causes are hypernatremia and marked hyperglycemia.

b. **Organ failure**

i. **Renal failure.** Usually with markedly elevated blood urea nitrogen.

ii. **Hepatic encephalopathy.** Seen in fulminant hepatitis and cirrhosis. Often precipitated by worsening hepatic function, gastrointestinal bleeding, spontaneous bacterial peritonitis, dehydration, azotemia, hypokalemic alkalosis, constipation, and medications such as sedatives.

iii. **Respiratory failure.** Hypoxia and/or hypercapnia.

c. **Endocrine**

i. **Pancreas.** Hypoglycemia (most often secondary to treatment of diabetes) or marked hyperglycemia resulting in a hyperosmolar state.

ii. **Pituitary.** Hypopituitarism secondary to tumor or apoplexy can lead to adrenal insufficiency and hypothyroidism.

iii. **Thyroid.** Thyrotoxicosis and hypothyroidism. Both may have associated mental status changes. Thyrotoxicosis is associated with agitation and nervousness. Hypothyroidism is associated with lethargy. A high index of suspicion is required for diagnosis in the elderly because mental status changes may be the only sign.

iv. **Parathyroid.** Either hyperparathyroidism resulting in hypercalcemia or hypoparathyroidism resulting in hypocalcemia can cause mental status alteration.

v. **Adrenal.** Cushing's syndrome can cause irritability, emotional lability, profound depression, confusion, and overt psychosis. Addisonian crisis can present with stupor or coma.

d. **Vitamin deficiencies**

i. **Thiamine (vitamin B_1).** Wernicke's encephalopathy is often seen in alcoholics but also occurs in hyperemesis gravidarum, AIDS, peritoneal dialysis, malnutrition, and eating disorders. Mental status changes range from mild confusion to coma. Patients presenting in coma with Wernicke's encephalopathy are often not diagnosed until autopsy. Ataxia, bilateral horizontal nystagmus, or other ophthalmoplegias are frequently present. Korsakoff's psychosis is a part of Wernicke's encephalopathy and is characterized by anterograde amnesia, impaired ability to learn, and confabulation. Recovery from Korsakoff's psychosis can be expected in only 50% of cases.

ii. **Cobalamin (vitamin B_{12}).** Symptoms include forgetfulness, dementia, irritability, and psychosis. Neurologic manifestations can precede macrocytic anemia.

iii. **Niacin (vitamin B_3).** In pellagra, fatigue and insomnia often precede an encephalopathic syndrome of memory loss, confusion, and psychosis. Other symptoms include dermatitis and diarrhea.

e. **Alteration in body temperature**

i. **Hypothermia.** See Section I, Chapter 43, Hypothermia, p 229. Occurs most commonly from exposure. Frequently observed in patients with alcohol or barbiturate intoxication, extracellular fluid deficit, sepsis, adrenal insufficiency, and myxedema.

ii. **Hyperthermia.** See Section I, Chapter 22, Fever, p 127. Most commonly seen from heat stroke. Also occurs with neuroleptic malignant syndrome in patients taking phenothiazines and as malignant hyperthermia secondary to inhaled anesthetics or succinylcholine. May be seen in hyperthyroidism (thyroid storm).

f. **Miscellaneous**

i. **Hepatic porphyria.** Anxiety, depression, disorientation, and hallucinations can occur in attacks of acute intermittent porphyria.

ii. **Reye's encephalopathy.** This rare syndrome can follow influenza or varicella upper respiratory infections in children less than 15 years old. Classically associated with salicylate use (salicylate use not necessary).

C. **Infection**

1. **Central nervous system infections.** Consider meningitis, encephalitis, tertiary syphilis, and stage 3 Lyme disease.
2. **Sepsis**
3. **Infections in the elderly.** Especially urinary or respiratory.

D. **Tumors**

1. **Primary or metastatic to CNS**
2. **Hypercalcemia from metastatic disease**
3. **Paraneoplastic syndromes.**

a. **Parathyroid hormone–related peptide.** Secretion by squamous cell bronchogenic carcinoma causes hypercalcemia.

b. **Syndrome of inappropriate antidiuretic hormone (SIADH).** Inappropriate secretion of antidiuretic hormone (ADH) by small cell lung cancer.

c. **Cushing's syndrome.** This can be due to ectopic adrenocorticotropic hormone (ACTH) production by small cell lung cancer or carcinoid.

d. **Paraneoplastic neurologic syndromes.** These include paraneoplastic encephalomyelitis and limbic encephalitis, both associated with small cell lung cancer.

E. **Psychiatric causes**

1. **Psychogenic coma.** In pseudocoma, patients appear unarousable and unresponsive but have no structural, metabolic, or toxic disorder.

2. **Catatonia.** State of muteness characterized by drastically decreased motor activity with preserved ability to sit, stand, and maintain body posture. Usually psychiatric in etiology (schizophrenia), but frontal lobe dysfunction and drug effects can mimic.
3. **Depression.** May mimic dementia or cause vegetative state, especially in the elderly.
4. **ICU psychosis**

F. **Miscellaneous**

1. **Hypotension.** See Section I, Chapter 42, Hypotension, p 224.
2. **Seizures.** Non–tonic-clonic seizures as well as postictal confusion.
3. **Cerebrovascular accident**
   a. **Ischemic infarction.** The most common causes include atherosclerosis with thromboembolism and cardiogenic embolism from mural thrombus or endocarditis. Also consider vasculitis and vasospasm.
   b. **Intracranial hemorrhage.** Causes include hypertension, trauma, ruptured aneurysm, arteriovenous malformation, coagulopathy, tumor, and cocaine.
4. **Locked-in syndrome.** In this de-efferented state, bilateral pontine lesions cause quadriplegia and lower cranial nerve palsies. Patients are alert and awake but mute.
5. **Hypertensive encephalopathy.** Blood pressure is markedly elevated. Funduscopic exam is notable for exudates, hemorrhages, and papilledema.
6. **Anoxic encephalopathy.** Can occur after resuscitation of sudden cardiac death.
7. **Syncope.** See Section I, Chapter 59, Syncope, p 315.
8. **Dementia.** Common causes include Alzheimer's disease, multi-infarct dementia, alcoholism, and Parkinson's disease. Also consider normal pressure hydrocephalus if ataxia and incontinence are present.
9. **Hyperviscosity syndrome.** This uncommon syndrome is associated with Waldenstrom's macroglobulinemia, multiple myeloma, leukemia, and polycythemia vera (see Section I, Chapter 55, Polycythemia, p 291). Somnolence, stupor, coma, and psychiatric illness can occur within a triad of bleeding, visual abnormalities, and neurologic deficits.

IV. **Database**

A. **Physical examination key points**

1. **Vital signs**
   a. **Blood pressure.** Hypotension can cause decreased cerebral perfusion and is a common finding in acute mental status changes due to ethanol or barbiturate intoxication, internal hemorrhage, myocardial infarction, dissecting aortic aneurysm,

Addison's disease, and gram-negative sepsis. Hypertension occurs with hypertensive encephalopathy, cerebral or brain stem infarction, subarachnoid hemorrhage, or increased intracranial pressure.

b. **Heart rate.** Tachycardia may be secondary to many causes of mental status alteration such as sepsis, pulmonary embolus, hypoglycemia, and myocardial infarction. Bradycardia in association with hypertension and respiratory irregularity may indicate increased intracranial pressure (Cushing's reflex).

c. **Respiratory rate and pattern.** Bradypnea may indicate ethanol, narcotic, or barbiturate intoxication. Tachypnea may indicate significant hypoxia or sepsis. Hyperpnea causing hyperventilation can be compensation for metabolic acidosis (*Kussmaul respiration*). A normal breathing pattern suggests the absence of brain stem damage. *Cheyne-Stokes respiration,* characterized by periods of waxing and waning hyperpnea alternating with shorter periods of apnea, implies an intact brain stem and may be present in bilateral hemispheric lesions or metabolic disturbance. Apneustic or ataxic breathing strongly suggests brain stem damage.

d. **Temperature.** In the comatose patient, temperature should be measured with a rectal probe. A fever suggests infection, thyroid storm, anticholinergic toxicity, heat stroke, malignant hyperthermia, or neurogenic hyperthermia due to subarachnoid hemorrhage or hypothalamic pathology. The elderly may not have a fever in response to an infection. Hypothermia suggests myxedema, cold exposure, intoxication with ethanol or barbiturates, or a posterior hypothalamic lesion.

2. **General.** An unkempt patient might be an alcoholic or schizophrenic. Cachexia points to malnutrition or malignancy. Emesis can indicate increased intracranial pressure. Decerebrate posturing occurs in bilateral midbrain or pontine lesions, bilateral supratentorial motor pathway lesions, and metabolic disturbances. Decorticate posturing can occur with any lesion above the brain stem.

3. **HEENT**

   a. **Head.** Look for evidence of trauma that may point to a subdural or epidural bleed or a cerebral contusion.

   b. **Eyes**

      i. **Pupils.** Pinpoint pupils (< 1 mm) may indicate narcotic use or a pontine lesion. A unilateral, fixed, and dilated pupil suggests ipsilateral temporal lobe herniation. Bilateral, fixed, and dilated pupils suggest anticholinergic poisoning, anoxia, or brain death. Pupils may be dilated or sluggish to direct and indirect light in hypothermia or hyperthermia.

      ii. **Fundus.** Conjunctival or fundal petechiae suggest fat embolism or endocarditis. Papilledema suggests a mass, intracranial bleed, or hypertensive encephalopathy. Subhyaloid hemorrhages may be seen trapped behind the vitreous humor at the edge of the optic disc, suggesting a sudden rise in intracranial pressure.

iii. **Ocular movements.** Assessment of unprovoked eye movements can be valuable. Smooth, fully conjugate, spontaneous eye movements (*roving*) in a comatose patient suggest an intact brain stem and a bihemispheric cause of coma. Nystagmus is seen with Wernicke's encephalopathy.

c. **Ears.** Blood behind the tympanic membrane suggests a traumatic basilar skull fracture. Otitis media could be a source of meningitis or brain abscess.

d. **Nasopharynx.** A fruity odor suggests diabetic ketoacidosis. A uriniferous smell implicates uremia. Fetor hepaticus points to hepatic encephalopathy. A burnt almond odor is found with cyanide toxicity. A garlic scent may be seen in arsenic poisoning.

e. **Neck.** Resistance to passive flexion of the neck without resistance to other neck movements is evidence for meningitis or subarachnoid bleed. Positive Kernig's and Brudzinski's signs indicate meningeal irritation. Thyroid enlargement points to hypothyroidism or hyperthyroidism. A bruit over an enlarged thyroid gland is pathognomonic of Graves' disease.

4. **Chest.** Findings of consolidation implicate pneumonia. A prolonged expiratory phase with rhonchi and wheezing suggests hypoxia and/or hypercapnia.

5. **Heart.** An irregularly irregular apical pulse (*atrial fibrillation*) points to embolization from a mural thrombus. A new murmur with fever and/or leukocytosis suggests endocarditis.

6. **Abdomen.** Splenomegaly, ascites, and stigmata of chronic liver disease suggest hepatic encephalopathy.

7. **Skin.** Jaundice, spider angiomata, and palmar erythema point to hepatic encephalopathy. Petechiae and ecchymoses may suggest a coagulation abnormality or thrombocytopenia. A maculohemorrhagic rash suggests meningococcal infection, staphylococcal endocarditis, or other infection. In carbon monoxide poisoning, the skin is usually cherry–red. Needle marks on extremities indicate possible drug abuse.

8. **Neurologic exam.** A thorough neurologic exam, including mental status evaluation, is essential. To avoid missing the locked-in syndrome, all patients should be asked to open the eyes and look up and down. Focal findings suggest an intracranial process. Hyperreflexia may be seen with upper motor neuron lesions or thyrotoxicosis. Clonus is absent with thyrotoxicosis and present in upper motor neuron lesions. Absent or sluggish reflexes are seen in hypothyroidism and hypothermia. The relaxation phase of the

reflex is delayed in hypothyroidism and increased in thyrotoxicosis. An extensor plantar reflex can be present in coma from any cause. The Glasgow Coma Scale is helpful in evaluating and following the comatose patient (see Appendix, Table A–3, p 619). Testing the oculocephalic reflex is also beneficial: Hold the eyes open and turn the patient's head quickly to one side. The eyes should move toward the midline as if staring at a fixed point (*positive* or *intact doll's eyes*). Movement of the eyes in the direction the head is turned (*absent doll's eyes*) suggests a brain stem lesion, bilateral labyrinth dysfunction, or drugs such as sedatives or anticonvulsants. Doll's eyes are not present in normal, alert persons.

B. Laboratory data

1. **Complete blood count with differential.** To evaluate for infection and anemia.
2. **Complete blood chemistry.** Includes electrolytes, glucose, blood urea nitrogen, creatinine, bilirubin, alkaline phosphatase, transaminases, calcium, and magnesium. Will rule out many organ-failure or metabolic causes. Serum glucose can be rapidly checked with a glucometer via a "finger stick."
3. **Arterial blood gases.** Along with serum bicarbonate, these measurements will uncover a metabolic or respiratory acid–base disturbance, which may point to the underlying cause. Also helpful to rule out hypoxemia.
4. **Osmolal gap.** This helpful diagnostic clue refers to the difference between measured and calculated (see Section II, Laboratory Diagnosis, p 370) serum osmolality. A gap greater than 10 implies the presence of a low molecular weight solute such as ethanol, methanol, isopropyl alcohol, ethylene glycol, ketones, or lactate.
5. **Platelet count and coagulation studies.** Especially if trauma is known or suspected, and the diagnosis of an intracranial hemorrhage is entertained.
6. **Thyroid-stimulating hormone (TSH) and thyroxine (T_4) levels.** To rule out suspected hypothyroidism or hyperthyroidism. Occasionally the T_4 will be normal with hyperthyroidism and only the triiodothyronine (T_3) will be elevated along with a low TSH.
7. **Urine and serum toxicology screening.** This is mandatory if the cause of the mental status alteration is uncertain or if there are medicolegal issues. Also important in the presence of an anion or osmolal gap.
8. **Blood and urine cultures.** If infection is suspected.
9. **Drug levels.** When appropriate, consider obtaining digoxin and phenytoin (Dilantin) levels.
10. **Miscellaneous labs.** Hyperammonemia is indicative of hepatic failure; however, not all patients with hepatic encephalopathy have an elevation. Creatine kinase levels should be assessed

serially for several days because of the high risk of rhabdomyolysis in the coma patient. When Addisonian crisis is suspected, an ACTH stimulation test should be performed and presumptive steroid therapy initiated.

C. Radiologic and other studies

1. **Chest x-ray.** Especially if an infectious or pulmonary source is suspected.
2. **CT scan of the head.** If there are any indications of a CNS etiology, especially in the presence of headache, vomiting, focal neurologic signs, or papilledema, or in the absence of any other etiology.
3. **Lumbar puncture** See Section III, Chapter 10, Lumbar Puncture, p 412. Should be performed in any patient with unexplained fever and mental status alteration.
4. **Electrocardiogram.** Look for myocardial infarction or atrial fibrillation. Myocardial infarction, especially in the elderly, may present with acute mental status changes.
5. **Electroencephalogram.** Diffuse theta and delta changes may be present with most metabolic causes. Often not diagnostic except for herpes encephalitis.

V. Plan

A. General. Although the therapy of altered mental status must be directed at the underlying cause, certain steps should be taken immediately: Ensure adequate airway, breathing, and circulation (the ABCs of basic life support). In the comatose patient with normal respiration, an oropharyngeal airway is usually adequate. However, intubation may be necessary to protect the airway. If trauma is known or suspected, stabilize the neck until radiographic clearance is obtained.

B. Metabolic causes. Treat the underlying defect. Refer to the specific abnormality in the index. Any patient in coma should receive thiamine 100 mg slow IV push. Empiric dextrose administration is controversial. Because the administration of D50 has been associated with a poorer outcome in patients with anoxic or ischemic coma, some experts recommend intravenous dextrose only if an immediate finger-stick glucose is low. If dextrose is given, it should be in conjunction with thiamine to avoid precipitation of acute Wernicke's syndrome.

C. Exogenous causes. Any suspicion of narcotic-induced somnolence can be safely treated with naloxone 0.4–0.8 mg IV push. A repeat dose may be necessary (up to 4–5 ampoules are commonly given in this situation). Consider gastric aspiration and lavage if toxic ingestion is suspected. If indicated, administer the appropriate antidote, such as ethanol for methanol or ethylene glycol ingestion, 100% FiO_2 for carbon monoxide poisoning, amyl nitrite and sodium nitrite followed by sodium thiosulfate for cyanide poisoning, and digitalis antibody for "digitalis delirium."

D. **Tumor.** Altered mental status in the presence of metastatic or primary CNS tumors can require emergent radiotherapy. Intracranial pressure should be acutely decreased with steroids, hyperventilation, and osmotic diuresis. Give dexamethasone 0.1–0.2 mg/kg IV bolus. The patient should be intubated to protect the airway and can be hyperventilated by increasing the ventilator rate to achieve a pCO_2 of 20–25 mm Hg. Osmotic diuresis with mannitol 50 g in a 20% solution over 20 minutes is also beneficial if there is associated cerebral edema.

E. **Infection.** Treat with appropriate antibiotics. Gram's stain may help direct initial antibiotic therapy prior to culture results.

F. **Cardiac syncope or low cardiac output.** Treat the underlying cardiac problem.

G. **Intracranial hemorrhage.** Consult neurosurgery immediately. Increased intracranial pressure should be emergently treated as outlined above.

REFERENCES

Adams RD, Victor M, Ropper AH: Coma and related disorders of consciousness. In: *Principles of Neurology.* 6th ed. McGraw-Hill;1997:344.

Adams RD, Victor M, Ropper AH: Delirium and other acute confusional states. In: *Principles of Neurology.* 6th ed. McGraw-Hill;1997:405.

Berger JR: Clinical approach to stupor and coma. In: *Neurology in Clinical Practice.* 3rd ed. Butterworth-Heinemann;2000:37.

Mendez Ashla MF: Delirium. In: *Neurology in Clinical Practice.* 3rd ed. Butterworth-Heinemann;2000:25.

14. CONSTIPATION

I. **Problem.** A 75-year-old bedridden woman from a nursing home was admitted with dehydration and a urinary tract infection. She has not had a bowel movement in 7 days.

II. **Immediate Questions**

A. **What are the patient's normal bowel habits?** Normal bowel habits vary from three stools per day to three stools per week.

B. **What medications is the patient taking?** Constipation is a side effect of many drugs. A careful medication history including use of vitamins and herbal products is necessary.

C. **Is the abdomen distended, tender, or tense?** Is the patient passing flatus or vomiting? Mechanical obstruction from sigmoid volvulus, intussusception, and hernia can lead to constipation. Mechanical obstruction often has other symptoms. Flatus signifies an intact, functioning gastrointestinal tract. Obstipation can result in tremendous abdominal distension.

D. **Does the patient have a history of hemorrhoids or rectal bleeding?** Rectal lesions, including hemorrhoids, proctitis, and fissures, may induce constipation. The patient suppresses bowel movements to avoid discomfort.

E. **Has the patient undergone any recent radiographic or surgical procedures?** Barium from radiologic studies can cause constipation. Many postoperative patients will have an ileus resulting in constipation.

F. **What is the patient's fluid status?** Decrease in fluid intake or increase of diuretic use, especially in the elderly patient, can cause constipation.

III. Differential Diagnosis

A. Systemic disorders

1. **Drugs.** Constipation is a side effect of many medications, including analgesics (inhibitors of prostaglandin synthesis, opiates); anticholinergics (antihistamines, antiparkinsonism agents, phenothiazines, tricyclic antidepressants); antacids containing aluminum hydroxide or calcium carbonate; barium sulfate; clonidine; diuretics (non-potassium sparing); calcium channel blockers (especially verapamil); ganglionic blockers; iron preparations; polystyrene sodium sulfonate, and $5HT_3$ receptor antagonists.
2. **Endocrine disorders.** Hypothyroidism, diabetes mellitus, and hyperparathyroidism are associated with constipation secondary to metabolic changes.
3. **Metabolic disorders.** Hypercalcemia, hypokalemia, and hypomagnesemia.
4. **Volume status.** Dehydrated patients, especially the elderly, can become constipated.

B. Gastrointestinal disorders

1. **Tumors.** Benign or malignant tumors can lead to constipation through obstruction by mass effect. This is of greater concern in the elderly.
2. **Inflammatory lesions.** With development of pain, the patient suppresses the urge to defecate, resulting in constipation. Common inflammatory disorders include diverticulitis, proctitis, hemorrhoids, fistula-in-ano, and inflammatory bowel diseases (IBD), in particular Crohn's disease. Diarrhea is a much more common symptom with IBD.
3. **Mechanical obstruction.** Constipation can be secondary to physical blockage from adhesions, incarcerated hernias, volvulus, ischemic strictures, or intussusception.

C. Neurologic conditions

1. **Spinal or pelvic trauma.** Results in colonic dysmotility or anal sphincter dysfunction.

2. **Autonomic neuropathy.** Results in colonic dysmotility and can even cause pseudo-obstruction.
3. **Cerebral vascular accident.** Constipation may develop via an associated decrease in activity level.

IV. Database

A. Physical examination key points

1. **Vital signs.** Fever suggests an inflammatory source such as diverticulitis. Orthostasis suggests dehydration.
2. **Abdomen.** Distension may result from obstruction. Evidence of prior surgery suggests adhesions. Listen for bowel sounds and quality to assess for ileus or obstruction. Absence of bowel sounds is consistent with any cause of complete obstruction. On palpation, assess for tenderness or rebound. Rebound suggests peritoneal inflammation. Feel for stool-filled colon.
3. **Rectum.** Rule out external lesions (hemorrhoids or fissures) as the cause. This will require anoscopy. Be sure the anal sphincter is not stenotic. Check the quality of sphincter tone. Absence of sphincter tone suggests a spinal cord lesion. Presence of blood suggests an inflammatory cause or a tumor.
4. **Neurologic exam.** Look for evidence of prior cerebrovascular accident or spinal injury, such as decreased motor function or asymmetric reflexes. A delay in the relaxation phase of the reflexes suggests hypothyroidism.

B. Laboratory data

1. **Electrolytes and calcium.** Check calcium level to rule out hypercalcemia. Hypokalemia or uremia can cause constipation.
2. **Complete blood count.** Elevated white blood cell count may indicate an inflammatory disorder. A low hemoglobin accompanies blood loss and can result from a variety of causes, such as tumors, diverticulitis, or IBD.
3. **Sedimentation rate or C-reactive protein (CRP).** With active inflammation, the sedimentation rate or CRP is elevated, but an elevated sed rate or CRP is not specific.
4. **Stool for occult blood.** Inflammatory disorders and tumors can result in blood loss.
5. **Thyroid function studies.** If history and physical examination are consistent with hypothyroidism, thyroid function studies (TSH, T_4) should be obtained.

C. Radiologic and other studies

1. **Acute abdominal series.** If acute obstruction is considered. This will assess the area of obstruction, the degree of intestinal distension, and the amount of stool in the colon.
2. **Proctosigmoidoscopy.** To further assess the colon for the presence of obstructing or inflammatory lesions.

3. **Barium enema.** This will demonstrate partial obstruction, or mass lesion, diverticulosis, or ischemic strictures.
4. **Colonoscopy.** The procedure of choice if colon carcinoma or colonic polyps are suspected.
5. **CT scan of abdomen.** To further evaluate for partial obstruction, inflammation, and lesions extrinsic to the colon.

V. Plan. Once the etiology is demonstrated, the underlying cause should be corrected. Medicines inducing constipation should be discontinued whenever possible. Electrolyte abnormalities should be corrected or obstruction relieved.

A. Prevention. Patients taking narcotics should receive stool softeners and bowel stimulants. Bedridden patients should also be given stool softeners. Place patients on high-fiber diets; encourage activity and adequate fluid intake.

B. Laxatives and enemas. There are several modalities from which to choose, depending on preference and etiology (Table 1–6). Use bulk laxatives (psyllium) and high-fiber diets for control and prevention of constipation. Surfactants or wetting agents, osmotic laxatives, and colonic stimulants for rapid action can also be used to relieve constipation. Suppositories or enemas, such as gentle tap-water or oil retention enemas, and glycerin suppositories are useful for rapid action.

TABLE I–6. LAXATIVES.

Type	Name	Dosage
Bulk—daily use	Effer-syllium	1 teaspoon (6–7 g) in fluid 1 or 2 times daily
	Metamucil	1 teaspoon (6–7 g) in fluid 1 or 2 times daily
Softeners/wetting agents—daily use	Docusate sodium (Colace)	50–200 mg 1 or 2 times daily Available: Capsules 50–100 mg Solution 10 mg/mL Syrup 25 mg/mL
	Docusate calcium (Surfak)	240 mg 1 or 2 times daily
	Lactulose (Chronuluc)	15–30 mL 1 or 2 times daily
	Mineral oil	14–45 mL; one-time dose
Stimulants—prn	Bisacodyl (Dulcolax	Oral 5–15 mg, 5-mg tablets Rectal 10 mg, 10-mg suppository
	Senna (Senokot)	1 tablet 1 or 2 times daily
	Glycerine suppository	3 g; 1 rectally
Osmotic—prn	Milk of Magnesia	15–30 mL 1 or 2 times daily
	Magnesium citrate	200 mL; one-time dose
Enema—prn	Fleet enema	120 mL rectally
	Oil retention enema	

C. **Disimpaction.** Digital disimpaction is occasionally required when hard stool will not pass through the rectum. This is more common in the elderly. After disimpaction, the patient should receive laxatives or preferably enemas to relieve the constipation. Use stool softeners or bulk laxatives to prevent recurrence.

D. **Other.** If obstructing or inflammatory lesions are demonstrated, they should be treated with surgery, anti-inflammatory medicines, or antibiotics.

REFERENCES

Camilleri M, Thompson WG, Fleshman JW et al: Clinical management of intractable constipation. Ann Intern Med 1994;121:520.

Floch MH, Wald A: Clinical evaluation and treatment of constipation. Gastroenterologist 1994;2:50.

Harari D, Gurwitz JH, Minaker KL: Constipation in the elderly. J Am Geriatr Soc 1993;41:1130.

Lange RL, DiPiro JT: Diarrhea and constipation. In: DiPiro JT, Talbert RL, Hayes PE et al, eds. *Pharmacotherapy: A Pathophysiologic Approach.* 2nd ed. Appleton & Lange;1993:566.

Lennard-Jones JE: Constipation. In: Feldman M, Scharschmidt BF, Sleisenger MH, eds. *Gastrointestinal and Liver Diseases: Pathophysiology/Diagnosis/Management.* 6th ed. Saunders;1998:174.

Wald A: Constipation in elderly patients. Drugs Aging 1993;3:220.

Wong P: How to deal with chronic constipation. Postgrad Med 1999;106:6.

15. COUGH

I. **Problem.** A nurse notifies you that one of your patients is unable to sleep because of a persistent cough.

II. **Immediate Questions**

A. **Is the cough acute or chronic?** Acute onset of cough most often results from infections such as the common cold, but can result from urgent conditions such as acute bronchospasm (see Section I, Chapter 63, Wheezing, p 341), pulmonary embolus (see Section I, Chapter 11, Chest Pain, p 57), aspiration (see Section I, Chapter 7, Aspiration, p 36), or decompensated congestive heart failure. A chronic cough is unlikely to represent a condition that is an immediate danger to the patient.

B. **Is the cough productive of sputum?** If so, what does the sputum look like? A productive cough implies an inflammatory condition such as infection. Blood in the sputum leads to consideration of several other causes. (See Section I, Chapter 30, Hemoptysis, p 170).

C. **Is the patient tachypneic or dyspneic?** Either of these suggests a significant underlying respiratory disease such as pulmonary embolus or pneumonia.

D. **Is the patient on an angiotensin-converting enzyme (ACE) inhibitor?** Cough is a side effect in 1–19% of patients on ACE inhibitors. The cough is nonproductive and persistent. It can begin 3–12 months after therapy initiation and remits 1–7 days after the drug is discontinued. There is a female predominance.

III. Differential Diagnosis. Cough reflex receptors are present throughout the respiratory tract and ear. Stimulation of these receptors can come from an array of sources.

A. Ear. Impacted cerumen, foreign body, or hair in the ear can produce cough.

B. Oropharynx/nasopharynx. Postnasal drip from allergic and nonallergic rhinitis or sinusitis is a common cause of cough. The common cold is a very frequent cause of cough.

C. Larynx. Acute viral laryngitis can produce cough.

D. Tracheobronchial tree. Any process irritating the mucosal receptors or preventing clearance of secretions can result in cough.

1. **Bronchospasm.** Asthma is a frequent cause of nonproductive cough, especially nocturnal cough. Wheezing may be absent.
2. **Bronchitis.** Both acute and chronic bronchitis can cause irritation of mucosal receptors and result in cough.
3. **Pneumonia.** Viral, bacterial, tuberculous, and fungal causes all should be considered, especially with any immunocompromised condition such as AIDS, immunosuppressive therapy, or lymphoproliferative or hematologic malignancy.
4. **Gastroesophageal reflux.** Aspiration of oropharyngeal and gastric contents can produce cough. Symptoms typically worsen at night or during meals.
5. **Inhaled irritants.** The most common cause of a chronic cough is tobacco smoke.
6. **Bronchogenic carcinoma.** Produces mechanical irritation of mucosal receptors. Chronic cough is common with bronchogenic carcinoma at some point in the illness.

E. Others. There are many other causes of cough; a few are listed here.

1. **Congestive heart failure.** A nocturnal cough may be the only manifestation of early congestive heart failure.
2. **Interstitial lung disease.** Includes interstitial fibrosis and granulomatous disease such as tuberculosis and sarcoidosis.
3. **Thoracic aneurysm.** Produces bronchial or tracheal compression.

IV. Database

A. Physical examination key points

1. **Vital signs.** Fever occurs with infection and pulmonary infarction. Tachypnea and use of accessory respiratory muscles suggest significant underlying pulmonary disease.
2. **Ears.** Examine for impacted cerumen, foreign body, or hair in the external auditory canal.

3. **Mouth.** Examine posterior pharynx for evidence of sinusitis or rhinitis (postnasal drip or cobblestoning resulting from lymphoid hyperplasia). Look for evidence of head and neck cancer.
4. **Sinuses.** Check for tenderness or opacification.
5. **Lungs**
   a. **Stridor.** This is a manifestation of upper airway obstruction resulting from laryngeal edema or epiglottitis.
   b. **Rhonchi.** Occur with bronchitis and inhalation injuries.
   c. **Signs of consolidation.** Peripheral bronchial breath sounds, egophony, and increased tactile fremitus occur with pneumonia.
   d. **Crackles.** Occur in congestive heart failure, pneumonia, and interstitial lung disease.
   e. **Wheezing.** Occurs in asthma. If localized, may signify a foreign body or obstructing neoplasm.
6. **Heart.** Jugular venous distension, laterally displaced point of maximal impulse, and left third heart sound (S_3) gallop indicate congestive heart failure.
7. **Lymph nodes.** Lymphadenopathy suggests metastatic carcinoma, a lymphoproliferative disorder, or a granulomatous disease such as sarcoidosis or tuberculosis.
8. **Extremities.** Clubbing occurs in patients with bronchiectasis, bronchogenic carcinoma, or idiopathic pulmonary fibrosis.

B. Laboratory data

1. **Hemogram.** Leukocytosis with left shift occurs with infectious diseases. Thrombocytosis may result from underlying malignancy.
2. **Arterial blood gases.** Important to evaluate in patients who appear dyspneic or cyanotic.

C. Radiologic and other studies

1. **Chest x-ray.** Look for congestive heart failure, neoplasm, pneumonia, interstitial lung disease, hilar adenopathy, and thoracic aortic aneurysm.
2. **Ventilation/perfusion ($\dot{V}/\dot{Q}$) scan.** Should be obtained if there is a high suspicion of pulmonary embolism.
3. **Sputum.** Examine for color, viscosity, odor, and amount. Perform Gram's stain.
4. **Purified protein derivative (PPD) skin test.** Should be performed if tuberculosis is considered.
5. **Pulmonary function tests.** A restrictive pattern occurs in interstitial lung disease. A *restrictive pattern* is a decrease in all lung volumes: forced expiratory volume at 1 second (FEV_1), forced vital capacity (FVC), total lung capacity (TLC), and other lung volumes. The FEV_1/FVC ratio is maintained near normal or may be high. A *reversible obstructive defect* (a decrease in the FEV_1 and FEV_1/FVC ratio) would suggest underlying emphysema or asthma. Bronchial provocation with methacholine may be necessary to di-

agnose occult asthma if baseline pulmonary function tests are normal.

6. **Bronchoscopy.** This is of value only if there is an abnormality on CXR, or a localized wheeze.

V. **Plan.** The treatment of cough is dependent on identifying the etiology, and then directing treatment toward that cause. Symptomatic cough suppression will often help the patient rest at night.

A. **Infectious conditions.** See Section VII for drug dosages.

1. **Community-acquired pneumonia.** Hospitalized patients should receive a third-generation fluoroquinolone such as levofloxacin (Levaquin) alone or an extended-spectrum cephalosporin (most commonly ceftriaxone or cefotaxime) in combination with a macrolide such as azithromycin (Zithromax). Severely ill hospitalized patients (those requiring intensive care unit admission) should receive a third-generation fluoroquinolone such as levofloxacin (Levaquin) or a macrolide such as azithromycin (Zithromax) in combination with ampicillin/sulbactam, piperacillin/tazobactam, ceftriaxone, or cefotaxime.
2. **Acute bronchitis.** Most often, acute bronchitis has a viral etiology; however, when mycoplasma or bacteria are suspected, trimethoprim-sulfamethoxazole, doxycycline, ampicillin, or a macrolide antibiotic can be given.
3. **Chronic bronchitis.** Most often occurs in smokers; cough resolves with cessation of smoking.

B. **Rhinitis/sinusitis.** In these instances, cough is best managed by treatment with an antihistamine and decongestant. Nasal ipratropium bromide may also have efficacy. Antibiotics are indicated if bacterial sinusitis is suspected.

C. **Asthma.** Inhaled bronchodilators such as albuterol represent the best treatment for those whose cough is due to asthma. Oral bronchodilators may be necessary for patients in whom inhalation therapy provokes cough; however, a trial with a spacer is warranted prior to changing to oral therapy. Spacers have been useful in eliminating the cough provoked by inhalation therapy in some patients. Initially, steroids (oral or inhaled) may be required to eliminate the cough.

D. **Gastroesophageal reflux.** These patients should have the head of their beds elevated and should not eat before retiring for bed. Antacids, histamine H_2 antagonists such as cimetidine (Tagamet), or proton pump blockers such as omeprazole (Prilosec) may also be required.

E. **General measures.** In patients with a nonproductive cough in whom infection is not a concern, cough suppression can provide much-needed symptomatic relief.

1. **Cough suppression**

a. Codeine phosphate is the most effective cough suppressant. The usual dose is 10–30 mg Q 4–6 hr (maximum dose is 120 mg/day). Other narcotics such as oxycodone may be likewise effective in those patients who are codeine intolerant.
b. Dextromethorphan, a codeine derivative, acts centrally and is the best nonnarcotic for cough suppression. The dose is 10–30 mg Q 4–8 hr or 60 mg Q 12 hours for sustained-action liquid (maximum dose 120 mg/day).
c. Diphenhydramine HCl acts centrally to suppress cough; the dose is 25 mg Q 4–6 hr (maximum 150 mg/day).

2. **Expectorants.** Have been shown to be of no value and should not be used.

REFERENCES

Bartlett JG, Dowell SF, Mandell LA et al: Practice guidelines for the management of community-acquired pneumonia in adults. Clin Infect Dis 2000;31:347.

Bryant BG, Lombardi TP: Cold, cough, and allergy products. In: Covington TR, Lawson LC, Young LL et al, eds. *The Handbook of Non-Prescription Drugs.* 10th ed. American Pharmaceutical Association;1993:89.

Irwin RS, Madison JM: The diagnosis and treatment of cough. N Engl J Med 2000;343:1715.

Irwin RS, Corrao WM, Pratter MR: Chronic persistent cough in the adult: Spectrum and frequency of causes and successful outcome of specific therapy. Am Rev Respir Dis 1981;123:413.

Poe RH, Harder RV, Israel RH et al: Chronic persistent cough: Experience in diagnosis and outcome using an anatomic diagnostic protocol. Chest 1989;95:723.

16. DELIRIUM TREMENS (DTS): MAJOR ALCOHOL WITHDRAWAL

I. **Problem.** A 55-year-old intoxicated man is admitted with abdominal pain and an elevated amylase. On the third hospital day, he is found talking incoherently and is markedly diaphoretic and very tremulous.

II. **Immediate Questions**

A. **What are the patient's vital signs?** Hypertension, tachycardia, and fever may represent signs of autonomic overactivity, common in DTs and minor alcohol withdrawal. A fever may also point to an infection as the cause of the delirium.

B. **What is the patient's mental status?** Altered levels of consciousness and impaired cognitive function define delirium. Hallucinations and confusion are common in major alcohol withdrawal. These, coupled with autonomic hyperactivity, are typical of DTs. Delirium tremens can also present as unresponsiveness. Most (80%) of the hallucinations occur after ethanol cessation and occur 12–24 hours after the last drink. The hallucinations may be visual (most common), auditory, olfactory, or tactile.

C. What is the patient's airway status? With an altered level of consciousness there is an increased risk of aspiration.

D. What medications or illicit drugs is the patient taking? Medications may cause disorientation. Likely offenders include narcotics (morphine, codeine, meperidine), phencyclidine (PCP), cocaine, barbiturates, amphetamines, atropine, scopolamine, H_2 blockers (cimetidine, ranitidine, famotidine, nizatidine) or aspirin; and especially in the elderly, digitalis, sedatives (benzodiazepines), tricyclic antidepressants, and steroids. Individuals who abuse one substance are more likely to abuse others. Ask specifically regarding the use of narcotics, sedatives, barbiturates, and atropine-like substances.

E. Is there a history of alcohol abuse? This is central to the diagnosis. Historical information may need to be obtained from family or friends because of the delirium.

F. Is there a previous history of DTs? Many times there is a past history of DTs. The absence of such a history does not exclude DTs.

G. Is there a history of alcohol withdrawal seizures? One-third of patients with a history of alcohol withdrawal seizures develop DTs, whereas only 5% of patients with minor alcohol withdrawal develop DTs. The seizures are tonic-clonic and occur 12–24 hours after ethanol cessation. Usually there is a single seizure, but there can be multiple seizures in a short period of time.

H. When was the patient's last drink? The length of time since the last drink will assist in the diagnosis of DTs. Minor alcohol withdrawal usually begins 6–8 hours after cessation of drinking, peaks at about 24 hours, and usually resolves within 48 hours. The onset of DTs is between days 2 and 10 after ethanol cessation.

III. Differential Diagnosis. DTs is a manifestation of diffuse cerebral dysfunction. Focal neurologic deficits point to a structural abnormality (stroke or brain tumor). The differential diagnosis of delirium is more extensive than given here and includes any cause of diffuse cerebral dysfunction. (See Section I, Chapter 13, Coma, Acute Mental Status Changes, p 72). Patients presenting with DTs may have a wide range of concomitant problems, any of which could cause delirium.

A. Withdrawal syndromes

1. **Minor alcohol withdrawal.** A less severe form of alcohol withdrawal, which occurs between 8 and 48 hours after the last drink. Disorientation is usually mild. Tachycardia, diaphoresis, insomnia, irritability, and tremor are often present. Seizures and hallucinations may occur.
2. **Barbiturate withdrawal.** Indistinguishable from DTs clinically.
3. **Opioid withdrawal.** Occurs up to 48 hours after cessation of agent (most rapid with heroin). Symptoms include restlessness, rhinorrhea, lacrimation, nausea, diarrhea, and hypertension.

B. **Metabolic abnormalities.** Multiple metabolic abnormalities can cause altered levels of consciousness and impaired cognitive function similar to DTs (see Section I, Chapter 13, Coma, Acute Mental Status Changes, p 72).

   1. **Wernicke's encephalopathy.** Results from nutritional deficiency of thiamine. Characterized by a triad of symptoms: (1) mental status changes (confusion to coma), (2) ataxia, and (3) ophthalmoplegia (most commonly lateral-gaze nystagmus from bilateral lateral rectus palsies).

C. **Endocrine abnormalities**

   1. **Hypoglycemia.** See Section I, Chapter 37, Hypoglycemia, p 202. Either from an insulin-secreting tumor or from intentional or accidental insulin overdose.
   2. **Hyperglycemia.** See Section I, Chapter 32, Hyperglycemia, p 180. Extreme hyperglycemia, especially in the elderly, can result in delirium.
   3. **Hyperthyroidism.** The signs/symptoms of hyperthyroidism may mimic alcohol withdrawal syndrome; there may be mental status changes, diaphoresis, tachycardia, tremor, and agitation. There is often a history of weight loss, hot weather intolerance, and hyperdefecation. The thyroid gland is often enlarged. The T_3 or T_4 will be elevated and the TSH level suppressed. The signs and symptoms of hyperthyroidism are usually more subacute or chronic; however, thyroid storm is manifested by thermoderegulation (hyperthermia) and mental status changes. There is usually an identifiable precipitating event such as an operation or infection).

D. **Hypertensive encephalopathy.** Encephalopathy induced by poorly controlled hypertension. Headache is common. Exudates and hemorrhages are present on funduscopic examination. Papilledema may be present.

E. **Central nervous system (CNS) infections.** In anyone with disorientation, consider CNS infection, including meningitis, brain abscess, and encephalitis. With bacterial causes, fever and leukocytosis with an increase in banded neutrophils are often present, as well as other signs (meningismus or papilledema). If there are focal findings or papilledema, a CT scan should be performed initially.

F. **Intracranial hemorrhage.** Symptoms and level of consciousness will vary depending on the location and size of the hemorrhage.

G. **Psychiatric disturbances**

   1. **ICU psychosis.** Secondary to unfamiliar setting; often seen in elderly patients. May be secondary to or aggravated by medications such as lidocaine and digoxin.
   2. **"Sundowning."** Nighttime agitation and confusion are common problems, especially in the elderly. The agitation and confusion resolve in the morning.

H. **Sepsis.** Sepsis can cause mental status changes. A fever and elevated white blood cell count with an increase in banded neutrophils is common. A source for sepsis is often evident, such as pyuria or an infiltrate on chest x-ray.

I. **Low cardiac output states.** From either ischemia or cardiomyopathy. Can cause confusion secondary to decreased cerebral perfusion and may cause agitation. Inquire about chest pain and congestive heart failure symptoms (orthopnea, paroxysmal nocturnal dyspnea, and dyspnea on exertion).

J. **Intoxications**

1. **Cocaine**
2. **Amphetamines**
3. **Anticholinergic toxicity**

IV. Database

A. Physical examination key points

1. **Vital signs.** Tachycardia, hypertension, and fever are common. Fever from DTs may be as high as 104°F (40°C). With severe hypertension and delirium, consider hypertensive encephalopathy. Fever may also be a manifestation of a localized infection or sepsis. Hypothermia could be associated with sepsis or could be the cause of the delirium. Carpal spasm with inflation of the blood pressure cuff between the diastolic and systolic blood pressure for 3 minutes (*Trousseau's sign*) is seen with hypocalcemia.
2. **Eyes.** Nystagmus suggests Wernicke's encephalopathy. Lid lag or proptosis suggests hyperthyroidism. Papilledema may be seen in meningitis or hypertensive encephalopathy, in CNS hemorrhage, or with a space-occupying lesion.
3. **Nose.** Look for rhinophyma (hypertrophy and follicular dilation).
4. **Neck.** Thyromegaly suggests hyperthyroidism as a cause of the delirium. Jugular venous distension points toward congestive heart failure.
5. **Chest.** Signs of congestive heart failure and other causes of pulmonary edema and hypoxia should be sought.
6. **Abdomen.** Check for bladder distension, a common cause of agitation in the elderly.
7. **Skin.** Profuse sweating is typical of DTs. Telangiectasias and gynecomastia are associated with chronic ethanol use and chronic liver disease.
8. **Neurologic exam.** Mental status changes define delirium. Hallucinations, confusion, and disorientation are typical. Tremulousness is a common sign of alcohol withdrawal. Reflexes will be exaggerated but symmetrical. Hyperreflexia is also seen in hyperthyroidism. Twitching at the corner of the mouth with tapping over the facial nerve (*Chvostek's sign*) is seen in hypocalcemia. Any

focal findings on motor, sensory, deep tendon, or cranial nerve examination point to a structural abnormality.

B. **Laboratory data.** Multiple electrolyte abnormalities may cause delirium or may be associated with heavy ethanol use.
   1. **Sodium.** Hyponatremia could be the etiology of the delirium.
   2. **Glucose.** Eliminate hypoglycemia or hyperglycemia as a cause of delirium; both may be associated with heavy ethanol ingestion.
   3. **Calcium.** May reveal hypocalcemia or hypercalcemia as the cause.
   4. **Potassium.** Hypokalemia often complicates heavy ethanol ingestion. Hyperkalemia may also cause delirium.
   5. **Blood urea nitrogen and creatinine.** May point to uremia/renal failure as the etiology of the delirium.
   6. **Liver function tests.** Transaminases (AST and ALT), total bilirubin, and alkaline phosphatase to rule out hepatic failure as a cause. Liver dysfunction is common with chronic alcohol use.
   7. **Arterial blood gases.** To eliminate hypoxemia as a cause.
   8. **Complete blood count with differential.** An elevated white blood cell count with an increase in banded neutrophils suggests a bacterial etiology. An elevated mean corpuscular volume may be from associated folate or vitamin B_{12} deficiency. Vitamin B_{12} deficiency can cause mental status changes. Anemia from a variety of causes is commonly seen in heavy ethanol use.
   9. **Thyroid function tests.** Thyroid-stimulating hormone (TSH) is suppressed and thyroxine is usually elevated with hyperthyroidism. Hypothyroidism may cause changes in mental status and result in an elevated TSH and a decrease in the thyroxine.
   10. **Phosphorus.** Hypophosphatemia is associated with heavy ethanol use and results from poor nutritional intake, diarrhea, vomiting, or refeeding after prolonged starvation.
   11. **Magnesium.** Hypomagnesemia is commonly seen with heavy ethanol use. Hypomagnesemia may result from poor intake, diarrhea, renal losses, and excessive sweating.

C. **Radiologic and other studies**
   1. **Chest x-ray.** May reveal cardiomegaly, pulmonary edema, or pneumonia.
   2. **Electrocardiogram.** To rule out myocardial ischemia as an etiology of delirium. Also tachyarrhythmias are associated with alcohol withdrawal (major or minor).
   3. **CT scan of head.** May be indicated if there are focal findings on examination, or seizures associated with DTs. Alcohol withdrawal seizures should occur before the onset of DTs.
   4. **Lumbar puncture.** Indicated in any patient with mental status changes and fever. It may be difficult to rule out meningitis in a patient with DTs without performing a lumbar puncture.

5. **Electroencephalogram.** May help diagnose encephalitis. Usually increased nonfocal activity with DTs. Rarely is an electroencephalogram needed.

V. Plan

A. Strategies. There are four treatment strategies for alcohol withdrawal (minor or moderate):

1. **Supportive care.** A calm environment with frequent assessment and nursing care is all that is required for many patients with *mild* alcohol withdrawal. Individuals with a history of alcohol withdrawal seizures or DTs, or a coexisting acute illness, will require medical management in addition to supportive care.
2. **Front-load dosing.** A long-acting benzodiazepine is given every 1–2 hours until symptoms abate; for example, diazepam (Valium) 10–20 mg PO every 1–2 hours (or 5 mg IV every 5 minutes) until symptoms subside; or lorazepam (Ativan) 2 mg IV or IM every 2 hours can be used. Symptoms are alleviated faster and the total dose of benzodiazepines required is less than the conventional scheduled dosing method.
3. **Symptom-triggered dosing.** The benzodiazepines are administered according to the patient's symptoms. This method requires frequent assessment and has been shown to require a lower amount of benzodiazepine than scheduled dosing regimens; moreover, the duration of treatment is shorter. Initially diazepam (Valium) 20 mg PO or chlordiazepoxide (Librium) 50 mg PO is given; or lorazepam (Ativan) 2 mg IM initially with additional doses every 1–2 hours if assessment indicates a need for more medication.
4. **Scheduled dosing.** A fixed dose of a benzodiazepine is given on a regular schedule and tapered over several days, for example, diazepam (Valium) 5–20 mg every 4–6 hours for 1–3 days, decreasing the dose by ½ every day. An as-needed dose of 10–20 mg every 2–4 hours is made available. Chlordiazepoxide (Librium) 100 mg every 6 hours can be given for 1–3 days, decreasing the dose by ½ every day with an additional 25–50 mg every 2–4 hours as needed. Lorazepam (Ativan) or oxazepam (Serax) PO or IM should be considered with moderate to severe hepatic dysfunction.

B. Delirium tremens

1. **ICU setting**
2. **Intravenous fluids.** May require 3–6 L per day; use D5 NS.
3. **Correction of electrolyte disorders**
   a. **Hypokalemia.** Replacement with potassium supplements either PO or IV. A total replacement dose of 100 mEq of potassium is required to raise a potassium of 3.0 mEq/L to 4.0 mEq/L. Intravenous replacement is generally 10–15 mEq per

hour. Oral replacement is 20–60 mEq per dose, and can be repeated in 2–4 hours.

b. **Hypophosphatemia.** IV replacement is reserved for severe, life-threatening hypophosphatemia (levels < 1.5 mg/dL). IV replacement is with 5–10 mmol over 4–6 hours. PO replacement can be with Neutra-Phos capsules (250 mg per capsule) or skim milk (1 quart contains 1 g of phosphorus, or about 30 mmol).

c. **Hypomagnesemia.** Replacement is generally either IV or IM. The oral route often causes diarrhea. Magnesium sulfate can be given 1 g IM in each hip or 1 g IV per hour for 4 hours. The magnesium level should be checked 1–2 hours after the fourth gram has been infused. This regimen may need to be repeated. Magnesium is mostly an intracellular cation. With extremely low levels of magnesium, often 10–15 g will be required.

4. **Thiamine replacement.** Thiamine 100 mg IV or IM should be given prior to the administration of any intravenous fluids containing glucose. Glucose can precipitate Wernicke's encephalopathy in a patient with marginal thiamine stores. Thiamine should be given for at least 3 days.
5. **Other vitamins.** Multivitamins and folate should be given daily either orally or intravenously.
6. **Restraints.** Are often needed to prevent injury.
7. **Benzodiazepines.** Diazepam (Valium) 5–10 mg intravenously every 5–10 minutes until sedated, or lorazepam (Ativan) 1–2 mg intravenously every 5–10 minutes. The dose of diazepam should not exceed 100 mg/hr or 250 mg over 8 hours.
8. **Other treatments.** Phenobarbital 100–200 mg IM or IV every 1–2 hours can be used if benzodiazepines cannot be used. Carbamazepine (800 mg/d, taper over 7 days) has been used for mild and moderate withdrawal as a single agent. Advantages are that it is nonaddictive and nonsedating, and metabolism is not affected by liver dysfunction.
9. **Adjunct therapy.** A beta-blocker, atenolol (Tenormin 50–100 mg/d) has been shown to be beneficial for mild to moderate withdrawal, in both outpatient and inpatient settings. Also, clonidine (Catapres) 0.1–0.2 mg PO bid can be used.
10. **Haloperidol (Haldol).** 2–10 mg PO, IV, or IM, can be used for hallucinations or for agitation not responding to benzodiazepines. Neuroleptics decrease the seizure threshold, however, and may precipitate alcohol withdrawal seizures. Butyrophenones are a better choice than phenothiazines.
11. **Antipyretics.** Acetaminophen 650–1000 mg or aspirin 650 mg and a cooling blanket may be required because of fever associated with DTs.

REFERENCES

Hall W, Zador D: The alcohol withdrawal syndrome. Lancet 1997;349:1897.

Kraus ML, Gottlieb LD, Horwitz RI et al: Randomized clinical trial of atenolol in patients with alcohol withdrawal. N Engl J Med 1985;313:905.

Mayo-Smith MF: Pharmacological management of alcohol withdrawal: A meta-analysis and evidence based practice guideline. JAMA 1997;278:144.

Olmedo R, Hoffman RS: Withdrawal syndromes. Emerg Med Clin North Am 2000;18:273.

Saitz R, Mayo-Smith MF, Roberts MS et al: Individualized treatment for alcohol withdrawal. JAMA 1994;272:519.

Schaffer A, Naranjo CA: Recommended drug treatment strategies for the alcoholic patient. Drugs 1998;56:571.

Shaw JM, Kolesar GS, Sellers EM et al: Development of optimal treatment tactics for alcohol withdrawal. I. Assessment and effectiveness of supportive care. J Clin Psychopharmacol 1981;1:382.

Turner RC, Lichstein PR, Peden JG et al: Alcohol withdrawal symptoms: A review of pathophysiology, clinical presentations, and treatment. J Gen Intern Med 1989;4:432.

Williams D, McBride AJ: The drug treatment of alcohol withdrawal symptoms: A systematic review. Alcohol Alcohol 1998;33:103.

17. DIARRHEA

I. **Problem.** A 50-year-old woman is admitted after having 36 hours of diarrhea.

II. **Immediate Questions**

A. **What are the patient's vital signs?** Hypotension suggests volume depletion or possible septic shock. Fever implies an infectious etiology. Diarrhea with associated hypotension or fever should be evaluated immediately.

B. **Is the diarrhea grossly bloody?** This usually is seen with ischemic bowel or infarction, invasive infections, neoplasms, or inflammatory bowel disease (IBD). Bloody diarrhea requires more active and immediate intervention.

C. **Is this an acute or chronic problem?** *Acute diarrhea* is usually a self-limited disease and can often be treated symptomatically. The most common cause of acute diarrhea in the outpatient setting is infection, and in the inpatient setting, drugs. *Chronic diarrhea* is defined as diarrhea that has been present 4–6 weeks or longer. Common causes include lactose intolerance, irritable bowel syndrome, IBD, postsurgical procedures, malabsorptive syndromes, drugs, and various infections. Some causes of chronic diarrhea can present with an acute exacerbation.

D. **Are there risk factors that suggest a specific cause?** Risk factors include drug-induced diarrhea, travel, homosexual relationships, abdominal surgery, vascular disease, and various endocrine disorders such as diabetes mellitus and Addison's disease.

E. **Is there associated abdominal pain?** Absence of pain makes inflammatory causes such as ischemic bowel disease or ulcerative colitis less likely.

F. **What is the volume of the stool? Does the patient have diarrhea (> 300 g stool per day) or just loose stools?** Large volumes suggest small bowel or right colon; small volumes suggest left colon.

G. **Has the patient participated in any recreational water activities?** Many outbreaks of gastroenteritis have been associated with recreational water activities (swimming pools, interactive water fountains at water parks, lakes, rivers, hot tubs). Offending agents include *Shigella sonnei* and *Cryptosporidium parvum.*

H. **Is there any reason to suspect laxative abuse (eg, a young woman with a history of bulimia)?** Testing the stool for laxatives may secure the diagnosis without an extensive workup.

I. **Does the diarrhea stop if the patient is not eating?** If the answer is yes, the etiology is likely an osmotic cause of diarrhea rather than a secretory cause, where the diarrhea will not vary with the oral intake.

III. Differential Diagnosis

A. Infection

1. **Viruses.** Viral syndromes usually resolve in a few days and can be treated symptomatically. Rotavirus and Norwalk virus are the most common viruses causing diarrhea.
2. **Bacteria.** *Shigella dysenteriae, Shigella sonnei, Salmonella typhimurium, Campylobacter jejuni, Yersinia* species, *Staphylococcus aureus, Vibrio cholerae, Vibrio parahaemolyticus, Escherichia coli, Bacillus cereus, Clostridium perfringens,* and *Clostridium difficile* all cause diarrhea by producing enterotoxins or by enteroinvasion. The spectrum of illness may range from asymptomatic to life threatening. *S aureus, B cereus,* and *C perfringens* are often associated with food poisoning. *C jejuni* and enterohemorrhagic *E coli* often cause a bloody diarrhea and may be associated with hemolytic-uremic syndrome in adults. *V cholerae* can cause severe life-threatening diarrhea, especially in patients with cirrhosis, and is associated with consumption of raw shellfish.
3. **Parasites.** *Giardia lamblia, Entamoeba histolytica,* and *Cryptosporidium. G lamblia* is often contracted by drinking contaminated water. *E histolytica* is seen in travelers to developing countries and in institutionalized patients. *Cryptosporidium* can cause a self-limited diarrhea in immunocompetent individuals working with livestock. *G lamblia, E histolytica,* and *Cryptosporidium* are common etiologic agents causing diarrhea in homosexual men. *Cryptosporidium* results in a severe, unremitting diarrhea in patients infected with human immunodeficiency virus (HIV).

B. Inflammatory diseases

1. **Ischemic bowel** secondary to thrombosis, embolism, or vasculitis such as polyarteritis nodosa or systemic lupus erythematosus can result in bloody or guaiac-positive diarrhea. Atrial fibrillation is a common source of embolism.
2. **Inflammatory bowel disease (IBD).** Ulcerative colitis (UC) begins in the rectum and spreads proximally in a continuous manner. Presenting complaints begin abruptly and usually include rectal bleeding and diarrhea. Crohn's disease presents with diarrhea; however, the onset of symptoms is more insidious than with UC, and the diarrhea is less often bloody.

C. Tumor

1. **Malignant carcinoid syndrome.** Flushing is also common.
2. **Colon carcinoma.** Bright red blood per rectum as well as occult blood loss or anemia is common.
3. **Medullary thyroid carcinoma**
4. **Lymphoma involving the bowel**
5. **Villous adenomas**
6. **Gastrinomas.** Usually a prior history of peptic ulcer disease or gastroesophageal reflux.

D. Endocrinopathies

1. **Hyperthyroidism.** Hyperdefecation (loose, frequent stools) rather than diarrhea. Diarrhea may be present with thyroid storm.
2. **Diabetes.** Associated with long-standing diabetes with neuropathy.
3. **Hypoparathyroidism**
4. **Addison's disease.** Nausea, vomiting, abdominal pain, weight loss, and lethargy along with diarrhea.

E. Drugs

1. **Laxatives.** Chronic laxative abuse causes chronic diarrhea.
2. **Antacids.** Magnesium-containing antacids can cause osmotic diarrhea.
3. **Lactulose.** Used to treat hepatic encephalopathy; should be titrated to two to three loose stools per day but can result in severe, life-threatening hypernatremia secondary to an osmotic diarrhea if not dosed properly.
4. **Cardiac agents.** Diarrhea is a common reason for discontinuation of quinidine. Digoxin may cause diarrhea.
5. **Colchicine.** In treatment of acute gout, diarrhea can occur with increasing doses.
6. **Antibiotics.** Antibiotics can produce diarrhea by altering gut flora. This leads to malabsorption or induction of *C difficile* overgrowth and toxin production, resulting in pseudomembranous colitis. Pseudomembranous colitis is most often secondary to antibiotics, especially broad-spectrum antibiotics such as clindamycin and the cephalosporins, and can occur as long as 4 months after antibiotic use.

7. **Antihypertensives.** Reserpine, guanethidine, methyldopa, guanabenz, and guanadrel all can cause diarrhea.
8. **Cholinergic agents.** Bethanechol, metoclopramide, and neostigmine all cause diarrhea.
9. **Metformin.** Many patients develop diarrhea, especially at higher doses.

F. **Abdominal surgery.** Can cause chronic diarrhea.
1. **Gastric surgery.** Vagotomy, resection, or bypass procedures.
2. **Cholecystectomy**
3. **Bowel resection**

G. **Malabsorption.** A common cause of chronic diarrhea that may result in deficiencies of fat-soluble vitamins A, D, E, and K; weight loss; and hypoalbuminemia.
1. **Chronic pancreatitis**
2. **Bowel resection**
3. **Bacterial overgrowth**
4. **Celiac or tropical sprue**
5. **Whipple's disease**
6. **Eosinophilic gastroenteritis**

H. **Lactose intolerance.** A common cause of chronic diarrhea resulting from lactase deficiency. Often associated with flatulence. Milk or milk products will exacerbate the diarrhea.

I. **Irritable bowel syndrome.** Intermittent diarrhea may alternate with constipation. Symptoms are aggravated by stress. Abdominal pain may be present. Physical examination and routine laboratory tests are normal.

J. **Fecal impaction.** Can present with diarrhea. Often occurs in older age group.

K. **Human immunodeficiency virus (HIV) infection.** Diarrhea is common in patients positive for HIV or with acquired immunodeficiency syndrome (AIDS). Parasitic infections mentioned in Section III.A.3. are common in homosexual men with or without HIV infection. *Isospora belli, Microsporidia,* and *Cyclospora* are three other parasites that can cause diarrhea in HIV patients. Other nonparasitic etiologies associated with HIV infection include *Salmonella typhimurium,* which often results in bacteremia; *Campylobacter jejuni, Mycobacterium avium-intracellulare,* and cytomegalovirus. Often the diarrhea is idiopathic and associated with fever and weight loss.

IV. Database

A. Physical examination key points

1. **General.** Cachexia suggests a chronic process such as carcinoma, AIDS, IBD, or malabsorption.
2. **Vital signs.** Hypotension or postural changes suggest sepsis or significant volume depletion. Tachycardia implies volume deple-

tion or infection, or could be secondary to pain. Tachypnea may indicate fever, anxiety, pain, or sepsis or may represent compensation for a metabolic acidosis from a variety of causes including sepsis and bowel infarction.

3. **HEENT.** Aphthous ulcers are associated with IBD. An enlarged thyroid suggests hyperthyroidism or medullary carcinoma.
4. **Abdomen.** Look for surgical scars. Distension may be from carbohydrate malabsorption. Absent bowel sounds suggest bowel infarction or associated peritoneal inflammation. Metastatic cancer can result in hepatomegaly.
5. **Rectum.** Rule out rectal carcinoma. Look for fissures suggesting UC. Fecal impaction can present with diarrhea.
6. **Musculoskeletal exam.** Arthritis is associated with IBD, Whipple's disease, and infection by *Yersinia enterocolitica.*
7. **Skin.** Hyperpigmentation can be seen with Addison's disease or celiac sprue. Erythema nodosum and pyoderma gangrenosum point to IBD. Dermatitis herpetiformis suggests celiac sprue, a rare cause of diarrhea.

B. Laboratory data

1. **Electrolytes.** With severe diarrhea, various electrolyte abnormalities can occur, including hypokalemia, metabolic acidosis, hypernatremia, and hyponatremia.
2. **Complete blood count with differential.** An elevated hematocrit suggests volume depletion. An anemia (see Section I, Chapter 5, Anemia, p 27) may be associated with IBD, carcinoma, or HIV infection. A microcytic anemia suggests chronic gastrointestinal blood loss or malabsorption of iron. Macrocytic anemia may be secondary to vitamin B_{12} deficiency after gastric surgery, or from malabsorption or folate deficiency.
3. **Sedimentation rate, C-reactive protein (CRP).** Expect to be increased in IBD, metastatic carcinoma, bowel ischemia, and systemic infections.
4. **Prothrombin time and partial thromboplastin time.** An elevated PT and PTT could be secondary to vitamin K deficiency from malabsorption or associated liver disease.
5. **Albumin.** Expect a low albumin in diarrhea secondary to malabsorption, IBD, and metastatic carcinoma.
6. **Calcium.** To rule out hypoparathyroidism as a cause. Hypocalcemia associated with vitamin D deficiency secondary to steatorrhea may also be seen.
7. **Endocrine tests.** Helpful as clinically indicated; include thyroid tests (thyroxine, thyroid-stimulating hormone), parathyroid hormone, Cortrosyn stimulation test, and gastrin.
8. **24- to 72-hour collection of stool for fecal fat.** Essential for workup of malabsorption. The patient should be on a 100-g fat diet before and during the stool collection.

9. **Stool for occult blood.** Follow with serial exams to increase sensitivity. Occult blood suggests UC, neoplasm, ischemic bowel, or various infections such as *C jejuni.*
10. **Stool for leukocytes.** Presence of fecal leukocytes suggests an inflammatory etiology such as infection, ischemia, or IBD. In the absence of fecal leukocytes, viruses, enterotoxic food poisoning, or parasites can be suspected, as can drugs, causes of malabsorption or endocrinopathies, cancer, irritable bowel, lactose intolerance, and abdominal surgery.
11. **Stool cultures.** Indicated for clinical dysentery (fever, abdominal cramps, fecal leukocytes), inflammatory causes, prolonged diarrhea (longer than 7–14 days), symptoms suggestive of acute proctitis, or a prolonged illness. Contact lab regarding special procedures to identify *Yersinia, Vibrio,* or *E coli* O157:H7 if clinically indicated.
12. **Stool for ova and parasites (O&P)**
    a. Parasitic infections often require a "fresh" specimen within several hours of collection.
    b. Amebic dysentery diagnosed with presence of trophozoites. Cysts suggest the carrier state in the absence of trophozoites. Serology may help in the diagnosis.
    c. Identification of *Giardia* cysts is diagnostic of active infection. A small bowel aspirate may be required to recover *Giardia.*
13. ***Clostridium difficile* toxin.** If antibiotics have been given in the last 4 months (usually 4–14 days). The presence of *C difficile* without the toxin should not cause diarrhea. Toxin-negative pseudomembranous colitis must also be considered.

C. Radiologic and other studies

1. **Proctosigmoidoscopy.** Indicated if pseudomembranous colitis is a possible etiology, if the patient remains ill with negative stool cultures, or if diarrhea is bloody. An unprepped study is useful in determining the presence of mucosal inflammation suggesting IBD, obtaining cultures and biopsies, and examining for masses or stool impaction. Enemas or suppositories may obscure the presence of disease.
2. **Colonoscopy.** Indicated if bleeding is seen coming from the proximal colon when examined by sigmoidoscopy.
3. **Barium enema.** May reveal carcinoma or IBD.
4. **Upper GI series with small bowel follow-through.** May suggest Crohn's disease, celiac sprue, Whipple's disease, or lymphoma.
5. **D-Xylose test.** Abnormal in diseases involving the small bowel mucosa such as Crohn's disease, celiac sprue, Whipple's disease, and lymphoma.

V. Plan. Symptomatic treatment with fluids, electrolytes, and antidiarrheal agents is usually all that is required for acute diarrhea. The initial use of antibiotic therapy should be avoided and implemented only in specific situations and guided by stool culture results. Many cases of diarrhea resolve by addressing the underlying cause (eg, discontinuation of a drug).

A. Fluid replacement. Essential in the early treatment.
   1. **Oral.** Helpful if given as hypoosmolar solution and with glucose to facilitate uptake of sodium and water.
   2. **Intravenous.** Necessary if the patient is markedly volume-depleted or has accompanying nausea and vomiting. Patient may need potassium replacement.

B. Diet. Place the patient on a lactose-free diet to prevent the development of diarrhea secondary to lactase deficiency, which may be transient as a result of acute gastroenteritis. Diarrhea could also be secondary to lactose intolerance. Administer a clear liquid diet for 24–48 hours, and then advance diet slowly.

C. Antidiarrheal agents. Often helpful but should not be used if invasive diarrhea is clinically suspected. Antimotility drugs are contraindicated in patients with pseudomembranous colitis or IBD because of the risk for precipitating toxic megacolon. Commonly used agents include bismuth subsalicylate (Pepto-Bismol) 30 mL or 2 tablets Q 30 min to 1 hr as needed up to 8 doses Q day; diphenoxylate with atropine (Lomotil 2.5 mg) 1–2 tablets qid, not to exceed 20 mg/day; and loperamide (Imodium) 4 mg initially, then 2 mg after each loose stool, not to exceed 16 mg Q day. Paregoric is an extremely effective agent (5 mL after each loose stool, up to 40 mL/d).

D. Antibiotics. Antibiotic treatment often does not shorten the duration of illness. It may select out resistant strains of organisms and may lead to pseudomembranous colitis.
   1. ***Salmonella.*** Does not usually require antibiotics unless the patient remains ill or is predisposed to developing complications (osteomyelitis, bacteremia), such as a patient with sickle cell disease. Treatment is chloramphenicol, ampicillin, trimethoprim-sulfamethoxazole (Bactrim or Septra), or ciprofloxacin.
   2. **Shigellosis.** Antibiotics are recommended to decrease duration of illness and fecal shedding. Antibiotic sensitivity is crucial because resistance is common. Treatment is ciprofloxacin, norfloxacin, trimethoprim-sulfamethoxazole, or ampicillin for 7 days.
   3. ***Clostridium difficile.*** Recommended treatment is metronidazole (Flagyl) 250–500 mg PO Q 6 hr for 10 days. If symptoms persist or recur, re-treatment with metronidazole is recommended. If a third course of treatment is needed, give vancomycin 125 mg PO Q 6 hr. Metronidazole is less expensive and is equally effective. Addition of cholestyramine (Questran) qid may help control diarrhea if given with antibiotics. If the patient cannot take medications orally or through a nasogastric tube, intravenous metronidazole can be used.

4. ***Campylobacter.*** Often self-limiting illness. With severe or persistent diarrhea, erythromycin or ciprofloxacin for 5–7 days is effective. Fluoroquinolone resistance has been reported.

REFERENCES

Aranda-Michel J, Giannella RA: Acute diarrhea: A practical review. Am J Med 1999;106:670.

Centers for Disease Control and Prevention: Outbreak of gastroenteritis associated with an interactive water fountain at a beachside park—Florida, 1999. MMWR 2000;49 (June 30):565.

Fine KD: Diarrhea. In: Feldman M, Scharschmidt BF, Sleisenger MH, eds. *Gastrointestinal and Liver Diseases: Pathophysiology/Diagnosis/Management.* 6th ed. Saunders;1998:128.

18. DIZZINESS

I. **Problem.** You are called by the nurse to evaluate a 65-year-old woman complaining of dizziness.

II. **Immediate Questions**

A. **What is the patient's description of the dizziness?** Asking open-ended questions and encouraging patients to give a detailed description of their dizziness enables you to classify dizziness into one of four specific categories (vertigo, pre-syncope, disequilibrium, or lightheadedness).

B. **What are the patient's vital signs?** Blood pressure and heart rate should be obtained lying and standing after 1 minute in all patients with dizziness. Orthostatic hypotension (a decrease in 10 mm Hg systolic) can often be attributed to drugs, volume depletion, or autonomic insufficiency. The heart rate will increase by 20 bpm (16 bpm in the elderly) in volume depletion, whereas with autonomic insufficiency the heart rate will not change. Consider an arrhythmia if the patient is tachycardic or bradycardic or has an irregular rhythm. Blood pressure and heart rate should be checked in both arms. A significant difference in systolic blood pressure (> 20 mm Hg) between the two arms may be suggestive of subclavian steal. Tachypnea may suggest hyperventilation or anxiety. Fever could represent an infectious etiology such as meningitis or otitis media.

C. **What are the patient's medications?** A thorough medication history is very helpful. New medications are a common cause of dizziness, which is easily reversible. Vasodilators, antihypertensives, and tricyclic antidepressants often cause orthostatic hypotension. Digoxin, beta-blockers, and calcium channel blockers (non-dihydropyridine calcium antagonists) can result in bradycardia and varying degrees of heart block. Antiarrhythmics such as quinidine, procainamide, and sotalol can induce ventricular arrhythmias. Aminoglycoside antibiotics (amikacin, gentamicin, streptomycin, tobramycin) and loop diuretics have been associated with ototoxicity and vertigo.

D. **What is the onset and duration of the dizziness?** Sudden onset of vertigo is suggestive of a peripheral vestibular disorder, whereas central vestibular disorders are associated with vertigo that is gradual in onset. In general, episodic symptoms occur with peripheral vestibular disorders and constant symptoms with central vestibular disorders. Knowing the duration of episodes can be helpful in differentiating benign positional vertigo (seconds), transient ischemic attack (minutes to hours), Ménière's disease (hours), and vestibular neuronitis/labyrinthitis (days). Common nonvestibular disorders (postural hypotension, vasovagal reactions, and cardiac arrhythmias) cause episodic dizziness usually lasting a few minutes. Chronic continuous dizziness is commonly caused by psychogenic factors and hyperventilation syndrome.

E. **Are there precipitating factors of the dizziness?** Dizziness related to position change can be attributed to vestibular and nonvestibular disorders. Positional vertigo is precipitated by changes in head position (turning/tilting head or rolling over in bed) or middle ear pressure (coughing, sneezing, or Valsalva maneuver). Postural hypotension is typically associated with a change in position (lying to standing). Generally, dizziness associated with exercise or stress is suggestive of a nonvestibular disorder.

F. **Are there other associated symptoms?** Hearing loss and tinnitus indicate a vestibular disorder, usually a peripheral disorder (eg, Ménière's disease). Nausea and vomiting are nonspecific findings often associated with vestibular disorders. Focal neurologic deficits usually represent a central nervous system disorder. Dyspnea, palpitations, and sweating occur with nonvestibular disorders, such as hyperventilation or cardiac disease.

III. **Differential Diagnosis.** Dizziness is a common complaint with an extensive differential diagnosis. A common approach is to categorize dizziness as vertigo, pre-syncope, disequilibrium, or lightheadedness. In general, the most common causes of dizziness are peripheral vestibular disorders, psychiatric disorders, and pre-syncope.

A. **Vertigo.** Vertigo is a symptom of vestibular dysfunction. It is a sensation of motion either of one's surroundings or of one's body, commonly described as a spinning or tilting sensation. If dizziness is attributed to vertigo, you must determine if it is due to a peripheral or central vestibular disorder.

1. **Peripheral vestibular disorders.** Due to disease of the inner ear or vestibular nerve (CN VIII).

   a. **Benign positional vertigo (BPV).** The most common cause of vertigo. Brief episodes of severe vertigo that are associated with changes of head position. Often occurs after ear trauma or infection.

b. **Vestibular neuronitis.** Sudden onset of severe vertigo associated with nausea and vomiting. Symptoms may persist for hours to days. Usually follows a viral upper respiratory infection.

c. **Labyrinthitis.** Similar to vestibular neuronitis except associated with hearing loss.

d. **Ménière's disease.** Characterized by episodic vertigo, tinnitus, aural fullness, and progressive sensorineural hearing loss.

e. **Ototoxic medications.** Aminoglycoside antibiotics, loop diuretics, aspirin, *cis*-platinum, alcohol.

f. **Other peripheral disorders.** Post-traumatic vertigo, acute/chronic otitis media, cholesteatoma, perilymphatic fistula, and acoustic neuroma.

2. **Central vestibular disorders.** Due to disease of brain stem or cerebellum. Usually vertigo is not the dominant manifestation of these disorders.

   a. **Cerebrovascular disease.** Ischemia involving the vertebrobasilar circulation often causes vertigo. Other signs of brain stem involvement such as diplopia, dysarthria, dysphagia, weakness, or numbness usually accompany vertigo due to brain stem ischemia. Cerebellar ischemia typically presents with vertigo and cerebellar signs; however, it may present with only vertigo. Altered mental status may indicate cerebellar infarction or hemorrhage with potential for herniation and progression to coma.

   b. **Tumors.** Brain stem, cerebellar, and cerebellopontine-angle tumors. *Acoustic neuromas,* which are benign tumors of the vestibular nerve, are the most common cerebellopontine-angle tumors. Tinnitus and hearing loss are common complaints, whereas vertigo is usually mild or absent.

   c. **Multiple sclerosis.** Vertigo is the presenting symptom in ~ 10% of patients. Up to one-third of patients with multiple sclerosis experience vertigo.

   d. **Subclavian steal syndrome.** Vertigo and other signs of vertebrobasilar insufficiency occur during arm exercise.

   e. **Other central disorders.** Temporal-lobe seizures, basilar artery migraines, meningitis, Friedreich's ataxia and related heredofamilial disorders, vasculitis.

B. **Pre-syncope.** A sensation of an impending faint, often described as "nearly fainting." Unlike syncope, there is no loss of consciousness. Typically lasts less than a minute. (See Section I, Chapter 59, Syncope, p 315).

1. **Vasovagal reaction.** Common in young patients and usually preceded by diaphoresis, pallor, and nausea. Frequently provoked by stressful, painful, or other noxious stimuli (ie, venipuncture).

2. **Orthostatic hypotension.** Hypovolemia, medications, or autonomic insufficiency.
3. **Cardiac disease.** Arrhythmias, valvular disease, atrial myxoma, cardiac ischemia, tamponade.
4. **Carotid sinus hypersensitivity.** Associated with head turning, tight collars, and shaving.
5. **Metabolic.** Hypoxia, hypoglycemia, hyponatremia, hypokalemia, hypocalcemia.

C. **Disequilibrium.** A sense of imbalance with ambulation. Typically not at rest.
1. **Multisensory deficit disorder.** The most common cause of disequilibrium in the elderly. It is due to any combination of peripheral neuropathy, visual impairment, vestibular disorder, or musculoskeletal disorder (ie, arthritis, cervical spondylosis). Often worsened by the patient's fear of falling.
2. **Altered visual input.** The elderly with vision loss and cataracts are prone to gait disturbances, particularly at night or in unfamiliar surroundings.
3. **Cerebellar disease**
4. **Parkinson's disease**
5. **Medications.** Psychotropics, benzodiazepines, anticonvulsants.

D. **Lightheadedness.** Dizziness that is difficult to define and not otherwise classifiable. The description given by the patient is often vague.
1. **Psychiatric.** Frequently nonspecific dizziness is a symptom of an underlying psychiatric disorder, including anxiety, depression, and panic disorder. The dizziness associated with anxiety is commonly associated with hyperventilation.
2. **Hyperventilation.** Dizziness is the most frequent symptom with hyperventilation syndrome. Dyspnea, palpitations, and paresthesias are associated symptoms. An abnormal pattern of breathing is often not recognized by the patient.

IV. Database

A. Physical examination key points
1. **Vital signs.** See Section II.B.
2. **Ears.** The external auditory canal should be evaluated for cerumen impaction or foreign body. The tympanic membrane should be examined for evidence of fluid, infection, or perforation. Do a simple assessment for hearing loss through whispered voice or finger rub. If hearing loss is suspected, then distinguish between sensorineural hearing and conductive hearing loss (Weber and Rinne tests). Sensorineural hearing loss is suggestive of Ménière's disease or an acoustic neuroma, whereas conductive hearing loss is often due to middle ear disease interfering with conduction, such as otitis media.

3. **Eyes.** Eyes should be examined for nystagmus, which is commonly associated with vertigo. Assess pupils and extraocular muscles for cranial nerve dysfunction, which may be due to a CNS lesion. Do a funduscopic exam to evaluate for papilledema (increased intracranial pressure). A quick check of visual acuity should also be done.
4. **Neck.** Auscultate for carotid/vertebral bruits, which may suggest possible cerebrovascular disease. Determine if head and neck movement precipitates dizziness.
5. **Cardiac.** Assess rate and rhythm, to determine presence of arrhythmia. Auscultate for heart murmurs suggestive of aortic stenosis or idiopathic hypertrophic subaortic stenosis (IHSS).
6. **Neurologic exam.** A careful neurologic exam is essential.
   a. **Mental status exam.** May give evidence of underlying psychiatric disorder. Altered mental status associated with nonvestibular dizziness may be attributed to drug toxicity, metabolic abnormalities, or CNS infection, whereas altered mental status with vertigo is often associated with life-threatening CNS disorders such as cerebellar hemorrhage or infarction.
   b. **Cranial nerves.** Cranial nerve abnormalities suggest a CNS disorder. Sensory: peripheral neuropathy, especially of lower extremities, contributes to disequilibrium.
   c. **Cerebellar.** Observe gait. Evaluate for limb ataxia and gait ataxia.

B. **Diagnostic physical tests**
1. **Nystagmus.** The presence of nystagmus suggests that dizziness is caused by vertigo. It may be the only objective finding in the examination of a patient with vertigo. Nystagmus associated with a peripheral lesion is different from that seen with a central lesion. Peripheral lesions cause only horizontal or rotary nystagmus; central lesions may cause nystagmus in any direction. Vertical nystagmus is only seen with central lesions. Visual fixation tends to suppress nystagmus that is due to peripheral but not central lesions. Changing the direction of gaze does not change the direction of nystagmus with peripheral lesions, but it may change the direction of nystagmus with central lesions.
2. **Nylen-Barany (Hallpike-Dix) maneuver.** Indicated with a history of vertigo. Will help differentiate peripheral positional vertigo from central vertigo. The physician moves the patient from a sitting to a supine position, with the head rotated 45° to one side and hanging off the table at 45°. The patient is then observed for vertigo and nystagmus. The maneuver is repeated with the head turned to the other side. With peripheral positional vertigo (BPV), the maneuver produces vertigo and rotary nystagmus after a latency of 2–20 seconds that diminishes in intensity within 30 seconds and fatigues with repetitive testing. Variation of these features often indicates a central disorder.

3. **Romberg test.** The patient stands with feet together, without support from arms. Monitor with eyes open and then closed. Pronounced imbalance with eyes closed compared to with eyes open suggests proprioceptive impairment. A *positive* Romberg test is common with disequilibrium.
4. **Hyperventilation maneuver.** The patient hyperventilates for 2–3 minutes. Monitor for reproduction of dizziness.

C. Laboratory data

1. **Complete blood count.** To rule out anemia or infection.
2. **Glucose.** To rule out hypoglycemia.
3. **Serum electrolytes.** To rule out electrolyte abnormalities such as hypokalemia or hypocalcemia.
4. **Thyroid function tests.** If hypothyroidism is suspected.
5. **Urine drug screen/drug levels.** If illicit drug use or drug toxicity is suspected.
6. **Serologic test for syphilis (RPR/VDRL).** If tertiary syphilis is suspected.

D. Special tests

1. **Brain imaging.** Not all patients with dizziness need neuroimaging. If a patient has findings on exam suggestive of a CNS disorder, neuroimaging is indicated. MRI is more sensitive than CT in diagnosing posterior fossa lesions and acoustic neuromas.
2. **Electronystagmogram (ENG).** Testing of vestibular function by evaluating nystagmus. This test is able to confirm nystagmus when the physical examination is equivocal. Detects peripheral and central vestibular disorders. Should be considered when etiology of vertigo is uncertain.
3. **Audiometry.** Should be considered with hearing complaints or with hearing loss on examination. May help with the diagnosis of peripheral vertigo (ie, Ménière's disease or acoustic neuroma).
4. **Brain stem evoked audiometry.** Very sensitive in the detection of acoustic neuromas.
5. **Electroencephalogram (EEG).** If seizures are suspected.
6. **Lumbar puncture.** If meningitis or multiple sclerosis is suspected.
7. **Electrocardiogram (ECG).** To rule out dysarrhythmia.
8. **Telemetry/Holter monitor/event recorder.** Useful in the evaluation of suspected arrhythmias.
9. **Echocardiogram.** If valvular heart disease or atrial myxoma is suspected.

V. Plan. Effective management of dizziness requires establishing the cause.

A. Vertigo. The management of central vertigo usually requires treatment of the underlying cause. The therapeutic goal of peripheral vertigo is to provide symptomatic relief from the vertigo as well as the nausea and vomiting. Most of the causes of peripheral vertigo are not life threatening, and most episodes should subside with conservative therapy (drug therapy and physical therapy).

1. **Drug therapy.** Antihistamines and anticholinergics are the drugs of choice. Phenothiazines and benzodiazepines are more sedating and usually reserved for patients with severe vomiting.
   a. **Antihistamines.** Meclizine (Antivert), 12.5–25 mg PO Q 6 hr; dimenhydrinate (Dramamine), 50 mg PO Q 6 hr; diphenhydramine (Benadryl), 25–50 mg PO/IM/IV Q 6 hr; promethazine (Phenergan), 25–50 mg PO/IM/IV Q 6 hr.
   b. **Anticholinergics.** Scopolamine (Transderm Scop), 0.5 mg/patch Q 3 days.
   c. **Phenothiazines.** Prochlorperazine (Compazine), 5–10 mg PO/IM/IV Q 6 hr.
   d. **Benzodiazepines.** Diazepam (Valium), 2–10 mg PO/IM/IV Q 6 hr.
2. **Physical therapy.** Vestibular rehabilitation often promotes recovery in patients with peripheral vertigo. Patients with vertigo tend to avoid head motion, which actually prolongs symptoms. Physical therapy forces them to perform exercises that may decrease the duration and severity of vertigo.
3. **Surgery.** Surgical intervention is reserved for refractory cases of vertigo. Endolymphatic shunts and labyrinthectomies have been performed for disabling cases of Ménière's disease.

B. **Pre-syncope.** See Section I, Chapter 59, Syncope, V, p 322.

C. **Disequilibrium**
1. **Treat any underlying treatable disorders.**
2. **Correct vision** if indicated.
3. **Advise to use cane or walker** when indicated.
4. **Consider physical therapy.**
5. **Assess environmental risks.** Prevent falls by eliminating hazards in environment.
6. **Avoid sedating medications.**

D. **Lightheadedness**
1. **Treat any underlying psychiatric disorder** (ie, give anxiolytics or antidepressants).
2. **Supportive psychotherapy.**
3. **Teach relaxation techniques.**
4. **Teach breathing techniques to relieve symptoms.**

REFERENCES

Branch WT: Approach to the patient with dizziness. In: Fletcher SW, Fletcher RH, Aronson MD, editors-in-chief. UpToDate [CD-ROM]. Version 8.2. Wellesley, MA;2000. www.uptodate.com

Hoffman RM, Einstadter D, Kroenke K: Evaluating dizziness. Am J Med 1999;107:468.

Warner EA, Wallach PM, Adelman HM et al: Dizziness in primary care patients. J Gen Intern Med 1992;7:454.

19. DYSPNEA

I. Problem. A patient admitted to the coronary care unit to rule out a myocardial infarction complains of difficulty breathing.

II. Immediate Questions

A. Was the onset of dyspnea acute or gradual? The differential diagnosis for acute dyspnea differs from subacute or chronic dyspnea. Causes of acute dyspnea include bronchospasm, pulmonary embolism (PE), pneumothorax, pulmonary infection, acute respiratory distress syndrome, diaphragmatic paralysis, myocardial ischemia, acute cardiogenic pulmonary edema, and anxiety. Chronic dyspnea can present with an acute exacerbation.

B. Are there other associated symptoms? The patient may focus on the shortness of breath and fail to disclose chest pain, pressure, or discomfort unless specifically asked. Qualify the chest pain; for example, pleuritic nature characterizes pneumothorax or PE with infarction. Bear in mind that dyspnea rather than angina may be the primary or the only symptom of acute myocardial ischemia. Determination of the effect of positional changes on dyspnea is important. *Orthopnea* (difficulty breathing when lying flat) suggests congestive heart failure, chronic pulmonary disease (COPD), asthma, or bilateral diaphragmatic dysfunction. *Platypnea* (difficulty breathing when sitting upright) invokes intrapulmonary or intracardiac shunting. *Trepopnea* (an inability to lie on one's side) implies pleural effusion or congestive heart failure. Assessment for precipitants, including exertion, exposure to chemicals, and other irritants is also helpful.

C. Is the patient cyanotic? Hypoxemia is a potentially lethal condition. If cyanosis (or evidence of hypoxia, such as by pulse oximetry) is noted, immediate oxygen therapy is indicated.

III. Differential Diagnosis. *Dyspnea* is the subjective sensation of difficult, labored, uncomfortable breathing. It may occur through increased respiratory muscle work, stimulation of neuroreceptors throughout the respiratory tract, or stimulation of peripheral and central chemoreceptors. Although many diseases produce dyspnea, two-thirds of the cases are caused by pulmonary or cardiac disorders.

A. Pulmonary

1. **Pulmonary embolism.** This diagnosis must be considered in any patient presenting with acute dyspnea. Also, recurrent pulmonary emboli can cause intermittent dyspnea at rest. This diagnosis should be especially considered with risk factors such as prolonged immobilization, recent operative procedure, obesity, malignancy (especially adenocarcinomas), venous trauma, known venous thrombosis, hypercoagulable risk factor (such as factor V resistance to activated protein C) or state (such as antiphospho-

lipid antibody syndrome), or high-dose estrogen therapy, especially in women over 35 years of age who take birth control pills and smoke.

2. **Pneumothorax.** This can occur after trauma, or spontaneously with bullous emphysema, or in young males with a tall, thin body habitus. Patients on ventilators are at increased risk. Iatrogenic pneumothoraces may occur after subclavian or internal jugular line placement or after bronchoscopy or thoracentesis.
3. **Asthma/chronic obstructive airway disease.** These patients usually have a prior history of dyspnea and known disease; however, anaphylaxis can also produce wheezing. (See Section I, Chapter 4, Anaphylactic Reaction, p 24). In addition to bronchospasm, these patients often demonstrate other evidence of anaphylaxis, such as stridor, wheezing, pruritus, hypotension, and urticaria.
4. **Aspiration.** See Section I, Chapter 7, Aspiration, III.H. Upper Airway Obstruction, p 37. An altered mental status is often present (eg, from intoxication, psychosis, delirium); also ask about dysphagia and muscle weakness suggesting an acute cerebral vascular accident.
5. **Pneumonia.** Characterized by fever, productive cough, radiographic infiltrates, and leukocytosis.
6. **Interstitial lung disease.** This usually produces progressive dyspnea, and is caused by diseases such as sarcoidosis, idiopathic pulmonary fibrosis, collagen vascular disease, and occupational lung disease.
7. **Pleural effusion.** More likely to cause chronic or subchronic dyspnea rather than acute dyspnea, except in the setting of significant parapneumonic effusion or in association with congestive heart failure or renal failure.
8. **Acute respiratory distress syndrome.** This is defined as acute bilateral lung injury and may be commonly associated with pneumonia, aspiration, sepsis, and severe trauma with shock and multiple transfusions.

B. Cardiac

1. **Acute myocardial infarction.** Myocardial ischemia can present primarily with dyspnea rather than chest pain. In addition, patients with acute myocardial infarction (MI) can develop acute PE or congestive heart failure with pulmonary edema.
2. **Congestive heart failure.** Accumulation of fluid in the interstitial spaces of the lung stimulates neuroreceptors, which produce a sensation of dyspnea often causing orthopnea and paroxysmal nocturnal dyspnea. Common etiologies include myocardial ischemia, hypertension, and viral infection.
3. **Pericarditis/pericardial tamponade.** Dyspnea and fatigue, as well as chest discomfort, are frequently significant complaints. Suspect pericardial effusion in a patient with a pulmonary malignancy.

4. **Arrhythmias.** Dyspnea may accompany tachyarrhythmias (eg, atrial fibrillation, supraventricular tachycardia, ventricular tachycardia) or bradyarrhythmias (eg, complete atrioventricular block, sinus bradycardia).
5. **Valvular and other cardiac diseases.** Aortic stenosis, aortic insufficiency, mitral stenosis, and mitral insufficiency, as well as intracardiac shunt and atrial myxoma, can cause dyspnea.

C. **Neuromuscular diseases.** Dyspnea can be caused by CNS disorders, myopathies, neuropathies, phrenic nerve and diaphragmatic disorders, spinal cord disorders, or systemic neuromuscular disorders.

D. **Other organic causes.** Anemia, gastroesophageal reflux, hyperthyroidism, hypothyroidism, metabolic acidosis (particularly diabetic ketoacidosis), renal failure (with concomitant pulmonary edema and/or uremic pericarditis), carbon monoxide poisoning, massive ascites (effectively resulting in restrictive lung disease), and deconditioning all can cause dyspnea.

E. **Psychogenic breathlessness.** Dyspnea associated with hyperventilation can be difficult to separate from dyspnea due to organic causes. Typically, anxiety, acral paresthesias, and lightheadedness are present. The dyspnea is often worse at rest and improves during exercise. Psychogenic breathlessness as a diagnosis should not be made until organic causes have been excluded. These patients often have an increased frequency of sighing.

IV. Database

A. Physical examination key points

1. **Vital signs.** Fever may signify infection, but also occurs with PE and MI. Tachypnea occurs in most cases of dyspnea; however, dyspnea can occur with a normal respiratory rate. Hypotension may result from a tension pneumothorax, anaphylaxis, pericardial tamponade, acute MI, or anemia from hemorrhage. Tachycardia is also seen in the above conditions. *Pulsus paradoxus* (inspiratory diminution in systolic pressure exceeding 10 mm Hg) may occur with acute exacerbation of asthma, COPD, constrictive pericarditis, or pericardial tamponade, and its significance is established only during normal cardiac rhythm and with respirations of normal rhythm and depth (*tidal breathing*). Bedside pulse oximetry is a valuable measurement.
2. **Lungs.** Observe the patient for accessory muscle use. Paradoxical abdominal movement during respiration suggests diaphragmatic and respiratory muscle fatigue. Palpate for tracheal deviation, which may be encountered in pneumothorax, large pleural effusion, or pulmonary mass. Percuss the lung fields to survey for asymme-

try of resonance, as found in pneumothorax. Listen for wheezes, stridor, crackles, friction rubs, and absent breath sounds.

3. **Heart.** Elevated jugular venous pressure, a displaced point of maximal impulse, or an S_3 gallop suggests decompensated heart failure. Jugular venous distension on inspiration, a nonpalpable apical impulse, and muffled heart tones evoke pericardial tamponade. Irregular heart beat and murmurs are also important signs.
4. **Extremities.** Examine for swelling or other evidence of deep venous thrombosis, which predisposes to pulmonary embolus. Also evaluate for pallor and peripheral cyanosis. Clubbing may be seen in the dyspneic patient with chronic suppurative lung disease, bronchial carcinoma, cyanotic heart disease, bacterial endocarditis, cirrhosis, or hyperthyroidism.
5. **Neurologic exam.** Confusion and impaired mentation may signify severe hypoxemia or may elucidate the etiology for dyspnea, such as infection.

B. Laboratory data

1. **Hemogram.** Leukocytosis with an increase in banded neutrophils occurs with pneumonia. Anemia can cause dyspnea on exertion and may precipitate myocardial ischemia in patients with established coronary heart disease.
2. **Arterial blood gases.** Should be obtained in any patient with significant dyspnea, or if hypoxemia is suspected based on a decreased percentage of oxygen saturation as measured by pulse oximetry. Assess for elevation of the alveolar-arterial (A-a) PO_2 gradient.
3. **Sputum Gram's stain and culture.** Obtain if pneumonia is suspected.
4. **Electrolytes and renal function tests.** Metabolic acidosis or renal failure may be discovered. Potential causes for cardiac arrhythmias (eg, hypocalcemia, hypokalemia, hypomagnesemia) or diaphragmatic dysfunction (hypophosphatemia) can be uncovered.
5. **Thyroid function tests.** Obtain if thyroid disease is considered.

C. Radiologic and other studies

1. **Chest x-ray.** Obtain a stat portable upright CXR if there is obvious distress. If the patient is unable to sit for an adequate film, obtain lateral decubitus films to rule out the possibility of a basilar pneumothorax. A clear CXR raises the possibility of airway obstruction or PE. An increased cardiac silhouette (implies either cardiomegaly from heart disease or pericardial effusion), pulmonary vascular congestion, infiltrates, pleural effusion, elevated diaphragm (seen in neuromuscular disorders), or pneumothorax may be discovered.
2. **Electrocardiogram.** Should always be obtained in evaluating acute dyspnea to rule out the possibility of myocardial ischemia or infarction (ST depression; ST elevation–convex upward; T wave

inversion; new Q waves); arrhythmia; pericarditis (PR depression; ST elevation–diffuse and concave upward; T wave inversion); pericardial effusion (low QRS amplitude, electrical alternans); or pulmonary embolism ($S_1Q_3T_3$; right-axis deviation; right bundle branch block; T wave inversion).

3. **Pulmonary function tests.** These are not applicable to the acute situation, but can assist in the evaluation of patients with obstructive or restrictive lung disease. Bronchoprovocation testing may help increase yield of pulmonary function testing. (See Section I, Chapter 15, Cough, Section IV.C.5., Pulmonary Function Tests, p 88).
4. **Ventilation/perfusion ($\dot{V}/\dot{Q}$) scan.** To evaluate for PE. With underlying cardiopulmonary disease, spiral computed tomography (CT) of the chest may be the preferred test because of the higher rate of ventilation defects, thus lowering the number of high-probability scans. Remember spiral CT is an excellent rule-in test, but a negative test does not rule out pulmonary embolus.
5. **Pulmonary angiogram.** In patients with a low or moderate probability ($\dot{V}/\dot{Q}$ scan or negative spiral CT) in whom there still exists a suspicion for PE, this test is the gold standard to diagnose PE. A venogram or impedance plethysmography and Doppler ultrasound of lower extremities may be helpful, potentially obviating the need for pulmonary angiogram if results are demonstrative of thrombosis.
6. **Echocardiogram.** Should be obtained emergently if there is a strong clinical suspicion for cardiac tamponade. Otherwise, an echocardiogram can be useful for assessing left ventricular function, valvular function, and whether or not cardiac disease is responsible for the dyspnea.
7. **Cardiopulmonary exercise testing.** It can be useful if the diagnosis is unclear, by helping to determine whether a cardiac or pulmonary abnormality exists.

V. Plan

A. Emergent therapy

1. **Oxygen supplementation.** The initial goal of treatment for acute dyspnea should be to ensure adequate oxygenation; thus, most patients should be treated with 100% oxygen therapy. In patients with a history of chronic obstructive airway disease in whom one is concerned about the possibility of suppression of their hypoxic ventilatory drive, therapy should be initiated with 24–28% oxygen by Venturi mask. In either case, an arterial blood gas (ABG) should be obtained to direct subsequent adjustments of the oxygen. Continuous oxygen saturation monitoring by pulse oximetry can be helpful.
2. **Stat portable CXR, ECG, and ABG.** Indicated in any patient who complains of acute dyspnea.

B. Asthma/acute exacerbation of chronic bronchitis

1. **Albuterol.** Request a stat nebulizer treatment with albuterol 0.5 mL in 2–3 mL normal saline or give 4 puffs albuterol by metered-dose inhaler (MDI) via a spacer device.
2. **Epinephrine.** For anaphylaxis or in young patients with acute asthma, epinephrine 0.25–0.4 mL of a 1:1000 concentration can be given SC.
3. **Methylprednisolone (Solu-Medrol).** 125 mg stat IV will provide relief of bronchospasm in 3–6 hours as the effectiveness of the albuterol dissipates.

C. **Anaphylaxis.** (See Section I, Chapter 4, Anaphylactic Reaction, V, p 26).

D. **Myocardial ischemia.** If initial assessment suggests myocardial ischemia, administer aspirin 325 mg (chewable) and nitroglycerin 0.4 mg SL, provided the systolic blood pressure is > 100. (See Section I, Chapter 11, Chest Pain, V, p 63).

E. **Acute congestive heart failure.** Furosemide (Lasix) 40–80 mg IV may be given, provided the patient is not hypotensive. Morphine sulfate 2–5 mg IV may also be helpful initially for acute pulmonary edema. Invasive monitoring via pulmonary artery catheter, IV inotropes, and angiotensin-converting enzyme (ACE) inhibitor therapy may be warranted.

F. **Pneumonia.** Treat with pulmonary toilet (bronchodilators, incentive spirometry, percussion and postural drainage) and antibiotics as directed by results of the sputum Gram's stain. Be mindful of nosocomial pathogens when beginning empiric antibiotic treatment.

G. **Pleural effusion.** Removal of pleural fluid by thoracentesis can often produce a significant improvement in a patient's dyspnea, particularly in the setting of an exudative process like malignancy (see Section III, Chapter 14, Thoracentesis, p 431).

H. **Aspiration.** (See Section I, Chapter 7, Aspiration, V, p 38).

REFERENCES

Burki NK: Acute dyspnea: Is the cause cardiac or pulmonary—or both? Consultant 2000;40:542.

DeGowin RL, Brown DD: *DeGowin's Diagnostic Examination.* 7th ed. McGraw-Hill;2000:247.

Gillespie DJ, Staats BA: Concise review for primary-care physicians: Unexplained dyspnea. Mayo Clin Proc 1994;69:657.

Mahler DA: Acute dyspnea. In: Mahler DA, ed. *Dyspnea.* Futura Publishing Co. (Mount Kisco, NY);1990:127.

Manning HL, Schwartzstein RM: Pathophysiology of dyspnea. N Engl J Med 1995;327:1547.

Salzman GA: Evaluation of dyspnea. Hosp Pract 1997;195 (March 15).

Ware LB, Matthay MA: Medical progress: The acute respiratory distress syndrome. N Engl J Med 2000;342:1334.

20. DYSURIA

I. **Problem.** A 36-year-old sexually active woman complains of pain with urination.

II. **Immediate Questions**

A. **How long have the symptoms been present?** Acute onset of symptoms of dysuria, frequency, and urgency within 1–2 days indicates lower urinary tract infection (UTI). Patients with symptoms for more than a week are more likely to have a more serious infection (upper tract involvement). A gradual onset of several days' duration suggests a chlamydial or gonorrheal infection. Prostatitis can also present with several days of symptoms.

B. **Are there any associated symptoms?** Fever, chills, nausea, vomiting, and back pain are often signs of upper UTIs such as pyelonephritis. Dysuria, frequency, urgency, and suprapubic pain are lower UTI signs/symptoms and can occur with cystitis, prostatitis, and urethritis. A vaginal discharge would suggest a vaginitis, such as caused by *Gardnerella vaginalis* in bacterial vaginosis, *Candida albicans,* or *Trichomonas vaginalis,* as a cause of dysuria. Also remember that other sexually transmitted diseases (STDs) such as chlamydia and gonorrhea can cause urethritis. In men, ask about a recent penile discharge.

C. **Does the patient have a prior history of urinary tract infection (UTI) or urologic abnormality?** Women and people with a urinary tract abnormality are predisposed to recurrent UTIs. Patients with recurrent UTIs (> 2 UTIs per year) are managed with longer courses of antibiotics and possibly prophylactic antibiotics. Bladder cancer can sometimes present with dysuria.

D. **Has the patient recently had a Foley catheter removed?** Catheter placement may result in an infection or transient urethral irritation.

E. **What types of contraception or sexual protection is used by the patient?** Use of diaphragm and spermicide enhance UTI susceptibility in females. In males, unprotected anal intercourse, intercourse with an infected partner, and an uncircumcised penis are all risk factors for UTIs.

III. **Differential Diagnosis.** The principal causes of dysuria differ for men and women.

A. **Women.** Women presenting with acute dysuria are likely to have one of seven conditions, each of which may require different management.

1. **Acute pyelonephritis.** Suggested by fever, rigors, flank pain, nausea, and vomiting with or without lower UTI symptoms.
2. **Complicated UTI.** Seen in patients with diabetes, immunosuppression, pregnancy, abnormal genitourinary tracts, resistant or-

ganisms, or history of relapsing infections. These patients can present with signs of only lower UTI and have an upper UTI as well (subclinical pyelonephritis).

3. **Lower UTI.** These patients have either cystitis or urethritis, with bacteria confined to either the bladder or urethra.
4. **Chlamydial urethritis.** This is characterized by a gradual onset over several days. The patient often reports intercourse with a partner with similar symptoms. An associated mucopurulent endocervical secretion may be noted on pelvic exam.
5. **Other urethral infections.** Urethritis may also be caused by *Neisseria gonorrhoeae* and *T vaginalis.*
6. **Vaginitis.** In contrast to the internal sensations of dull pain associated with dysuria caused by cystitis, vaginitis causes external burning pain as the urine stream flows over the inflamed labia. The most common causes include bacterial vaginosis, candida vulvovaginitis, and trichomoniasis.
7. **No recognized pathogen.** These patients have no pyuria and no evidence of infection. The most common cause is atrophic vaginitis. Consider bladder or urethral carcinoma. "Urethral syndrome" is seen in some women who may be exquisitely sensitive to pH changes in the urine.

B. Men

1. **Acute pyelonephritis.** Presents with the same symptoms and signs as in women. Requires further anatomical workup once infection is resolved.
2. **Lower UTI.** Presents with the same signs and symptoms as in women. If an isolated event, no further workup is needed presuming the patient is cured with treatment. Recurrent UTIs require workup.
3. **Urethritis.** Always keep in mind that chlamydia and gonorrhea often coexist.
   a. **Nongonococcal.** The most common etiologic agent is *Chlamydia trachomatis.* Discharge occurs 8–21 days after exposure and is typically thin and clear.
   b. **Gonococcal.** In contrast to nongonococcal urethritis, the discharge associated with this condition is heavy and purulent. Symptoms occur 2–6 days after exposure.
4. **Prostatitis.** Symptoms include dysuria, frequency, hesitancy, and vague groin and/or back pain. Associated fever, chills, and malaise suggest acute prostatitis. Chronic bacterial prostatitis is less common and associated with recurrent UTIs in men. Nonbacterial prostatitis is the most common and is sometimes referred to as "prostatodynia."
5. **Cancer.** Think of bladder, prostate, and urethral cancer.
6. **Benign conditions.** Urethral stricture, meatal stenosis, and benign prostatic hypertrophy.

IV. Database

A. Physical examination key points

1. **Vital signs.** Check for fever, tachycardia, or hypotension, which suggest upper tract involvement and, in the case of hypotension, urosepsis.
2. **Abdomen/back.** Examine for evidence of suprapubic tenderness or costovertebral angle tenderness.
3. **Genitalia.** In women who present with acute dysuria and also complain of a vaginal discharge, pelvic exam is mandatory to rule out vaginitis, cervicitis, and pelvic inflammatory disease. In men with a history of urethral discharge, penile stripping may be necessary to produce a discharge. Examine for evidence of epididymitis or orchitis.
4. **Prostate.** In acute prostatitis, the gland is swollen, tender, and boggy. In patients presenting with acute prostatitis, digital exam of the prostate can result in bacteremia, so vigorous massage of the prostate is contraindicated. In patients with chronic prostatitis, examination of the prostate may be unremarkable.

B. Laboratory data

1. **Urinalysis.** Pyuria, which can be quickly detected by testing the urine for the presence of leukocyte esterase, is present in almost all cases of UTI (sensitivity 90%, specificity 95%). Bacteriuria, which can be detected using the nitrite test (except for the following uropathogens: *Enterococcus, Staphylococcus saprophyticus,* and *Acinetobacter* species that do not split nitrates to nitrites), confirms a bacterial cause. It is important to remember that false-negative nitrite results may occur in patients who consume a low-nitrate diet or who take diuretics. Also examine for white blood cell casts with microscopy, which indicates pyelonephritis. Hematuria occurs with cystitis and pyelonephritis but is seldom seen with urethritis. A Gram's stain of uncentrifuged urine is also helpful in assessing the presence of bacteria and may help direct therapy, especially if gram-positive bacteria are seen.
2. **Urine culture.** Although useful in determining a bacterial cause of dysuria, a urine culture is usually indicated only in women if acute pyelonephritis or complicated UTI is suspected; or if the patient is presenting with a relapse from a UTI. In men, a urine culture should always be obtained to confirm and direct subsequent treatment.
3. **Blood cultures.** Should be ordered in all patients who appear septic and are admitted for presumed acute pyelonephritis.
4. **Complete blood count with differential.** Leukocytosis and a left shift are seen with acute pyelonephritis and sometimes with acute prostatitis. They are seldom seen in urethritis, cystitis, or chronic prostatitis.
5. **Urethral discharge.** In both men and women, the discharge should be gram-stained and cultured on Thayer-Martin medium.

The presence of intracellular gram-negative diplococci on Gram's stain is sufficient presumptive evidence of gonorrhea in men and warrants therapy. In women with endocervical discharge, cultures for gonorrhea should be obtained. Discharge should also always be sent for DNA probe for *C trachomatis* as well.

6. **Urine test for gonorrhea and chlamydia.** There is a new urine test called the *ligase chain reaction,* which tests the urine for the presence of both gonorrhea and chlamydia. This test amplifies the DNA of the organisms, a lot like polymerase chain reaction (PCR) tests did in the past.
7. **Vaginal discharge.** Wet mount to look for *T vaginalis,* which have flagella and, when viewed on a wet mount, move rapidly and erratically. *Clue cells,* or activated squamous cells coated with bacteria, indicate bacterial vaginosis. The presence of hyphae, indicating infection with *C albicans,* should be assessed on a slide of vaginal discharge treated with 2–3 drops of 10% potassium hydroxide. Cervical swabs can also be sent for culture, DNA probe, or ligase chain reaction tests for chlamydia and gonorrhea.

C. **Radiologic and other studies.** Full urologic evaluation is indicated in men with pyelonephritis, recurrent infections, or other complicating factors. Women who have had more than two recurrences of pyelonephritis, as well as women in whom complicating factors such as anatomic abnormalities are suspected, should also undergo full urologic evaluation. An ultrasound, CT scan, or intravenous pyelography should be obtained in patients admitted for acute pyelonephritis if they remain febrile after 2–3 days of treatment with an appropriate antibiotic. An ultrasound or pelvic CT should also be obtained in patients with acute prostatitis who do not improve after 3 days of an appropriate antibiotic.

V. Plan

A. Acute pyelonephritis

1. **Suspected sepsis or intolerance to oral medications.** Administer a fluoroquinolone IV (Cipro 200–400 mg IV Q 12 hr). A third-generation cephalosporin such as ceftriaxone 1 g IV Q 24 hr is an alternative. If you suspect *Enterococcus* (more commonly with recurrence or in the presence of structural abnormalities), use ampicillin 1.5–2.0 g Q 4–6 hr and gentamicin 1.5–2.0 mg/kg IV loading dose; then give about 1.5 mg/kg IV Q 8–24 hr depending on renal function (see Aminoglycoside Dosing, Table 7–18, p 614). Once antibiotic susceptibility tests are known, the patient can be switched to oral medications after being afebrile for 24–48 hours. Duration of therapy should be 14 days.
2. **Hospitalization indications.** Include dehydration; inability to tolerate oral medications; concern about compliance; uncertainty about diagnosis; and severe illness with high fever, severe pain, and marked debility.

3. **Acute uncomplicated pyelonephritis.** A 14-day outpatient course of a fluoroquinolone antibiotic such as ciprofloxacin 500 mg PO bid. Other possibilities include amoxicillin/potassium clavulanate (Augmentin) and oral cephalosporins. Bactrim has fallen out of favor due to the high rate of resistance.
4. **Follow-up.** Urine cultures should be checked 2–3 weeks after therapy is completed.

B. **Complicated UTI.** These patients should be treated with a 7- to 14-day course of the same oral or IV agents as described above for uncomplicated pyelonephritis.

C. **Lower UTI.** In patients presenting with acute dysuria who are noted to have pyuria and bacteriuria on urinalysis, but do not have the clinical picture of acute pyelonephritis, an uncomplicated lower UTI (most likely cystitis) can be presumed and treated. A urine culture is not required in these patients. Studies indicate that trimethoprim-sulfamethoxazole (Bactrim) is the most efficacious treatment. A 3-day regimen of Bactrim DS, 1 tablet PO bid, is sufficient for uncomplicated lower UTIs in women. A 7-day regimen should be considered for patients with diabetes mellitus, > 7 days of symptoms, a recent UTI, UTI with associated use of a diaphragm or spermicide, and UTIs in men. Alternative antibiotics for patients with a history of intolerance to sulfa are trimethoprim 100 mg PO bid for 3 days or nitrofurantoin 100 mg qid for 7 days. Ciprofloxacin and other fluoroquinolones are reserved as second-line agents for patients who have recurrences and treatment failures. A follow-up culture is also **not** necessary for acute uncomplicated lower UTIs unless they occur frequently.

D. **Vaginitis.** Therapy is directed to the specific cause of the vaginitis. For patients with bacterial vaginosis, metronidazole 500 mg PO bid for 7 days or 2 g, as a single dose, is effective. For candida vaginitis, miconazole (Monistat) cream topically for 7 days is effective. An alternative is a single 150-mg oral dose of fluconazole (Diflucan). For trichomonal vaginitis, metronidazole 2 g PO in a single dose is recommended for the sex partner as well as the patient. Alternatively, treatment can be metronidazole 500 mg PO bid for 7 days. Topical Premarin cream is effective for atrophic vaginitis. The cream should be applied daily for 1 week and then 2–3 times a week thereafter.

E. **Chlamydial urethritis.** This should be suspected when dysuria and pyuria but no bacteriuria is present, and when the partner has symptoms. Doxycycline 100 mg bid for 7 days is effective. An alternative therapy is azithromycin 1 g PO in a single dose or ofloxacin 300 mg PO bid for 7 days. The partner should be evaluated and treated. Verify that women are not pregnant before prescribing doxycycline.

F. **Gonococcal urethritis.** With the emergence of penicillin resistance, ceftriaxone 125 mg IM or ofloxacin 400 mg PO is now recommended. Because of the frequent coexistence of chlamydial urethritis, azithromycin 1 g PO 1 dose or doxycycline 100 mg PO twice a day for 7 days should also be given. The patient's partner(s) should be evaluated and treated.

G. **Acute prostatitis.** Patients who are septic should be admitted and broad antibiotic coverage administered IV. If Gram's stain shows gram-positive cocci in chains, patients should be treated with intravenous ampicillin and gentamicin to cover *Enterococcus.* Patients with gram-negative rods in their urine should be treated with intravenous ceftriaxone and either a fluoroquinolone (PO or IV) or an aminoglycoside. Once the patient has been afebrile for 24–48 hours, the patient may be switched to oral antibiotics for a total of 4–6 weeks. Outpatient management usually involves either a fluoroquinolone PO or trimethoprim-sulfamethoxazole DS PO for 4 weeks pending results of the urine culture. Nonsteroidal anti-inflammatory drugs (NSAIDs) can be given to relieve pain, speed clearing of inflammation, and liquefy prostatic secretions.

H. **Chronic prostatitis.** Patients may respond to an oral agent such as a fluoroquinolone (ciprofloxacin) or Bactrim DS for 4–12 weeks. Many patients have nonbacterial prostatitis and should be referred for urologic evaluation if symptoms do not resolve on a course of antibiotics.

I. **Urethral syndrome.** Identify foods or medications that cause symptoms. Alkalinization of urine may help some patients.

REFERENCES

Claudius HI: Dysuria in adolescents. West J Med 2000;172:201.

Gilbert DN, Moellering RC, Sande MA: *The Sanford Guide to Antimicrobial Therapy.* 30th ed. Antimicrobial Therapy, Inc. (Hyde Park, VT);2000:15.

Hooton TM, Stamm WE: Diagnosis and treatment of uncomplicated urinary tract infection. Infect Dis Clin North Am 1997;11:551.

Lipsky BA: Urinary tract infections in men. Ann Intern Med 1989;110:138.

Orenstein R, Wong ES: Urinary tract infections in adults. Am Fam Physician 1999;59:1225.

Pappas PG: Laboratory in the diagnosis and management of urinary tract infections. Med Clin North Am 1991;75:313.

Ronald AR, Nicolle LE, Harding GKM: Standards of therapy for urinary tract infections in adults. Infection 1992;20:S164.

Stamm WE, Hooton TM: Management of urinary tract infection in adults. N Engl J Med 1993;329:1328.

21. FALLS

I. **Problem.** You are called to evaluate an 84-year-old female patient with pneumonia who has fallen on her way to the bathroom.

II. **Immediate Questions**

A. **What were the circumstances of the fall?** Determine, if possible, exactly how the fall occurred: What activity was the patient doing and how did the patient feel at the time of the fall? Causes of falls can be characterized as *intrinsic* (due to some condition of the patient, such as orthostatic hypotension) or *extrinsic* (due to some environmental cause, such as a slippery floor). In many cases, the causes are intermingled.

B. What symptoms (if any) does the patient have? Determine whether premonitory symptoms such as dizziness, palpitations, dyspnea, chest pain, weakness, confusion, incontinence, loss of consciousness, or tongue biting occurred. In addition, inquire about pain involving the head, neck, ribs, arms, back, or hips.

C. What are the vital signs? Hypotension and tachycardia may be associated with many conditions such as acute infection, dehydration, or acute myocardial infarction (MI). Tachypnea may be noted with the above conditions or with a pulmonary embolus. Fever or hypothermia may be indicative of infection.

D. What medical conditions does the patient have? Many conditions predispose to dizziness. Diabetes mellitus may be associated with autonomic dysfunction leading to orthostatic hypotension; hyperglycemia can cause osmotic diuresis and lead to volume depletion. Parkinson's disease results in gait imbalance. Dementia is associated with an increased risk of falls.

E. What medications is the patient taking? Medication-related side effects such as dizziness, hypotension, or confusion may predispose to falls. Vasodilators and diuretics commonly cause hypotension and dizziness. Anxiolytics, antidepressants, sedatives, and anticholinergics have also been associated with increased risk of falls.

III. Differential Diagnosis. With younger patients, the cause of the fall may be easily apparent. However, the differential diagnosis with an older patient may be quite extensive. The elderly frequently have multiple contributing causes of a fall.

A. Extrinsic causes. These result from the environment.

1. **Slippery floors.** From water or urine.
2. **Inadequate lighting.** Older patients may have cataracts or other ophthalmologic problems that impair vision.
3. **Transfers.** A weakened patient attempting to make a transfer from the bed to a wheelchair may fall.
4. **Bed side rails.** If side rails are placed up, a delirious patient attempting to climb over them can fall.
5. **Walking aids not available.** Often a hospitalized patient will not have his or her cane or walker immediately available and may attempt to walk to the bathroom unaided.

B. Intrinsic causes

1. **"Normal" aging.** Such as visual impairment (eg, presbyopia or cataracts). Patients with visual or hearing loss may be unable to move well in a new environment.

2. **Neurologic**
   a. **Cerebrovascular accident with hemiparesis.** May have decreased mobility.
   b. **Parkinson's disease.** May have decreased mobility.
   c. **Dementia.** From any number of causes such as multi-infarct dementia, Alzheimer's disease, or hypothyroidism. The patient with dementia may have poor judgment about his or her ability to move in a new environment.
   d. **Seizures.** Usually functioning normally after the episode; look for evidence of tongue biting or urinary incontinence.
   e. **Carotid sinus hypersensitivity**
   f. **Peripheral neuropathy.** Vitamin B_{12} deficiency is more common among the elderly. Also consider in a patient with a history of diabetes mellitus or alcohol abuse.
   g. **Vestibular dysfunction.** Inner ear problems may have associated attacks of vertigo, affecting balance.
3. **Cardiovascular.** See Section I, Chapter 59, Syncope, p 315.
   a. **Orthostatic hypotension.** Should be considered with dehydration, acute infections, gastrointestinal bleeding, or autonomic dysfunction (diabetes mellitus).
   b. **Arrhythmias.** Tachyarrhythmias or bradyarrhythmias should be considered—especially in the elderly or if there is a history of heart disease. (See Section I, Chapter 60, Tachycardia, p 323; and Section I, Chapter 8, Bradycardia, p 39).
   c. **Angina or myocardial infarction (MI).** Syncope or hypotension can be a sign of ischemic heart disease.
   d. **Vagal response disorders.** Valsalva (due to defecation, micturition, or other cause) may cause an increase in vagal tone, resulting in a decrease in heart rate and blood pressure, which then may result in a fall.
4. **Fluid/volume loss.** From any cause, including diuretic use, diarrhea, vomiting or nasogastric suction, GI hemorrhage, high fever, or decreased oral intake.
5. **Musculoskeletal disorders.** Degenerative joint disease or osteoarthritis is very common in the elderly. Deconditioning can be a problem, especially during hospitalization. In addition, a fall can cause a hip fracture, predisposing the patient to fall again. Proximal muscle weakness is common in the elderly.
6. **Metabolic disorders**
   a. **Hyperthyroidism.** Associated arrhythmias (such as atrial fibrillation) may affect function.
   b. **Hypoglycemia.** There may be associated diaphoresis, tachycardia, or syncope.
   c. **Electrolyte imbalance.** Hypokalemia or hypomagnesemia can lead to muscle weakness or arrhythmias. Hypercalcemia can cause confusion.
   d. **Diabetes mellitus.** Uncontrolled diabetes mellitus can cause an osmotic diuresis leading to volume depletion. Peripheral

neuropathy and autonomic insufficiency causing orthostatic hypotension can result from long-standing diabetes mellitus.

e. **Metabolic encephalopathy.** Uremia and hepatic failure can cause confusion.

7. **Psychological factors**
   a. **Refusal of assistance or ancillary devices.** Some patients may feel that they do not need a walker or assistance with transfer.
   b. **Disorientation.** From any number of causes, including dementia, acute bacterial infection, "sundowning," and intensive care unit psychosis. (See Section I, Chapter 13, Coma, Acute Mental Status Changes, p 72).
   c. **Depression.** Depression may present as dementia. These patients may become increasingly immobile or less likely to notice obstacles or changes in their environment.
8. **Medications.** See II.E. above. Also, medications that may affect the vestibular system at either normal or toxic doses include aminoglycosides (gentamicin, tobramycin), aspirin, furosemide (Lasix), quinine, quinidine, and alcohol.
9. **Congestive heart failure.** Exercise tolerance may be quite limited, leading to a fall upon overexertion.
10. **Infection.** Any infection may be associated with a change in mental status, particularly in the elderly. Also, infections (eg, pneumonia) may cause weakness during hospitalization, and the patient may be unable to move about safely unassisted.

IV. Database

A. Physical examination key points

1. **Vital signs.** Look for hypotension, tachycardia or bradycardia, tachypnea, or an increase or decrease in the temperature from baseline. Check for orthostatic changes, a decrease in systolic blood pressure of 10 mm Hg, and/or an increase in heart rate of 20 bpm (16 bpm in the elderly), 1 minute after going from supine to a standing position.
2. **HEENT.** Look for evidence of trauma from the fall, such as soft tissue swelling and tenderness. Look for cataracts, which may impair vision.
3. **Extremities.** Look for evidence of fractures, such as an externally rotated and flexed hip, deformity of long bones, or swelling over these sites.
4. **Neurologic exam.** Examine for evidence of peripheral neuropathy or movement disorder (eg, Parkinson's disease). Perform a brief mental status exam and check for localizing findings to assess for possible subdural hematoma.

B. Laboratory data. If there are obvious clues from the history and/or physical examination, an extensive laboratory evaluation may not be indicated.

1. **Complete blood count.** To evaluate for infection and anemia.
2. **Electrolytes.** Include blood urea nitrogen, creatinine, and glucose. Hypokalemia or hypomagnesemia can cause arrhythmias; hypercalcemia can cause confusion.
3. **Urinalysis.** Rule out infection, especially in older patients.
4. **Liver function tests.** Aspartate aminotransferases (AST), alanine aminotransferases (ALT), total bilirubin, and alkaline phosphatase or γ-glutamyltransferase (GGT) to rule out hepatic dysfunction.

C. **Radiologic and other studies**
1. **Skeletal x-rays.** In elderly patients, the most common sites for significant fractures would be hip, humerus, distal radius, and ulna (Colles' fracture).
2. **Computed tomography scan of head.** Perform if the patient has new neurologic deficits or confusion not explained by routine evaluation.
3. **Electrocardiography.** Look for evidence of ischemia, infarction, tachyarrhythmia, or bradyarrhythmia. Check the QT interval, especially if the patient is taking any medications that prolong the QT interval, such as amiodarone, sotalol, quinidine, or procainamide. A prolonged or a shortened QT interval can be secondary to hypocalcemia or hypercalcemia, respectively.

V. Plan

A. **Prevention.** Preventive measures can greatly reduce the number of falls and are essential for good patient care. Environmental modifications include avoidance of restraints if possible and removal of obstacles that interfere with patient movement. Assistive devices used routinely, such as a walker, cane, or hearing aid, should be made available if possible.

B. **Medication modification.** Review all medications and reduce or eliminate those that may contribute to mental status changes or orthostatic hypotension or that may limit mobility.

C. **Treat potential underlying causes.** Including but not limited to infection, cerebrovascular accident, myocardial ischemia or infarction, and gastrointestinal bleeding.

D. **Observation.** The patient who has had a head injury should undergo a thorough neurologic examination by the physician and be monitored by neurologic checks by the nursing staff. Patients with abnormal vital signs should be monitored more frequently than the usual once per nursing shift. Patients should also be monitored for complaints of pain (eg, neck, back, arm, or hip) not present during the initial evaluation.

E. **Physical therapy.** If the patient has gait imbalance or weakness, consult a physical therapist for a thorough gait and balance assessment and strengthening exercises.

REFERENCES

Coogler CE, Wolf SL: Falls. In: Hazzard WR, Bierman EL, Blass JP et al, eds. *Principles of Geriatric Medicine and Gerontology.* 4th ed. McGraw-Hill;1999:1535.

Fuller GF: Falls in the elderly. Am Fam Physician 2000;61:2159.

Kiel DP: The evaluation of falls in the emergency department. Clin Geriatr Med 1993;9:591.

Mahoney JE: Immobility and falls. Clin Geriatr Med 1998;14:699.

Tinetti M, Speechley M: Prevention of falls among the elderly. N Engl J Med 1989;320:1055.

22. FEVER

I. **Problem.** You are called to see a 57-year-old man who has been hospitalized for 3 days and now has a fever of 39.5°C (103.1°F).

II. **Immediate Questions**

A. **Was the patient febrile on admission, implying community-acquired illness, or did the fever develop in the course of hospitalization (nosocomial)?** It is important to know if this elevation in temperature signals the abrupt onset of fever or represents the gradual worsening of a prior fever. Fever above 40.0°C (104.0°F) requires immediate action.

B. **Does the patient have any other pertinent medical illnesses, or is he or she immunocompromised?** Such information is vital before you can properly assess the patient. Review should include all medical illnesses as well as previous surgeries. For example, a history of trauma that resulted in splenectomy places that patient at higher risk of infection with encapsulated organisms such as *Streptococcus pneumoniae.* Is there an underlying malignancy? Has the patient recently received chemotherapy? Is the patient taking or has he or she recently taken any other immunosuppressive medications such as prednisone or azathioprine? Also see Section I, Chapter 23, Fever in the HIV-Positive Patient, p 135.

C. **Are any indwelling catheters in place?** Indwelling Foley catheters, intravenous access sites, nasogastric tubes (which can predispose to sinusitis), and central venous catheter sites are frequent sources of nosocomial fever.

D. **Are there any associated symptoms?** The symptoms to ascertain include chills, rigors, rash, myalgias, arthralgias, cough, sputum production, postnasal drainage, chest pain, headache, dysuria, abdominal pain, nausea, vomiting, pain at an intravenous site, diarrhea, night sweats, and change in mental status. Such questions may point toward a specific cause.

E. **What medications is the patient taking?** Ask if the patient is taking any antipyretics or antibiotics. If the patient has been on antibiotics in the past 4 months, consider the possibility of *Clostridium difficile* colitis. Also consider a drug-induced fever and review all medications.

F. **Have any recent procedures such as bronchoscopy been done, or has the patient recently received blood?** A fever to 38.3°C (101°F) is common after bronchoscopy and transfusions.

G. **Are there any factors relating to the patient's psychosocial history that need to be assessed?** Inquire about recent travel, especially to countries with poor sanitation; HIV risk factors (intravenous drug use; homosexual or bisexual male; promiscuous sexual activity; or sexual intercourse with a prostitute, a person with AIDS, or HIV-positive persons); exposure to dogs, cats, birds, ticks, and cattle; and health of family members.

H. **Does the patient have significant valvular heart disease including a prosthetic valve?** Significant valvular heart disease predisposes the patient to bacterial endocarditis. Be sure to inquire about recent procedures, including dental work.

III. **Differential Diagnosis.** An exhaustive list is extraordinarily long; only the major categories are presented here:

A. **Infections**
   1. **Bacterial**
   2. **Viral**
   3. **Mycobacterial**
   4. **Fungal**
   5. **Parasitic**
   6. **Protozoal**
   7. **Rickettsial**

B. **Neoplasms.** Solid tumors, especially with metastasis to the liver; lymphoma; Hodgkin's disease; multiple myeloma; leukemia; myelodysplastic syndromes. Fever with leukemia is often due to infection but may be caused by the primary disease, especially in chronic myelogenous leukemia. Solid tumors causing fever include renal cell and hepatocellular carcinoma, osteogenic sarcoma, and atrial myxoma.

C. **Connective tissue disease**
   1. **Acute rheumatic fever**
   2. **Rheumatoid arthritis**
   3. **Adult Still's disease**
   4. **Systemic lupus erythematosus (SLE)**
   5. **Vasculitis.** Including hypersensitivity vasculitis, polymyalgia rheumatica, temporal arteritis, and polyarteritis nodosa.

D. **Thermoregulatory disorders.** Heat stroke, malignant hyperthermia, thyroid storm, and malignant neuroleptic syndrome. Thyroid storm may be a postoperative complication in a hyperthyroid patient. Features of malignant neuroleptic syndrome include hyperthermia, hypertonicity of skeletal muscle, mental status changes, and autonomic nervous system instability in patients on neuroleptics.

E. **Drug-induced fever.** Potential culprits include antibiotics (especially beta lactams, sulfonamides), methyldopa, quinidine, hydralazine, procainamide, phenytoin, chlorpromazine, carbamazepine, anti-inflammatory agents such as ibuprofen, antineoplastic agents, and allopurinol. Other agents that may cause fever include steroids, antidopaminergic neuroleptic agents, sympathomimetics, cocaine, LSD, hallucinogens, ecstasy or MDMA (3,4-methylenedioxymethamphetamine), phencyclidine, and tricyclic antidepressants (increase thermoset point via action at the anterior hypothalamus). Withdrawal from ethanol, barbiturates, benzodiazepines, and sedative hypnotics also increases thermoset point via action at the anterior hypothalamus, as well as producing excessive muscular activity with consequent increased heat production. Dystonic reactions due to butyrophenones, phenothiazines, and metoclopramide can stimulate excess muscular activity as well. Salicylate toxicity can cause increased heat production. Parasympatholytic agents (anticholinergics, antihistamines, antiparkinsonism agents, phenothiazines, and tricyclic antidepressants) decrease sweating, with consequent decreased heat dissipation.

F. **Miscellaneous disorders.** Including pulmonary embolus with infarction, myocardial infarction, inflammatory bowel disease, and Addisonian crisis. Deep venous thrombosis, hematoma formation, alcoholic hepatitis, Jarisch-Herxheimer reaction, or central fever due to CNS process.

G. **Fever of unknown origin (FUO).** Manifested by fever > 38.3°C (101.0°F) on several occasions for a duration of at least 3 weeks, with no definite etiology. When an etiology is uncovered for an FUO, it usually falls into one of three categories: infection, malignancy, or autoimmune process.

H. **Unknown source.** 18% in one series of inpatients.

I. **Factitious (self-induced) fever**

IV. Database

A. Physical examination key points

1. **General appearance.** This factor can help determine whether the patient should receive empiric antibiotic therapy based on the most likely etiology.
2. **Vital signs.** Take both oral and rectal temperatures. Neutropenia is a contraindication to taking rectal temperature. A rectal temperature should be taken to make sure the oral temperature is not falsely elevated secondary to recent consumption of a hot liquid or smoking. The rectal temperature is usually 1°F higher than the oral temperature. Check pulse and blood pressure to make sure the patient is hemodynamically stable. Hypotension suggests sepsis or volume depletion, possibly secondary to the fever. (The heart rate should increase 9 bpm for each 1°F increase in temperature.) If the heart rate does *not* increase

(*pulse-temperature dissociation*), consider psittacosis (*Chlamydia psittaci*), brucellosis, typhoid fever (*Salmonella typhi*), atypical pneumonia (*Mycoplasma, Chlamydia pneumoniae, Moraxella catarrhalis, Legionella pneumophila*), and malaria.

3. **Skin.** Check IV sites, if any. Examine skin for rashes; if a rash involves the palms and soles, consider Rocky Mountain spotted fever, secondary syphilis, and Stevens-Johnson syndrome (hypersensitivity drug reaction). Look for splinter hemorrhages under the fingernails, Osler nodes, and Janeway lesions, which suggest endocarditis.
4. **HEENT.** Look for evidence of conjunctivitis, sinusitis (can be caused by an indwelling nasogastric tube), otitis, and pharyngitis. Cotton-wool spots and flame hemorrhages on funduscopic examination could indicate systemic candidiasis, endocarditis, or cytomegalovirus. Conjunctival hemorrhages are seen with endocarditis as well as severe thrombocytopenia.
5. **Neck.** Check for meningeal signs, including Kernig's and Brudzinski's signs.
6. **Lymph nodes.** Including cervical, supraclavicular, epitrochlear, axillary, and inguinal nodes. May suggest cause of fever such as lymphoma or focus the examination to a particular area.
7. **Lungs.** A unilateral increase in tactile fremitus, dullness to percussion, bronchial breath sounds, inspiratory crackles, egophony, and whispered pectoriloquy suggest pneumonia.
8. **Heart.** A murmur, especially a new regurgitant murmur, suggests endocarditis.
9. **Abdomen.** Listen for bowel sounds; palpate and percuss for signs of tenderness. Check for *Murphy's sign* (while palpating the right upper quadrant, tenderness is elicited and there is inspiratory arrest with deep inspiration), which is seen in cholecystitis. Examine for costovertebral angle tenderness suggesting pyelonephritis.
10. **Genitourinary system.** Exclude pelvic inflammatory disease (PID) or tubo-ovarian abscess in a female and epididymitis or orchitis in a male. Also check prostate for tenderness.
11. **Extremities.** Check intravenous sites for erythema and tenderness. Look for joint effusions or tenderness.

B. Laboratory data

1. **Complete blood count with differential.** An elevated WBC count and left shift suggest an infectious etiology. Eosinophilia suggests drug reaction or parasitic infection. A low WBC count may suggest overwhelming sepsis, a collagen vascular disease such as SLE, a viral infection, or a process that has replaced the normal bone marrow (lymphoma, carcinoma, or a granulomatous disease such as tuberculosis or histoplasmosis).
2. **Blood cultures.** Usually two sets; three sets if endocarditis is suspected.

3. **Culture tips of central lines.** If a patient with a central venous catheter becomes febrile and diagnostic evaluation fails to reveal a source of infection, the venous catheter is assumed to be the culprit and must be removed. Be sure to culture the tip of the catheter. One may try to treat prior to removing the catheter in patients with indwelling intravenous catheters (eg, Hickman and Groshong catheters).
4. **Sputum Gram's stain.** Request a Gram's stain if there is a productive cough.
5. **Urinalysis and culture.** Rule out cystitis, prostatitis, or pyelonephritis. Sterile pyuria suggests tuberculosis or, if the WBCs are eosinophils (interstitial nephritis), possibly a drug reaction.
6. **Miscellaneous tests.** In certain circumstances if clinically indicated: liver function tests, erythrocyte sedimentation rate, C-reactive protein (CRP), hepatitis serologies, PPD and anergy screen, culture for acid-fast bacillus and fungus, examination of peripheral blood smear, *Legionella* titers, viral titers, fungal serologies, rapid plasma reagin (RPR), DFA stains for *Pneumocystis* and *Legionella, Legionella* urine antigen, *Histoplasma* urine antigen, stool stains for fecal leukocytes, enteric pathogens, *C difficile* toxin, antistreptolysin-O (ASO) titer, antinuclear antibody (ANA), lumbar puncture.

C. Radiologic and other studies

1. **Chest x-ray.** CXR should be obtained with a fever of unknown source.
2. **Sinus CT.** If sinus tenderness or discharge is present or if a nasogastric tube has been in place.
3. **Acute abdominal series.** Should be obtained if peritoneal signs are present or if bowel or viscus obstruction or perforation is suspected.
4. **Ultrasound.** To assess the gallbladder and biliary tree. Can also be used to detect abdominal, renal, and pelvic masses.
5. **HIDA scan.** If acute cholecystitis is suspected.
6. **Bone scan/MRI.** If osteomyelitis is suspected.
7. **CT scans.** To detect subphrenic, abdominal, pelvic, and intracranial lesions.
8. **Echocardiogram.** Especially if blood cultures are positive. Sensitivity is not high enough that a normal transthoracic echocardiogram rules out endocarditis; however, transesophageal echocardiography has a 90% sensitivity.
9. **Lumbar puncture.** In any patient with fever and unexplained mental status changes as well as any patient with suspected meningitis (see Section III, Chapter 10, Lumbar Puncture, p 412).
10. **Thoracentesis.** Should be performed with unexplained fever and a pleural effusion or with pneumonia and a pleural effusion (see Section III, Chapter 14, Thoracentesis, p 431).

V. Plan. The plan depends on the clinical setting. Many of the previously mentioned tests should be obtained only in certain circumstances, and only if a previous workup has been unrevealing. The initial workup of a febrile patient late at night will not be as exhaustive as a more leisurely performed FUO evaluation.

A. Initial assessment

1. **Rule out hemodynamic instability.**
2. **Review medications.** Especially looking for any recent changes.
3. **Obtain appropriate cultures.** Blood from at least two different sites if possible.
4. **Reduce patient's temperature.** Give antipyretics such as acetaminophen 650 mg PO or PR. If the patient has underlying cardiac disease, the temperature should be brought down quickly to avoid cardiac decompensation.
5. **Monitor for dehydration.** Insensible losses will increase with a fever.
6. **Consider antibiotics.** If the patient is *hemodynamically stable* and there is no apparent source of infection, *it is often prudent to withhold antibiotics.* As noted in the differential, the causes of fever are many and often nonbacterial. Unneeded empiric antibiotics will confuse the issue in many cases.

B. Fever with hypotension. *Septic shock is a medical emergency.* Begin fluid resuscitation with normal saline through a large-bore IV or central line, place the patient in Trendelenburg position, begin appropriate antibiotics, and transfer to an ICU. The antibiotics chosen should provide coverage for gram-positive and gram-negative aerobic and anaerobic bacteria unless the source of the sepsis is obvious. If the patient's blood pressure fails to respond to fluids, begin a dopamine infusion at 2–5 μg/kg/min. The use of IV steroids is not warranted unless you suspect Addisonian crisis.

C. IV catheter infection. Remove the offending peripheral IV, apply local heat, use anti-inflammatory agents if it is a peripheral site, and administer antibiotics. A first-generation cephalosporin (cephalothin or cephalexin) or nafcillin can be used. Vancomycin should be reserved for use in suspected or culture-proven methicillin-resistant *Staphylococcus aureus* (MRSA) infection or *Staphylococcus epidermidis.* If you feel a warm, tender, swollen vein or the patient has a history of IV drug abuse, suspect septic thrombophlebitis. Obtain a surgery consult immediately and begin antibiotics. If a central line is in place, change all line(s) to different site(s), culture the catheter tip(s), and begin antibiotics. Gram-positive organisms are likely causes.

D. Pneumonia. Initial treatment of pneumonia should be based on results of Gram's stain and the clinical picture. Recent guidelines suggest that community-acquired pneumonia in a normal host requiring hospitalization should be treated with a fluoroquinolone (such as levofloxacin) alone OR a third-generation cephalosporin (ceftriaxone or cefotaxime) PLUS a macrolide combination OR a beta-lactam/beta-lactamase inhibitor (such as Unasyn or Zosyn) PLUS a macrolide. With a severe community-acquired pneumonia (altered mental status, pulse > 125 bpm, respiratory rate > 30 per minute, SBP < 90, temperature < 35°C or > 40°C), treatment should consist of a macrolide OR fluoroquinolone PLUS a third-generation cephalosporin OR beta-lactam/beta-lactamase inhibitor combination; if *Pseudomonas aeruginosa* is suspected (as in a patient with cystic fibrosis), then empiric therapy should provide double coverage consisting of an antipseudomonal cephalosporin (ceftazidime or cefepime) OR antipseudomonal penicillin such as ticarcillin or piperacillin, OR a carbapenem (imipenem) AND an aminoglycoside OR a fluoroquinolone. Hospital-acquired pneumonia or pneumonia in an immunocompromised host also requires broader coverage. Antipseudomonal coverage as outlined above must be considered. Caution is advised when administering aminoglycosides to patients with renal insufficiency. A Gram's stain can also be helpful in guiding therapy. If there are gram-positive cocci in clusters, the chosen antibiotic regimen should include vancomycin until the possibility of MRSA is excluded. Be sure to adjust the dose of vancomycin with renal insufficiency.

E. **Febrile, neutropenic patient.** If there is evidence of infection or fever with an absolute neutrophil count (ANC) below 500/μL, the patient should be immediately pancultured (body fluid cultures as indicated, eg, blood and urine) and broad-spectrum antibiotics initiated. The specific pathogens found are almost always pyogenic or enteric bacteria or certain fungi. These are usually endogenous to the patient and include *Staphylococcus* from skin and gram-negative organisms from the GI or urinary tract. In febrile neutropenic patients who were bacteremic, one study found that 46% of the isolated organisms were gram-positive (as high as 60–70% in one reference), 42% were gram-negative, and 12% were polymicrobial. Antibiotic coverage should therefore include both gram-positive and gram-negative bacteria. One may treat with one drug, such as ceftazidime, imipenem, cefepime, or meropenem; or two drugs, such as an aminoglycoside (amikacin, gentamicin, or tobramycin) plus an antipseudomonal beta lactam (ceftazidime, piperacillin, ticarcillin, ticarcillin plus clavulanate). An aminoglycoside may be added, depending on how toxic the patient's condition appears. Vancomycin should be added if the patient is at high risk (serious catheter-related infections, significant mucosal damage from chemotherapy, use of prophylactic quinolone antibiotics, septic shock or cardiovascular compromise, colonization with penicillin or cephalosporin-resistant *Streptococcus pneumoniae* or with MRSA, and positive blood cultures for gram-positive bacteria prior to determination of antibiotic susceptibility). An antifungal agent (amphotericin B) should be added on day 5–7 if the absolute neutrophil count remains $< 500/\text{mm}^3$ and the patient remains febrile despite antibiotics. Neutropenia with infection is a medical emergency requiring immediate investigation and treatment.

F. **Meningitis.** *Meningitis is a medical emergency.* A lumbar puncture should be done as quickly as possible, especially if there is no history of a bleeding disorder and no focal neurologic deficits or papilledema and you have no reason to suspect an intracranial abscess. Begin giving antibiotics as you are doing the lumbar puncture. If for any reason there is a delay in performing the lumbar puncture (such as obtaining a CT scan of the head because of papilledema), the antibiotics should be administered immediately and not delayed until after the procedure. A third-generation cephalosporin such as cefotaxime (Claforan) or ceftriaxone (Rocephin) should be given for meningitis of unknown etiology. Empiric therapy for meningitis should also cover for *Listeria monocytogenes* (ampicillin) if the patient is immunocompromised or over 50 years old. Vancomycin should be included if there is a high rate of penicillin-resistant pneumococcus in the community. Vancomycin and ceftazidime would be recommended for patients with a CNS shunt, recent neurosurgery, or head trauma. Otherwise, antibiotic therapy should be adjusted based on the Gram's stain. Acyclovir should be added if herpes simplex virus meningoencephalitis is suspected.

G. **Cholecystitis.** Obtain an ultrasound and/or HIDA scan, begin antibiotics (ticarcillin/clavulanate or gentamicin plus ampicillin plus metronidazole, *or* imipenem/cilastatin) and consult surgery.

H. **Drug-induced fever.** Discontinue all drugs possibly causing a drug fever and substitute appropriate alternatives.

I. **Thyroid storm.** Treat with hydration, apply cooling blanket, and give saturated solution of potassium iodide (SSKI), beta-blockers (specifically propranolol), propylthiouracil, and glucocorticoids.

J. **Addisonian crisis.** Treat immediately with IV steroids such as dexamethasone 4 mg for 1 dose, perform Cortrosyn stimulation test, and then begin a glucocorticoid (hydrocortisone 100 mg IV push, then 100 mg IV Q 6–8 hr). Dexamethasone will not interfere with the Cortrosyn stimulation test.

K. **Malignant neuroleptic syndrome.** Treatment consists of discontinuation of the neuroleptics, general supportive measures, and consideration of dantrolene (Dantrium) 50 mg PO Q 12 hr.

L. **Uncertain or unknown diagnosis.** Remember to consider pulmonary infarction and myocardial infarction.

REFERENCES

Bohr D: Fever of unknown origin. In: Fletcher SW, Fletcher RH, Aronson MD, editors-in-chief. UpToDate [CD-ROM]. Version 8.1. Wellesley, MA;2000. www.uptodate.com

Hughes WT, Armstrong D, Bodey GP et al: 1997 Guidelines for the use of antimicrobial agents in neutropenic patients and unexplained fever. Clin Infect Dis 1997;25:551.

Infectious Diseases Society of America: Practice guidelines for the management of community-acquired pneumonia in adults. Clin Infect Dis 2000;31:347.

Mackowiak PA: Temperature regulation and the pathogenesis of fever. In: Mandell GL, Bennett JE, Dolin R, ed. *Principles and Practice of Infectious Diseases.* 5th ed. Churchill Livingstone;2000:604.

O'Grady NP, Barie PS, Bartlett JG et al: Practice guidelines for evaluating new fever in critically ill adult patients. Clin Infect Dis 1998;26:1042.

Quagliarello VJ, Scheld MW: Treatment of bacterial meningitis. N Engl J Med 1997;336:708.

23. FEVER IN THE HIV-POSITIVE PATIENT

I. Problem. A 35-year-old man presents to the emergency room with a fever to 102.5°F for 2 days. The patient is known to be HIV-positive but has not yet had an AIDS-defining illness.

II. Immediate Questions

A. Have there been any constitutional symptoms, including headache, anorexia, weight loss, fatigue, or malaise? Any of these can occur periodically through the course of HIV, and may occur more frequently in the late stages of the disease. Night sweats are sometimes reported but are most often secondary to an infectious process or lymphoma.

B. What is the fever history? When did it start? How high has the temperature risen? HIV-related fever is usually no higher than 102.0°F. Symptoms such as chills and rigors are uncommon with HIV-related fever, and are more often associated with bacterial infections. Elevation of temperature above 102°F strongly suggests an opportunistic infection. Remember, however, that nonopportunistic pathogens (eg, *Streptococcus pneumoniae, Haemophilus influenzae*) are potential causes of pneumonia in an HIV patient, and should be considered as etiologic agents along with opportunistic pathogens.

C. Are there any specific symptoms? Your physical examination and further laboratory testing will be directed by specific symptoms, such as a history of visual problems, dysphagia, cough and dyspnea, diarrhea, focal neurologic symptoms, mental status changes, or skin lesions. Headache may be a constitutional symptom or a symptom associated with specific central nervous system (CNS) diseases. About one-half of patients with *Toxoplasma gondii* infections of the CNS complain of headache.

D. Does the patient have AIDS? What was the last CD4 count? If the patient has AIDS, what was the indicator disease? This presentation could be a recurrence since many of the infectious agents associated with AIDS recur, such as *Pneumocystis carinii, Salmonella typhi, Cryptococcus neoformans,* and *T gondii.* Certain infections do not occur until the CD4 count is very low (< 50/mL), such as *Mycobacterium avium-intracellulare* (MAI).

III. Differential Diagnosis. There are multiple causes of fever in this setting. The HIV-positive patient is a special problem because you must consider not only opportunistic infections seen frequently in this population but also other causes of fever that occur in non–HIV-positive patients. (See Section I, Chapter 22, Fever, p 127). Most opportunistic infections occur when the CD4 count is < 200/mL; they are especially common when the CD4 count is < 50/mL.

A. Drug fever. Antiretroviral agents rarely cause a fever, but zidovudine (AZT) and zalcitabine (ddC) may cause fever. Antimicrobials, such as sulfonamides, are common causes of fever.

B. Sinusitis. Bacterial sinusitis may occur at any time during the course of HIV infection but is more severe in the later stages. Presentation may include headache, fever, or congestion. Likely pathogens include *S pneumoniae, H influenzae,* and *Staphylococcus aureus.*

C. Eye disease. Retinitis can occur at low CD4 counts, especially < 50/mL. The most common etiology is cytomegalovirus (CMV). Presentation includes floaters, blurred vision, and visual field defects. Pain is not a symptom of CMV retinitis; fever is nonspecific and frequently absent. Patients with the above symptoms should immediately be seen by an ophthalmologist. CMV retinitis characteristically has a "spaghetti and cheese" appearance (whitish exudate with surrounding edema and hemorrhage). Other organisms that cause retinitis include Varicella-zoster virus, *Toxoplasma,* and *P carinii.* Other eye diseases include optic neuritis, conjunctival Kaposi's sarcoma, and herpetic keratitis.

D. Oral disease. Oral disease rarely causes fever but may signify more widespread disease. For example, darkly pigmented nodular lesions on the hard palate suggest widespread Kaposi's sarcoma.

E. Pulmonary disease. Pulmonary disease with fever can be caused by a wide variety of bacteria, fungi, viruses, protozoa, and tumors.

1. **Bacterial pneumonia.** Common organisms include *S pneumoniae* and *H influenzae.* In addition to fever, cough, pleuritic chest pain, sputum production, an increased white blood cell (WBC) count may be present. Focal infiltrates are usually seen on chest x-ray (CXR).
2. **Acid-fast organisms.** Consider *Mycobacterium tuberculosis* (TB) if fever has been present for > 2 weeks. Remember that HIV patients may present more frequently with extrapulmonary signs and symptoms. TB occurs most frequently at CD4 counts < 500/mL, but can occur at any time during the course of the disease regardless of the CD4 count. A negative PPD does not rule out TB, especially at low CD4 counts. CXR findings vary from the classical apical cavitary lesion to hilar adenopathy, nodules or infiltrates in any lung field, or a normal CXR (14% in one series). MAI may also cause diarrhea as well as fever and pulmonary disease.

Often MAI occurs very late in the course of the disease (CD4 counts < 50/mL).

3. **Parasitic infections.** *Pneumocystis carinii* pneumonia (PCP) tends to have a prodromal illness for 1–2 weeks. PCP is the most common indicator disease for AIDS. Progressive dyspnea, nonproductive cough, and fever are common symptoms. Diffuse bilateral interstitial pulmonary infiltrates are frequently seen on CXR. An increased lactate dehydrogenase level may be present.

F. **Cardiac disease.** Consider endocarditis, especially if a new murmur is present.

G. **Gastrointestinal disease**

1. **Esophagitis** generally presents with dysphagia. *Candida* esophagitis may or may not present with fever. Other common causes of esophagitis are CMV and herpes simplex virus (HSV).
2. **Diarrhea.** Often fever and abdominal pain accompany low-volume diarrhea and mucoid stools. Depending on the etiologic agent, blood may be present. *S typhi* often causes recurrent bacteremia and diarrhea. Other bacterial pathogens may include *Campylobacter jejuni, Shigella flexneri, Clostridium difficile,* and MAI, as well as enterotoxigenic *Escherichia coli.* CMV and a variety of parasites including *Cryptosporidium, Isospora belli,* and *Microsporidia* may cause diarrhea and fever. *Histoplasma capsulatum* can also cause diarrhea.

H. **Hepatobiliary/pancreatic disease**

1. **Sclerosing cholangitis-like syndrome.** Fever, RUQ pain, and progressive cholangitis have been described in patients with CMV and *Cryptosporidium* involving the biliary tract.
2. **Hepatitis B or C**
3. **Cholestatic hepatitis.** Secondary to MAI, TB, *H capsulatum, C neoformans.*
4. **Pancreatitis.** May occur as a result of an opportunistic infection, increased triglycerides, or drug toxicity (eg, pentamidine).

I. **Skin.** Bacillary angiomatosis thought to be secondary to *Bartonella* (*Rochalimaea*) *henselae* causes firm purplish-to-reddish papules, subcutaneous nodules, or cellulitis-like plaques. HSV type I or II may cause primary or recurrent erythematous/vesicular lesions with ulceration.

J. **Neurologic disease.** Many agents can cause a variety of neurologic complications, including meningitis, encephalitis, and mass lesions.

1. **Meningitis.** HIV can initially cause an aseptic meningitis. *C neoformans* is a common cause of meningitis; presenting symptoms include fever, night sweats, and headaches. *M tuberculosis* as well as *S pneumoniae, H influenzae,* and *Neisseria meningitidis* need to be considered as etiologic agents.
2. **Encephalitis.** *T gondii* causes altered mental status, headache, fever, and focal neurologic findings.

3. **Mass lesions** can be caused by a variety of infectious agents (*T gondii, M tuberculosis, Nocardia asteroides, C neoformans, H capsulatum*) and noninfectious agents (primary CNS lymphoma, metastatic lymphoma, and Kaposi's sarcoma).

K. **Malignant disease.** Malignancies, including B-cell non-Hodgkin's lymphoma, Kaposi's sarcoma, and Hodgkin's lymphoma, may have associated fever.

L. **Gynecologic complications.** Gynecologic complications, including sexually transmitted disease (*Neisseria gonorrhoeae, Chlamydia trachomatis*), can cause fever as well as a vaginal discharge and pain.

IV. Database

A. Physical examination key points

1. **General appearance.** First, determine whether the patient appears ill or septic.
2. **Vital signs.** Should be evaluated for hypotension and tachycardia, either of which may be a sign of sepsis.
3. **HEENT.** Perform ophthalmologic exam to check for papilledema and signs of retinitis. Palpate sinuses for tenderness; inspect oral cavity for signs of candidiasis or hairy leukoplakia.
4. **Neck.** Check for neck stiffness as a sign of meningitis; however, meningeal signs are often absent in AIDS patients with meningitis. Palpate for lymphadenopathy. Check the jugular veins for distension to help assess fluid status.
5. **Lungs.** Percuss the lungs for dullness, which may occur with a focal infiltrate. Dullness at one base may indicate a pleural effusion. Auscultate for inspiratory crackles as a sign of consolidation.
6. **Heart.** Determine rate and note any murmurs.
7. **Abdominal exam.** Note any hepatomegaly or splenomegaly, and look for signs of peritoneal inflammation.
8. **Extremities/skin.** Note general appearance of the skin; look for any rashes, papules, or nodules.
9. **GU/rectal.** Inspect genitalia, noting presence and characteristics of any discharge. Examine the rectum for perineal abscess.
10. **Neurologic exam.** Should be *thorough,* including mental status examination.

B. Laboratory data.

Proceed with your workup based on findings from the history and physical examination. Many times specific aspects of the patient's history and physical will point you to a specific organ system. When only constitutional symptoms are present, diagnostic testing should include complete blood count and differential, electrolytes, liver function tests, and blood for bacterial, acid-fast bacteria (AFB), and fungal cultures. A CXR should also be obtained.

1. **Complete blood count with differential.** An elevated WBC count with an increase in banded neutrophils suggests a bacterial

infection. The total WBC and lymphocyte count will often decrease, especially late in HIV disease. In addition, many medications (eg, AZT) can suppress the WBC count.

2. **Liver function tests** (AST, ALT, bilirubin, GGT, alkaline phosphatase). Look for abnormalities suggesting hepatitis, cholangitis, or liver involvement from a systemic disease.
3. **Arterial blood gases (ABG).** Essential in the evaluation of cough and dyspnea. Hypoxemia is almost universally present with PCP.
4. **Urinalysis.** Pyuria with bacteria suggests a urinary tract infection. Sterile pyuria could result from *M tuberculosis* or fungal involvement of the urinary tract.
5. **Electrolytes, blood urea nitrogen (BUN), and creatinine.** To help assess volume status.

C. Other studies

1. **Stool tests.** If diarrhea is present, you need to obtain stool for WBCs, culture for enteric pathogens, *C difficile* toxin, fungal smear and culture, and AFB stain and culture. In addition, stool will need to be carefully examined for parasites such as *Cryptosporidium.*
2. **Sputum studies.** Expectorated sputum should be sent for Gram's stain, culture and sensitivity, AFB stain and culture, and fungal stain and culture. *P carinii* can be diagnosed in about 10% of cases via a silver stain of expectorated sputum. Sputum for AFB smear and culture should be obtained in an HIV patient with a fever and cough even if the CXR is normal.
3. **Blood cultures.** Essential in the evaluation of an HIV patient with a fever. Fungi and mycobacteria as well as bacteria are potential isolates.
4. **Serum cryptococcal antigen test.** Order this test if meningitis is suspected; 70–90% of patients with cryptococcal meningitis have a positive serum cryptococcal antigen test. May also be helpful in a patient with a fever without neurologic symptoms or signs. Also consider if CD4 count is < 50/mL.
5. **Lumbar puncture.** Should be performed with mental status change, meningeal signs, or focal neurologic findings. An imaging study should be done first to rule out a space-occupying lesion. Be sure to obtain cerebrospinal fluid (CSF) for cryptococcal antigen. The sensitivity of the AFB smear of CSF for diagnosing *M tuberculosis* will increase with larger amounts of fluid and with repeated lumbar punctures.
6. **Chest x-ray.** Essential in the initial evaluation of an HIV patient with a fever or cough and dyspnea. Look for infiltrates, pleural effusions, or cavitary lesions.
7. **CNS imaging.** Necessary with mental status changes and symptoms or signs of CNS disease such as papilledema. Look for a space-occupying lesion, which may be secondary to primary lymphoma, metastatic lymphoma, Kaposi's sarcoma, *T gondii,* or

M tuberculosis. Magnetic resonance imaging is more sensitive than computerized tomography scans and is the preferred modality to image the CNS in this setting.

8. **Bronchoscopy.** With brushings and bronchoalveolar lavage. Essential in the evaluation of an HIV patient with an infiltrate on CXR whose sputum does not reveal the etiology.

V. **Plan.** The treatment of various causes of fever in the HIV patient is beyond the scope of this book. Refer to references specific to this topic. Discussed below are the treatments for the more common causes of fever in the HIV patient and salient points.

A. **General.** See Section I, Chapter 22, Fever, V, p 132.

B. **Specific infectious causes**

1. ***Pneumocystis carinii* pneumonia**. First line of treatment is trimethoprim (TMP)-sulfamethoxazole (SMX) PO or IV (15–20 mg/kg/d TMP and 75–100 mg/kg/d SMX in 3–4 divided doses q day). Pentamidine 4 mg/kg/day q day, or dapsone 100 mg/d with TMP, can be used. Atovaquone 750 mg bid is reserved for patients who cannot tolerate TMP-SMX or pentamidine. Corticosteroids (prednisone 40 mg bid for 5 days followed by a taper) should be given if the initial pO_2 is < 70 mm Hg.
2. ***Mycobacterium tuberculosis*.** Four first-line drugs should be used initially, including isoniazid (INH) 300 mg once q day; rifampin 600 mg once q day; pyrazinamide (PZA) 20–35 mg/kg/d, once q day; and ethambutol 25 mg/kg or streptomycin 0.5–1 g q day to 1 g twice weekly. There is an increasing incidence of multi-drug resistant tuberculosis, especially in HIV-infected patients. Strict respiratory isolation must be observed. Consider use of corticosteroids (prednisone 60 mg PO q day for 1–2 weeks followed by a taper) with tuberculous meningitis.
3. **Cytomegalovirus retinitis.** Give ganciclovir or foscarnet.
4. **Cryptococcal meningitis.** Amphotericin B, 0.5–0.7 mg/kg/d with or without flucytosine 150 mg/kg/day in divided doses every 6 hr.
5. ***Toxoplasma gondii** infection.* Pyrimethamine and sulfadiazine or clindamycin. Will also need folinic acid to prevent myelosuppression from the pyrimethamine.

REFERENCES

Bissuel F, Leport C, Perronne C et al: Fever of unknown origin in HIV-infected patients: A critical analysis of a retrospective series of 57 cases. J Intern Med 1994;236:529.

Carrier J: MAC infections in HIV infected patients. In: Fletcher SW, Fletcher RH, Aronson MD, editors-in-chief. UpToDate [CD-ROM]. Version 8.1. Wellesley, MA;2000. www.uptodate.com

Falloon J: Pulmonary manifestations of human immunodeficiency virus infection. In: Mandell GL, Bennett JE, Dolin R, eds. *Principles and Practice of Infectious Diseases.* 5th ed. Churchill Livingstone;2000:1415.

Holloway RG, Kieburtz KD: Neurologic manifestations of human immunodeficiency virus infection. In: Mandell GL, Bennett JE, Dolin R, eds. *Principles and Practice of Infectious Diseases.* 5th ed. Churchill Livingstone;2000:1432.

Sande M, Volberding P: *Medical Management of AIDS.* 4th ed. Saunders;1995.

Sepkowitz K, Talzak E, Carrow M et al: Fever among outpatients with advanced human immunodeficiency virus infection. Arch Intern Med 1993;153:1909.

Sulkowski MS, Chaisson RE: Gastrointestinal and hepatobiliary manifestations of human immunodeficiency virus infection. In: Mandell GL, Bennett JE, Dolin R, eds. *Principles and Practice of Infectious Diseases.* 5th ed. Churchill Livingstone;2000:1426.

Vander Els N: Clinical features and diagnosis of TB in HIV infected patients. In: Fletcher SW, Fletcher RH, Aronson MD, editors-in-chief. UpToDate [CD-ROM]. Version 8.1. Wellesley, MA;2000. www.uptodate.com.

24. FOLEY CATHETER PROBLEMS

(See also Section III, Chapter 4, Bladder Catheterization, p 394).

I. **Problem.** The Foley catheter is not draining in a patient admitted 2 days previously for congestive heart failure.

II. **Immediate Questions**

A. **What has the urine output been?** If the urine output has slowly tapered off, then the problem may be oliguria rather than a nonfunctioning Foley catheter. A Foley catheter that has never put out urine may not be in the bladder.

B. **Is the urine grossly bloody; are there any clots in the tubing or collection bag?** Clots or tissue fragments, such as those present after prostate or bladder resection, can obstruct the flow of urine in a Foley catheter.

C. **Is the patient complaining of any pain?** Bladder distension often causes severe lower abdominal pain; bladder spasms are painful and may cause urine to leak out around the catheter rather than through the catheter.

D. **Was any difficulty encountered in catheter insertion?** Problematic urethral catheterization should raise the possibility that the catheter is not in the bladder. Patients with known pathologic conditions (urethral structure, benign prostatic hypertrophy, prostate cancer, etc) may be at higher risk of faulty catheter placement.

III. **Differential Diagnosis**

A. **Low urine output.** It may be a result of dehydration, hemorrhage, or acute renal failure, as well as a host of other causes (see Section I, Chapter 51, Oliguria/Anuria, p 266).

B. **Obstructed Foley catheter**

1. **Kinking of catheter or tubing**
2. **Clots, tissue fragments.** Most common after transurethral resection of the prostate or bladder. Grossly bloody urine suggests a clot

has formed. "Tea"-colored or "rusty" urine suggests an organized clot may be present even though the urine is no longer grossly bloody. Bleeding will often accompany "accidental" catheter removal with the balloon still inflated and with a coagulopathy.

3. **Sediment/stones.** Chronically indwelling catheters (usually > 1 month) can become encrusted and obstructed. Calculi can lodge in the catheter.

C. **Improperly positioned Foley catheter.** These problems are much more common in males. In traumatic urethral disruption associated with a pelvic fracture, the catheter can pass into the periurethral tissues. Strictures or prostatic hypertrophy may cause the end of the catheter to be positioned in the urethra and not the bladder. Improper catheter placement technique can cause a false passage.

D. **Bladder spasms.** The patient may complain of severe suprapubic pain or pain radiating to the end of the penis. With a spasm, urine may leak around the sides of the catheter. Spasms are common after bladder or prostate surgery or surgery near the bladder. Spasms may be the only catheter complaint or may be so severe as to obstruct the flow of urine.

E. **Bladder disruption.** Resulting from blunt abdominal trauma or operative complication, or caused by severe distension secondary to a blocked catheter.

F. **Inability to deflate Foley balloon.** Rare with modern catheters. All catheters should be test inflated and deflated before insertion.

IV. Database

A. Physical examination key points

1. **Vital signs.** Check for tachycardia or hypotension, which is characteristic of hypovolemia and may explain the low urine output.
2. **Abdominal exam.** Determine if the bladder is distended (suprapubic dullness to percussion with or without tenderness); may be indicative of an obstructed Foley catheter. Percuss the bladder to help identify distension.
3. **Genital exam.** Bleeding at the meatus suggests urethral trauma or partial removal of the catheter with the balloon inflated.
4. **Rectal exam.** A "floating prostate" suggests urethral disruption.
5. **General.** Look for signs of hypovolemia causing low urine output, such as poor skin turgor (which may be a normal variant in the elderly) and dry mucous membranes.

B. **Laboratory data.** Most problems are usually mechanical in nature, so laboratory data are somewhat limited in this setting.

1. **Blood urea nitrogen (BUN), serum creatinine.** Elevations may be seen with cases of renal insufficiency. An elevated BUN-to-creatinine ratio (> 20:1) suggests volume depletion.
2. **Coagulation studies.** Especially if bleeding is present. See Section I, Chapter 12, Coagulopathy, p 66.

C. **Radiologic and other studies.** In the acute setting of a Foley catheter problem, radiologic studies are usually not needed. Ultrasound may demonstrate hydronephrosis in cases of obstructive uropathy, or ultrasound may be used to guide puncture of the balloon as a last resort.

V. **Plan**

A. **Be sure the catheter is functioning.** A rule of thumb is that a catheter that will not irrigate is in the urethra and not in the bladder. Start by gently irrigating the catheter with aseptic technique using a catheter-tipped 60-mL syringe and sterile normal saline. This may dislodge any clots obstructing the catheter. If sterile saline cannot be satisfactorily instilled and completely aspirated, the catheter should be replaced. Catheter irrigation or changing the catheter in any patient who has undergone bladder or prostate surgery should not be done without input from the surgical team that performed the procedure.

B. **If the catheter irrigates freely, evaluate the patient for anuria.** See Section I, Chapter 51, Oliguria/Anuria,V, p 273.

C. **Bladder spasms.** Can be treated with oxybutynin (Ditropan), propantheline (Pro-Banthine), or belladonna and opium (B&O) suppositories. (See Section VII, Therapeutics, p 555, 565, 485 for dosing). Be sure to discontinue these medications before removing the catheter to allow normal bladder function.

D. **Techniques to deflate a balloon that will not empty**

1. Injection of 5–10 mL mineral oil into the inflation port will cause balloon rupture in latex catheters in 5–10 minutes. Follow-up cystoscopy is needed to make sure there are no retained fragments. (*Note:* Hyperinflation of the balloon to rupture it should not be done.)
2. Cut off the valve; if this does not work, thread a 16 Fr central venous catheter or 0.38 guide wire into the inflation channel, which may bypass the obstruction or perforate and deflate the balloon.
3. As a last resort, ultrasound-directed transvesical needle puncture of the balloon may be needed.

REFERENCE

Shahbandi M, Parulkar BG: Foley catheter problems. In: Gomella LG, ed. *5 Minute Urology Consult.* Lippincott Williams & Wilkins;2000:50.

25. HEADACHE

I. **Problem.** You are called to the emergency room to evaluate a 58-year-old man who complains of a severe headache that has lasted for several hours.

II. **Immediate Questions**

A. **Has the patient experienced similar headaches before?** If the headache is similar to previous tension or migraine headaches, then the situation is unlikely to be urgent; however, if the headache is new or deviates from a previous pattern, several potentially serious conditions should be considered, including acute glaucoma, sinusitis, subarachnoid hemorrhage, meningitis, neoplasm, and early hypertensive encephalopathy.

B. **What are the patient's vital signs?** Although essential hypertension by itself is an infrequent cause of headache, it may exacerbate a preexisting vascular or tension headache. Diastolic blood pressures > 140 mm Hg can cause severe headache. A fever should alert the clinician to the possibility of subarachnoid hemorrhage, meningitis, temporal arteritis, or acute sinusitis.

C. **Is the patient taking any anticoagulants?** Is there a predisposition to bleeding? Aspirin or coumadin increases the risk for an intracranial hemorrhage, especially with minor head trauma. Spontaneous intracranial bleeding occurs with platelet counts of less than 20,000/μL.

III. **Differential Diagnosis.** A detailed, well-focused history is the most important tool for evaluating headache. The great majority of headaches are secondary to either tension-type or migraine headaches. A headache may also be the only symptom of a more serious condition, such as an intracranial mass, temporal arteritis, meningitis, and subarachnoid hemorrhage.

A. **Tension-type headache**

1. **Episodic tension-type headache.** This is frequently described as a squeezing, "bandlike" tightness that is usually felt bilaterally. It may occur in the occipital, frontal, or bitemporal regions. Occasionally, patients with tension-type headaches may describe a "throbbing" pain. This form of headache may last minutes to days; it is generally described as having a mild to moderate intensity.
2. **Chronic tension-type headache.** This headache is similar to the acute tension-type in quality but its duration may be months or even years. Depression, personality problems, and a history of narcotic abuse are common in these patients.

B. **Migraine headache.** Although the precise pathophysiology has not been fully ascertained, it is thought to be secondary to cerebral vasoconstriction followed by vasodilation. The initial vasoconstriction may be associated with a variety of neurologic deficits including visual disturbances (scotoma, zig-zag lines, bright lights), dysarthria, hemiparesis, and hemianesthesia. Of these, the visual phenomena are most common. These neurologic features generally last 5–30 minutes and are then followed by headache. The headache is usually pounding or throbbing but may be dull and boring. It is usually unilateral but may also occur bilaterally in any location. Anorexia, nausea, and vomiting are frequently associated. The attack may last several hours to 2–3 days and occasionally longer. Migraines are much more common in women. Three characteristic migraine patterns are recognized:

1. **Migraine without aura (common migraine).** This vascular headache is not preceded by neurologic deficits or visual disturbances. It is the most common type, especially in women.
2. **Migraine with aura (classic migraine).** The headache is preceded by visual deficits such as scotomata and field deficits, but can affect somatic sensation, speech, and motor function.
3. **Complicated migraine.** The headache is accompanied by neurologic symptoms including hemiplegia and ophthalmoplegia.

C. **Cluster headaches.** Cluster headaches are excruciating, usually unilateral, and frequently associated with ipsilateral nasal congestion, lacrimation, and conjunctival injection. Nausea, vomiting, photophobia, and phonophobia are absent in cluster headaches. Each headache typically lasts < 2 hours; however, multiple attacks can occur within a 24-hour period.

Onset shortly after falling asleep is common. Unlike migraine, cluster headaches most often affect men between the ages of 20 and 40. They are not familial.

D. **Temporal arteritis.** Temporal arteritis should be considered in any patient older than 50 years presenting with a recent history of headache. Other symptoms such as malaise, weight loss, fever, and myalgias are frequently present. Jaw claudication is a classic symptom. It is especially important to ask about any new visual problems such as double or blurred vision. Temporal arteritis can cause sudden blindness as a result of inflammation of the ophthalmic artery. Early diagnosis and treatment with steroids are necessary to prevent this complication.

E. **Trigeminal neuralgia.** This condition is more common in the elderly. The pain is described as brief, but severe and jabbing. The pain is usually unilateral and localized to one or more divisions of the trigeminal nerve. Precipitants include talking, chewing, or having physical pressure exerted on a specific trigger area. Etiology is unknown.

F. **Cerebrovascular disease.** Headache can be a presenting complaint in some patients experiencing an acute stroke. When the internal carotid is involved, the headache is usually located in the frontal region; involvement of the vertebrobasilar system generally yields an occipital headache. The headache of a cerebrovascular accident may precede or follow focal neurologic symptoms.

G. **Sinusitis.** Headache is usually dull, aching, and located frontally. Pain is frequently worse in the morning when the patient awakens but improves as the sinuses drain during the day. If the patient displays an altered mental status or complains of a stiff neck, a complicated sinus infection should be suspected (brain abscess, meningitis, septic cavernous sinus thrombosis).

H. **Eye disease.** Glaucoma, keratitis, and uveitis all may cause headaches. The pain is usually dull and located in the periorbital or retroorbital regions.

I. **Dental disease.** The teeth are innervated by the second and third divisions of the trigeminal nerve; thus, disease involving these structures may cause pain referred to the face or head. Secondary muscle spasm may result.

J. **Temporomandibular joint disease.** Headache is usually unilateral on the side of face and head. It is described as "aching" in quality and is worsened with jaw movement.

K. **Mass lesions.** Both neoplasm and brain abscess can produce headache as a result of either increased pressure or distension of local structures. Any new neurologic deficit such as visual or motor loss or change in mental status should alert the clinician to the possibility of a mass lesion. Onset of new headache in a patient greater than 50 years old suggests a mass lesion. Nonspecific features of headache resulting from a mass lesion include progressive worsening despite administration of analgesics; early-morning headache; headache exacerbated by coughing or sneezing; anorexia; and vomiting without nausea. It is important to note that these features also occur frequently with other types of headache, including chronic tension headache, migraine headache, cluster headache, and sinus headache.

L. **Subarachnoid hemorrhage.** The rupture of a cerebral aneurysm is associated with acute onset of a violent headache. The typical patient with a subarachnoid hemorrhage has a sudden onset of severe headache (frequently described as the worst headache of his or her life) that develops during exertion. Transient loss of consciousness or buckling of the legs often accompanies the headache. Vomiting soon follows. Between 20% and 50% of patients with documented subarachnoid hemorrhage report a distinct, unusually severe headache in the days or weeks before the index episode of bleeding, referred to as a *warning headache.*

These so-called *thunderclap headaches* develop in seconds, achieve maximal intensity in minutes, and last hours to days.

The differential diagnosis includes subarachnoid hemorrhage, acute expansion, dissection, or thrombosis of unruptured aneurysms; cerebral venous sinus thrombosis, brief headaches during exertion and sexual intercourse, and benign thunderclap headaches. The physical exam may show retinal hemorrhages, restlessness, a diminished level of consciousness, and focal neurologic signs. Blood in the subarachnoid space may induce fever and nuchal rigidity resembling acute meningitis. Sentinel leaks (warning leaks) from a cerebral aneurysm are more subtle and frequently precede subsequent rupture. These headaches may be difficult to distinguish from tension headaches and may cause nonspecific symptoms such as myalgias or a stiff neck, which may be erroneously attributed to an acute viral illness.

M. **Carotid or vertebral artery dissection.** Unilateral head, face or neck pain, and a partial *Horner's syndrome* (miosis and ptosis without anhidrosis) with subsequent retinal or cerebral ischemia is the classic presentation of carotid artery dissection. The headache may be similar to the headache associated with subarachnoid hemorrhage ("thunderclap headache") but the onset is usually insidious. Unilateral facial or orbital pain is common. Transient ischemic attacks or transient monocular blindness occurs hours to days after the onset of the pain. An occipital headache or neck pain followed by unilateral arm pain or weakness suggests vertebral artery dissection.

N. **Acute febrile illness.** Fever may cause a vascular-type throbbing headache that remits as the illness resolves. Any febrile patient in whom headache is a major complaint should also be suspected of having meningitis, especially if nuchal rigidity or other signs of meningeal irritation are present.

IV. Database

A. Physical examination key points

1. **Vital signs.** See II.B.
2. **HEENT**
   a. **Scalp.** Patients with both migraine and chronic tension headaches frequently complain of scalp tenderness, which may also suggest temporal arteritis.
   b. **Temporal arteries.** A diminished pulse or tender temporal arteries suggests arteritis; however, temporal arteries may feel normal to palpation in 30–40% of patients with temporal arteritis.
   c. **Eyes.** Examine for injected conjunctivae and excessive lacrimation, which occur with cluster headaches. Miosis and ptosis suggest carotid artery dissection as the cause of the headache. Examine the fundi for any signs of papilledema or optic nerve atrophy resulting from an intracerebral mass. Retinal hemorrhage may be observed after subarachnoid hemorrhage. Subhyaloid hemorrhages may be seen trapped behind the vitreous humor at the edge of the optic disc, suggesting a sudden rise in intracranial pressure.
   d. **Sinuses.** Palpate or percuss the maxillary and frontal sinuses for tenderness.
   e. **Ears.** Examine the ears for any signs of otitis media.
   f. **Mouth.** Examine dentition for painful teeth and the temporomandibular joint for any crepitus, pain, or limited jaw opening.
3. **Neck.** Examine for any resistance to passive flexion of the neck, which would suggest meningeal irritation from either subarachnoid hemorrhage or meningitis.
4. **Neurologic exam.** A detailed exam is mandated in any patient with a complaint of headache to identify localizing signs that

would suggest a CNS mass lesion, meningitis, intracerebral hemorrhage, or carotid or vertebral artery dissection.

B. **Laboratory data**
   1. **Complete blood count.** An elevated leukocyte count could suggest infection such as sinusitis or meningitis.
   2. **Erythrocyte sedimentation rate (ESR).** Almost always greater than 50 mm/h with temporal arteritis; however, on occasion the ESR may be normal. If clinical suspicion is high, a temporal artery biopsy should never be deferred simply because of a normal ESR.
   3. **Prothrombin time (PT), partial thromboplastin time, (PTT), and platelets.** If you suspect or if the patient has an intracranial hemorrhage.

C. **Radiologic and other studies**
   1. **Sinus films or CT with coronal images.** If sinusitis is suspected.
   2. **Head CT scan.** Should be obtained in any patient with a chronic headache pattern that has recently changed in frequency or severity, progressive worsening of a headache despite appropriate therapy in any patient greater than 50 years old with a new onset of headache, or if the neurologic exam reveals any focal findings. Additionally, a head CT scan should be obtained in any patient with onset of headache that is exacerbated with exertion, cough, or sexual activity; or in any patient with orbital bruit.

      Helical CT angiography is useful in diagnosing carotid artery dissection and intracranial aneurysms.
   3. **MRI.** Preferable when posterior fossa lesions or craniospinal abnormalities (eg, Arnold-Chiari malformation) are suspected. MR angiography is replacing conventional angiography as the test of choice in diagnosing carotid or vertebral artery dissection and can be used to diagnose intracranial aneurysms.
   4. **Lumbar puncture.** If meningitis is suspected, lumbar puncture should be performed and not delayed for a CT scan when papilledema is absent and the neurologic examination is nonfocal. Lumbar puncture should be performed when subarachnoid hemorrhage is suspected and CT results are negative, equivocal, or technically inadequate.

V. **Plan.** The initial goal in the management of headache is to exclude rare but potentially serious causes, such as brain tumor, subarachnoid hemorrhage, brain abscess, and meningitis. When these conditions have been excluded, treatment can be directed according to the type of headache. Only the management of tension-type headache, migraine headache, and cluster headache is discussed here.

A. **Episodic tension-type headache**
   1. **Nonsteroidal anti-inflammatory drugs (NSAIDs).** Relief of pain can usually be obtained with simple analgesics like aspirin, acetaminophen, or NSAIDs.

2. **Avoid analgesic combinations.** Such as ergotamines, caffeine, butalbital, and codeine.

B. **Chronic tension-type headache.** This condition is notoriously difficult to manage. As with episodic tension-type headache, avoid the chronic use of narcotic analgesics, which may result in narcotic dependence. Also inquire about the possibility of overused drugs, because withdrawal of daily analgesics enhances the effect of prophylactic drugs.

1. **A tricyclic antidepressant.** Amitriptyline (Elavil) 75 mg HS is one of the most useful agents for treating chronic tension headache. This medication should be used regardless of whether depression is overtly present.
2. **Nonsteroidal anti-inflammatory drugs (NSAIDs).** Aspirin 325–650 mg PO Q 6 hr, naproxen 275–550 mg Q 12 hr, or ibuprofen 400–600 mg PO Q 6 hr may be beneficial.
3. **Massage of the neck and local application of heat.** When occipital, suboccipital, or cervical muscle spasm is present.
4. **Psychotherapy, relaxation therapy, and biofeedback.** May be used if preceding measures fail.

C. **Migraine headache.** Several different medications are now administered in the management of acute migraine.

1. **NSAIDs.** For an early mild attack, treatment with a NSAID such as ibuprofen 400–600 mg Q 4–6 hr or naproxen (Naprosyn) 550 mg Q 12 hr may be effective. Metoclopramide (Reglan) 10 mg PO can be given at this time to increase drug absorption and reduce nausea and vomiting. In addition, ketorolac, a parenteral NSAID, has been shown to be effective at 60 mg IM.
2. **Ergot alkaloids**
   a. **Ergotamine tartrate (Cafergot) 1 mg.** Two tablets PO at onset of the headache followed by one tablet Q 30 min to a maximum of six tablets in 24 hours (most effective if taken early in an attack).
   b. **Dihydroergotamine 1 mg.** IV/IM/SC Q hour for three doses can also be administered. This regimen is especially useful in patients whose headache has been present for several hours or who cannot tolerate oral drugs because of nausea.
   c. ***Caution:*** Avoid administration of ergotamines in patients with peripheral vascular disease (PVD), coronary artery disease, hypertension, renal failure, hepatic disease, and hyperthyroidism, and in pregnant patients. Because ergot alkaloids decrease cerebral blood flow, they should be avoided in patients with complicated migraine.
3. **Sumatriptan (Imitrex) 6 mg SC.** (Other regimens and routes are available). Sumatriptan has been found to be effective in relieving the headache and accompanying symptoms (nausea, vomiting, and photo- and phonophobia). It is effective even when taken late

during an attack. A second dose is usually not effective. ***Caution:*** The triptans are contraindicated in patients with known or suspected ischemic heart disease, a history of angina, ischemic or vasospastic (Prinzmetal's) angina, uncontrolled hypertension, peripheral vascular disease, recent monoamine oxidase inhibitor therapy, severe liver disease, and hemiplegic or basilar artery migraine. The safety of the triptans during pregnancy is unclear. Use with ergotamines is contraindicated.

4. **Zolmitriptan (Zomig) 2.5 mg.** Give 1 tablet PO at the onset of headache. Repeat at 2 hours if the headache returns, not to exceed 10 mg in 24 hours. One study has found zolmitriptan, 2.5 mg and 5 mg, to be at least as effective as sumatriptan, 25 mg or 50 mg, in the acute treatment of migraine. ***Caution:*** See above for triptans.
5. **Isometheptene 65 mg/dichloralphenazone 100 mg/acetaminophen 325 mg (Midrin).** Give 2 capsules at onset of headache followed by 1 capsule Q 1 hour to maximum of 5 capsules in 24 hours.
6. **Prochlorperazine (Compazine) 25 mg IV.** This medication has been shown in some controlled trials to be superior to dihydroergotamine in migraine relief.
7. **Lidocaine intranasally.** May provide rapid relief of migraine headache. However, relapse of headache is common and occurs early after treatment.
8. **Prophylactic therapy.** Several medications can be used for prophylaxis of migraine, including propranolol (Inderal), amitriptyline (Elavil), and verapamil (Calan). These medications are less useful in the management of an acute migraine and will not receive further discussion here. In addition, naproxen (Naprosyn) has been shown to be effective in migraine prophylaxis.

D. Cluster headaches

1. **Oxygen.** Inhalation by face mask at 7 L/min for 10 minutes has been reported to be successful in aborting a cluster headache. Greatest benefit is obtained in patients younger than 50 years of age with episodic cluster headache.
2. **Sumatriptan.** Found to be effective in aborting cluster headache in some patients and is administered as described above for migraine headaches.
3. **Lidocaine.** Locally applied 1 cc of 4% lidocaine nasal drops has been reported to be effective. Patients lie supine with the head tilted backward toward the floor at 30 degrees and turned to the side of the headache. Fifteen minutes after the initial dose, the dose may be repeated once.
4. **Prophylactic therapy.** The mainstay of therapy and involves the use of such medications as ergotamine, verapamil, prednisone in a tapering dose, lithium carbonate, methysergide (Sansert), and valproate. Prophylactic therapy should be started early. The pa-

tient should use medications daily until he or she is headache free for at least 2 weeks, and then taper the medications.

REFERENCES

Abramowicz M, ed: Drugs for migraine. Med Lett Drug Ther 1995;37:17.
Bartleson JD: Treatment of migraine headaches. Mayo Clin Proc 1999;74:702.
Dalessio DJ: Diagnosing the severe headache. Neurology 1994;44:S6.
Edlow JA, Caplan LR: Avoiding pitfalls in the diagnosis of subarachnoid hemorrhage. N Engl J Med 2000;342:29.
Gallagher RM, Dennish G, Spierings ELH et al: A comparative trial of zolmitriptan and sumatriptan for the acute oral treatment of migraine. Headache 2000;40:119.
Kumar KL, Cooney TG: Headaches. Med Clin North Am 1995;79:261.
Maizels M, Scott B, Cohen W et al: Intranasal lidocaine for treatment of migraine: A randomized, double-blind, controlled trial. JAMA 1996;276;4.
Matthew N: Cluster headache. Semin Neurol 1997;17;4.
Schievink WI: Intracranial aneurysms. N Engl J Med 1997;336:28.
Schievink WI: Spontaneous dissection of the carotid and vertebral arteries. N Engl J Med 2001;344:898.
Welch KMA: Drug therapy for migraine. N Engl J Med 1993;329:1476.

26. HEART MURMUR

I. **Problem.** You are asked to see a 50-year-old man complaining of acute shortness of breath. The nursing staff notes a loud murmur.

II. **Immediate Questions**

A. **Is the murmur itself responsible for the problem, or is it a sign of some other underlying problem?** Acute aortic or mitral regurgitation from endocarditis or acute mitral regurgitation resulting from rupture of a papillary muscle after a myocardial infarction (MI) could explain the patient's condition. Underlying medical conditions such as severe anemia, hyperthyroidism, and pregnancy can also have associated "innocent" flow murmurs related to increased cardiac output.

B. **Does the patient have known valvular disease?** Progression of valvular dysfunction may be the cause of deterioration in such a patient.

C. **Does the patient have known congenital heart disease?** In a patient with a history of a murmur, bicuspid aortic valve, atrial septal defect (ASD), ventricular septal defect (VSD), patent ductus arteriosus (PDA), and pulmonic stenosis (PS) should always be considered. Often, patients with mild PS or a small ASD will be asymptomatic.

D. **Has the deterioration been chronic or acute?** Acute decompensation would suggest an acute process such as endocarditis or myocardial ischemia. Chronic deterioration would suggest increasing ventricular dysfunction from preexisting valvular disease.

E. **Is there a history of IV drug abuse, recent dental work, invasive procedures such as a sigmoidoscopy or cystoscopy, evidence**

of embolism such as stroke, or a history of fever or chills? These factors would suggest endocarditis.

F. **Does the patient have any chest pain?** If so, it is important to characterize the chest pain. Chest pain is often seen with angina, aortic dissection, and pericarditis. (See Section I, Chapter 11, Chest Pain, p 57). Angina is one of the three presenting symptoms (syncope and dyspnea secondary to congestive heart failure [CHF]) of hemodynamically significant aortic stenosis.

G. **Does the patient have coronary artery disease, and if so, is this the etiology of the murmur?** A recent MI with papillary muscle dysfunction or rupture may result in acute mitral regurgitation. An acute VSD or free wall rupture following an MI can cause a new murmur. Hypertrophic obstructive cardiomyopathy (also called idiopathic hypertrophic subaortic stenosis [IHSS]) and aortic dissection can cause angina.

III. Differential Diagnosis

A. Murmur aggravated by an underlying problem

1. **Flow murmur.** A flow murmur may be caused by or aggravated by a significant anemia or thyrotoxicosis and resultant high-outflow CHF.
2. **Congestive heart failure with "secondary" mitral regurgitation.** Can result from a variety of etiologies, most notably severe dilated cardiomyopathy.
3. **Murmur of aortic insufficiency with possible aortic dissection.** Always consider an underlying connective tissue disorder such as Marfan syndrome as well as severe hypertension.
4. **Noncardiac murmur.** Thyroid or carotid bruits, subclavian artery stenosis, venous hums, and pericardial or pleural friction rubs all can be mistaken for a cardiac murmur.
5. **A new murmur in a patient with known bacteremia or sepsis.** An ominous finding and requires emergent evaluation.

B. Coronary artery disease

1. **Acute ischemia/injury with papillary muscle dysfunction.** Can cause reversible mitral regurgitation.
2. **Recent myocardial infarction**
   a. **Acute severe mitral regurgitation secondary to ruptured chordae tendineae or head of a papillary muscle**
   b. **Acute VSD**
   c. **Acute rupture of the ventricular wall**
3. **Acute ischemia.** Leading to immediate, severe left ventricular dysfunction with pulmonary edema and new or worsening mitral regurgitation.

C. Valvular heart disease

1. **Mitral valve prolapse with ruptured chordae/papillary muscle head and CHF.** Arrhythmias (ventricular or atrial) may lead to decompensation.

2. **Mitral stenosis.** New-onset atrial fibrillation can lead to decompensation.
3. **Aortic stenosis.** With progression may result in angina, left ventricular dysfunction, syncope, or arrhythmias (especially ventricular).
4. **Hypertrophic obstructive cardiomyopathy.** Arrhythmias, angina, and dyspnea are common. Sudden death can occur and is often related to exertion.
5. **Prosthetic valve dysfunction.** A regurgitant murmur is an alarming finding in a patient with a prosthetic valve.
6. **Severe stenosis or regurgitation of any valve (especially mitral or aortic).** Can lead to left ventricular dysfunction and associated symptoms.

D. **Congenital heart disease**
1. **ASD/VSD with right-to-left shunt, causing systemic hypoxemia.** Results in pulmonary hypertension or Eisenmenger's syndrome.
2. **New dysrhythmias in a patient with previously stable congenital defects.** Can cause acute deterioration, especially atrial fibrillation.

E. **Atrial myxoma.** A rare cause of a murmur; may present with CHF, chest pain, syncope, arrhythmias, constitutional symptoms (eg, fever, weight loss) or an embolic event, mimicking endocarditis, collagen vascular disease, or occult malignancy.

IV. Database

A. **Physical examination key points**
1. **General.** Inability to lie flat suggests pulmonary edema, pericarditis, or pericardial effusion.
2. **Vital signs**
   a. **Temperature.** Elevated temperature might indicate infection (endocarditis), although postinfarct patients can have a moderate fever for up to a week. A fever from any etiology can cause or intensify a flow murmur.
   b. **Heart rate and rhythm.** Tachycardia (see Section I, Chapter 60, Tachycardia, p 323) is often associated with CHF, pain, infection, pericarditis, and perhaps arrhythmias. Irregular rhythm (see Section I, Chapter 45, Irregular Pulse, p 238) may suggest the presence of atrial fibrillation or frequent premature atrial or ventricular beats as well as second-degree atrioventricular block.
   c. **Blood pressure.** Hypertension or hypotension is often associated with angina or MI. Hypotension could reflect sepsis or hemodynamic collapse. A widened pulse pressure may suggest aortic insufficiency. *Pulsus paradoxus* (a difference of 10 mm Hg in systolic blood pressure between tidal inspiration and expiration) points to pericardial tamponade.

d. **Tachypnea.** Suggests CHF, or decreased perfusion or hypoxia from any cause such as a VSD with a right-to-left shunt.

3. **Neck**

a. **Elevated jugular venous distension.** Suggests right-sided ventricular failure or pericardial tamponade.

b. **A decrease in the carotid upstroke.** Suggests significant aortic stenosis. Also, the murmur of aortic stenosis radiates to the carotids bilaterally and should not be confused with bilateral carotid bruits, a venous hum, or a thyroid bruit.

4. **Cardiovascular.** Careful cardiac examination is essential. Palpate the carotid pulsations and for displacement of the apical impulse or a cardiac thrill. First (S_1) and second (S_2) heart sounds and splitting of S_2 must be characterized. The presence of a fourth heart sound (S_4) may suggest a recent MI, hemodynamically significant aortic stenosis, or long-standing hypertension. A third (S_3) heart sound is consistent with ventricular dysfunction.

a. **Flow murmur.** A mid-systolic murmur with normal carotid upstroke is present.

b. **Aortic insufficiency.** A diastolic blowing murmur *is* heard best at the right second intercostal space down to the left lower sternal border with the patient leaning forward in full expiration. This may occur with acute aortic dissection or acute bacterial endocarditis, or may be chronic. The aortic component of S_2 may be soft or absent. The murmur of acute aortic insufficiency is usually soft in intensity and short in duration, is heard best at the left lower sternal border, and can easily be missed. The carotid upstroke is sharp, followed by a rapid downstroke (*Corrigan's,* or *water-hammer, pulse*).

c. **Aortic stenosis.** This systolic murmur is crescendo-decrescendo and harsh; it is heard best at the right second intercostal space. Critical aortic valve stenosis is characterized by the absence of the aortic component of S_2, a palpable S_4 gallop at the apex, late peaking of the maximal intensity of the murmur, a palpable carotid thrill (usually over the left carotid artery), and a diminished and delayed carotid upstroke (*pulsus parvus et tardus*).

d. **Mitral regurgitation.** It is heard best as a blowing pansystolic murmur at the apex, radiating to the axilla and occasionally into the midback. An intermittent murmur of mitral regurgitation might suggest intermittent papillary muscle dysfunction secondary to ischemia or other causes. The murmur of acute, severe mitral regurgitation may be short in duration and soft in intensity. Other findings associated with severe mitral regurgitation include an S_3 gallop, tachycardia, pulmonary rales, and signs of poor peripheral perfusion.

e. **Mitral valve prolapse.** A mid-systolic click followed by a late systolic murmur suggests mitral valve prolapse. A click or murmur may be present together or singly. Squatting delays the onset of the click and murmur.

f. **Mitral stenosis.** This mid-diastolic murmur is heard best in the left lateral decubitus position with the bell of the stethoscope positioned over the apical impulse. An opening snap may be heard between S_2 and the diastolic rumble. Mitral stenosis is often missed, particularly in a sick patient. It is always an important consideration; a confirmatory echocardiogram is usually indicated. An otherwise stable patient with mitral stenosis will decompensate quickly when atrial fibrillation develops. Control of the heart rate to permit adequate diastolic filling is beneficial.

g. **Hypertrophic cardiomyopathy.** Characteristically it causes a systolic murmur that might be confused with aortic stenosis, but actually represents reversible left ventricular outflow tract obstruction secondary to hypertrophy of the interventricular septum. The murmur is a crescendo-decrescendo systolic murmur that increases in intensity with the Valsalva maneuver and standing, and decreases in intensity with squatting. The murmur is best heard at the apex and left lower sternal border. An S_4 gallop is usually present. A bisferiens contour to the carotid pulse is characteristic (double peaking of the pulse). Again, rapid decompensation occurs in the face of new onset atrial fibrillation.

h. **Atrial septal defect/ventricular septal defect.** An ASD murmur may be difficult to hear. Widely fixed splitting of S_2 is a clue to the presence of an ASD. VSDs are usually heard over the entire precordium; the murmur is holosystolic and a thrill is frequently present.

i. **Atrial myxoma.** An apical diastolic or systolic murmur will be encountered more commonly than a third heart sound (*tumor plop*).

5. **Extremities.** Examine distal pulses, for a pulse deficit that might suggest the presence of dissection or embolic phenomena. Clubbing is seen in cyanotic heart disease and bacterial endocarditis. *Quincke's sign* (a to-and-fro movement seen in the capillary bed of the fingers when light pressure is applied to the distal fingertip) is seen in chronic severe aortic insufficiency.
6. **Neurologic exam.** Focal neurologic deficits may occur with subacute bacterial endocarditis, myxoma, and thrombus formation with embolus. Funduscopic exam should be done to survey for stigmata of embolic disease (*Roth spots*).
7. **Skin.** Look for any evidence of IV drug use or embolic phenomena, like subcutaneous nodules at the fingertips (*Osler nodes*), splinter hemorrhages under the fingernails, and petechiae (particularly of the conjunctivae and mucous membranes), that might suggest bacterial endocarditis.

B. **Laboratory data.** Clearly, these depend on the history and exam. The order in which laboratory data are acquired depends on the clinical picture.

1. **Complete blood count with differential.** Anemia can cause high-output CHF. A significantly elevated WBC count with an increase in the percentage of banded neutrophils indicates the presence of a bacterial infection. An elevated WBC count can accompany an acute MI.
2. **Blood culture.** Should be obtained if there is any question of endocarditis. Three sets of two cultures should be obtained over several hours if the patient is stable. If the patient is unstable, at least one set of blood cultures should be obtained before antibiotic therapy is initiated.
3. **Arterial blood gases.** Acidosis (see Section I, Chapter 2, Acidosis, p 9) and hypoxia suggest the presence of significant left ventricular compromise and pulmonary congestion in an ill patient with a new murmur.
4. **Thyroid function tests, electrolytes including magnesium, renal function tests.** These may determine the etiology as well as reflect the effects of a disease process.

C. **Radiologic and other studies**

1. **Electrocardiogram.** The most useful test to screen for myocardial ischemia, MI, or dysrhythmia, particularly atrial fibrillation. Keep in mind that the abrupt onset of atrial fibrillation in a person with compensated CHF, stable hypertrophic cardiomyopathy, or stable valvular disease may cause rapid decompensation.
2. **Chest x-ray.** The cardiac silhouette may give a clue to valvular disease, such as left atrial enlargement in mitral stenosis. Increased vascularization, pleural effusion, Kerley A and B lines, and confluent alveolar densities are radiographic evidence of pulmonary edema. Other signs to look for are cardiac chamber enlargement and mediastinal widening, and presence of prosthetic valves.
3. **Echocardiogram.** In evaluating an acutely ill patient with a murmur that is not easily identified, the echocardiogram may be the single best source of information. It can accurately determine the presence and degree of valvular stenosis or regurgitation. The etiology of the valvular problem can also be suggested. Atrial and ventricular septal defects can be detected.
4. **Swan-Ganz catheterization.** From a diagnostic standpoint, one can obtain right atrial and pulmonary artery blood samples to diagnose a stepup in oxygen saturation, confirming the diagnosis of acute VSD. Acute or severe mitral regurgitation can be suggested by the presence of significant V waves in the pulmonary capillary wedge pressure tracing.

V. **Plan.** Treatment is generally aimed at the condition that is either causing the murmur (MI, papillary muscle dysfunction, VSD, aortic insufficiency in the face of aortic root dissection) or aggravating the condition for which the murmur is a secondary finding (hyperthyroidism, new-onset atrial fibrillation, endocarditis, thrombus on a mechanical valve or anemia). While one is initiating therapy, consultation should be considered. When a patient is symptomatic from a cardiac murmur, a cardiology consult is appropriate.

A. **Relieve angina.** This may result in prompt improvement in cases of recurrent pulmonary edema secondary to ischemia. See Section I, Chapter 11, Chest Pain, V, p 63.

B. **Maintain hemodynamic support**
   1. **Dopamine.** Can be used if an arterial vasoconstricting agent is needed. See Section I, Chapter 42, Hypotension, V., p 227.
   2. **Dobutamine.** Should be used if a positive inotropic drug is required.

C. **ICU monitoring.** Certain pathologic conditions may require arterial pressure monitoring (see Section III, Chapter 1, Arterial Line Placement, p 390) or continuous monitoring of right heart pressures and pulmonary wedge pressure (see Section III, Chapter 12, Pulmonary Artery Catheterization, p 421).

D. **Treatment of acute myocardial infarction**
   1. **Pain relief.** Relieve pain with nitroglycerin, IV beta-blockers, and morphine sulfate. (See Section I, Chapter 11, Chest Pain, Section V, p 63; or Section VII, Therapeutics, pp 551, 601, and 546 respectively, for doses.)
   2. **Thrombolysis.** If indicated and if the patient is an appropriate candidate.

E. **Treatment of suspected endocarditis after obtaining three sets of blood cultures.** Initiate empiric antibiotic therapy, being mindful of the presence of bioprostheses (eg, valves, hips), IV drug abuse, or infective focus.

F. **Arrange for invasive evaluation if warranted.** The evaluation of an unknown heart murmur in a critically ill patient can be extremely complex. The basic goal is to determine the possible etiologies as quickly as possible. Emergent evaluation with an echocardiogram, aortic root contrast injection, or surgical consultation may be indicated depending on the patient's condition.

REFERENCES

Banning AP: Valvular disease: The GP's key role. Practitioner 1999;243:740.

Braunwald E, Perloff JK: Physical examination of the heart and circulation. In: Braunwald E, Zipes DP, Libby P, eds. *Heart Disease: A Textbook of Cardiovascular Medicine.* 6th ed. Saunders;2001:45.

DeGowin RL, Brown DD: *DeGowin's Diagnostic Examination.* 7th ed. McGraw-Hill;2000:247.

27. HEMATEMESIS, MELENA

I. **Problem.** A 56-year-old male is admitted to the hospital because of pneumonia; you are called because he "vomited blood."

II. **Immediate Questions**

A. **What are the patient's vital signs?** Is there supine hypotension (indicates 30% volume loss)? Is there resting tachycardia (indicates 20% volume loss)? Are there orthostatic changes in pulse or blood pressure (indicates 10% volume loss)? If the patient has supine hypotension or resting tachycardia, fluid resuscitation must begin immediately.

B. **Does the patient have adequate IV access?** With no indication of hemodynamic instability, one 16- to 18-gauge IV with D5 NS at KVO is adequate. In the presence of hemodynamic compromise, two large-bore (14–16 gauge) IVs should be in place.

C. **Is there a prior history of gastrointestinal problems? Is there a history of peptic ulcer disease (PUD), liver disease, or esophageal varices?** A previous history of these disorders may indicate the etiology; however, in only 50% of patients with known esophageal varices can upper GI bleeding be attributed to variceal bleeding. Has the patient ever been evaluated or treated for *Helicobacter pylori?*

D. **Is the patient taking any medications?** Review medications. Note particular use of nonsteroidal anti-inflammatory drugs (NSAIDs), aspirin, steroids, and anticoagulants. Anticoagulants may unmask significant pathology or aggravate insignificant lesions.

E. **Does the patient smoke, or have a family history of PUD?** Both are risk factors for PUD.

F. **Does the patient have a history of alcohol abuse?** This suggests gastritis or varices as the source of bleeding. Ethanol alone is not an etiologic factor for peptic ulcer disease, unless there is accompanying cirrhosis. Alcohol use is also a risk factor for a Mallory-Weiss tear.

G. **Is there a previous hematocrit?** It will be important to establish a baseline with which to monitor the patient.

H. **Is there a history of abnormal liver function studies?** Suggests occult liver disease.

I. **What is the volume of hematemesis?** Ask the nurse to save the emesis. This is important to establish the volume of hematemesis as well as to validate the presence of blood. A large amount indicates more urgency. Indiscriminate use of Hemoccult to document blood is not recommended. The visual appearance is much more reliable.

J. **Has there been any melena or bright red blood per rectum?** Acute upper GI tract blood loss of about one unit results in melena; two units may cause hematochezia.

III. Differential Diagnosis

A. Peptic ulcer disease. PUD accounts for 50% of upper GI hemorrhages. The use of NSAIDs is the single most important risk factor for PUD and bleeding.

B. Esophageal varices. Accounts for 10% of upper GI bleeding. Esophageal varices have the highest morbidity and mortality of all causes of upper GI bleeding. (See Section I, Chapter 28, Hematochezia, p 162).

C. Mallory-Weiss tear. Causes ~ 5–15% of upper GI bleeding. Associated with recent heavy alcohol intake in 30–60% of cases. Vomiting often precedes the hematemesis.

D. Acute hemorrhagic gastritis. Accounts for 15% of community-acquired upper GI hemorrhage. Often associated with alcohol, NSAID use, and stress (severely ill ICU patients).

E. Carcinoma. Very seldom the cause of acute bleeding; almost always found in patients over 50 years old.

F. Aortoenteric fistula. A rare cause of upper GI hemorrhage, but can be quite dramatic. Should be suspected in patients who have had aortic bypass graft surgery. Of these fistulae, 75% communicate with the duodenum (3rd portion). Generally preceded by a self-limited episode of bleeding ("herald bleed").

IV. Database

A. Physical examination key points

1. **Vital signs.** Including orthostatic blood pressure and heart rate. *Orthostatic changes* are a decrease in systolic blood pressure of 10 mm Hg and/or an increase in heart rate of 20 bpm 1 minute after changing from supine to standing position. Vital signs need to be checked frequently until the patient is stable.
2. **Skin.** Spider telangiectasia, palmar erythema, and jaundice indicate underlying cirrhosis and possible varices. Poor skin turgor and absent axillary sweat may indicate volume depletion. Acanthosis nigricans and Kaposi's sarcoma are associated with GI malignancy.
3. **Eyes.** Scleral icterus suggests liver disease.
4. **Chest.** Gynecomastia suggests cirrhosis.
5. **Abdomen.** An increase in bowel sounds suggests upper GI bleeding. Hepatomegaly or splenomegaly suggests cirrhosis or cancer. An abdominal mass points to cancer. Tenderness in the epigastrium or LUQ suggests PUD. Ascites may be seen with cirrhosis and associated esophageal varices.
6. **Genitourinary system.** Rectal examination to look for melena or bright red blood per rectum. Testicular atrophy may be secondary to cirrhosis/chronic liver disease.

B. Laboratory data

1. **Stat complete blood count.** This can be done by phlebotomy before your arrival. Differential is not necessary.
2. **Type and cross-match.** At least four units of packed red blood cells (PRBCs).
3. **A nasogastric tube for gastric lavage.** This procedure is essential for accurate diagnosis. The possibility of varices is not a contraindication. Lavage until clear or at least only pink-tinged.
4. **Hematocrit.** Serial hematocrits are helpful; however, in acute hemorrhage the hematocrit may not reflect the amount of blood loss. The hematocrit may fall precipitously after aggressive fluid resuscitation.
5. **BUN and creatinine.** An increased BUN/creatinine ratio is seen in upper GI bleeding and volume depletion.
6. **PT, PTT, platelet count.** An elevated PT, PTT, or thrombocytopenia can interfere with stabilization of the patient. An elevated PT may be seen in chronic liver disease. Platelets and clotting factors are lost with rapid bleeding.

C. Radiologic and other studies. The source of bleeding must be identified so that specific therapy can be instituted.

1. **Upper GI endoscopy (EGD).** This is the cornerstone to diagnose upper GI tract bleeding; it should be performed as soon as possible after hemodynamic stabilization and adequate lavage.
   a. The optimal timing of EGD is not well established. Most experts believe that EGD should be performed within 24 hours. With the multitude of available therapeutic interventions, however, earlier endoscopy is considered preferable. Urgency of procedure is based on severity and/or ongoing nature of bleeding.
   b. It is important in patients with known alcoholic liver disease to distinguish varices from other sources of UGI bleeding and to direct therapy.
   c. Endoscopic appearance predicts outcome (active bleeding—55% rebleeding and 11% mortality; visible vessel—43% rebleeding and 11% mortality; adherent clot—22% rebleeding and 7% mortality; flat pigmented lesion—10% rebleeding and 3% mortality, and clean base—< 5% rebleeding and 2% mortality).
2. **Colonoscopy.** Should be performed if EGD is entirely negative and the patient has melena. Necessary to rule out a right-sided colonic lesion.
3. **Technetium-labeled bleeding scan.** Should be done if the upper GI endoscopy and colonoscopy are negative.

V. Plan

A. Monitoring. The first step in management is to determine whether the patient should be monitored in an ICU. The following are guidelines for admission to the ICU.

1. Clearly documented frank hematemesis.
2. Coffee-ground emesis *and* either melena or hematochezia.
3. Hemodynamic instability, either hypotension, tachycardia, or orthostatic hypotension.
4. A drop in hematocrit of 5 points after fluid resuscitation.
5. A significant unexplained increase in the BUN when GI bleeding is suspected.
6. High-risk patient: advanced age, inpatient status at time of bleed, recurrent or evidence of persistent bleeding, major comorbidity (hepatic, renal, pulmonary, or cardiac disease).

B. Volume resuscitation. If massive bleeding is evident, place two large-bore (14- or 16-gauge) IV lines. Begin IV fluids containing normal saline at a rate to maintain hemodynamic stability. Transfuse PRBCs when available for massive bleeding to keep the hematocrit above 30%. With massive bleeding, consider transfusing typed-uncrossmatched blood.

C. Surgical consult. Essential in the management of upper GI tract hemorrhage; should be obtained within the first few hours of the patient's arrival. If hemodynamic stability cannot be achieved, immediate surgical intervention may be necessary.

D. Specific treatment. The management of various sources of upper GI hemorrhage is dependent on the diagnosis.

1. **Peptic ulcer disease.** Pharmacologic therapy with proton pump inhibitors has recently been shown to help prevent rebleeding. The dose of omeprazole (Prilosec) is 40–60 mg per day. Omeprazole may require 24–48 hours to become maximally effective. H_2 receptor antagonists (Zantac, Tagamet, Pepcid) are not recommended for acute hemorrhage. Endoscopic therapies are effective to control bleeding and to prevent rebleeding. They include thermal probe, injection therapy, electrocoagulation, and laser.
2. **Acute hemorrhagic gastritis or esophagitis.** Acid reduction therapy. (See V.D.1.)
3. **Mallory-Weiss tear.** No specific therapy beyond supportive care. Thermal or electric probes have been used successfully.
4. **Esophageal varices.** Give octreotide bolus of 25–50 μg, followed by a continuous infusion of 25 μg/hr. If octreotide fails, then balloon tamponade should be considered. Endoscopic therapies include band ligation (preferred) and injection sclerotherapy.
5. **Aortoenteric fistula.** Surgical intervention is necessary.

REFERENCES

Besson I, Ingrand P, Person B et al: Sclerotherapy with and without octreotide for acute variceal bleeding. N Engl J Med 1995;333:555.

Cappell MS, ed: High risk gastrointestinal bleeding, Part I. Gastroenterol Clin North Am 2000;29:1.

Cappell MS, ed: High risk gastrointestinal bleeding, Part II. Gastroenterol Clin North Am 2000;29:275.

Consensus Conference: Therapeutic endoscopy and bleeding ulcers. JAMA 1989;262:1369.

Khuroo MS, Yattoo GN, Javid G et al: A comparison of omeprazole and placebo for bleeding peptic ulcer. N Engl J Med 1997;336:1054.

Laine L: Acute and chronic gastrointestinal bleeding. In: Feldman M, Scharschmidt BF, Sleisenger MH, eds. *Gastrointestinal and Liver Diseases: Pathophysiology/Diagnosis/Management.* 6th ed. Saunders;1998:198.

Laine L, Cook D: Endoscopic ligation compared with sclerotherapy for treatment of esophageal variceal bleeding: A meta-analysis. Ann Intern Med 1995;123:280.

Rockall TA, Logan RF, Devlin HB et al: Risk assessment after acute upper gastrointestinal hemorrhage. Gut 1996;38:316.

28. HEMATOCHEZIA

I. **Problem.** A 38-year-old man comes to the emergency room and states, "I have just passed a lot of blood from my bowels."

II. **Immediate Questions**

A. **What are the patient's vital signs?** Is there supine hypotension (indicates 30% volume loss)? Is there resting tachycardia (indicates 20% volume loss)? Are there orthostatic changes in pulse or blood pressure (indicates 10% volume loss)? If the patient has supine hypotension or resting tachycardia, resuscitation must begin immediately.

B. **Does the patient have IV line access?** With no indication of hemodynamic instability, one 16- to 18-gauge IV with D5 NS at KVO is adequate. In the presence of hemodynamic compromise, two large-bore IVs should be in place.

C. **Is there a history of previous gastrointestinal (GI) bleeding?** Ask about a history of diseases associated with lower GI bleeding, such as diverticular disease, colon polyps or carcinoma, inflammatory bowel disease, hemorrhoids, and other anal diseases. Inquire about prior upper GI bleeding and also peptic ulcer disease (PUD).

D. **What medications is the patient taking?** Ask specifically about steroids, nonsteroidal anti-inflammatory drugs (NSAIDs), and anticoagulants.

E. **Does the patient have a history of alcohol abuse?** This suggests the possibility of an upper GI source of bleeding such as varices or gastritis.

F. **What is the most recent hematocrit?** Obtain this information from previous visits. This will establish the baseline value with which to compare future hematocrits.

G. **What is the volume of bright red blood per rectum?** Ask the nurse to save the specimen or specimens for your inspection. This is important for establishing the presence and volume of blood loss. A large volume of blood suggests need for immediate action.

H. Has there been hematemesis? Acute severe upper GI blood loss may result in hematochezia.

III. Differential Diagnosis

A. Hemorrhoids. These account for 98% of all episodes of hematochezia. Usually not brought to the attention of a physician. Rarely significant but may be of concern in the presence of portal hypertension.

B. Diverticular disease. Causes up to 70% of significant lower GI bleeding.

C. Angiodysplasia. This condition is much more common in the elderly, causing approximately 10% of significant lower GI bleeding. Also seen with renal failure.

D. Upper GI bleeding. See Section I, Chapter 27, Hematemesis, Melena, p 158. UGI sources are responsible for 10% of hematochezia. Hematochezia from an upper GI bleed represents at least a two-unit bleed and is almost always associated with hemodynamic instability. *Always an indication for ICU monitoring.* Must be ruled out before surgical exploration for hematochezia.

E. Neoplasia including carcinoma and polyps. Causes 1–2% of significant lower GI tract bleeding.

F. Inflammatory bowel disease (IBD). Infrequent cause of significant lower GI tract bleeding. Bleeding is more likely with ulcerative colitis than with Crohn's disease. Bleeding from IBD is more common in younger patients.

G. Ischemic colitis. Seen in elderly patients, often with previous history or signs of vascular disease, such as a history of surgery for peripheral vascular disease or an abdominal bruit or history of atrial fibrillation.

IV. Database

A. Physical examination key points

1. **Vital signs.** Including orthostatic blood pressure and heart rate. A decrease in systolic blood pressure of 10 mm Hg, or an increase in the heart rate by 20 bpm 1 minute after movement from a supine position to standing, indicates volume depletion. May need to recheck frequently. An irregularly irregular pulse suggests ischemic colitis caused by emboli secondary to atrial fibrillation.
2. **Skin.** Telangiectasias or melanotic lesions on palms or soles suggest Osler-Weber-Rendu disease and Peutz-Jeghers syndrome, respectively. Look for peripheral stigmata of chronic liver disease

and lesions associated with GI cancer (acanthosis nigricans, Kaposi's sarcoma).

3. **HEENT.** Vascular malformations on lips or buccal mucosa suggest angiodysplasia or Osler-Weber-Rendu disease. Scleral icterus suggests chronic liver disease.
4. **Heart.** Aortic stenosis is associated with angiodysplasia.
5. **Abdomen.** Bruits suggest atherosclerosis and thus possible ischemic colitis. Hyperactive bowel sounds may indicate upper GI tract bleeding. Check for masses (cancer) or tenderness (midepigastric area: PUD). Hepatomegaly and splenomegaly suggest portal hypertension (varices) or cancer.
6. **Rectum.** Check for hemorrhoids, for a mass and to document blood in the rectal vault (melena, bright red blood, or guaiac-positive stools).

B. **Laboratory data**

1. **Nasogastric (NG) tube placement.** Obtain a quick aspirate for coffee-ground material (testing for occult blood should *not* be performed if coffee-ground material is not aspirated).
2. **Stat complete blood count; type and cross-match.** These can be done before you arrive if phlebotomy is available. Changes in the indices may also be helpful in differentiating acute from chronic bleeding.
3. **Serial hematocrits.** Can be spun without phlebotomy. Helpful, but the hematocrit does not always reflect the amount of blood loss because equilibration with extravascular fluid may take several hours.
4. **Type and cross-match.** At least four units of packed red blood cells (PRBCs).
5. **BUN, creatinine.** An increased BUN/creatinine ratio is seen in upper GI bleeding or volume depletion.
6. **PT, PTT, platelet count.** An elevated PT, PTT, or thrombocytopenia can interfere with stabilization of the patient. An elevated PT may be seen in chronic liver disease. Platelets and clotting factors decrease with brisk bleeding and massive transfusions.

C. **Radiologic and other studies**

1. **Anoscopy and flexible sigmoidoscopy.** Look for bleeding hemorrhoids or rectal mass. Frequently provides the diagnosis.
2. **Colonoscopy.** Preferred evaluation if flexible sigmoidoscopy is negative. Colonoscopy should be performed after large-volume oral preparation. Colonoscopy allows for both diagnosis and possible therapeutic intervention.
3. **Nasogastric tube.** For gastric lavage. Should be done if the NG aspirate is positive for blood.
4. **Upper GI endoscopy.** An upper GI source must be ruled out prior to surgery. In upper GI bleeds, 10% will have a negative nasogastric aspirate.

5. **Technetium-labeled bleeding scan.** The next examination to be ordered if upper and lower endoscopies are normal. Can detect very slow bleeding (0.5 mL/min). Localization is only fair and needs to be documented with endoscopy or angiography.
6. **Angiography.** Localization is very good but patients must be bleeding fairly rapidly (2 mL/min) to detect the source. Can also treat with selective intra-arterial infusion of pitressin.

V. Plan

A. Monitoring. The primary question in managing bleeding patients is the necessity of ICU monitoring. The following are guidelines for admission to the ICU:

1. Clearly documented frank hematochezia (> 100 mL).
2. Coffee-ground emesis or positive NG aspirate and hematochezia.
3. Any indication of hemodynamic instability (tachycardia, hypotension, or orthostasis).
4. Drop in hematocrit > five percentage points after fluid resuscitation.
5. Significant increase in BUN when GI bleeding is suspected.
6. High-risk patient: advanced age, inpatient status at time of bleed, recurrent or evidence of persistent bleeding, major comorbidity (hepatic, renal, pulmonary, or cardiac disease).

B. Volume resuscitation. If massive bleeding is evident, place two large-bore (14- or 16-gauge) peripheral or central lines. Begin IV fluids containing NS at a rate to maintain hemodynamic stability. With massive bleeding, transfuse PRBCs when available. Blood should be given to maintain a hematocrit above 30%.

C. Surgical consultation. Contact early in the management, especially if brisk bleeding is encountered.

D. Establish source of bleeding. The source of bleeding must be identified in order to institute specific therapy.

1. If bleeding is brisk, start with NG aspirate. If positive, evaluate for upper GI source. If negative, proceed with anoscopy and flexible sigmoidoscopy. If endoscopy is negative and bleeding remains brisk, proceed to bleeding scan and angiography. If all tests fail to reveal the site, and the bleeding remains brisk, then the patient will require laparotomy.
2. If the bleeding has stopped and the nasogastric aspirate is negative, proceed first with colonoscopy after prep. Colonoscopy is rarely helpful during brisk bleeding. If the colonoscopy is negative, do an upper GI endoscopy and then angiography. Remember, if at any point the patient becomes unstable and difficult to stabilize with IV fluids and blood, surgery is indicated.
3. The tempo of the evaluation is dictated by the rate of the patient's bleeding and overall stability.

REFERENCES

Cappell MS, ed: High risk gastrointestinal bleeding, Part I. Gastroenterol Clin North Am 2000;29:1.

Cappell MS, ed: High risk gastrointestinal bleeding, Part II. Gastroenterol Clin North Am 2000;29:275.

Jansen DM, Machicado GA, Jutabha R et al: Urgent colonoscopy for the diagnosis and treatment of severe diverticular hemorrhage. N Engl J Med 2000;340:78.

Laine L: Acute and chronic gastrointestinal bleeding. In: Feldman M, Scharschmidt BF, Sleisenger MH, eds. *Gastrointestinal and Liver Diseases: Pathophysiology/ Diagnosis/Management.* 6th ed. Saunders;1998:198.

29. HEMATURIA

I. **Problem.** A 51-year-old male patient has red blood cells noted on urinalysis 3 days after undergoing a total hip replacement.

II. **Immediate Questions**

A. **Is there a history of gross hematuria?** Microscopic hematuria may have been present for a long time without the patient's being aware of it, suggesting a chronic or acute process. Gross hematuria will not have gone unnoticed by the patient and likely represents an acute process or a process that has previously been evaluated.

B. **Does the patient have a Foley catheter in place?** Irritation of the bladder mucosa by a Foley catheter is a common cause of hematuria, as are trauma during placement and manipulation of the catheter by the patient. Other causes should be investigated if the hematuria does not completely clear after removal of the catheter.

C. **Has the patient had recent abdominal surgery?** This raises the question of an injury to the urinary tract, and would usually be apparent the night of surgery.

D. **Does the patient have abdominal pain or fever?** Abdominal pain may suggest an inflammatory or infectious cause. Colicky pain radiating from the flank to the groin suggests a renal stone. Infection is often accompanied by fever.

E. **Has there been a significant change in urine output?** A sudden decrease in urine output may indicate acute oliguric renal failure, obstruction, or renal vein thrombosis. See Section I, Chapter 51, Oliguria/Anuria, p 266.

F. **Does the patient have symptoms suggestive of urinary tract infection (UTI)?** Dysuria, frequency, and urgency are common symptoms associated with a UTI.

G. **Is the patient taking anticoagulant medication?** Anticoagulation therapy may cause hematuria by unmasking significant urinary tract pathology.

H. **Has the patient been treated with antineoplastic agents such as cyclophosphamide (Cytoxan)?** Complications of cyclophosphamide therapy are hemorrhagic cystitis or secondary genitourinary tract tumors.

I. **Is there a history of urologic conditions?** A history of nephrolithiasis, genitourinary surgery, bladder cancer, or benign prostatic hypertrophy should be determined.

III. Differential Diagnosis

A. Blood

1. **Coagulopathy.** See Section I, Chapter 12, Coagulopathy, p 66. Inheritable defects such as hemophilia, severe liver dysfunction, and pharmacologic anticoagulation are potential etiologies.
2. **Hemoglobinopathy.** Sickle cell disease with crisis is frequently associated with gross hematuria.

B. Kidneys

1. **Glomerular disease**
   a. **Primary.** Red cell casts characterize poststreptococcal glomerulonephritis, IgA nephropathy, Goodpasture's syndrome, idiopathic rapidly progressive glomerulonephritis.
   b. **Secondary.** Vasculitis associated with systemic lupus erythematosus (SLE), scleroderma, Wegener's granulomatosis, polyarteritis, hypersensitivity vasculitis, subacute bacterial endocarditis.
   c. **Hereditary.** Alport's syndrome, associated with sensorineural hearing loss and ocular abnormalities.
2. **Interstitial disease**
   a. **Consequence of systemic diseases.** Diabetic nephrosclerosis, accelerated hypertension, SLE.
   b. **Consequence of pharmacologic therapy.** Analgesic nephropathy, heavy metals, heroin nephropathy.
3. **Infections**
   a. **Pyelonephritis**
   b. **Tuberculosis.** Characterized by sterile pyuria.
4. **Malformations**
   a. **Cystic.** Familial polycystic kidney disease, ruptured solitary cysts, medullary sponge kidney.
   b. **Vascular.** Suggested by findings of hemangiomas or telangiectasias elsewhere.
5. **Neoplasms.** Particularly renal cell carcinoma and more rarely transitional cell carcinoma.
6. **Ischemia**
   a. **Embolism.** Aortic atherosclerosis, cardiac arrhythmias, manipulation of the aorta (aortography, coronary angiography).
   b. **Thrombosis.** Nephrotic syndrome, neoplastic disease, coagulation disorders (antithrombin III, protein C, or protein S deficiencies).
7. **Trauma**

C. **Postrenal**
   1. **Mechanical**
      a. **Kidney stones.** Nephrolithiasis and urolithiasis.
      b. **Obstruction.** Prostatic hypertrophy (common cause in men over 50 years), posterior urethral valves, retroperitoneal fibrosis, ureteropelvic junction abnormalities, strictures.
   2. **Inflammatory.** Infection or regional inflammation.
      a. **Periureteritis.** Diverticulitis, pelvic inflammatory disease.
      b. **Cystitis.** Infectious or inflammatory, such as cyclophosphamide-induced hematuria, which is a medical emergency.
      c. **Prostatitis**
      d. **Urethritis**
   3. **Neoplasm.** Transitional cell carcinoma, adenocarcinoma of the prostate, squamous cell carcinoma of the penis.
   4. **Exercise.** Especially in marathon runners.

D. **False hematuria**
   1. **Vaginal/rectal bleeding**
   2. **Factitious.** Most common in patients demonstrating drug-seeking behavior and requesting narcotics for nephrolithiasis.

IV. Database

A. **Physical examination key points**
   1. **Abdomen.** Examine for palpable masses indicative of tumors, polycystic kidneys, or diverticular abscess. Tenderness will accompany infection, infarction, sickle cell crisis, inflammatory processes, and obstruction.
   2. **Urethral meatus.** Look for gross blood, especially in trauma patients, and evidence of recent instrumentation or superficial lesions.
   3. **Rectum.** Is critical in the trauma patient when a "free-floating" prostate may be found, signifying urethral disruption. More commonly, prostatitis or prostatic carcinoma is uncovered. Attention should also be given to possible hemorrhoids.
   4. **Pelvis.** Check for another source of bleeding such as vaginitis, cervicitis, and menorrhagia.
   5. **Skin.** Ecchymoses, petechiae, and rash are suggestive of vasculitis or a coagulation disorder.

B. **Laboratory data**
   1. **Urinalysis.** Red cell casts are seen only with glomerulonephritis. White blood cells or bacteria suggest an infectious cause; WBC casts suggest pyelonephritis. Crystals may be seen in association with stones. Red discoloration without red blood cells should suggest myoglobinuria; urine should be checked for myoglobin and a serum creatine phosphokinase (CK).
   2. **Coagulation studies.** Prothrombin time, partial thromboplastin time, platelets.

3. **Hemogram.** An elevated WBC count will suggest an infectious or inflammatory process. Microcytic anemia may suggest chronic blood loss; however, hematuria is an unusual cause of microcytic anemia.
4. **Urine culture.** Rule out bacterial infection. Cultures for acid-fast bacilli should be done if there is pyuria and bacteria cultures are sterile (assuming the patient is not receiving antibiotics). An acid-fast stain may be helpful; however, some common saprophytes are acid-fast staining.
5. **BUN and creatinine.** To be used for baseline evaluation of renal function or to assess any change in renal function.
6. **Sickle cell screen.** Useful if the patient's status was previously unknown and this is being entertained as a cause of the hematuria.
7. **Urinary cytology.** May diagnose transitional cell carcinoma.

C. Radiologic and other studies

1. **Abdominal plain x-ray (kidney/ureter/bladder [KUB]).** 80% of urinary calculi are radiodense. Also, the KUB may show an inflammatory process (ileus or loss of psoas shadow).
2. **Excretory urography (IV pyelography) or other contrast imaging.** A part of the evaluation in all patients without an active infection who can receive IV contrast without undue risk. The evaluation of painful hematuria in many centers includes spiral CT scanning, which is highly sensitive for demonstrating nephrolithiasis. In the evaluation of painless hematuria, a CT IV pyelogram is often used instead of an excretory urogram.
3. **Retrograde urethrogram/cystogram.** Second-line study to be used in cases in which tumor, vesicoureteral reflux, posterior urethral valves, or traumatic disruption is suspected.
4. **Further studies.** Should be directed by clinical suspicion and the results of initial studies. Further studies may include a CT scan of the abdomen, ultrasound, angiography, cystoscopy, and renal biopsy. With normal renal imaging, patients with hematuria should have cystoscopy. With proteinuria, red cell casts, or suggestion of upper tract disease, if the renal imaging is normal, a renal biopsy may be indicated.

V. Plan. Treatment depends on the etiology. Keep in mind that apart from gross hematuria with or without clots (trauma, severe coagulopathy, cyclophosphamide-induced hematuria), the causes of hematuria are rarely emergencies; a thoughtful and careful evaluation can therefore be pursued over several days.

A. Urinary tract infection. See Section I, Chapter 20, Dysuria, V, p 120. The infection must be eradicated and a repeat urinalysis performed to rule out continued hematuria. If hematuria persists, further evaluation is necessary.

B. Urolithiasis. If the stone is expected to pass spontaneously (usually < 1 cm) and there are no complicating factors (infection, obstruction), expectant therapy with analgesics and hydration is appropriate. The urine should be strained.

C. **Neoplasms.** A complete urologic evaluation is recommended for assessing gross hematuria.

D. **Tuberculosis.** Treat appropriately with antibiotics. Initial therapy is usually with isoniazid (INH) 300 mg PO Q day, rifampin 600 mg PO Q day, and pyrazinamide 15–30 mg/kg with a maximum dose of 2 g Q day and ethambutol 15–25 mg/kg/day. The American Thoracic Society and the Centers for Disease Control and Prevention recommend a four-drug regimen for treatment until the results of drug susceptibility studies are available; or unless there is < 4% primary resistance to INH within the community. If so, an initial three-drug regimen is recommended. Long-term follow-up with IV pyelograms is necessary, because strictures are late sequelae and can lead to obstruction.

E. **Collecting system abnormality.** Usually requires surgical referral and repair.

F. **Coagulopathy.** Correct clotting factor deficiencies or adjust anticoagulant dose. Frequently the coagulopathy will induce bleeding from a preexisting abnormality. A thorough evaluation is usually indicated in a patient who has hematuria and a coagulopathy.

G. **Glomerulonephritis.** Most cases require a biopsy for definitive diagnosis, with therapy as appropriate for the underlying illness.

H. **Hemorrhagic cystitis.** Treat with continuous saline irrigation and occasionally a 1% alum irrigation. Also, hyperbaric oxygen can be used. The primary treatment is prevention, which includes hydration (oral or intravenous) and mesna (Mesnex).

REFERENCES

Copley JB: Isolated asymptomatic hematuria in the adult. Am J Med Sci 1986;291:101.

Miller OF, Rineer SK, Reichard SR et al: Prospective comparison of unenhanced spiral computed tomography and intravenous urogram in the evaluation of acute flank pain. Urology 1998;52:982.

Topham PS, Harper SJ, Furness PN et al: Glomerular disease as a cause of isolated microscopic haematuria. Q J Med 1994;87:329.

30. HEMOPTYSIS

I. **Problem.** A 60-year-old male smoker comes to the emergency room complaining of "spitting up blood" for 1 week.

II. **Immediate Questions**

A. **Is the patient truly experiencing hemoptysis?** Blood from a nasal, oral, or gastric source may be aspirated to the larynx and then expectorated.

B. What is the volume of the hemoptysis? Massive hemoptysis (> 600 mL/24 hr) connotes a life-threatening problem that demands immediate ICU admission as well as a rapid diagnostic evaluation.

C. Has this happened before? If so, how frequently? Patients with recurrent acute bronchitis or with mitral stenosis may have had multiple episodes of minor hemoptysis.

D. What is the smoking history? The higher the pack-years, the more likely the patient has chronic bronchitis or bronchogenic carcinoma.

E. Is there a history of productive cough preceding the hemoptysis? If the answer is yes, then the problem may be an infection such as acute bronchitis or bronchiectasis.

F. Has there been any accompanying chest pain? Pleuritic chest pain may be a symptom of pneumonia or a pulmonary embolism with infarction. Hemoptysis may accompany pulmonary edema from any number of causes.

III. Differential Diagnosis

A. Pulmonary sources

1. **Infection**
   a. **Acute or chronic bronchitis.** Most common cause of hemoptysis.
   b. **Pneumonia.** A necrotizing gram-negative or staphylococcal pneumonia are the usual types of pneumonia to have associated hemoptysis. Symptoms are acute.
   c. **Lung abscess.** Often produces foul-smelling sputum.
   d. **Bronchiectasis.** Seen in patients with recurrent episodes of respiratory infections, voluminous sputum production, and intermittent hemoptysis.
   e. **Tuberculosis.** Usually apical infiltrates on chest x-ray. Symptoms often chronic or subacute.
   f. **Mycetoma (fungus ball).** A ball of *Aspergillus* fungus may form in a previously formed cavity. Look for the "crescent sign" on the CXR.
2. **Neoplasm**
   a. **Bronchogenic carcinoma.** Usually the CXR is abnormal, but it may be normal in up to 13% of patients with early lung cancer and hemoptysis.
   b. **Bronchial adenoma**
   c. **Metastatic disease.** A history of cancer should be uncovered during the history. The CXR will be abnormal.
3. **Vascular**
   a. **Pulmonary embolism (PE) with infarction.** Only 10% of PEs present with hemoptysis, but pulmonary emboli are very common and should not be missed.
   b. **Mitral stenosis.** May arise either from rupture of the pulmonary veins or from frank pulmonary edema.

c. **Cardiogenic pulmonary edema.** Surprisingly common, especially now that most cardiac patients are on some form of anticoagulation.

d. **Arteriovenous malformation**

B. **Trauma**

1. **Pulmonary contusion**
2. **Bronchial or vascular tear**
3. **Retained foreign body.** Teeth and fillings sometimes find their way down into the bronchi.

C. **Systemic diseases**

1. **Anticoagulation**

a. **Drugs.** Warfarin (Coumadin), heparin, aspirin, streptokinase (Streptase), urokinase (Abbokinase), tissue plasminogen activator (TPA), and APSAC (anisoylated plasminogen streptokinase activator complex) or antistreplase (Eminase).

b. **Uremia**

c. **Thrombocytopenia.** Drugs, idiopathic thrombocytopenic purpura, cancer.

d. **Disseminated intravascular coagulation (DIC)**

e. **Liver disease.** Severe liver disease can result in thrombocytopenia, and also a decreased production of coagulation factors.

2. **Autoimmune diseases**

a. **Wegener's granulomatosis.** Look for renal changes (red cell casts, hematuria, proteinuria) and sinus disease. The CXR often is abnormal. Bilateral nodular densities and cavitation are common.

b. **Goodpasture's syndrome.** This disease also involves the kidney. Proteinuria, hematuria, and red cell casts may be present. Diffuse alveolar infiltrates are often present.

c. **Systemic lupus erythematosus (SLE).** Lupus more frequently involves the pleura, but patients may develop life-threatening hemoptysis from lupus pneumonitis.

IV. Database

A. Physical examination key points

1. **Vital signs.** Look particularly for fever and signs of impending respiratory failure: breath rate above 30 per minute, abdominal paradox with inspiration and accessory muscle use.
2. **HEENT.** Look carefully for a nasal or oropharyngeal source of bleeding.
3. **Chest.** Inspect and palpate for signs of trauma such as rib or clavicle fractures. Listen for a pleural rub, localized rales, or signs of consolidation.
4. **Heart.** An irregularly irregular pulse signifies atrial fibrillation and suggests mitral stenosis as a possible cause. Pulmonary embolus can also cause atrial fibrillation. An S_3 and jugular venous

distension suggest congestive heart failure as a possible etiology. Always listen carefully for the low diastolic rumble of mitral stenosis at the apex with the bell.

5. **Abdomen.** Palpate the epigastrium, liver, and spleen. Peptic ulcer disease or alcoholic liver disease could certainly cause GI bleeding, which might mimic hemoptysis.
6. **Extremities.** Examine lower extremities for signs of deep venous thromboses or edema. Look for cyanosis and clubbing. Clubbed fingers associated with hemoptysis would generally implicate either bronchiectasis or a pulmonary neoplasm.
7. **Skin.** Inspect the skin for petechiae, ecchymoses, angiomata, and rashes.

B. Laboratory data

1. **Complete blood count.** May reveal an anemia that could be caused by the hemoptysis or, more likely, is related to the hemoptysis. A normocytic anemia with a normal or low reticulocyte count may be secondary to anemia of chronic disease (eg, cancer). An elevated reticulocyte count indicates a hemolytic anemia possibly secondary to SLE. An iron deficiency may indicate Goodpasture's syndrome.
2. **Platelet count, prothrombin time, and partial thromboplastin time.** All are indicated to rule out coagulopathy as a cause. See Section I, Chapter 12, Coagulopathy, p 66. If platelet dysfunction is suspected, a bleeding time will be prolonged in the presence of a normal platelet count.
3. **BUN, creatinine, and urinalysis.** For rapid evaluation of "pulmonary-renal" syndromes (Goodpasture's syndrome, Wegener's granulomatosis, SLE, and vasculitis).
4. **Anti-neutrophil cytoplasmic antibodies (ANCA) and anti-glomerular basement membrane (anti-GBM) antibody.** May indicate Wegener's (especially cytoplasmic-staining ANCA or C-ANCA) and anti-GBM Ab is positive in 85% of patients with Goodpasture's syndrome.
5. **Arterial blood gases.** Check for adequate ventilation and oxygenation. If there is underlying pulmonary disease, respiratory failure may be precipitated by hemoptysis.
6. **Sputum examination.** Gram's stain, acid-fast bacillus stain and culture, and cytology all are imperative.
7. **PPD skin test. To help rule out tuberculosis.**

C. Radiologic and other studies

1. **Chest x-ray.** First and most important test after the history and physical. The pattern and location of any infiltrate, coupled with the history and physical examination, will dictate the remainder of your workup.
2. **Ventilation/perfusion ($\dot{V}/\dot{Q}$) lung scan.** If pulmonary embolism is highly suspected, a $\dot{V}/\dot{Q}$ scan must be done.

3. **Angiography.** If PE is suspected and $\dot{V}/\dot{Q}$ scans are not clearly positive or negative, then pulmonary angiography is indicated. Angiography may also be indicated for the diagnosis of pulmonary arteriovenous malformations.
4. **Chest computerized tomography (CT) scan including CT angiography.** This will provide a much better anatomic view of pulmonary pathology compared with chest radiographs and will also reveal lesions not seen previously; however, the CT scan is only indicated acutely when looking for an aortic dissection and PE. CT angiography (helical or spiral and electron-beam) are about 90% sensitive and 90% specific for detecting proximal (main, lobar, and segmental) pulmonary artery emboli. CT angiography is poor at detecting sub-segmental emboli.
5. **Electrocardiogram.** May show atrial fibrillation. A right axis shift and/or right bundle branch block may suggest a PE. Classically, a PE produces an S wave in lead I, and a Q wave and inverted T wave in lead III (S_1-Q_3T_3).
6. **Bronchoscopy.** Patients with unclear sources of hemoptysis, massive hemoptysis, or the suspicion of a neoplasm require fiberoptic bronchoscopy. The earlier it is done, the more likely the source of bleeding will be identified.

V. Plan

A. Intensive care unit

1. **Massive hemoptysis**
2. **Present or impending hypoxemic or hypercarbic respiratory failure**

B. Establish IV access. Death comes from asphyxia rather than hemorrhage, but IV medications will be needed.

C. Always protect the airway. This may require early intubation.

D. Correct any coagulopathy. See Section I, Chapter 12, Coagulopathy, V, p 70.

E. Fiberoptic bronchoscopy. Arrange early if the diagnosis is in doubt or hemoptysis continues.

F. Consult. Obtain a thoracic surgery consultation if the patient has massive or continuous hemoptysis. Medical management of massive hemoptysis is associated with a high mortality rate.

G. Cough suppression. Retard the cough reflex with codeine-based drugs, and place the patient on quiet bed rest.

H. Treat the underlying disease state

1. **Lung cancer.** Can be treated surgically if there are no metastases and the pulmonary reserve is adequate. Otherwise, radiation or laser therapy can rapidly control bleeding.
2. **Infections.** Treat with antibiotics as dictated by Gram's stain and clinical picture.

3. **Pulmonary emboli.** Treat acutely with heparin. See Section I, Chapter 11, Chest Pain, V, p 63.
4. **Diffuse alveolar hemorrhage or a pulmonary-renal syndrome.** 1000 mg methylprednisolone (Solu-Medrol) IV may control bleeding, pending definitive workup.
5. **Nonsurgical patients with localized bleeding.** Bronchial arteriography followed by embolism may be lifesaving. However, collateral circulation to the spinal arteries or carotids must be excluded prior to embolization.

REFERENCES

Cahil BC, Ingbar DH: Massive hemoptysis-assessment and management in clinics. Clin Chest Med 1994;15:147.

Ryu JH, Swensen SJ, Olson EJ et al: Diagnosis of pulmonary embolism with use of computed tomographic angiography. Mayo Clin Proc 2001;76:59.

31. HYPERCALCEMIA

I. **Problem.** A 60-year-old man is admitted for severe diffuse bone pain and is found to have a calcium of 5.5 mEq/L or 2.75 mmol/L (normal: 4.2–5.1 mEq/L or 2.10–2.55 mmol/L).

II. **Immediate Questions**

A. **What other symptoms are present?** The classic presentation of primary hyperparathyroidism is “stones, bones, moans, and groans” from renal calculi, osteitis fibrosa, constipation, and neuropsychiatric problems, respectively. Renal calculi and osteitis fibrosa are seldom associated with hypercalcemia of malignancy because both result from long-standing hypercalcemia. Hypercalcemia causes a variety of nonspecific symptoms including fatigue, weakness, polyuria, polydipsia, bone pain, constipation, nausea, vomiting, anorexia, and mental status changes ranging from confusion to coma.

B. **Does the patient have any condition that could be related to hypercalcemia?** Hypertension, peptic ulcer, and nephrolithiasis are associated with hyperparathyroidism.

C. **Is the patient on any medications that might cause hypercalcemia?** Thiazide diuretics, vitamin D, and exogenous sources of calcium are possible causes.

D. **Is there a family history of hypercalcemia?** One cause is familial hypocalciuric hypercalcemia. There are also three syndromes of multiple endocrine neoplasia (MEN) that are inherited in an autosomal dominant pattern. *MEN I* includes primary hyperparathyroidism, hypersecretion of pancreatic islet hormones, pituitary adenoma, and possibly other endocrine tumors. *MEN IIA* consists of primary hyperparathyroidism, medullary carcinoma of the thyroid, and pheochromocytoma. Hyperparathyroidism is rare in *MEN IIB.*

E. **Has the patient been noted to have elevated calcium in the past?** Long-standing hypercalcemia suggests primary hyperparathyroidism. Malignant disease is usually associated with recent-onset hypercalcemia.

III. Differential Diagnosis

A. **Primary hyperparathyroidism.** About 20% of patients with hypercalcemia have hyperparathyroidism, usually from a single hyperfunctioning adenoma. An elevated calcium, a low phosphate, and elevated or relatively elevated parathyroid hormone are characteristic findings. Most patients in whom hyperparathyroidism is diagnosed are asymptomatic.

B. **Malignant disease.** From bony metastasis or more often from humoral factors produced by a tumor.

1. **Metastatic carcinoma to bone.** Breast, lung, and renal cell carcinoma.
2. **Hematologic malignancies.** Direct bone involvement with multiple myeloma and lymphoma.
3. **Humoral factors.** Prostaglandins, parathyroid hormone-related protein, and osteoclast-activating factor (OAF). These factors are most commonly seen with squamous cell, renal cell, and transitional cell carcinomas, lymphomas, and multiple myelomas.

C. **Medications**

1. **Thiazide diuretics.** These agents increase renal reabsorption of calcium.
2. **Vitamin D intoxication.** A fat-soluble vitamin that increases intestinal absorption, increases mobilization from bone, and increases renal reabsorption of calcium.
3. **Vitamin A intoxication.** Another fat-soluble vitamin that is a rare cause of hypercalcemia; causes increased bone reabsorption.
4. **Exogenous calcium.** For example, calcium carbonate, which is found in certain antacids.

D. **Granulomatous diseases—Sarcoidosis.** These conditions are marked by increased sensitivity to vitamin D.

E. **Milk-alkali syndrome.** From increased intake of calcium and alkali. Results in hypercalcemia, hypocalciuria, hyperphosphatemia, renal failure, and metastatic calcifications.

F. **Immobilization.** Prolonged bed rest increases bone reabsorption, resulting in hypercalcemia and osteoporosis.

G. **Recovery from acute renal failure.** Thought to be from secondary hyperparathyroidism.

H. **Endocrinopathies**

1. **Hyperthyroidism.** Bone reabsorption induced by thyroid hormone.
2. **Acromegaly**
3. **Adrenal insufficiency**

I. **Paget's disease.** The calcium level is usually normal but may increase with immobilization.

J. **Familial hypocalciuric hypercalcemia.** An autosomal dominant condition causing lifelong hypercalcemia with normal urinary calcium excretion.

IV. Database

A. Physical examination key points

1. **Vital signs.** There may be associated hypertension.
2. **Skin.** Excoriations may occur as a result of pruritus from metastatic calcifications in the skin.
3. **Lymph nodes.** Lymphadenopathy suggests carcinoma, hematologic malignancy, or sarcoidosis.
4. **HEENT.** An enlarged thyroid gland suggests hyperthyroidism.
5. **Chest.** Look for evidence of lung carcinoma.
6. **Abdomen.** An enlarged liver or spleen suggests metastatic carcinoma, a hematologic cancer, or sarcoidosis.
7. **Musculoskeletal exam.** Bone pain with palpation or percussion points to carcinoma or Paget's disease. Myopathy from hypercalcemia can cause proximal muscle weakness.
8. **Neurologic exam.** Impaired mentation, weakness, and hyporeflexia may result from hypercalcemia.

B. Laboratory data

1. **Repeat levels for calcium along with a serum albumin or obtain an ionized calcium level.** Always confirm an elevated calcium and the severity of the hypercalcemia before initiating therapy. Keep in mind that a high normal total calcium may signify hypercalcemia in the presence of marked hypoalbuminemia. A calcium value must be corrected in the presence of hypoalbuminemia. Normally, the total calcium decreases by 0.2 mmol/L, or 0.4 mEq/L, for every 1 g/dL decrease in the serum albumin from normal levels (4.0 g/dL) without changing the ionized calcium level. Symptoms of hypercalcemia usually develop at 6.5–7.0 mEq/L, or 3.25–3.5 mmol/L.
2. **Phosphorus.** The phosphorus level is low in primary hyperparathyroidism; it is elevated in vitamin D intoxication.
3. **Arterial blood gases.** A decrease in the pH will increase the ionized calcium mostly by displacing calcium bound to albumin. A metabolic acidosis may also be seen with adrenal insufficiency, a potential cause of hypercalcemia. An increase in the pH is seen in milk-alkali syndrome and possibly with thiazide diuretics if there is associated volume depletion.
4. **Alkaline phosphatase.** This value is increased in primary hyperparathyroidism and Paget's disease and with bony metastases.
5. **BUN and creatinine.** Renal insufficiency will exacerbate hypercalcemia or may be secondary to hypercalcemia.

6. **Total protein and albumin.** An increased total protein-to-albumin ratio suggests multiple myeloma. If there is an elevated total protein-to-albumin ratio, then quantitative immunoglobulins and serum and urine protein electrophoresis should be ordered.
7. **Amylase and lipase.** Hypercalcemia can cause pancreatitis. If abdominal pain is present, pancreatitis should be ruled out.
8. **Urinalysis.** Hematuria may arise from renal cell carcinoma or secondary to nephrolithiasis.

C. **Radiologic and other studies**

1. **Chest x-ray.** Bilateral hilar adenopathy implies sarcoidosis. Also, carcinoma or lymphoma may be detected by CXR. Osteopenia of the vertebral column may be evident on the lateral film.
2. **Abdominal x-rays.** May reveal renal calcifications as a result of hypercalcemia; other findings may suggest carcinoma.
3. **Bone films.** These are especially useful if there is localized bone pain; they may reveal osteolytic/osteoblastic lesions from carcinoma or the osteolytic lesions of multiple myeloma. If lesions are present, a bone scan would be helpful to reveal extent of the disease. A bone scan will be negative with multiple myeloma because of the absence of associated osteoblastic activity.
4. **Skull films and skeletal survey.** Obtain if multiple myeloma is suspected. Classically reveals multiple punched-out lesions. May also be helpful in detecting subperiosteal resorption resulting from primary hyperparathyroidism, especially evident on hand films.
5. **Electrocardiogram.** Associated shortening of QT interval and lengthening of PR interval.

V. **Plan.** Lower the calcium level and then treat the underlying disorder. Treat more aggressively with severe hypercalcemia > 7.0 mEq/L, or 3.5 mmol/L, or when the patient is symptomatic. Treatment is directed at decreasing the release of calcium from bone or increasing deposition in bone, decreasing absorption from the gastrointestinal tract, and increasing excretion renally or through chelation.

A. **Restrict calcium intake and encourage mobilization**

B. **Treat underlying causes**

C. **Institute saline diuresis.** Patients with moderate to severe symptomatic hypercalcemia are frequently volume-depleted. It is essential to restore the patient's volume and then to maintain a urine output of at least 2 L/d. Sodium increases calcium excretion by inhibiting proximal tubule reabsorption. Administration of large volumes of normal saline can be hazardous in the elderly or in patients with renal failure or with left ventricular dysfunction.

D. **Administer medications**

1. **Furosemide (Lasix).** Dosage is 20–80 mg IV Q 2–4 hours. You frequently administer the furosemide concomitantly with normal saline. Furosemide is a calciuric agent; however, calcium excretion is not promoted if volume depletion develops. You must fol-

low urinary output closely as well as monitor the volume of normal saline administered and daily weights. Older patients with tenuous cardiac conditions may need hemodynamic monitoring in an ICU if vigorous saline diuresis is attempted. Potassium chloride should be added to the saline solution after rehydration to maintain normokalemia. Also, monitor for hypomagnesemia and correct if necessary. ***Caution:*** Thiazide diuretics should *never* be used because they may actually worsen the hypercalcemia through enhanced distal tubular reabsorption of calcium.

2. **Bisphosphonates.** These agents inhibit osteoclastic activity. Pamidronate disodium (Aredia) is superior to etidronate (Didronel), the first drug in this class approved to treat hypercalcemia. Pamidronate 60–90 mg is given intravenously over 4–24 hours. Hypokalemia, hypomagnesemia, and hypophosphatemia can occur. Calcium levels decline in 2 days, with nadir at 7 days and duration of action of approximately 2 weeks. Use in combination with calcitonin if rapid reduction is desired.
3. **Plicamycin (Mithramycin).** Give 25 μg/kg in 1 L of normal saline over 3–6 hours. This agent inhibits bone reabsorption; effect may not manifest for 12–24 hours, with a peak action at 48–96 hours. The dose can be repeated at 24–48 hours for 3–4 total doses. Nausea and renal, hepatic, and bone marrow toxicity (thrombocytopenia) can occur.
4. **Calcitonin.** This agent is rapid-acting, but weak; it inhibits bone reabsorption and increases urinary excretion of calcium. Usually only a temporary measure because resistance to the calcium-lowering effect often develops. An effective dose is 4 U/kg every 12 hours IM or SC (salmon calcitonin). Side effects include nausea, vomiting, flushing, and allergic reactions.
5. **Corticosteroids.** Hydrocortisone 50–75 mg every 6 hours decreases calcium absorption from the GI tract and inhibits bone reabsorption. Also may inhibit growth of lymphoid cancers. Effective for treating hypercalcemia associated with sarcoidosis, vitamin D intoxication, and hematologic cancers (multiple myeloma, lymphoma, leukemia).

   Note: Onset of action is relatively slow.
6. **Intravenous phosphates.** These drugs work by increasing deposition of calcium in bone and soft tissues and decreasing bone reabsorption. Can result in metastatic calcification, renal failure, and death. Their use is contraindicated in patients with renal insufficiency. Should be reserved for life-threatening hypercalcemia resistant to other measures.

E. Dialysis. This is a treatment of last resort.

REFERENCES

Edelson GW, Kleerekoper M: Hypercalcemic crisis. Med Clin North Am 1995;79:79.

Popovtzer MM, Knochel JP, Kumar R: Disorders of calcium, phosphorus, vitamin D and parathyroid hormone activity. In: Schrier RW, ed. *Renal and Electrolyte Disorders.* 5th ed. Lippincott-Raven;1997:241.

Marx SJ: Hyperparathyroid and hypoparathyroid disorders. N Engl J Med 2000;343:1863.

32. HYPERGLYCEMIA

I. **Problem.** A 44-year-old man is admitted because of chest pain. His glucose is 428 mg/dL, or 23.79 mmol/L.

II. **Immediate Questions**

A. **What are the patient's vital signs?** Fever may indicate sepsis, which can exacerbate hyperglycemia. Hypotension or tachycardia may indicate volume depletion common in diabetic ketoacidosis (DKA) and hyperosmolar syndromes. Tachypnea may be due to Kussmaul respirations in DKA.

B. **Is the patient known to be diabetic?** A history of diabetes should make the clinician consider factors such as noncompliance with medication/diet, sepsis, acute stress, glucocorticoid use, and myocardial infarction (MI), which can result in poor control of hyperglycemia. The absence of a prior history of diabetes should make one consider all of the preceding factors as unmasking latent carbohydrate intolerance, as well as the possibility of laboratory error.

C. **If the patient is diabetic, what medications is he or she taking and when was the last meal in relation to the time of phlebotomy?** Before one modifies the regimen, it is important to know whether the patient is receiving large or small amounts of insulin, or whether he or she is receiving oral hypoglycemic agents. In addition, it is important to know whether the blood sugar was drawn randomly (and therefore could be postprandial) or whether it represents a fasting level.

III. **Differential Diagnosis**

A. **Diabetes mellitus**

1. **Type 1 (previously called juvenile diabetes or insulin-dependent diabetes).** Patients with Type 1 diabetes require insulin even when not eating, although in lower doses. They are more likely to be thin or normal in weight, young, and "brittle," and are prone to DKA. *Diabetic ketoacidosis* may be defined as a blood sugar level > 300 mg/dL (16.68 mmol/L), urine ketones that are strongly positive, and a serum bicarbonate < 17 mmol or a pH < 7.30.
2. **Type 2 (previously called adult-onset diabetes or non–insulin-dependent diabetes mellitus).** Patients with Type 2 diabetes tend to be obese and older, and are more prone to hyperosmolar hyperglycemic syndromes than to ketoacidosis. Weight loss may normalize carbohydrate metabolism initially. Some patients can be managed with diet and exercise alone, although data from the United Kingdom Prospective Diabetes Study indicate that Type 2 diabetes usually progresses to require oral agents and eventually insulin.
3. **Gestational diabetes.** Glucose intolerance associated with pregnancy. Close monitoring and tight control are important to improve outcome of mother and infant.

B. Acute stress. With mild carbohydrate intolerance, acute events such as sepsis, MI, trauma, and surgery may cause relatively marked hyperglycemia. Some patients will not require therapy once the acute event has resolved.

C. Exogenous glucose load. Hyperalimentation and peritoneal dialysis.

D. Medications. Exogenous or endogenous glucocorticoids (Cushing's syndrome), thiazide diuretics, and other agents may cause hyperglycemia or unmask latent carbohydrate intolerance.

E. Pancreatic disease. Severe acute pancreatitis or long-standing chronic pancreatitis with endocrine pancreatic insufficiency.

F. Spurious hyperglycemia. Drawing blood above an IV line that contains dextrose; mislabeling; or inadvertently switching blood from different patients, inaccurate finger-stick glucoses. When in doubt, immediately repeat the test before treating.

IV. Database

A. Physical examination key points

1. **Vital signs.** Include orthostatic blood pressure and pulse to evaluate volume status. A decrease in systolic blood pressure of 10 mm Hg and/or an increase in heart rate of 20 bpm suggest volume depletion in younger patients. In patients over 75 years there may be up to 25 mm systolic orthostatic drop normally, and a pulse increase of 16 bpm signifies volume depletion. Fever implies sepsis. *Kussmaul respirations* (deep, regular respirations, whether slow or fast) suggest DKA.
2. **HEENT.** Fruity odor on breath suggests ketones and DKA. Funduscopic exam may show diabetic retinopathy, which suggests long-standing disease and increases the likelihood of other diabetic complications such as nephropathy and neuropathy.
3. **Lungs.** Evaluate for signs of pneumonia. Follow-up lung exams for rales are important in assessing volume.
4. **Heart.** Listen for associated findings of ischemia/MI, such as a third (S_3) or fourth (S_4) heart sound, or murmur of mitral insufficiency.
5. **Peripheral vascular system.** Listen for bruits.
6. **Abdomen.** Evaluate for cause of sepsis. Rebound tenderness suggests peritonitis. A positive Murphy's sign (see Section I, Chapter 1, Abdominal Pain, p 1) suggests acute cholecystitis, which is more common in diabetics.
7. **Extremities.** Check for foot ulcers and cellulitis.
8. **Neurologic exam.** A clouded sensorium suggests more severe disease (ketoacidosis or hyperosmolar syndrome).

B. Laboratory data

1. **Serum glucose.** Significantly elevated finger-stick glucose should be further evaluated with a serum glucose.

2. **Complete blood count.** Leukocytosis with a left shift suggests the presence of infection. An elevated WBC count may be seen in DKA without an associated infection or sepsis, but a left shift, toxic granulation, and vacuolization suggest a bacterial infection.
3. **Serum electrolytes, BUN and creatinine, phosphorus, calcium, magnesium, amylase.**
   a. Even though serum potassium may be normal or even high, total body potassium is often depleted and potassium repletion is indicated. Initially normal or elevated potassium will decrease with insulin administration and with correction of acidosis if present.
   b. Serum sodium is spuriously lowered by hyperglycemia. Originally, a correction factor of 1.6 mmol/L for each 100 mg/dL (5.56 mmol/L) rise in glucose concentration was proposed; however, a more recent study suggests that a correction factor of 2.4 mmol of Na^+ per 100 mg/dL increase in serum glucose is more accurate.
   c. Serum bicarbonate is low and the anion gap is elevated in DKA.
   d. Creatinine may be falsely elevated in the presence of serum ketones. Both BUN and creatinine may be elevated as a result of profound volume depletion or diabetic nephropathy.
   e. Phosphate may fall with treatment and should be monitored, although routine prophylactic treatment with phosphate is not recommended.
   f. Calcium may be low with acute pancreatitis.
   g. Magnesium may be low, especially in DKA. Magnesium deficiency may contribute to relative insulin resistance.
   h. An elevated amylase or lipase may indicate pancreatitis; ketone bodies may factitiously elevate the serum amylase.
4. **Arterial blood gases.** To evaluate the degree of acidemia. A careful look at the pH, pCO_2, and serum bicarbonate often reveals more than one acid–base disorder. (See Section I, Chapter 2, Acidosis, p 9).
5. **Urine or serum for ketones.** This helps to distinguish between DKA and hyperosmolar coma. Acetoacetate is the ketone that is measured on standard tests; however, β-hydroxybutyrate is the predominant ketone in DKA. Initially, the level of ketones may not decrease or may actually increase as β-hydroxybutyrate is metabolized to acetoacetate.
6. **Cultures.** If sepsis is suspected, appropriate cultures should be ordered.

C. **Radiologic and other studies**
   1. **Chest x-ray.** To evaluate for pneumonia and congestive heart failure (CHF).
   2. **Electrocardiogram.** To rule out MI as a cause of difficult-to-control diabetes.

3. **Miscellaneous studies.** Depending on clinical suspicion; for example, CT of the abdomen if intra-abdominal abscess is suspected.

V. **Plan.** Management depends on the clinical setting and severity of hyperglycemia. This section is divided into three parts on the basis of severity.

A. **Type 2 diabetes with a serum glucose** < 450 mg/dL, or 25.0 mmol/L (no ketones, no metabolic acidosis, and probably asymptomatic)

1. **Insulin.** Initially, may use sliding scale regular insulin Q 6 hr based on results of finger-stick glucoses. For a typical regimen, see Table 1–7. Patients already receiving insulin may be continued on their usual dose with supplemental sliding scale insulin or have their usual dose increased.
2. **Oral hypoglycemic agents.** Some patients with Type 2 diabetes mellitus may be managed with oral hypoglycemic agents, especially when the glucose is below 300 mg/dL (16.68 mmol/L).
   a. **Metformin.** An excellent drug, with a low risk of hypoglycemia. It is the only oral agent shown to reduce macrovascular complications. However, metformin should be avoided if the serum creatinine is > 1.4. Some diabetologists avoid using metformin in the inpatient setting or in unstable patients due to the risk of lactic acidosis. Caution is advised with CHF and ethanol abuse. Metformin should be held for 48 hours after intravenous contrast and after surgery.
   b. **Sulfonylureas.** These are often used for first-line treatment; generic sulfonylureas are less expensive.
   c. **Thiazolidinediones.** Thiazolidinediones such as pioglitazone (Actos) and rosiglitazone (Avandia) potentiate the action of insulin by decreasing insulin resistance. The thiazolidinediones need to be monitored for potential hepatic toxicity. In fact, the prototypic agent troglitazone was removed from the market for this reason. Obtain baseline serum transaminases, then every 2 months for the first year and periodically thereafter.
   d. **Other drugs.** Acarbose may be considered for mild hyperglycemia. Combination therapy with different classes of oral agents and/or bedtime insulin is becoming more common.

TABLE I–7. SLIDING SCALE OF INSULIN DOSAGE FOR HYPERGLYCEMIA.

Glucose Level	Insulin (Short-Acting/Regular)
<180 mg/dL (10.00 mmol/L)	0 U SC
180–240 mg/dL (10.00–13.34 mmol/L)	3–5 U SC
240–400 mg/dL (13.34–22.23 mmol/L)	8–10 U SC
>400 mg/dL (>22.23 mmol/L)	10–15 U SC[1]

[1]Follow with a stat serum glucose and notify the house officer of result.
SC = subcutaneous.

3. **Diet.** In the short term, an 1800-calorie American Diabetes Association (ADA) diet is useful, although other modified diets may be appropriate in certain settings. The importance of diet is controversial. A nutritious diet low in simple sugars and fat will usually suffice. If there is a complicating condition such as a foot ulcer that requires positive nitrogen balance for resolution, be sure the patient receives adequate calories and protein.

B. **Hyperosmolar, hyperglycemic nonketotic syndrome, glucose > 600 mg/dL, or 33.35 mmol/L (no ketones, no metabolic acidosis)**

1. **Aggressive management.** The ICU is often required. Depressed mental status is a marker of a more serious situation.
2. **Saline**
   a. **Rate of administration.** Depending on the degree of volume depletion, 500–1000 mL of NS is given in the first hour, after which the rate is decreased to 250–500 mL/hr until signs of volume depletion resolve. Obviously, caution is indicated, particularly in smaller or older individuals and those with limited cardiac and renal reserve. These patients need frequent (every 1–2 hours) assessment of volume status with orthostatic blood pressure and pulse, and auscultation for a S_3 and rales. Some patients will need monitoring with a pulmonary artery catheter for optimal fluid management.
   b. **Concentration.** Some authors prefer switching from NS to half-normal saline after the first liter, or alternating half-normal saline with NS. When the blood sugar reaches 250–300 mg/dL (13.90–16.68 mmol/L), IV fluids are switched to D5 half-normal saline at a rate based on volume assessment.
3. **Potassium.** If serum potassium is < 5.5 mmol/L, add 20–30 mEq/L at a rate not to exceed 10–15 mEq/hr. Follow levels Q 4 hr. Keep serum potassium at 4.0–5.0 mmol/L.
4. **Insulin.** There are many ways of giving insulin. Continuous IV infusion drip of short-acting (regular) insulin is preferred. An initial dose of 0.15 U/kg of short-acting (regular) insulin is given as a bolus and is followed immediately by a continuous infusion drip at 0.1 U/kg/hr. This should be adjusted to ensure that blood glucose is falling at least 10% per hour.
5. **Lab work.** Serum glucose measurements are needed Q 1–2 hr. Magnesium should be checked initially and repeated if there are signs of magnesium deficiency. Potassium should be checked Q 4–6 hr, and phosphorus Q 6–12 hr.
6. **Dextrose in IV fluids.** When glucose falls to the range 250–300 mg/dL (13.89–16.68 mmol/L), then the insulin drip may need to be decreased and the IV fluids changed to D5 half-normal saline, with the goal of maintaining the glucose at 100–200 mg/dL (5.56–11.12 mmol/L).

C. **Diabetic ketoacidosis.** Hyperglycemia with ketonuria and low serum bicarbonate. This is a medical emergency, often requiring management in the ICU setting. In the setting of profound ketoacidosis, patients are less responsive to insulin and larger doses are required. Volume repletion is essential.

1. **IV fluids.** One liter of NS in the first hour followed by 200 mL to 1 L per hour until volume status improves. The same volume assessment parameters should be followed as in hyperosmolar coma, described earlier (see V.B.2.a.). Some authors prefer switching or alternating half-normal saline with NS. When serum glucose levels reach 250–300 mg/dL (13.89–16.68 mmol/L), change to D5 half-normal saline at a rate based on volume assessment.
2. **Insulin.** The American Diabetes Association, in its recent guidelines, recommends a bolus of 0.15 U/kg of regular insulin followed by a continuous infusion of 0.1 U/kg/hr with a desired decrease in glucose by 50–75 mg/dL/hr. If the glucose does not decrease by at least 50 mg/dL/hr, the rate of the continuous infusion is doubled every hour until the glucose decreases by the desired rate. When the glucose is 250–300 mg/dL, the continuous infusion of insulin is decreased to 0.05–0.1 U/kg/hr and the intravenous fluids are changed to include 5% dextrose. A continuous infusion of insulin is maintained until the metabolic acidosis in DKA resolves (ketones are cleared) or until mental status changes and hyperosmolarity resolves in hyperosmolar hyperglycemia.
3. **Potassium.** If serum potassium is < 5.5 mEq/L, potassium 20–30 mEq /L is given in IV fluids at a rate not to exceed 15 mmol/hr unless the patient's rhythm is being continuously monitored. Potassium 10–15 mEq/hr is given to maintain serum potassium at 3.0–5.0 mmol/L. Doses of potassium > 15 mEq/hr should not be administered without continuous cardiac monitoring.
4. **Bicarbonate.** Its use is controversial and most authors are more conservative than in the past. One approach is to use bicarbonate to correct the pH to 7.00. For pH 6.90–7.00, give 44 mmol over 1–2 hr; for pH < 6.90, give 88 mmol of sodium bicarbonate over 1–2 hr.
5. **Lab work.** Glucose should be repeated Q 1–2 hr, and electrolytes Q 4–6 hr. Magnesium should be checked initially, and phosphate initially and after 6–12 hr. An ABG should be obtained Q 2–4 hr if acidosis is severe, or if the patient requires sodium bicarbonate. Serum/urine ketones may be of some use, although increasing ketones may be spurious (see IV.B.5, p 184).
6. **Associated conditions.** Treat any associated condition such as sepsis, MI, or stress appropriately.

D. **Guidelines for management of hyperglycemia in diabetes.** Accumulating evidence suggests that close management ("tight" control) of diabetes will lower the incidence of complications. Current recommendations for patients with diabetes are to maintain the glucose before meals of 80–120 mg/dL and a hemoglobin A_{1c} level < 6.5%. Such tight control frequently necessitates self-monitoring of fingerstick glucoses and multiple insulin injections per day.

REFERENCES

American Diabetes Association: Clinical practice recommendations. Diabetes Care 2001;24(suppl 1).

American Diabetes Association: Standards of medical care for patients with diabetes mellitus. Diabetes Care 2000;23(suppl 1):S32.

DeFronzo RA: Pharmacologic therapy for type 2 diabetes mellitus. Ann Intern Med 1999;131:281.

Hillier TA, Abbott RD, Barrett EJ: Hyponatremia: Evaluating the correction factor for hyperglycemia. Am J Med 1999;106:399.

Kitabchi AE, Wall BM: Diabetic ketoacidosis. Med Clin North Am 1995:79:9.

Lorber D: Nonketotic hypertonicity in diabetes mellitus. Med Clin North Am 1995;79:39.

The Diabetes Control and Complications Trial Research Group: The effect of intensive treatment of diabetes on the development and progression of long-term complications in insulin-dependent diabetes mellitus. N Engl J Med 1993;329:977.

33. HYPERKALEMIA

I. **Problem.** A 64-year-old man with diabetes admitted for a myocardial infarction is found to have a potassium (K^+) of 7.1 mmol/L.

II. **Immediate Questions**

A. **What are the patient's vital signs?** Hyperkalemia can result in life-threatening ventricular arrhythmias. Obtain an electrocardiogram (ECG) immediately.

B. **What is the urine output?** Acute oliguric renal failure is the most common cause of potentially fatal hyperkalemia. Evaluate urine output and renal function tests.

C. **Is the patient receiving potassium in an intravenous solution?** Supplemental potassium administration is the most common cause of severe hyperkalemia in hospitalized patients, and the risk is greater with intravenous potassium. Often standard IV solutions contain 20–40 mEq/L potassium; hyperalimentation solutions may contain more. Stop all exogenous potassium until the problem is resolved.

D. **Is the patient on any medications that could elevate the potassium?** Potential causes include potassium-sparing diuretics such as spironolactone (Aldactone), triamterene (Dyrenium), and amiloride (Midamor); nonsteroidal anti-inflammatory drugs (NSAIDs); angiotensin-converting enzyme (ACE) inhibitors, and trimethoprim-sulfamethoxazole.

E. **Is the lab result correct?** If hyperkalemia is unexpected or inconsistent after the preceding questions are answered, consider pseudohyperkalemia, especially if the ECG shows no changes of hyperkalemia. There are several causes of factitious hyperkalemia, the most common being from the tourniquet used to draw blood. A tight tourniquet around an exercising extremity can elevate the potassium as much as 2.0 mmol/L. Hemolysis of a blood sample prior to the chemical determination is another frequent source of error. Extreme leukocytosis (> 70,000) or thrombocytosis (> 1,000,000) can also elevate the serum potassium. If there is a question, obtain a plasma potassium.

III. **Differential Diagnosis.** In general, true hyperkalemia results from one of two mechanisms: a shift of potassium from intracellular to extracellular space; or impaired renal excretion of potassium.

A. **Acidosis.** With acidosis, potassium moves out of the cells and hydrogen ions move into the cells. A common example is diabetic ketoacidosis. Although insulin deficiency per se is probably not a cause of hyperkalemia, it may increase the degree of hyperkalemia in response to either an endogenous or an exogenous potassium load.

B. **Tissue breakdown.** Any condition associated with rapid destruction of cells results in the release of potassium into the extracellular fluid. Examples include rhabdomyolysis, burns, massive hemolysis, and tumor lysis.

C. **Digitalis intoxication.** A massive overdose of digitalis is a rare cause of hyperkalemia. This results from inhibition of the sodium/potassium-dependent ATPase pump and intracellular potassium is lost.

D. **Succinylcholine.** Mild increases in serum potassium occur with this commonly used muscle relaxant. In patients with tissue destruction or neuromuscular disease, life-threatening hyperkalemia may occur. Succinylcholine causes cell membrane depolarization, resulting in intracellular-to-extracellular shifts in potassium.

E. **Hyperosmolality.** Administration of hypertonic mannitol or saline results in major increases in serum osmolality, and thus may cause hyperkalemia.

F. **Arginine hydrochloride.** Intravenous administration of arginine hydrochloride, whether used diagnostically to assess growth hormone reserves, or therapeutically in the treatment of metabolic alkalosis, may lead to hyperkalemia. This is probably due to an arginine-potassium exchange.

G. **Hyperkalemic periodic paralysis.** This rare, inherited disorder is characterized by spontaneous episodes of hyperkalemia and muscle weakness.

H. **Chronic renal failure.** Most patients with chronic renal failure maintain normal potassium balance until renal function is severely impaired. However, when this condition is challenged with a potassium load or potassium-sparing diuretics (spironolactone, triamterene, amiloride), ACE inhibitors (enalapril, lisinopril), or NSAIDs (indomethacin, ibuprofen), the patient's adaptive mechanisms are inadequate to prevent hyperkalemia.

I. **Acute renal failure.** Hyperkalemia complicates oliguric renal failure because of the flow-dependent distal tubular potassium secretion. Acute renal failure often occurs in the setting of increased potassium load (trauma, blood transfusions, or postoperative hypercatabolic state).

J. **Adrenal insufficiency.** Adrenal insufficiency, in particular hypoaldosteronism, results in reduced renal ability to excrete potassium.

K. **Hyporeninemic hypoaldosteronism.** Hyperchloremic metabolic acidosis (type IV renal tubular acidosis) as well as hyperkalemia is present. Mild renal insufficiency secondary to diabetic nephropathy or interstitial nephropathy is also seen. May be aggravated by administration of NSAIDs or potassium-sparing diuretics.

L. **Heparin.** Long-term anticoagulation with heparin may lead to hyperkalemia, probably through the inhibition of aldosterone synthesis.

M. **Potassium-sparing diuretics.** Hyperkalemia secondary to triamterene or spironolactone is usually seen with underlying renal insufficiency. But there have been cases, especially in diabetics, in which patients with normal renal function developed hyperkalemia.

N. **NSAIDs.** See III.H.

O. **ACE inhibitors.** See III.H.

P. **Systemic lupus erythematosus (SLE), renal transplant, sickle cell disease.** Patients with these disorders may demonstrate an isolated defect in renal potassium excretion thought to be secondary to aldosterone resistance.

Q. **Increased exogenous intake.** High-potassium foods, potassium salts (salt "substitutes"), or large doses of potassium penicillin are examples of exogenous sources of potassium. Hyperkalemia in this setting usually occurs in patients on potassium-sparing diuretics, ACE inhibitors, or NSAIDs.

R. **Trimethoprim-sulfamethoxazole (TMP-SMX).** High-dose TMP-SMX therapy used for the treatment of *Pneumocystis carinii* pneumonia in HIV-infected patients may result in life-threatening hyperkalemia. Standard-dose TMP-SMX has subsequently been shown to increase serum potassium when used to treat various infections, especially with concomitant renal insufficiency. Trimethoprim acts like amiloride to block sodium channels in the distal nephron, decreasing renal potassium excretion.

IV. Database

A. Physical examination key points

1. **Cardiovascular exam.** The conduction system of the heart is most vulnerable to hyperkalemia, which may result in bradycardia, ventricular fibrillation, or asystole.
2. **Neuromuscular exam.** Skeletal muscle paralysis may occasionally dominate and result in weakness, tingling, and hyperactive deep tendon reflexes.

B. Laboratory data

1. **Electrolytes.** A low bicarbonate may indicate a metabolic acidosis. A low sodium may result from aldosterone deficiency.
2. **Plasma potassium.** Obtain if the serum level is in doubt.
3. **BUN and creatinine.** Assess renal function.
4. **Arterial blood gases.** Along with a serum bicarbonate, an ABG is essential in establishing the acid–base status.
5. **Platelets and white blood cell count.** Marked elevations may cause factitious hyperkalemia.
6. **Serum creatine phosphokinase (CK).** To detect rhabdomyolysis.
7. **Digoxin level.** If indicated.
8. **Serum aldosterone level.** Indicated after initial workup. Lack of stimulation with volume depletion is consistent with mineralocorticoid deficiency.

C. Other studies.

An ECG is **a must!** The cardiac abnormalities that occur with hyperkalemia are initially tall, peaked T waves in the precordial leads, followed by decreased amplitude of the R wave, widened QRS complex, prolongation of the PR interval, and then decreased amplitude and disappearance of the P wave. Finally, the QRS blends into the T wave, forming the classic sine wave. Ventricular fibrillation and asystole may follow.

V. Plan.

Hyperkalemia should be treated as an emergency if the serum potassium has reached 7 mmol/L, although cardiac or neuromuscular symptoms may mandate urgent treatment at lower potassium levels.

A. Acute treatment

1. Calcium is the initial treatment. Calcium antagonizes the membrane effects of hyperkalemia and restores normal excitability within 1–2 minutes. 10% calcium chloride 5–10 mL or 10% calcium gluconate 10–20 mL should be given IV over 3–5 minutes.
2. Potassium can be quickly shifted into cells by the administration of alkali or glucose plus insulin.
   a. Sodium bicarbonate (one ampoule [44 mmol] of bicarbonate) may be administered IV over several minutes.
   b. A 50-g ampoule of dextrose and 15 U of IV regular insulin may be given (3 g glucose for every 1 U of regular insulin).

B. Further treatment. It should be noted that calcium, alkali, glucose, and insulin do not lower the total body potassium. Once the patient is stabilized, the total body potassium needs to be reduced.

1. Potassium-binding resins may be used when the immediate life-threatening cardiac manifestations are under control. Kayexalate may be given orally, 40 g in 25–50 mL of 70% sorbitol every 2–4 hours; or rectally, 50–100 g in 200 mL water as a retention enema for 30 minutes every 2–4 hours.
2. Hemodialysis and peritoneal dialysis are definitive measures for controlling hyperkalemia in renal failure.

REFERENCES

Acker CG, Johnson JP, Palevsky PM et al: Hyperkalemia in hospitalized patients. Arch Intern Med 1998;158:917.

Black RM: Disorders of acid-base and potassium balance. Scientific American 1999;Sect 10: *Nephrology*.

Greenberg S, Reiser IW, Chou S-Y et al: Trimethoprim-sulfamethoxazole induces reversible hyperkalemia. Ann Intern Med 1993;119:291.

Perazella MA: Drug-induced hyperkalemia: Old culprits and new offenders. Am J Med 2000;109:307.

Perazella MA, Mahnensmith RL: Hyperkalemia in the elderly. J Gen Intern Med 1997;12:646.

Velazquez H, Perazella MA, Wright FS et al: Renal mechanism of trimethoprim induced hyperkalemia. Ann Intern Med 1993;119:296.

34. HYPERNATREMIA

I. Problem. The clinical chemistry lab calls to tell you that the 65-year-old female patient admitted with pneumonia has a serum sodium of 155 mmol/L (normal: 136–145 mmol/L).

II. Immediate Questions

A. Is the patient awake, alert, and oriented? Or is the patient lethargic and confused? The major signs and symptoms of hypernatremia are lethargy, which may lead to coma or convulsions; and neuromuscular irritability, including tremors, rigidity, and hyperreflexia. Mortality and symptoms are related to the level and the acuity of the hypernatremia. Mortality in adults is increased with the sodium levels above 160 mmol/L.

B. What medications is the patient taking? Mannitol can cause an osmotic diuresis, resulting in hypernatremia with low total body sodium. Exogenous steroids and salt tablets can cause an increase in the total body sodium.

C. What are the intake/output values for the past few days? A loss of total body water by fluid deprivation (inadequate thirst mechanism or inadequate administration of fluids) or from sweating can cause hypernatremia.

D. Are there any underlying medical conditions? Certain diseases, such as diabetes insipidus (DI) (central or nephrogenic), hyperaldosteronism, and Cushing's syndrome, are associated with hypernatremia. Recent cerebral trauma or neurosurgery can be a cause of central DI.

E. Does the patient have a condition that prevents access to water? Dehydration can result from inadequate access to water secondary to being bedridden or inadequate thirst mechanism from CNS dysfunction.

F. Is the lab value accurate? As with any lab result that is unexpected, the abnormal laboratory value could be an error. It may be prudent to repeat the test.

G. What is the composition of fluids administered? Check sodium content of fluids; hypertonic solutions (eg, hypertonic dialysate) can cause hypernatremia. If the patient is on tube feedings, be sure there is adequate free water (300 cc/day).

H. Is there a history of polyuria and polydipsia? Diabetes mellitus and DI can cause hypernatremia.

III. Differential Diagnosis. The differential diagnosis is best considered in light of the possible causes of hypernatremia: a loss of water and sodium, a loss of total body water, and, rarely, an increase in total body sodium.

A. Water and sodium loss. Significant sodium loss with even greater loss of water.

1. **Renal losses** (urine $[Na^+] > 20$ mmol/L)
   a. **Osmotic diuresis**
      i. **Mannitol**
      ii. **Hyperglycemia**
      iii. **Urea**
   b. **Diuretics.** For example, thiazide diuretics and furosemide.
   c. **Postobstructive diuresis.** Caused by relief of long-standing bilateral ureteral (nephrolithiasis, cervical carcinoma) and bladder outlet obstruction (prostatic hypertrophy).
   d. **Acute tubular necrosis.** Polyuric phase.
   e. **Intrinsic renal disease**
2. **Extra-renal losses** (urine $[Na^+] < 20$ mmol/L)
   a. **Cutaneous losses**
      i. **Fever.** Losses of 500 mL/24 hr for each degree centigrade increase above 38.3°C (101°F).
      ii. **Burns**
      iii. **Profuse sweating**
   b. **Gastrointestinal losses**
      i. **Vomiting**
      ii. **Nasogastric suction**

- *iii.* **Diarrhea.** Hypotonic diarrhea in children. Also, with the use of lactulose when the number of stools per day exceeds the recommended 2–3.
- *iv.* **Fistulae**

B. **Water losses without loss of sodium** (urine [Na^+] is variable)
   1. **Renal losses**
      a. **Central diabetes insipidus.** Results from failure to produce adequate amounts of antidiuretic hormone (ADH). If thirst mechanism is intact and patient has free access to water, hypernatremia may be minimal. May be idiopathic or caused by CNS surgery, trauma, infection, or tumor (metastatic or primary).
      b. **Nephrogenic.** ADH is not effective. May be congenital or caused by sickle cell disease, hypokalemia, hypercalcemia, polycystic kidney disease; or by drugs (lithium, alcohol, phenytoin, and glyburide).
   2. **Extra-renal losses**
      a. **Pulmonary losses.** Insensible losses, especially in intubated patients who are not receiving adequate humidification or with increased respiratory rates.
      b. **Cutaneous losses.** Fever or sweating.

C. **Increase in total body sodium without a change in total body water** (urine [Na^+] > 20 mmol/L).
   1. **Increase in mineralocorticoids or glucocorticoids**
      a. **Exogenous steroids** (eg, prednisone)
      b. **Primary aldosteronism**
      c. **Cushing's syndrome.** Cushing's disease, bilateral adrenal hyperplasia, or ectopic adrenocorticotropin (ACTH) production.
      d. **Exogenous steroids**
   2. **Administration of hypertonic sodium**
      a. **Sodium chloride tablets**
      b. **Hypertonic dialysate**
      c. **Hypertonic sodium bicarbonate.** Given during resuscitation after cardiopulmonary arrest.
      d. **Hypertonic sodium chloride fluids** ("hot salt," 3% NaCl)
      e. **Improper mixed formulas or tube feedings**
      f. **Ingestion of sea water**
      g. **Hypertonic saline enemas**
      h. **Sodium chloride–rich emetics**
      i. **Intrauterine injection of hypertonic saline**

IV. Database

A. **Physical examination key points**
   1. **Vital signs.** Check for orthostatic changes in blood pressure and heart rate. A decrease in systolic blood pressure of 10 mm Hg and/or an increase in heart rate of 20 bpm 1 minute after moving

from a supine to a standing position points to volume depletion. Also a decrease in weight suggests volume depletion.

2. **Skin.** Check turgor; poor turgor suggests volume depletion. Remember poor skin turgor can be a normal variant in the elderly.
3. **Mouth.** Dry mucous membranes suggest volume depletion.
4. **Neurologic exam.** Look for signs of irritability, muscle twitching, hyperreflexia, or seizures. A thorough neurologic examination needs to be done since CNS trauma, infection, or tumor can cause DI.

B. **Laboratory data**

1. **Serum sodium.** Normal 136–145 mmol/L. Follow closely, especially if sodium is > 160 mmol/L.
2. **Urine osmolality.** > 700 mOsm/L suggests insufficient water intake with or without extra-renal water losses or an osmoreceptor defect. A urine osmolality between 700 mOsm/L and the serum osmolality suggests partial central DI, osmotic diuresis, diuretic therapy, acquired (partial) nephrogenic DI, or renal failure. A urine osmolality < serum osmolality suggests complete central DI or nephrogenic DI.
3. **Spot urine sodium.** In hypernatremia with water and sodium loss, a level < 20 mmol/L suggests extra-renal loss. In hypernatremia with water loss without loss of sodium, the spot sodium in extra-renal losses is variable.
4. **Water deprivation/vasopressin.** If you suspect DI. The patient is fluid-deprived until the plasma osmolality is 295 mOsm/kg or greater; or on three consecutive hourly urines, the osmolality does not increase; or the patient loses 3% to 5% of his or her body weight. Five units of aqueous vasopressin is then given, either IM or SC.
   a. **Normal subjects.** Urine concentrates with fluid deprivation and no change occurs with vasopressin.
   b. **Complete central DI.** Urine does not concentrate with fluid deprivation. There is a significant increase in urine osmolality after vasopressin.
   c. **Nephrogenic DI.** Urine does not concentrate with deprivation and there is no change in urine osmolality with vasopressin.

C. **Radiologic and other studies.** A CT scan of the head to rule out a CNS lesion may be helpful if central DI is suspected.

V. **Plan.** The overall plan is to slowly decrease the serum sodium toward normal. Only hyperacute hypernatremia (hypernatremia < 12 hr) may be treated rapidly. Too rapid a correction of the sodium in hypernatremia may result in cerebral edema, seizures, and herniation, leading to death. The rate of correction of the sodium should not exceed 0.7 mmol/L/hr or about 10% of the serum sodium concentration per day. Specific treatment depends on whether there is a loss of sodium and water, a loss of water, or an increase in total body sodium.

A. **Water and sodium loss.** Represents significant volume depletion. With shock, replenish volume with normal saline. If patient is hemodynamically stable, replace volume with hypotonic saline (half-normal saline).

B. **Water loss without loss of sodium.** Calculate the free water deficit: weight (kg) × 0.60 = total body water. Water deficit = total body water × (1 – [desired $[Na^1]$ / measured $[Na^+]$]). Give ½ of the calculated free water deficit in the first 12 hours and the remainder in the next 24 hours. Include maintenance fluids.

C. **Increase in total body sodium.** Remove excess sodium, either by giving free water and diuretics, or by dialysis with hypotonic dialysate.

D. **Treatment of underlying cause**
   1. **Central DI.** After correction of free water deficit, begin vasopressin.
   2. **Diabetes mellitus.** Treat with insulin and IV fluids. (See Section I, Chapter 32, Hyperglycemia, V, p 183).
   3. **Nephrogenic DI.** After correction of free water deficit, begin thiazide diuretic and low-salt diet. Remove offending agent if appropriate.

REFERENCES

Adrogue HJ, Madias NE: Hypernatremia. N Engl J Med 2000;342:1493.

Berl T, Schrier RW: Disorders of water metabolism. In: Schrier RW, ed. *Renal and Electrolyte Disorders.* 5th ed. Lippincott-Raven;1997:1.

Palvevsky PM, Bhagrath R, Greenberg A: Hypernatremia in hospitalized patients. Ann Intern Med 1996;124:197.

35. HYPERTENSION

I. **Problem.** A 37-year-old woman complains of a severe occipital headache for the past 6 hours. Her blood pressure is 220/140.

II. **Immediate Questions**

A. **Is there a past history of hypertension?** You want to know if she is being treated for hypertension and regularly sees a physician. Previously, what was the highest blood pressure?

B. **What is the patient's medical regimen?** You want to know all the medications the patient is taking and whether she is compliant. For example, she may have stopped taking clonidine (Catapres) or a short-acting beta-blocker such as propranolol (Inderal), which can cause severe rebound hypertension. Hypertensive crisis can occur in people taking a monoamine oxidase inhibitor (MAOI) who ingest certain cheeses or wine containing tyramine. Ingestion of street drugs such as cocaine or amphetamines can also cause hypertensive crisis.

C. **Is the patient experiencing any other symptoms besides headache?** A patient with severe hypertension who has a headache with mental status changes may have hypertensive encephalopathy, which is a medical emergency. Hypertensive encephalopathy is more common in patients whose blood pressure suddenly rises, as with toxemia of pregnancy. Other manifestations of end-organ damage from malignant hypertension include myocardial infarction, angina, dyspnea (left ventricular dysfunction), dissecting aortic aneurysm, visual loss, nausea, vomiting, seizures, focal neurologic deficits, and a decrease in urinary output.

III. **Differential Diagnosis.** Hypertension can be classified as essential or secondary (describes the cause); and as accelerated or malignant (describes urgency). Patients with malignant hypertension often have a secondary cause of hypertension. With malignant hypertension the first concern is to lower the blood pressure.

A. **Essential.** Comprises 90–95% of all hypertension. No underlying cause.

B. **Secondary**

1. **Renovascular.** From fibromuscular dysplasia (usually women 20–30 years old) and atherosclerosis (usually men older than 50).
2. **Primary aldosteronism.** Hypertension with unexplained hypokalemia.
3. **Cushing's disease.** Characteristic findings include moon facies, truncal obesity, purple striae, a buffalo hump, hirsutism, and easy bruising. Hypernatremia and hypokalemic metabolic alkalosis are common.
4. **Pheochromocytoma.** Usually episodic hypertension. The hypertension often has associated diaphoresis, palpitations, pallor, and headache.
5. **Coarctation of the aorta.** Should be suspected in anyone young presenting with hypertension. Blood pressures are often higher in the right arm and femoral pulses are often absent.
6. **Primary renal disease**
7. **Hyperthyroidism.** Systolic hypertension.
8. **Hypothyroidism.** Diastolic hypertension.
9. **Heavy ethanol use or withdrawal.** May cause or aggravate underlying hypertension. Hypertension associated with withdrawal is secondary to hyperadrenergic state.
10. **Drugs**
    a. **Estrogens**
    b. **Other prescription medications.** Cyclosporine, nonsteroidal anti-inflammatory drugs, corticosteroids, and erythropoietin can occasionally cause hypertension.
    c. **Over-the-counter medications containing sympathomimetics.** For example, decongestants (pseudoephedrine) and weight loss medications (ephedrine and ephedra) may elevate the blood pressure.
    d. **Illicit drugs.** Phencyclidine (PCP), amphetamines, and cocaine.

11. **Postoperative conditions.** Multifactorial, including hypoxia, pain, anxiety, volume overload, hypothermia, and medications.
12. **Gestational**
13. **Hyperparathyroidism**

C. **Miscellaneous diseases.** Other diseases can cause a marked elevation in blood pressure; or may be the consequence of long-standing, poorly controlled hypertension.
   1. **Cerebrovascular accident.** If the patient has had a stroke resulting in marked elevation of blood pressure, the physician is not quite as aggressive in lowering the blood pressure. A sudden marked drop in blood pressure can extend a stroke.
   2. **Subarachnoid hemorrhage.** Patients classically complain of the worst headache of their life.
   3. **Aortic dissection.** "Tearing" chest pain, often with radiation to the back, and most severe at onset. Usually a previous history of hypertension.
   4. **Congestive heart failure/pulmonary edema**
   5. **Angina pectoris/myocardial infarction.** See Section I, Chapter 11, Chest Pain, p 57.

D. **Accelerated hypertension.** Markedly elevated blood pressure with no current life-threatening problem secondary to the hypertension.

E. **Malignant hypertension.** Usually a markedly elevated blood pressure with an associated serious complication, such as hypertensive encephalopathy, angina, myocardial infarction, aortic dissection, or cerebrovascular accident; proteinuria, hematuria, and red blood cell casts may be present.

IV. Database

A. Physical examination key points

1. **Vital signs.** Take blood pressure in both arms; feel both radial pulses and check for a radial-femoral pulse lag. Such maneuvers may point to aortic dissection or coarctation.
2. **Eyes.** Look for evidence of papilledema, hemorrhages, exudates, severe arteriolar narrowing, and arteriovenous nicking. Papilledema is usually present with malignant hypertension but can occur in other conditions with increased intracranial pressure.
3. **Lungs.** Presence of rales may indicate congestive heart failure.
4. **Heart.** Palpate the apical impulse for displacement. Listen for a third heart sound (S_3) indicative of left ventricular dysfunction; a fourth heart sound (S_4) often seen with long-standing hypertension or a recent myocardial infarction; and for a murmur of aortic insufficiency, which can occur in aortic dissection.
5. **Neurologic exam.** Assess the patient's mental status and look for any focal deficits that may indicate a cerebrovascular accident. Confusion and somnolence progressing to coma are hallmarks of

hypertensive encephalopathy. Be sure to check reflexes; unilateral hyperreflexia may indicate an intracranial event.

B. Laboratory data

1. **Electrolytes, BUN, glucose, and creatinine.** To rule out evidence of renal insufficiency, hypokalemia, or hyperglycemia. Hypokalemia occurs in Cushing's disease, primary hyperaldosteronism, and renovascular hypertension. Hyperglycemia can be a manifestation of a pheochromocytoma, Cushing's disease, or stress. Mild renal insufficiency points toward hypertensive nephropathy, whereas marked renal insufficiency potentially suggests a secondary cause of hypertension.
2. **Urinalysis.** To look for proteinuria, hematuria, and red cell casts for evidence of a secondary cause or hypertensive nephropathy.
3. **Complete blood count and examination of peripheral blood smear.** Red blood cell fragments, or *schistocytes,* occur in microangiopathic hemolytic anemia resulting from malignant hypertension.

C. Radiologic and other studies

1. **Chest x-ray.** To look for cardiomegaly, congestive heart failure, and mediastinal widening suggesting proximal aortic dissection. Rib notching and obliteration of the aortic knob suggest coarctation of the aorta.
2. **Electrocardiogram.** To look for ischemic changes and left ventricular hypertrophy.
3. **CT scan.** If patient has mental status changes or focal neurologic findings, a CT scan must be performed to exclude a thromboembolic stroke or subarachnoid hemorrhage.

V. Plan

A. Hypertensive emergency. Treatment must be initiated within minutes if possible.

1. **Admission to an ICU.** Intravenous and arterial lines should be placed.
2. **Appropriate therapy.** Initiated once therapeutic goals are established. The goal of immediate therapy is to reduce mean arterial blood pressure by no more than 25% within minutes to 2 hours. Overly aggressive reduction of blood pressure beyond these levels can lead to cerebral hypoperfusion and worsening neurologic deficits. This is particularly important in patients who have a stroke or a transient ischemic attack, who are more susceptible to abrupt falls in blood pressure.
   a. Nitroprusside is commonly used in hypertensive crises. It reduces preload and afterload when given in a dose of 0.25–10 μg/kg/min as a continuous IV infusion. It has the advantage of immediate onset and is easily titrated. Disadvantages include the need for constant monitoring; also, prolonged use is asso-

ciated with thiocyanate toxicity. ***Caution:*** Avoid use in the presence of azotemia.

b. Intravenous labetalol, an alpha- and beta-blocker, is infused at 20 mg IV over 2 minutes followed by 40–80 mg at 10-minute intervals, to a total dose of 300 mg; **OR** 2 mg/min IV as a constant infusion. Potential disadvantages include beta-blocking side effects. ***Caution:*** Avoid use in the presence of acute heart failure.

c. Intravenous enalaprilat (1.25–5 mg every 6 hours) can be used. Onset of action is 15–30 minutes. Especially useful with acute left ventricular failure. ***Caution:*** Avoid using in the presence of acute myocardial infarction; enalaprilat may cause a precipitous decrease in blood pressure, especially with high-renin state.

d. For suspected pheochromocytoma, IV labetalol, phentolamine, or phenoxybenzamine can be used.

e. Hypertension associated with aortic dissection should be controlled with IV labetalol, esmolol, or verapamil (see Section I, Chapter 11, Chest Pain, V, p 63).

3. Treatment of accelerated hypertension. Can be treated with oral medications. Clonidine 0.1 mg PO can be used; repeat the dose every 1–2 hours. You may just want to increase the patient's current medications and follow him or her closely. ***Caution:*** Calcium channel–blocking agents other than sustained-release formulations have fallen into disfavor because of the increased mortality associated with their long-term use. Other oral agents such as beta-blockers and angiotensin-converting enzyme inhibitors can also be used. It is imperative that you closely monitor the blood pressure to avoid wide fluctuations in blood pressure and avoid hypotension.

4. Treatment of hypertension. A thorough discussion of hypertension is beyond the scope of this book. Please refer to any number of references including those listed here.

REFERENCES

Coates ML, Rembold CM, Farr BM: Does pseudoephedrine increase blood pressure in patients with controlled hypertension? J Fam Pract 1995;40:22.

Joint National Committee on Detection, Evaluation, and Treatment of High Blood Pressure: The Sixth Report of the Joint National Committee on Detection, Evaluation, and Treatment of High Blood Pressure. Arch Intern Med 1997;157:2413.

Kaplan NM: *Clinical Hypertension.* 6th ed. Williams & Wilkins;1994.

36. HYPOCALCEMIA

I. Problem. A 54-year-old man admitted for an acute myocardial infarction (MI) has a calcium of 3.5 mEq/L, or 1.75 mmol/L (normal: 4.2–5.1 mEq/L, or 2.10–2.55 mmol/L).

II. Immediate Questions

A. **Are there any symptoms relevant to the low calcium?** Asymptomatic hypocalcemia usually does not require emergent treatment. Signs and symptoms of hypocalcemia may include peripheral and perioral paresthesias, Trousseau's *and/or* Chvostek's signs (see IV.4.a. and b.), confusion, muscle twitching, laryngospasm, tetany, and seizures.

B. **Does the low calcium level represent the true ionized calcium?** Most laboratories report the total serum calcium, but it is the ionized calcium level that is important physiologically. The total serum calcium level decreases by 0.2 mmol/L, or 0.4 mEq/L, for every 1 g/dL decrease in the serum albumin level without changing the ionized calcium level. Calculate the adjusted total calcium level or order an ionized calcium level.

C. **Is there a past history of neck surgery?** Surgical removal or infarction of the parathyroid glands is one of the more common causes of hypocalcemia. Look for a scar on the neck.

III. Differential Diagnosis.

The causes of low ionized serum calcium can be categorized as parathyroid hormone deficits, vitamin D deficits, and loss or displacement of calcium.

A. **Parathyroid hormone (PTH) deficits**
   1. **Decreased PTH level**
      a. **Surgical excision or injury.** Including thyroid surgery.
      b. **Infiltrative diseases of the parathyroid gland.** For example, hemochromatosis, amyloid or metastatic cancer.
      c. **Idiopathic**
      d. **Irradiation.** To the neck to treat lymphoma.
   2. **Decreased PTH activity**
      a. **Congenital.** Pseudohypoparathyroidism: resistance to PTH at the tissue level.
      b. **Acquired.** Hypomagnesemia.

B. **Vitamin D deficiency**
   1. **Malnutrition**
   2. **Malabsorption**
      a. **Pancreatitis**
      b. **Postgastrectomy**
      c. **Short gut syndrome**
      d. **Laxative abuse**
      e. **Sprue**
      f. **Hepatobiliary disease with bile salt deficiency**
   3. **Defective metabolism**
      a. **Liver disease.** Failure to synthesize 25-hydroxyvitamin D.
      b. **Renal disease.** Failure to synthesize 1,25-dihydroxyvitamin D.
      c. **Anticonvulsant treatment with phenobarbital or phenytoin (Dilantin).** Possibly from an increase in the metabolism of vitamin D in the liver leading to a vitamin D deficiency.

C. **Calcium loss or displacement**
   1. **Hyperphosphatemia.** Increases bone deposition of calcium.
      a. **Acute phosphate ingestion**
      b. **Acute phosphate release by rhabdomyolysis or tumor lysis**
      c. **Renal failure**
   2. **Acute pancreatitis**
   3. **Osteoblastic metastases.** Especially breast and prostate cancer.
   4. **Medullary carcinoma of the thyroid.** Increased calcitonin.
   5. **Decreased bone resorption.** Overuse of actinomycin, calcitonin, or mithramycin.
   6. **Miscellaneous disorders.** Sepsis, massive transfusion, hungry bone syndrome, toxic shock syndrome, and fat embolism.

IV. Database

A. **Physical examination key points**
   1. **Skin.** Dermatitis with chronic hypocalcemia.
   2. **HEENT.** Cataracts with chronic hypocalcemia. Laryngospasm is rare but life-threatening. Look for surgical scars on the neck.
   3. **Neuromuscular exam.** Confusion, spasm, twitching, facial grimacing, and hyperactive deep tendon reflexes all indicate symptomatic hypocalcemia.
   4. **Specific tests for tetany of hypocalcemia**
      a. **Chvostek's sign.** Present in 5% to 10% of normocalcemic patients. Tapping on the facial nerve near the zygoma will elicit a twitch in hypocalcemic patients.
      b. **Trousseau's sign.** Inflate a blood pressure cuff above the systolic pressure for 3 minutes and watch for carpal spasm.

B. **Laboratory data**
   1. **Serum electrolytes.** Particularly calcium, phosphate, potassium, and magnesium. Calcium must be interpreted in terms of the serum albumin (see II.B., p 199). Hypomagnesemia and hyperkalemia may potentiate the effects of hypocalcemia.
   2. **Serum albumin.** As mentioned earlier.
   3. **BUN and creatinine.** To rule out renal failure.
   4. **Parathyroid hormone level.** A low normal level is inappropriately low in the presence of true hypocalcemia.
   5. **Vitamin D levels.** 25-hydroxyvitamin D and 1,25-dihydroxyvitamin D.
   6. **Urinary cyclic AMP.** May indicate evidence of PTH resistance.
   7. **Fecal fat.** To evaluate for steatorrhea.

C. **Radiologic and other tests**
   1. **Electrocardiogram.** A prolonged QT interval and T wave inversion can occur with marked hypocalcemia, as can various arrhythmias.

2. **Bone films.** May show bony changes of renal failure or osteoblastic metastases.

V. **Plan.** Assess for tetany, which can potentially progress to laryngeal spasm or seizures, and requires immediate treatment. Otherwise, establish the diagnosis by testing blood for calcium, albumin, magnesium, phosphate, and PTH levels, and begin appropriate oral therapy.

A. **Emergency treatment.** Emergency treatment is usually needed for a calcium level below 1.5 mmol/L (3 mEq/L) to prevent fatal laryngospasm. Give 100–200 mg of elemental calcium IV over 10 minutes in 50–100 mL of D5W; follow with a 1–2 mg/kg/hr infusion for 6–12 hours. Use caution in patients on digoxin because calcium may potentiate the effect of digoxin, resulting in heart block.

1. **10% calcium gluconate.** One 10-mL ampoule contains 23.25 mmol (93 mg) of calcium. Give 10–20 mL initially; follow with the infusion.
2. **10% calcium chloride.** One 10-mL ampoule contains 68 mmol (272 mg) of calcium. Give 5–10 mL IV, being careful to avoid extravasation, which can cause skin to slough; then start an infusion.
3. **10% calcium gluceptate.** One 5-mL ampoule contains 90 mg of elemental calcium. One can deliver 900 mg of calcium in 500 mL of fluid by adding 10 ampoules to 450 mL of D5W.

B. **Chronic therapy.** With primary PTH deficiency the goal is to give 2–4 g of oral calcium daily in four divided doses, adding vitamin D as necessary. With vitamin D disorders, vitamin D must always be supplemented.

1. **Calcium carbonate.** There is 240 mg of calcium per 600-mg tablet.
2. **Calcium citrate and lactate tablets and calcium glubionate syrup are available.**
3. **Vitamin D.** Ergocalciferol (vitamin D_2) 50,000 U/d or dihydrotachysterol (vitamin D_2 analogue) 100–400 μg/d or calcitriol (1, 25-dihydroxy-vitamin D_3) 0.25–1.0 μg/d.
4. **Magnesium.** Patients on parenteral nutrition need at least 4–7 mg/kg/d of magnesium.

C. **Magnesium deficiency.** See Section I, Chapter 39, Hypomagnesemia, V, p 212.

1. In an emergency, one can give 10–15 mL of $MgSO_4$ 20% solution IV over 1 minute, followed by 500 mL of $MgSO_4$ 2% solution in D5W over 4–6 hours.
2. More typically, 6 g (49 mEq, or 24.5 mmol) of $MgSO_4$ in 1000 mL of D5W is given IV over 4 hours, followed by 6 g every 8 hours × 2, followed by 6 g every day.

REFERENCES

Reber PM, Heath H: Hypocalcemic emergencies. Med Clin North Am 1995;79:93.
Bushinsky DA, Monk RD: Calcium. Lancet 1998;352:306.

37. HYPOGLYCEMIA

I. **Problem.** A 33-year-old woman was admitted for diabetic ketoacidosis (DKA) 24 hours ago. The patient's finger-stick glucose is now 50 mg/dL, or 2.78 mmol/L.

II. **Immediate Questions**

A. **What are the patient's vital signs?** Is the patient symptomatic? Assessment of current status and vital signs allows the house officer to evaluate the urgency of the situation; that is, is there time for a repeat finger-stick or blood glucose, or should therapy be instituted immediately? Patients with hypoglycemia can have multiple symptoms. Early symptoms include headache, hunger, palpitations, tremor, and diaphoresis. As hypoglycemia progresses, abnormal behavior (such as combativeness) and slurred speech mimicking ethanol intoxication is followed by loss of consciousness, seizures, and even death. Beta-blockers can mask the early adrenergic symptoms of hypoglycemia (but diaphoresis, a cholinergic response, may still be present). Patients with long-standing diabetes mellitus may also lose the ability to perceive hypoglycemia.

B. **What medications is the patient taking?**

1. The dose, route, and type of insulin are important in determining the timing and severity of the hypoglycemia. Patients on intermediate-acting insulin (NPH or Lente) generally have a peak effect between 6 and 16 hours, whereas those on rapid-acting insulin (regular) given subcutaneously peak at 2–6 hours. Ultra-short-acting insulin (Humalog, Humulin) has an onset of action of 15 minutes and peaks at 1 hour. Only regular insulin is used intravenously. IV bolus insulin produces its maximum effect in 30 minutes. Patients on continuous IV infusion insulin drips and continuous SC insulin (by insulin pump) can show very rapid decreases in their serum glucose although the total dose received may be relatively small.
2. Some patients have different responses to rapid-acting and intermediate-acting insulin such that the peak effect is extended to 18–24 hours for intermediate-acting insulin and to 6–12 hours or longer for regular insulin.
3. Knowing the amount, type, and route for administration of insulin will help determine the likelihood of the hypoglycemia's worsening or recurring after treatment, as well as necessary changes in the insulin regimen. If a patient is on an oral hypoglycemic agent, it is important to know which one. Longer-acting agents increase the risk of recurrent hypoglycemia for hours or even a day, especially if the patient is fasting.

C. **Is there IV access?** It is necessary to determine that IV access is available to administer D50 if needed and to ascertain whether the patient is receiving intravenous fluids containing dextrose.

D. **When was the patient's last meal or snack?** If the patient has eaten a meal within the hour since the finger-stick was obtained, the situation will be less urgent since the meal may be treating the hypoglycemia.

III. Differential Diagnosis

A. Medications

1. **Insulin.** Check for accidental overdose, as when insulin is given to the wrong patient; or administration of the wrong type of insulin or by the wrong route; or intentional overdose (eg, Munchausen's syndrome).
2. **Oral hypoglycemic agents.** Especially chlorpropamide (Diabinese) in elderly patients.
3. **Other medications.** Acetaminophen (Tylenol), pentamidine (Pentam), haloperidol (Haldol), quinine, and salicylates can cause hypoglycemia.
4. **Ethanol.** Ethanol intoxication may cause hypoglycemia; in addition, many alcoholics may be glycogen-depleted prior to alcohol consumption due to inadequate food intake.
5. **Drug interactions.** The activity of oral hypoglycemic agents is increased when taken with nonsteroidal anti-inflammatory drugs, sulfonamides, or monoamine oxidase inhibitors.

B. **Reactive hypoglycemia.** This is a form of hypoglycemia that occurs after eating. It is found in 5–10% of patients who have undergone partial to complete gastrectomies, as well as de novo in the general population.

C. **Severe liver disease.** With massive liver destruction, glycogen stores are easily depleted.

D. **Insulinoma.** Pancreatic islet cell tumor; may be malignant. Serum insulin or C-peptide levels are helpful in establishing the diagnosis.

E. **Endocrinopathies.** These include Addison's disease, pituitary insufficiency, and myxedema.

F. **Renal disease.** This usually occurs in the setting of combined uremia and malnutrition. Insulin clearance decreases with renal failure.

G. **Sepsis.** Hypoglycemia is more likely in the setting of septic shock.

H. **Malnutrition/prolonged fasting.** Hypoglycemia is common in protein calorie malnutrition (kwashiorkor).

I. **Abrupt discontinuation of total parenteral nutrition (TPN).** This diagnosis is more likely if the TPN solution contains insulin.

J. **Factitious hypoglycemia.** This may occur as a result of either a marked elevation in the white blood cell count (*leukocyte metabolism*) or prolongation of contact of serum with red blood cells. Be suspicious of self-induced hypoglycemia if the patient has access to insulin or sulfonylurea drugs.

K. **Neoplasms.** Retroperitoneal sarcoma, hepatocellular carcinoma, and small cell (oat cell) carcinoma can cause hypoglycemia by production of insulin-like hormone, impaired glycogenolysis, or glucose consumption.

L. **Other causes.** These include glycogen storage disease, hereditary fructose intolerance, carnitine deficiency, anorexia nervosa, and ackee-fruit poisoning.

IV. Database

A. Physical examination key points

1. **Vital signs.** Hypertension and tachycardia may be caused by increased catecholamines as a response to hypoglycemia. This response may be eliminated in the presence of a beta-blocker.
2. **Skin.** Diaphoresis is a common cholinergic response to hypoglycemia that is not generally eliminated by beta-blockers.
3. **Neurologic exam.** The patient's sensorium and orientation are often altered. (See Section I, Chapter 13, Coma, Acute Mental Status Changes, p 72). Tremor at rest and with intention may be present. Unconsciousness and seizures indicate need for urgent treatment. Hypoglycemia occasionally presents with focal neurologic findings.

B. Laboratory data

1. **Serum glucose.** This is the most critical test; in general, a glucose level below 50 mg/dL and the presence of symptoms are diagnostic of hypoglycemia. Finger-stick values should always be confirmed by serum glucose measurements because they are prone to error secondary to strips that have been exposed to air, inappropriate preparation of the finger with Betadine, presence of alcohol on the finger, incorrect timing, or an uncalibrated machine. In the presence of symptoms, blood should be obtained immediately, but treatment should not be withheld pending results or a delay in obtaining blood.
2. **Electrolytes, BUN and creatinine, liver function studies, complete blood count, urinalysis.** In the setting of hypoglycemia with no history available, obtain to evaluate for common causes listed in the differential diagnosis.
3. **Drug screens.** Look specifically for oral hypoglycemics as well as for ethanol, salicylates, acetaminophen, and antipsychotics (eg, haloperidol).
4. **Serum insulin.** Results may indicate either exogenous insulin administration or insulinoma.
5. **C-peptide.** Will help to differentiate between insulinoma and exogenous insulin administration. The C-peptide level will be elevated with an insulinoma and low with the administration of exogenous insulin.

C. Radiologic and other studies. These may be indicated in specific circumstances to rule out infection, insulinoma, malignancy, or pituitary lesion.

V. Plan

A. Administer glucose. Do not wait for the results of the serum glucose if you strongly suspect the diagnosis. It is best to draw blood before administering glucose; however, you should proceed with treatment if there will be a significant delay before blood can be obtained and the patient is markedly symptomatic. If the patient is awake, and able and willing to take fluids, glucose should be given orally. Otherwise, administer IV glucose.

1. Orange juice with added sugar is usually readily available. Specific glucose-containing liquids are stocked on most hospital floors and may be substituted for orange juice. For mild hypoglycemia, 8 ounces of 2% milk or a package of saltines with juice may be adequate and not result in "overshoot" hyperglycemia.
2. Give one ampoule of 50% dextrose (D50) IV push; repeat in 5 minutes if no response. If there is no response after the second ampoule, the diagnosis should be seriously questioned and other causes for the symptoms should be considered, such as hypoxia, transient ischemic attack, and ethanol or drug intoxication or overdose.
3. If the patient is unable to take glucose PO, and IV access is not immediately available, give glucagon 0.5–1 mg IM or SC (may induce vomiting; be prepared to protect the patient's airway).
4. Start maintenance IV fluids with D5W at 75–100 mL/hr, especially if the hypoglycemia may recur, such as that resulting from chlorpropamide use or sepsis.
5. Follow serial glucoses frequently. Depending on the severity of the hypoglycemia, repeat glucose after treatment and again in 1–2 hours according to the results.

B. Adjust medications. Review schedule and dosing of insulin and/or oral hypoglycemics. Consider use of metformin (Glucophage) for Type 2 diabetics (less likely to cause hypoglycemia). See Section VII, Therapeutics, pp 597, 610 and 541.

C. Miscellaneous. If the patient is not taking hypoglycemic agents, then consider other causes listed in the differential diagnosis and evaluate accordingly.

REFERENCES

Bailey CJ: Biguanides and NIDDM. Diabetes Care 1992;15:755.

Campbell PJ: Mechanisms for prevention, development and reversal of hypoglycemia. Adv Intern Med 1988;33:205.

Service FJ: Hypoglycemia. Med Clin North Am 1995;79:1.

Service FJ: Hypoglycemic disorders. N Engl J Med 1995;332:1144.

38. HYPOKALEMIA

I. **Problem.** A 72-year-old woman with hypertension develops profound muscle weakness after 3 days of vomiting and diarrhea. Her serum potassium is 2.5 mmol/L (2.5 mEq/L).

II. **Immediate Questions**

A. **What are the patient's vital signs?** Although cardiac arrhythmias rarely occur with hypokalemia without underlying heart disease, even mild to moderate hypokalemia can induce cardiac arrhythmias in the presence of cardiac ischemia, congestive heart failure, or left ventricular hypertrophy. Premature atrial contractions (PACs), premature ventricular contractions (PVCs), or ventricular arrhythmias may be suggested by examination of the pulse.

B. **What medications is the patient taking?** The most common cause of hypokalemia is medications. Medications, especially diuretics, can cause renal potassium wasting. Also, digitalis toxicity is potentiated by hypokalemia.

C. **Has the patient had vomiting, diarrhea, nasogastric suction, or excessive sweating?** Gastrointestinal sources are possible causes of potassium loss. A prolonged, elevated temperature or delirium tremens can result in hypokalemia from sweating.

III. **Differential Diagnosis.** In general, hypokalemia is caused by cellular shifts or by renal or gastrointestinal losses.

A. **Hypokalemia resulting from cellular shifts**

1. **Alkalosis.** Both respiratory alkalosis and metabolic alkalosis are associated with hypokalemia. Hyperventilation during surgical anesthesia can cause acute respiratory alkalosis and produce significant hypokalemia.
2. **Familial periodic paralysis.** This rare, inherited disease is characterized by intermittent attacks of varying severity, ranging from muscle weakness to flaccid paralysis.
3. **Barium poisoning.** Ingestion of soluble barium salts may cause profound hypokalemia, muscle paralysis, and cardiac arrhythmias, probably as a result of intracellular shifts, although associated vomiting and diarrhea may contribute.
4. **Treatment of megaloblastic anemia.** Treatment of severe pernicious anemia (HcT $< 20\%$) with vitamin B_{12} causes an acute reduction in serum potassium as a result of the rapid uptake of potassium because of the marked increase in bone marrow activity.
5. **Leukemia.** Hypokalemia may be produced by sequestration of potassium ions by rapidly proliferating blast cells.
6. **Transfusions.** Administration of previously frozen washed red blood cells may cause hypokalemia due to the uptake of potassium by these cells.

7. **Drugs.** Drugs with β_2-sympathomimetic activity, including decongestants (pseudoephedrine), bronchodilators (albuterol), and inhibitors of uterine contractions (terbutaline), can cause hypokalemia. The standard dose of albuterol reduces the serum potassium by 0.2–0.4 mmol/L, and a second dose within 1 hour reduces it by almost 1 mmol/L. Theophylline, caffeine, verapamil intoxication, chloroquine intoxication, and insulin overdose may produce clinically significant hypokalemia.
8. **Hyperthyroidism.** Severe hypokalemia can occur rarely in association with hyperthyroidism. Results in sudden onset of severe muscle weakness and paralysis and is most commonly seen in patients of Asian descent.

B. Hypokalemia resulting from abnormal losses

1. **Diarrhea.** Diarrhea from virtually any cause may result in hypokalemia. But severe hypokalemia secondary to diarrhea is suggestive of colonic villous adenoma or non–insulin-secreting pancreatic islet cell tumors.
2. **Excessive sweat.** The sweat glands contain an aldosterone-dependent sodium/potassium exchange mechanism.
3. **Clay ingestion.** Reported to be relatively common in the southeastern United States. Clay binds potassium, resulting in potassium being excreted in stool.

C. Hypokalemia resulting from renal losses

1. **Diuretics.** The most common cause of hypokalemia is diuretic therapy. Loop diuretics, thiazides, and acetazolamide (Diamox) all may cause hypokalemia.
2. **Vomiting**
   a. Although gastric contents contain some potassium ions, the major loss through vomiting occurs in the urine. The loss of gastric hydrogen ions generates metabolic alkalosis, which stimulates potassium ion secretion. The sodium and water losses from vomiting cause volume depletion and stimulate aldosterone secretion.
   b. In cases of surreptitious vomiting (*bulimia*), hypokalemia, metabolic alkalosis, volume depletion, and a low urine chloride suggests the diagnosis.
3. **Renal losses caused by excess mineralocorticoid**
   a. **Primary aldosteronism.** Should be suspected in hypertensive patients who are hypokalemic prior to institution of diuretic therapy, or in those who become profoundly hypokalemic (< 2.5 mmol/L) with diuretics.
   b. **Cushing's syndrome.** Fifty percent of patients with Cushing's syndrome have hypokalemia. Hypertension and metabolic alkalosis are also seen.
   c. **Ectopic ACTH production.** Most commonly seen with small-cell carcinoma of the lung.

d. **Adrenogenital syndrome.** *11-Hydroxylase deficiency* is manifested by virilization in the female, precocious puberty in the male, hypokalemia, metabolic alkalosis, and hypertension. *17-Hydroxylase deficiency* is a rare form of congenital hyperplasia of the adrenal glands associated with hypokalemia and hypertension.

e. **Licorice ingestion.** Natural licorice contains glycyrrhizic acid, which has potent mineralocorticoid activity. These patients clinically resemble those with primary aldosteronism.

f. **Hyperreninemic states.** Hypokalemia is accompanied by hypertension and metabolic alkalosis in renal vascular hypertension, malignant hypertension, and renin-producing tumors. It is distinguished from primary aldosteronism by an elevated plasma renin.

g. **Bartter's syndrome.** A rare disorder characterized by hypokalemia, metabolic alkalosis, elevated renin and aldosterone levels, and normal blood pressure.

h. **Liddle's syndrome.** A rare disorder characterized by hypokalemia, hypertension, metabolic alkalosis, low plasma renin, and low urinary aldosterone.

i. **Type I (distal) renal tubular acidosis.** Characterized by hyperchloremic metabolic acidosis and hypokalemia. Results from an inability to maintain a hydrogen ion gradient.

j. **Type II (proximal) renal tubular acidosis.** Impaired proximal bicarbonate reabsorption results in distal delivery of bicarbonate and urinary loss of potassium ions as well as bicarbonate.

k. **Antibiotics.** Carbenicillin and ticarcillin, administered as sodium salts, enhance potassium ion excretion. Amphotericin B alters distal tubule permeability, resulting in hypokalemia.

l. **Magnesium depletion.** This may increase mineralocorticoid activity, but the pathophysiology is unknown.

m. **Ureterosigmoidostomy.** Hypokalemic hyperchloremic metabolic acidosis occurs because of an exchange mechanism in the colon. Ureteral implantation into a loop of ileum is now performed.

IV. Database

A. Physical examination key points

1. **Cardiovascular.** Irregular pulse may represent an arrhythmia (PACs or PVCs), or digitalis toxicity.
2. **Abdomen.** Look for distension and presence of bowel sounds. Ileus secondary to hypokalemia may be present. Abdominal examination may reveal a cause of vomiting.
3. **Neurologic exam.** Weakness, blunting of reflexes, paresthesias, and paralysis may be seen.

B. Laboratory data

1. **Serum electrolytes.** Hypomagnesemia may coexist or cause the hypokalemia.

2. **Arterial blood gases.** Look for alkalosis.
3. **Urine potassium, chloride, and sodium.** If the patient is not taking diuretics, a low urine sodium or chloride indicates volume depletion. A relatively high urine potassium in the face of hypokalemia indicates renal losses.
4. **Digoxin level.** A must if the patient is on digoxin. Hypokalemia may potentiate digoxin toxicity.

C. **Radiologic and other studies.** An electrocardiogram may show digitalis effect or manifestations of hypokalemia ranging from PACs and PVCs to life-threatening ventricular arrhythmias. A U wave is a common finding.

V. **Plan.** The degree of hypokalemia cannot be used as a rigid determinant of the total potassium ion deficit. It has been estimated that in a normal adult, a decrease in serum potassium from 4 to 3 mmol/L corresponds to a 100- to 200-mmol decrement in total body potassium. Each additional fall of 1 mmol/L in serum potassium represents an additional deficit of 200–400 mmol.

A. **Parenteral replacement**
1. **Indications.** Should be considered in the following situations: digoxin toxicity or significant arrhythmias, severe hypokalemia (< 3.0 mmol/L), and inability to take oral replacements (NPO, ileus, nausea, and vomiting). Ideally, parenteral solutions should be administered through a central venous catheter. In most other cases, hypokalemia can be safely corrected in a slow, controlled fashion with oral supplementation. Unfortunately, supplemental potassium administration is also the most common cause of severe hyperkalemia in hospitalized patients, and the risk is greatest with intravenous potassium.
2. **Implementation.** The maximum concentration of potassium chloride used in peripheral veins should generally not exceed 40 mmol/L because of the sclerosing effect of potassium (especially high concentrations) on the veins, although in an emergent situation 60 mmol/L can be attempted. Potassium chloride 20 mmol diluted in 50–100 mL D5W or normal saline can be infused over 1 hour through a central line safely, with doses repeated as needed when severe depletion or life-threatening hypokalemia is present. Special care must be taken to ensure slow infusion of high doses. For lesser degrees of hypokalemia that require parenteral replacement, 10–15 mmol/hr can be infused peripherally.
3. **Monitoring.** With large total replacement doses, check serum potassium every 2–4 hours to avoid hyperkalemia. Cardiac monitoring in an ICU is required if arrhythmias are present, or for rapid infusions of potassium chloride. ***Caution:*** Cardiac monitoring is required for rates that exceed 10–15 mmol/hr.

B. **Oral replacement.** Generally indicated for asymptomatic, mild potassium depletion (potassium usually > 3.0 mmol/L). Oral replacements include liquids and powder. Slow-release pills typically contain 8–10 mmol per tablet and thus are not usually appropriate for repletion therapy. The replacement rate should be 40–120 mmol/d in divided doses, depending on the patient's weight and level of hypokalemia. Maintenance therapy, if needed, should be given in doses of 20–80 mmol daily, using the preparation best tolerated by the patient. With normal renal function, it is difficult to induce hyperkalemia through the oral administration of potassium. An important exception is the use of potassium supplements with potassium-sparing diuretics or with angiotensin-converting enzyme (ACE) inhibitors.

C. **Replacement of ongoing losses.** Large amounts of nasogastric aspirate should be replaced milliliter for milliliter, with D5 half-normal saline with 20 mmol/L potassium chloride every 4–6 hours.

D. **Refractory cases.** Rarely, hypokalemia may not be correctable because of concomitant hypomagnesemia (see Section I, Chapter 39, Hypomagnesemia, V, p 212).

REFERENCES

Black RM: Disorders of acid-base and potassium balance. In: Rubenstein E, ed. Scientific American 1999;Sect 10: *Nephrology.*

Gennari FJ: Hypokalemia. N Engl J Med 1998;339:451.

39. HYPOMAGNESEMIA

I. **Problem.** A 40-year-old male complaining of chest pain is admitted to rule out myocardial infarction. A magnesium level returns at 0.8 mEq/L (normal: 1.5–2.1 mEq/L).

II. **Immediate Questions**

A. **What are the patient's vital signs?** Magnesium deficiency is associated with cardiac arrhythmias, including atrial fibrillation, supraventricular tachycardia, ventricular tachycardia, and ventricular fibrillation. Determining that the patient is not in any immediate distress and does not have hypotension or a tachyarrhythmia is essential.

B. **Is the patient tremulous or currently having a seizure?** Tremor, tetany, muscle fasciculations, and seizures all are associated with magnesium deficiency. Determining the presence or absence of these neurologic symptoms will help guide the urgency of treatment.

III. **Differential Diagnosis.** The diagnosis of magnesium deficiency, in general, rests on a high degree of suspicion, clinical assessment, and measurement of serum magnesium. It is important to recognize that serum magnesium levels do not always correlate well with intracellular magnesium levels. Thus, it is possible to have total body or intracellular magnesium depletion with normal (or even high) serum magnesium levels. For this reason, some experts have suggested that an initial 24-hour urine collection for magnesium, or a 24-hour urine magnesium retention test after parenteral administration of magnesium, be done to determine whether magnesium depletion is truly present. Although such tests may be useful in specific settings, an acutely ill patient is generally treated based on the serum level and good clinical judgment.

A. **Hypocalcemia.** The signs and symptoms of hypocalcemia are similar to those of hypomagnesemia, and both problems often coexist. Hypocalcemia that does not correct with IV supplementation suggests the presence of magnesium deficiency.

B. **Hypokalemia.** Potassium depletion often coexists with hypomagnesemia and can cause arrhythmias and muscle weakness, similar to hypomagnesemia. Hypokalemia that does not correct with potassium repletion suggests magnesium depletion.

C. **Lab error.** More likely if a colorimetric assay is used. When in doubt, ask the lab to repeat the test and controls.

D. **Causes of hypomagnesemia**
   1. **Increased excretion**
      a. **Medications.** Especially diuretics, antibiotics (ticarcillin, amphotericin B), aminoglycosides, *cis*-platinum, and cyclosporin may cause hypomagnesemia.
      b. **Alcoholism.** Very common cause; results from decreased intake and renal magnesium wasting.
      c. **Diabetes mellitus.** Commonly seen in diabetic ketoacidosis.
      d. **Renal tubular disorders.** With magnesium wasting.
      e. **Hypercalcemia/hypercalciuria**
      f. **Hyperaldosteronism/Bartter's syndrome**
      g. **Excessive lactation**
      h. **Marked diaphoresis**
   2. **Reduced intake/malabsorption**
      a. **Starvation.** A common cause.
      b. **Bowel bypass or resection**
      c. **Total parenteral nutrition without adequate magnesium supplementation**
      d. **Chronic malabsorption syndrome.** Such as pancreatic insufficiency.
      e. **Chronic diarrhea**
   3. **Miscellaneous**
      a. **Acute pancreatitis**
      b. **Hypoalbuminemia**
      c. **Vitamin D therapy.** Resulting in hypercalciuria.

IV. Database

A. **Physical examination key points**
   1. **Vital signs.** Blood pressure and pulse to evaluate for hypotension and tachyarrhythmias. While taking blood pressure, leave cuff in-

flated above the systolic blood pressure for 3 minutes to check for carpal spasm (*Trousseau's sign*).

2. **HEENT.** Check for *Chvostek's sign* (tapping over the facial nerve produces twitching of the mouth and eye). Nystagmus may be present.
3. **Heart.** Check for rate and regularity of rhythm.
4. **Abdomen.** Evaluate for evidence of pancreatitis, such as absent bowel sounds and tenderness. Stigmata of chronic liver disease such as hepatosplenomegaly, caput medusae, ascites, spider angiomas, and palmar erythema suggest chronic alcohol abuse.
5. **Neurologic exam.** Hyperactive reflexes, muscle fasciculations, seizures, and tetany can occur. Hyperactive reflexes may also be seen with alcohol withdrawal.
6. **Mental status.** Psychosis, depression, and agitation may be present.

B. **Laboratory data**

1. **Serum electrolytes, glucose, calcium, and phosphorus.** Hypomagnesemia frequently accompanies other electrolyte abnormalities, especially hypocalcemia, hypokalemia, and alkalosis. If the patient is an alcoholic, then hypophosphatemia is also likely. Patients with diabetes are prone to develop hypomagnesemia (especially with diabetic ketoacidosis).
2. **24-hour urine for magnesium.** May be helpful if the diagnosis is in question, or if there is a suspicion of renal magnesium wasting.
3. **Magnesium retention test.** Using either parenteral or oral magnesium. May be helpful in certain subsets of patients in whom either the diagnosis is in question or malabsorption is suspected.
4. **Miscellaneous.** As indicated. Liver function studies in alcoholics and serum amylase if pancreatitis is suspected.

C. **Radiologic and other studies.** Electrocardiographic findings may include prolongation of the PR, QT, and QRS intervals as well as ST depression and T-wave changes. Rhythm disturbances include supraventricular arrhythmias (especially atrial fibrillation) as well as ventricular tachycardia and ventricular fibrillation. Arrhythmias may be particularly common if the patient is taking digoxin.

V. **Plan.** The urgency of treatment depends on the clinical setting. The patient who is having neurologic or cardiac manifestations should be treated urgently with parenteral IV therapy. Asymptomatic individuals may be treated with oral magnesium, although many clinicians treat magnesium levels < 1.0 mEq/L with parenteral magnesium even though there is not always a good correlation between serum levels and intracellular levels.

A. **IV magnesium sulfate.** Magnesium sulfate 1 g (2 mL of a 50% solution of $MgSO_4$) equals 98 mg of elemental magnesium, which is equal to 8 mEq $MgSO_4$ or 4 mmol Mg^{++}. With tetany, status epilepticus, or significant cardiac arrhythmias, then 2 g of magnesium sulfate (16 mEq) can be given IV over 10–20 min. For slightly less urgent situations, 1–2 g/hr (not to exceed 12 g in the first 12 hours) may be given with close hemodynamic and electrocardiographic monitoring including checking of deep tendon reflexes Q 3–4 hr. Deep tendon reflexes (DTRs) will typically decrease with replacement; toxicity is suggested by diminished or absent DTRs. Magnesium should be administered only in life-threatening situations with renal insufficiency; monitoring of DTRs is required every hour. For less urgent replacement, the infusion can be slowed so that the patient receives approximately 10 g of magnesium sulfate in the first 24 hours as long as signs and symptoms of hypomagnesemia are improving. Selected patients may require more or less magnesium. Subsequently, 5–6 g of magnesium sulfate may be given Q 24 hr to replenish body reserves for the next 3–4 days.

In the setting of acute myocardial infarction, some authors feel that therapeutic (rather than replacement) administration of magnesium may prevent arrhythmias, limit damage from reperfusion injury, and have a favorable impact on hemodynamics. Other authors dispute these claims. Protocols for administration vary, but one popular protocol is to give 2 g magnesium sulfate IV over 5 min followed by 16 g over 24 hr as a constant infusion. Patients often experience a flushing sensation with rapid infusions. An overdose of magnesium may occur in the setting of renal failure and also accidentally. (Several formulations are available in different concentrations.) Magnesium overdose complicated by respiratory arrest, shock, or asystole should be initially treated with 1–2 g IV calcium gluconate (100–200 mg elemental calcium) over 3 min followed by 15 mg/kg over 4 hr. Physostigmine 1 mg given over 1 min has also been used. Initial treatment can be followed with dialysis, or saline and furosemide diuresis.

B. IM magnesium sulfate. Give 1–2 g IM Q 4 hr for five doses during the first 24 hours (following the patient's clinical status and serum levels as described earlier). This can then be followed by 1 g IM Q 6 hr for 2–3 days. Many patients complain about pain with the injections.

C. Magnesium oxide PO (20 mEq of magnesium per 400-mg tablet). Give 1–2 tablets per day for chronic maintenance therapy (may cause diarrhea, especially at higher doses).

D. Miscellaneous. Treat other electrolyte disorders, especially hypocalcemia (see Section I, Chapter 36, Hypocalcemia, V, p 201), hypokalemia (see Section I, Chapter 38, Hypokalemia, V, p 209) and hypophosphatemia (see Section I, Chapter 41, Hypophosphatemia, V, p 222), as well as other underlying illnesses.

REFERENCES

Heesch CN, Eichorn EJ: Magnesium in acute myocardial infarction. Ann Emerg Med 1994;24:1154.

McLean R: Magnesium and its therapeutic uses: A review. Am J Med 1994;96:63.

40. HYPONATREMIA

I. **Problem.** A 50-year-old man is admitted for evaluation of a right pulmonary hilar mass. The serum sodium is 118 mmol/L (normal: 136–145 mmol/L).

II. **Immediate Questions**

A. **Is the patient symptomatic from the hyponatremia?** Patients with hyponatremia may be asymptomatic, or there may be central nervous system (CNS) changes ranging from lethargy, anorexia, nausea, vomiting, agitation, and headache to marked disorientation, seizures, and death. Muscle cramps, weakness, and fatigue are also common.

B. **Are there any recent sodium levels to document the chronicity of the hyponatremia?** The rate of development and magnitude of hyponatremia correlates directly with the severity of the symptoms. Acute changes in sodium levels are more likely to produce more severe symptoms.

C. **Is there any evidence of volume depletion?** Orthostatic changes in blood pressure and heart rate suggest volume depletion.

D. **Does the patient have a history of vomiting or diarrhea?** Vomiting and diarrhea can cause wasting of sodium and extracellular fluid, resulting in hyponatremia.

E. **Is there any history of renal disease, congestive heart failure (CHF), cirrhosis, or nephrotic syndrome?** Any of these edematous states suggests an excess of sodium accompanied by an even greater excess of total body water.

F. **Is there any history of hypothyroidism or adrenal insufficiency?** Hypothyroidism and hypoadrenalism cause renal wasting of sodium, even in the face of hyponatremia.

G. **Is the patient taking any medications that could cause the hyponatremia?** Diuretics can cause hyponatremia by inducing sodium deficits in excess of water deficits. Chlorpropamide, clofibrate, nicotine, narcotics, cyclophosphamide, vincristine, nonsteroidal anti-inflammatory drugs (NSAIDs), antipsychotic medications (eg, haloperidol and thioridazine), tricyclic antidepressants, selective serotonin reuptake inhibitors (SSRIs), and anticonvulsants such as carbamazepine (Tegretol) may cause hyponatremia. Mannitol used to treat elevated intracranial pressure or glaucoma can cause a low serum sodium by shifting water from the intracellular space to the hypertonic extracellular space.

H. **Is there any pulmonary disease?** Pneumonia, tuberculosis, lung carcinoma, and other pulmonary pathology may cause the syndrome of inappropriate antidiuretic hormone secretion (SIADH).

I. **Is there any CNS disease?** Meningitis, encephalitis, brain abscess, tumors, trauma, and a variety of other diseases can cause SIADH.

J. **Is there a history of weight loss, cough, and hemoptysis?** SIADH has been associated with bronchogenic carcinoma as well as several other cancers.

K. **Is there any history of hyperlipidemia or hyperproteinemia?** Either can cause a low serum sodium without extracellular fluid hypertonicity. This condition is also called pseudohyponatremia.

L. **Is there a history of diabetes?** A markedly elevated glucose can lower the serum sodium. The serum sodium is diluted by water moving from the intracellular space to the hypertonic extracellular space. Correction of the hyperglycemia will correct the hyponatremia.

M. **Has the patient undergone a colonoscopy recently?** In a recent study of 40 patients undergoing colonoscopy, 10 had elevated levels of serum arginine vasopressin and 3 patients developed hyponatremia of 130 mmol/L or lower.

N. **Is the lab value correct?** If the sodium level is unexpected, repeat the test.

III. **Differential Diagnosis.** The initial differentiation is between true hyponatremia with hypotonicity and laboratory artifact (*pseudohyponatremia*), as well as dilutional effects that result in isotonic or hypertonic hyponatremia. True hyponatremia may be classified according to the volume status of the patient: hypovolemic, euvolemic, or hypervolemic (see IV.A).

A. **Laboratory error.** If the serum sodium concentration is unexpected, laboratory error should always be considered as a potential cause.

B. **Pseudohyponatremia due to space-occupying compounds.** Lipids are the most common cause. For every increase in triglycerides of 1 g/dL, sodium will falsely decrease by 1.7 mmol/L. The lab can ultracentrifuge the specimen to find the correct plasma sodium level. Proteins are also a common cause of pseudohyponatremia, such as in Waldenström's macroglobulinemia and multiple myeloma. For accumulation of every 1 g/dL of protein, sodium will be falsely lowered by 1 mmol/L, plus some true reduction that occurs via the accumulation of cationic proteins in multiple myeloma.

C. **Dilutional.** This is not a true pseudohyponatremia but rather a hypertonic hyponatremia resulting from the intracellular-to-extracellular movement of water. Diabetes mellitus is the most common cause. The expected decrease in serum sodium is 2.4 mmol/L for each 100 mg/dL of glucose > 100 mg/dL. Other nonglucose solutes that can cause the same effects are mannitol or glycerol. If the calculated serum osmolality differs from the measured serum osmolality by > 10 mOsm/kg, then it can be inferred that another solute is present.

D. **Essential hyponatremia.** This is an uncommon congenital disorder where the osmostat is set for a serum sodium that is lower than the normal range. However, it is normal for the patient. It is a benign condition that does not require treatment. Previous serum sodium values and the exclusion of other conditions causing the hyponatremia are required to diagnose.

E. **Acute water intoxication (hypotonic hyponatremia).** Occurs when the water intake exceeds maximal urinary free water excretion. Urine osmolality should be < 120 mOsm/kg (specific gravity < 1.003) if maximal urinary dilution is present. This can occur by inappropriate administration of IV fluids or tube feedings, extensive use of tap water enemas, excessive swallowing of water during swimming or bathing, or abnormal water consumption (eg, in psychiatric patients). Treated by restricting water intake.

F. **Hypovolemic hyponatremia**
   1. **Extra-renal losses** (spot urinary sodium < 10 mmol/L)
      a. **GI fluid losses.** Occur through vomiting, diarrhea, drainage tubes, and fistulae. In surreptitious or bulimic vomiting, the urinary chloride is usually < 10 mmol/L.
      b. **Third-space fluid loss.** May occur in pancreatitis, peritonitis, muscle trauma, effusions, or burns.
      c. **Skin.** Fluid may be lost through burns, cystic fibrosis, or heat stroke. Sweating secondary to vigorous exercise can cause marked losses of water and sodium. Resulting increases in antidiuretic hormone will lead to retention of ingested water.
   2. **Renal losses** (spot urinary sodium > 20 mmol/L)
      a. **Diuretic usage.** Caused by thiazides and loop diuretics; often associated with hypokalemia and metabolic alkalosis. With surreptitious diuretic use, urine chloride is > 20 mmol/L.
      b. **Renal disorders.** Renal tubular acidosis, medullary cystic disease, polycystic disease, and chronic interstitial nephritis can cause hyponatremia.
      c. **Addison's disease.** Characterized by mineralocorticoid deficiency. Hyperkalemia, low urinary potassium, and metabolic acidosis are present.
      d. **Osmotic diuresis.** Most commonly caused by hyperglycemia or mannitol.
      e. **Cerebral salt wasting.** Inappropriate renal sodium wasting associated with a CNS disorder, most commonly subarachnoid hemorrhage, also seen in bacterial and tuberculous meningitis. Mediated through atrial natriuretic hormone or cerebral natriuretic peptide.

G. Euvolemic hyponatremia

1. **SIADH.** The diagnosis is based on the findings of low serum osmolality, elevated urine sodium (> 20 mmol/L), and concentrated urine (osmolality near normal) after ruling out hypothyroidism and hypoadrenalism and confirming euvolemia.
   a. **Carcinoma.** Small-cell lung carcinoma is the most common, but many others can also cause SIADH.
   b. **Pulmonary disease.** Pneumonia, tuberculosis, tumor, atelectasis, and pneumothorax.
   c. **CNS disorders.** Include trauma, tumors, infections (eg, meningitis and encephalitis), cerebrovascular accidents, and psychoses.
   d. **Stress.** Including perioperative stress.
   e. **Drugs.** See II.G. There are reports of SSRIs causing SIADH, especially in the elderly, as well as ACE inhibitors.
   f. **Postoperative conditions.** Anesthesia, stress from surgery, and postoperative pain as well as narcotics cause an increase in antidiuretic hormone.
   g. **After colonoscopy.** May cause transient hyponatremia.
2. **Hypothyroidism**
3. **Glucocorticoid deficiency**
4. **Hypopituitarism**
5. **Psychogenic polydipsia and beer potomania.** Differentiated from G.1.–G.4. in that psychogenic polydipsia and beer potomania have a low urine osmolality, whereas the others have an inappropriately high urine osmolality.

   Note: In addition to the above, there is a new postulated cause of hyponatremia seen after intracranial surgery. The proposed mechanism involves an extracellular-to-intracellular shift of sodium in exchange for potassium.

H. Hypervolemic hyponatremia

1. **CHF.** Urine sodium is < 10 mmol/L.
2. **Cirrhosis.** Urine sodium is < 10 mmol/L.
3. **Renal disease**
   a. **Chronic renal failure.** Urine sodium > 20 mmol/L.
   b. **Nephrotic syndrome.** Urine sodium < 10 mmol/L.

IV. Database

A. Physical examination key points. Assessment of volume status is essential.

1. **Vital signs.** Evaluate for orthostatic blood pressure and heart rate changes. A decrease in systolic blood pressure of 10 mm Hg, and/or an increase in heart rate of 20 bpm 1 minute after changing from a supine to a standing position points to volume depletion. Tachypnea may suggest volume overload and pulmonary edema.

2. **Skin.** Tissue turgor will be diminished and mucous membranes may appear dry with volume depletion. Poor skin turgor can be a normal variant in the elderly. Edema suggests volume overload. Jaundice, spider angiomas, and caput medusae suggest cirrhosis.
3. **HEENT.** Evaluate the internal jugular veins. Determine the jugular venous pressure. When the patient's bed is elevated at 30 degrees, the veins will be flat with volume depletion and markedly engorged with volume overload.
4. **Lungs.** Crackles may be heard with CHF. Noncardiogenic pulmonary edema is seen in marathon runners with hyponatremia and is thought to be secondary to the resulting cerebral edema.
5. **Heart.** An S_3 gallop suggests CHF.
6. **Abdomen.** Hepatosplenomegaly and ascites suggest cirrhosis. A hepatojugular reflux may be present in CHF.
7. **Neurologic exam.** Decreased deep tendon reflexes (DTRs), altered mental status, confusion, coma, or seizures may be present after a rapid fall in the serum sodium or from a chronically low serum sodium. If hyponatremia is chronic, the neurologic and mental status exams may be normal, even with levels < 120 mmol/L. A delay in the relaxation phase of DTRs is seen in hypothyroidism.
8. **Extremities.** Clubbing may be present with lung cancer.

B. Laboratory data

1. **Electrolytes.** Other abnormalities may coexist. Hypokalemia can potentiate hyponatremia as sodium shifts into cells in exchange for potassium. Hypokalemia and an increase in serum bicarbonate are seen with diuretic use. Hyperkalemia and a decrease in serum bicarbonate are seen in Addison's disease.
2. **Spot urine electrolytes and creatinine.** Obtain prior to any diuretic treatment.
3. **Urine and serum osmolality.** Serum osmolality will be normal in cases of laboratory artifact but decreased in true hyponatremia. Serum osmolality will be increased in hypertonic hyponatremia secondary to mannitol or glucose. Serum osmolality will be low with SIADH.
4. **Liver function tests.** To detect liver disease.
5. **Thyroid function.** Hypothyroidism must be ruled out prior to diagnosing SIADH.
6. **Cortisol levels, ACTH stimulation test.** Glucocorticoid deficiency must be ruled out prior to diagnosing SIADH.
7. **Cultures. Cultures and stains as indicated.**

C. Radiologic and other studies

1. **Chest x-ray (CXR).** Look for CHF, lung cancer, pneumonia, or tuberculosis. Noncardiogenic pulmonary edema is seen in marathon runners with hyponatremia.
2. **Head CT scan.** If indicated.

V. Plan. The etiology and the presence and severity of symptoms guide therapy. Aggressive treatment of severe symptoms (eg, coma) is discussed below, as are specific therapies for certain diagnoses.

A. Emergency treatment. Usually for severe CNS symptoms (eg, seizures or coma).

1. Normal saline (NS) and furosemide 1 mg/kg. Use a combination of NS and diuretics to achieve a net negative free water deficit in hyponatremia associated with euvolemic or hypervolemic conditions. Use NS by itself if the hyponatremia is associated with volume depletion. Carefully document fluid intake and output. Supplement fluids with potassium as needed. Too rapid correction of sodium can be deleterious, resulting in central pontine myelinolysis. Correct sodium level *rapidly* (> 1.0 mmol/L/hr) to 120–125 mmol/L; then *slowly* correct sodium level (< 0.5 mmol/L/hr) over the next 24–48 hr to normal.

For hypovolemic states, calculate the total amount of sodium required to increase the sodium to a desired level, use the following formula:

$$\text{Sodium required (mmol)} = (\text{desired sodium [Na]} - \text{actual serum [Na]}) \times \text{TBW}$$

$$\text{TBW} = \text{weight (kg)} \times 0.60$$
$$\text{TBW} = \text{total body water}$$

To estimate the increase in serum sodium concentration for a given amount of saline administered, the following equation can be used:

$$\text{Increase in serum [Na}^+\text{]} = \frac{(\text{IV fluid [Na}^+\text{]} - \text{serum [Na}^+\text{]}) \times \text{IV fluid volume}}{\text{TBW}}$$

$$\text{TBW} = \text{weight (kg)} \times 0.60$$
$$\text{TBW} = \text{total body water}$$

2. Hypertonic saline. (3%: contains 513 mEq of Na per liter). This preparation is rarely needed. Hypertonic saline can replace NS in the above treatment regimens. Extreme care must be taken in using hypertonic saline because of the potential for serious complications (eg, pulmonary edema and central pontine myelinolysis) secondary to overly rapid correction of hyponatremia.

B. Hypovolemic hyponatremia

1. Treat by replacing volume and sodium. Give NS IV.

2. Potassium. In cases of diuretic abuse, repletion of lost body potassium is also necessary.

C. Euvolemic hyponatremia. (Patient is not edematous.) In cases of SIADH, restrict patient's water intake to 800–1000 mL daily. Give demeclocycline (300–600 mg bid PO) for chronic SIADH, such as that resulting from neoplasms. Onset of medication action may take up to a week.

D. **Hypervolemic hyponatremia.** (Patient is edematous.) Restrict IV and oral fluids.
   1. **CHF.** Treat with digoxin, diuretics (eg, furosemide), angiotensin-converting enzyme (ACE) inhibitors, and sodium restriction.
   2. **Nephrotic syndrome.** Give steroids (if the cause is steroid-responsive), restrict sodium and water intake, increase patient's protein intake. Furosemide is commonly used.
   3. **Cirrhosis.** Treat with restriction of sodium and water, and diuretics. Initially, give spironolactone 100 mg PO Q day, increasing dose Q 2–3 days up to 400 mg Q day. Furosemide 40 mg is often used with spironolactone especially if edema is present. A portosystemic shunt is needed in only 5–10% of patients to control ascites.
   4. **Renal failure.** Treat with sodium and water restriction, loop diuretics, and dialysis if indicated.

REFERENCES

Adrogue HJ, Madias NE: Hypernatremia. N Engl J Med 2000;342:1493.

Ayus CJ, Varon J, Arieff AI: Hyponatremia, cerebral edema, and noncardiogenic pulmonary edema in marathon runners. Ann Intern Med 2000;132:711.

Bell T, Schrier RW: Disorders of water metabolism. In: Schrier RW, ed. *Renal and Electrolyte Disorders.* 5th ed. Lippincott-Raven;1997:1.

Cohen CD, Keuneke C, Schiemann U et al: Hyponatremia as a complication of colonoscopy. Lancet 2001;357:282.

Van Amelsvoort T, Bakshi R, Devaux CV et al: Hyponatremia associated with carbamazepine and oxcarbazepine therapy: A review. Epilepsia 1994:35:181.

Weisberg LS: Pseudohyponatremia: A reappraisal. Am J Med 1989;86:315.

41. HYPOPHOSPHATEMIA

I. **Problem.** A 26-year-old male with Type 1 diabetes was admitted 6 hours ago for treatment of diabetic ketoacidosis (DKA) and now has a serum phosphate level of 1.0 mg/dL.

II. **Immediate Questions**

A. **Are there any symptoms related to the low phosphate?** Serum phosphate levels below 1.0 mg/dL require prompt treatment regardless of symptoms. Above that level, one should check for symptoms related to low phosphate, such as numbness or tingling, muscle weakness, anorexia, confusion, irritability, seizures, and skeletal pain. Muscle weakness, mental status changes, and hematologic abnormalities are common findings.

B. **What treatment is the patient receiving?** Hypophosphatemia usually results from phosphate shifts within the body. This is most often a consequence of medical treatment, such as hyperalimentation, correction of DKA, or refeeding of malnourished or alcoholic patients. Antacids also can cause hypophosphatemia by binding phosphate in the gut.

C. **Does the patient consume alcohol?** Chronic alcoholism is a common cause of hypophosphatemia secondary to poor intake and possible increased renal excretion, especially if hypomagnesemia is also present.

III. **Differential Diagnosis.** A low serum phosphate level usually results from a combination of increased renal loss, increased intestinal loss, or intracellular shift of phosphate, the latter being the most common.

A. **Intracellular shift of phosphate.** Alkalosis from any etiology. See Section I, Chapter 3, Alkalosis, p 18.

B. **Increased intestinal phosphate loss**
   1. **Phosphate-binding antacids**
   2. **Malabsorption, vomiting, diarrhea, malnutrition**

C. **Increased renal phosphate loss**
   1. **Acidosis.** Including untreated DKA.
   2. **Hyperparathyroidism, renal tubular disease, hypokalemia, hypomagnesemia, diuretics**

D. **Multifactorial**
   1. **Alcoholism and liver disease.** All three mechanisms.
   2. **Vitamin D deficiency or resistance.** Renal and intestinal loss.
   3. **Treatment of DKA and severe burns.** Renal and intracellular shift.

IV. **Database**

A. **Physical examination key points**
   1. **Vital signs**
      a. **Temperature.** Heat stroke can cause hypophosphatemia from intracellular shifts. Sepsis occurs with greater frequency with hypophosphatemia because of leukocyte dysfunction.
      b. **Respiratory rate.** Hyperventilation with resulting alkalosis is a cause of extracellular-to-intracellular shifts of phosphate.
   2. **HEENT.** Check for thyromegaly. Thyrotoxicosis can also cause extracellular-to-intracellular shifts of phosphate.
   3. **Heart.** A reversible congestive cardiomyopathy may result from hypophosphatemia. Look for a laterally displaced apical pulse and third heart sound (S_3).
   4. **Lungs.** Listen for rales as evidence of cardiomyopathy. Acute hypophosphatemia can also result in acute respiratory failure.
   5. **Neurologic exam.** Confusion and coma may be present. Sensory examination may be abnormal secondary to related paresthesias.
   6. **Musculoskeletal exam.** Check for diffuse muscle weakness. Tenderness suggests rhabdomyolysis; however, the phosphate may increase to extremely high levels secondary to rhabdomyolysis.

B. Laboratory data

1. **Serum electrolytes.** Especially bicarbonate and potassium. An elevated bicarbonate may suggest a metabolic alkalosis; a low bicarbonate may represent compensation for a chronic respiratory alkalosis. Alkalosis results in extracellular-to-intracellular shifts of phosphate. Hypokalemia can cause hypophosphatemia.
2. **Arterial blood gases and pH.** Alkalosis (either metabolic or respiratory) results in intracellular shifts of phosphate. A metabolic acidosis with an increased anion gap and an elevated glucose suggests DKA, which can have associated hypophosphatemia. An elevated pCO_2 also suggests respiratory failure, which can occur as a result of hypophosphatemia.
3. **Calcium, magnesium, and glucose levels.** A low calcium may suggest vitamin D deficiency or osteomalacia. A high calcium suggests hyperparathyroidism or thiazide diuretic use, which can cause hypophosphatemia. Hypomagnesemia results in increased phosphate excretion.
4. **Glucose.** There is increased urinary excretion of phosphate in DKA.
5. **Uric acid.** Hypophosphatemia can be seen with acute gout; however, the uric acid level may be high, normal, or low in acute gout.
6. **Liver enzymes, albumin, bilirubin, and creatine phosphokinase (CK).** Hypophosphatemia may cause liver dysfunction. A CK should be checked to rule out rhabdomyolysis from severe hypophosphatemia, especially if muscle tenderness is present or develops.
7. **Complete blood count with differential.** An elevated white blood cell (WBC) count with a left shift suggests a bacterial infection. As a result of WBC dysfunction, patients with hypophosphatemia are more susceptible to bacterial infections.
8. **Peripheral smear.** Severe hypophosphatemia can cause hemolysis.
9. **Platelet count.** Thrombocytopenia and platelet dysfunction can result.

C. Radiologic and other studies

1. **Bone films.** May show pseudofractures.
2. **Chest x-ray.** Possible complications of hypophosphatemia such as congestive cardiomyopathy and respiratory failure are indications for a CXR.
3. **Electroencephalogram.** An EEG may be needed to evaluate seizures or encephalopathy, which are possible complications.

V. Plan. If the phosphate level is < 1.0 mg/dL, start IV replacement therapy immediately. If the level is 1.0–1.5 mg/dL and the patient is symptomatic, start IV replacement therapy. Otherwise, oral treatment is usually sufficient.

A. Intravenous treatment

1. If the hypophosphatemia is recent and uncomplicated, give 0.08 mmol/kg (2.5 mg/kg) intravenously over 6 hours. Sodium phosphate and potassium phosphate IV solutions both contain 3 mmol of phosphate per milliliter.
2. If the hypophosphatemia is long-standing or complicated, give 0.16 mmol/kg (5.0 mg/kg) IV over 6 hours.
3. In either case, consider using 25% to 50% higher doses if the patient is symptomatic, but do not exceed 0.24 mmol/kg (7.5 mg/kg) or 16.9 mmol (525 mg) for a 70-kg patient.
4. Recheck the phosphate level promptly after the 6-hour infusion, and reassess need for further replacement.

B. Oral replacement

1. Neutra-Phos tablets contain 250 mg phosphorus (8 mmol) per tablet; Neutra-Phos powder contains 0.1 mmol of phosphate per milliliter.
2. Milk contains modest amounts of phosphate. Skim milk has slightly more phosphate and may be better tolerated for those who are lactose intolerant (Table 1–8).
3. Fleet enema solution and Fleet Phospho-Soda contain buffered sodium phosphate. Can be administered orally. Fleet enema solution contains 1.4 mmol/mL, administer 15–30 mL, tid–qid (50–150 mmol/24 hr). Fleet Phospho-Soda contains 4.15 mmol/mL of phosphate. It is estimated that two-thirds of orally administered phosphate is absorbed.

C. Precautions

1. It may be necessary to give calcium supplements to hypocalcemic patients who are being given phosphate.
2. Do not give calcium and phosphate through the same IV line.
3. Beware of causing hyperphosphatemia, hypotension, hyperkalemia, osmotic diuresis, and hypernatremia.

TABLE I–8. AMOUNT OF PHOSPHATE IN AN 8-OZ SERVING OF MILK.

Milk	Phosphorus[1] (mg/8-oz. serving)
Skim	247
Whole	227

[1]250 mg of elemental phosphorus = 8 mmol phosphate.

REFERENCES

Subramanian RMB, Khardori R: Severe hypophosphatemia: Pathophysiologic implications, clinical presentations, and treatment. Medicine 2000;79:1.

Weisinger JR, Bellorin-Font E: Magnesium and phosphorus. Lancet 1998;352:391.

42. HYPOTENSION (SHOCK)

I. **Problem.** A 70-year-old man is admitted for nausea, abdominal pain, and weakness. Blood pressure is 70/50.

II. **Immediate Questions**

A. **What are all of the patient's vital signs?** Confirm the blood pressure in both arms manually. An arterial line may be useful. Severe bradycardia or tachycardia can be either the primary problem or a tachycardia can be secondary to the hypotension. Fever suggests sepsis, but hypothermia can also be seen in sepsis, myxedema, or Addisonian crisis. Tachypnea may be seen in cardiogenic shock, pulmonary embolus (PE), and sepsis.

B. **What is the patient's mental status?** This is an indicator of adequate perfusion of vital organs.

C. **What are the patient's usual medications and when were they last taken? Have any medications been started recently?** Many medications such as angiotensin-converting enzyme (ACE) inhibitors, direct vasodilators, and central-acting antihypertensive agents such as clonidine significantly lower blood pressure, especially in the setting of volume depletion or with concomitant use of diuretics. Other IV medications with similar effects include nitroprusside, nitroglycerin, α_1-blockers such as terazosin (Hytrin), and phenytoin. Anaphylaxis should be considered, especially if there is respiratory distress. Diuretics rarely cause sufficiently significant volume depletion to cause hypotension.

D. **Are there any accompanying symptoms?** A history of bleeding, vomiting, diarrhea, polyuria, polydipsia, dysuria, cough, chest pain, or abdominal pain may suggest the underlying cause. Chest discomfort and dyspnea suggest PE or myocardial ischemia/infarction. Dyspnea may be the only symptom of cardiac ischemia/infarction.

III. **Differential Diagnosis.** *Hypotension* is a relative term and must be individualized to the patient. An elderly hypertensive patient may not tolerate a systolic blood pressure (SBP) of 100 mm Hg, but in others, a SBP of 90 mm Hg may be normal. *Shock* is a condition in which the blood pressure is inadequate to provide required tissue perfusion. The following are subcategories of shock.

A. **Hypovolemic**

1. **Hemorrhagic**

a. **Traumatic.** Trauma patients may lose a large volume of blood internally (chest, abdomen, and pelvis), which may not be readily apparent.

b. **Postoperative or postprocedural.** Hemorrhage may occur after percutaneous biopsy (liver, kidney, lung) or following central venous line placement, angiography, or cardiac catheterization.

c. **Miscellaneous.** Gastrointestinal bleeding, ruptured aneurysm, ruptured ovarian cyst, or ectopic pregnancy.

2. **Fluid losses.** From severe vomiting, diarrhea, perspiration, extensive burns, diuresis, and "third-space losses" (peritonitis or pancreatitis).

B. **Vasogenic.** Inappropriate loss of vascular tone may develop as a result of sepsis, anaphylaxis, adrenal insufficiency, acidosis, CNS injury, and certain medications, or postprandial (especially in the elderly).

C. **Cardiogenic.** Acute pump failure most commonly occurs as a result of acute myocardial infarction (MI) or profound ischemia, and may occur with decompensated congestive heart failure (CHF). Cardiac arrhythmia (supraventricular, ventricular, or various degrees of heart block), tension pneumothorax, pericardial tamponade, and PE can cause hypotension.

D. **Neurogenic.** An increase in vagal stimulation from a variety of causes, including spinal cord injury and pain.

IV. Database

A. Physical examination key points

1. **Vital signs.** Temperature, blood pressure, pulse, respiratory rate, including orthostatic blood pressure and heart rate. A decrease in SBP of 10 mm Hg and/or an increase in heart rate of 20 bpm from the supine to the standing position after 1 minute are indicative of volume depletion.
2. **Skin.** Poor skin turgor suggests volume depletion, but may be a normal variant in the elderly. Cool, clammy skin indicates cardiogenic or hypovolemic shock, whereas warm, moist skin signifies vasodilation (sepsis).
3. **Neck.** Jugular venous distension (JVD) and pulsations may be helpful in determining volume status and cardiac rhythm, as well as in diagnosing cardiac tamponade or tension pneumothorax. JVD with the latter two conditions does not decrease with inspiration.
4. **Chest.** Tracheal deviation suggests tension pneumothorax. Wheezing or stridor may indicate anaphylaxis. (See Section I, Chapter 4, Anaphylactic Reaction, p 24). Rales and wheezes point to cardiac failure. Chest percussion may help diagnose pneumothorax, pleural effusion, hemothorax, or pneumonia.
5. **Heart.** Auscultate for a murmur and palpate for a thrill or a change in the apical impulse. A new thrill may indicate a ventricular septal defect (VSD) or papillary muscle dysfunction complicating an acute MI. Loss of a palpable apical pulse suggests a pericardial effusion. A new systolic murmur suggests acute mitral regurgitation or a VSD. A third heart sound (S_3) is heard with left ventricular failure; a new fourth heart sound (S_4) suggests an acute MI.

6. **Abdomen.** Rebound tenderness or positive Murphy's sign and absence of bowel sounds suggest sepsis from an abdominal source. (See Section I, Chapter 1, Abdominal Pain, p. 1.) Absent bowel sounds and tenderness may be present with a large GI bleed. A pulsatile mass suggests a leaking aortic aneurysm. Ecchymoses may be seen with retroperitoneal bleeding from a variety of causes such as hemorrhagic pancreatitis.
7. **Rectum.** Presence of hematochezia or occult blood may indicate acute GI blood loss.
8. **Female genitalia.** A gynecologic exam in young females is mandatory to rule out a ruptured ectopic pregnancy.
9. **Extremities.** Instability of pelvis or femurs suggests a fracture, which can result in significant bleeding into either the pelvis or the thigh. Edema may indicate volume overload or venous/lymphatic obstruction. Inspect for inflammation of vascular access sites suggesting iatrogenic infection/sepsis.
10. **Neurologic exam.** Altered mental status may indicate inadequate cerebral hypoperfusion as well as suggest possible etiologies (cerebrovascular accident).

B. Laboratory data

1. **Complete blood count.** Serial hematocrits may indicate blood loss. Acute blood loss may not be reflected by an immediate drop in the hematocrit, but will fall as intravascular volume equilibrates. The white blood cell count and differential may indicate sepsis. A low platelet count may point to disseminated intravascular coagulation (DIC), suggesting sepsis.
2. **Serum electrolytes.** A low serum bicarbonate could be caused by a lactic acidosis secondary to decreased perfusion. Severe acidosis or hypokalemia may cause an arrhythmia. Refractory lactic acidosis most often suggests an abdominal catastrophe such as bowel infarction.
3. **Prothrombin time, partial thromboplastin time.** A coagulopathy may indicate DIC, hepatic dysfunction, or excessive anticoagulation.
4. **Arterial blood gases.** Early sepsis may produce a respiratory alkalosis, and a metabolic acidosis will develop with progression of the infection. Metabolic acidosis also develops in shock as a result of poor tissue perfusion. Severe acidosis ($pH < 7.20$) may inhibit the effectiveness of vasopressors and cause arrhythmias. Hypoxemia may also require ventilatory support.
5. **Creatine phosphokinase (CK) with isoenzymes and troponin-I and troponin-T.** Obtain if MI or myocarditis is suspected, as well as to rule out myocardial injury secondary to the hypotension.
6. **Type and cross-match.** Blood should be made ready for transfusion if hemorrhage is suspected.
7. **Pregnancy test.** To rule out ectopic pregnancy in women of childbearing age.

8. **Blood, sputum, urine, and other cultures as indicated.** If sepsis is suspected.
9. **Nasogastric (NG) aspirate.** To assess for upper GI bleeding. A negative NG aspirate does not rule out upper GI bleeding since a small percentage of duodenal bleeding does not reflux into the stomach.

C. Radiologic and other studies

1. **Chest x-ray.** May indicate source of sepsis or identify CHF. May be diagnostic for pneumothorax or hemothorax.
2. **Electrocardiogram.** Myocardial infarction/ischemia or arrhythmias can be detected.
3. **Pulmonary artery catheter (Swan-Ganz).** Very helpful in evaluating and treating shock. Hemodynamic measurements may be used to aid the diagnosis and management of the hypotensive patient (see Table 3–3, p 423). Also useful when ruling out cardiac tamponade where there is equalization of pressures. The right atrial pressure equals the elevated right ventricular diastolic pressure.
4. **Angiography.** Pulmonary angiograms may reveal a PE. Abdominal angiograms may be helpful in detecting the source of GI bleeding, particularly in lower GI bleeding.
5. **Nuclear scans.** A ventilation/perfusion ($\dot{V}/\dot{Q}$) lung scan may aid in diagnosing PE. Radiolabeled red blood cell scans may help identify sources of GI bleeding.
6. **Echocardiogram.** A noninvasive test to evaluate global ventricular function and valvular function, and to rule out mechanical defects such as VSD or ruptured papillary muscle. Pericardial effusion resulting in tamponade can also be identified.
7. **Paracentesis, thoracentesis, culdocentesis, pericardiocentesis.** As indicated.
8. **CT of the abdomen.** If ruptured abdominal aortic aneurysm or intra-abdominal infection is suspected.

V. Plan. Establish adequate tissue perfusion as soon as possible. Generally, a systolic blood pressure > 90 mm Hg is adequate. Signs of adequate perfusion include an improved mental status and a urine output of 0.5–1.0 mL/min.

A. Emergency management

1. Control external hemorrhage with direct pressure.
2. Establish venous access, preferably two large-bore (14–16 gauge) peripheral intravenous lines or a central venous line (jugular or femoral).
3. Trendelenburg position (supine with feet elevated) or pneumatic antishock garment (PASG or MAST) may be useful in hypovolemic shock.
4. Insert Foley catheter to monitor urinary output.
5. Administer supplemental oxygen and ventilatory support as needed.

6. Severe metabolic acidosis (pH < 7.10) should be corrected with intravenous sodium bicarbonate to a pH > 7.20 or a serum bicarbonate > 12 mmol/L. Remember, an ampoule of sodium bicarbonate is hyperosmolar. After several ampoules, it is prudent to start an isotonic bicarbonate drip for persistent acidosis. A bicarbonate drip is made by adding 2.5 ampoules of sodium bicarbonate (50 mEq/50 mL) to 1 L of D5W. Respiratory acidosis can be corrected by improving minute ventilation (V_e) to reduce pCO_2.
7. Central venous pressure or Swan-Ganz catheterization will aid in the differential diagnosis of shock as well as with fluid management.

B. Hypovolemic shock

1. Administer fluids (intravenous normal saline or lactated Ringer's) and administer packed red blood cells if HcT < 30%, using blood pressure, urine output, and central filling pressures as a guide for further therapy. Give intravenous fluid bolus of 250–500 cc followed by either a second fluid bolus or maintenance intravenous fluids at 200–250 cc/hr.
2. Use vasopressor agents such as norepinephrine and dopamine, if hypotension persists despite a fluid challenge sufficient to achieve adequate filling pressures (PCWP 16–18 mm Hg). If systolic BP is 70–90 mm Hg, begin dopamine at a dose of 2.5–5.0 μg/kg/min and increased up to 20 μg/kg/min. If the systolic BP < 70, then begin norepinephrine, 1–20 μg/min.

C. Neurogenic shock

1. Institute moderate IV fluid administration See V.B. Avoid volume overload.
2. Low-dose vasopressors may be necessary. Use an alpha agent such as phenylephrine (Neo-Synephrine) 100–180 μg/min initially; the usual maintenance dose is 40–60 μg/min. Or use norepinephrine (see V.B.).

D. Vasogenic shock

1. **Septic shock.** Identify and treat the source of the infection.
   a. Administer intravenous fluids and vasopressors as indicated.
   b. Broad-spectrum antibiotics are generally used if a specific source cannot be readily identified. Gram's stain of infected fluid will guide antibiotic choice. See Section I, Chapter 22, Fever, V, p.127.
2. **Anaphylactic shock.** See Section I, Chapter 4, Anaphylactic Reaction, p 24.
   a. Remove precipitating agent as soon as possible.
   b. Immediately administer epinephrine 0.3 mL of 1:1000 SC or IM. Depending on the BP, the onset of action may be delayed by the subcutaneous route. For intravenous resuscitation, 10 cc of 1:10,000 (10 mg) is administered. If epinephrine is given by a peripheral IV, the IV line should be subsequently flushed

with 20 cc of fluid. If IV access is not available, epinephrine can be delivered via an endotracheal tube. The dose for this route should be twice the IV dose.

   c. Maintain an adequate airway.
   d. An antihistamine such as diphenhydramine (Benadryl) 25 mg IM or IV, and corticosteroids such as hydrocortisone 100–250 mg IV, can also be given.

3. **Addisonian crisis.** Give hydrocortisone 100 mg IV bolus, then 100 mg IV every 6 hours, if this diagnosis is suspected. Obtain a cortisol level before instituting therapy.

E. Cardiogenic shock

1. This form of shock is usually complicated and more difficult to manage; therefore, consider hemodynamic monitoring with a Swan-Ganz catheter.
2. Initial priority should be given to establishing an adequate perfusion pressure (SBP > 90 mm Hg) while hemodynamic monitoring catheters are placed.
3. Once cardiac hemodynamics have been evaluated, appropriate use of diuretics (IV furosemide, bumetanide), cardiac inotropes (dopamine, dobutamine, amrinone, milrinone), vasopressors (dopamine, norepinephrine; see V.B.2.), antiarrhythmics, and intra-aortic balloon counterpulsation can be instituted.
4. Pericardiocentesis is indicated if there is hemodynamic compromise secondary to pericardial tamponade.
5. If a tension pneumothorax is present, a 14- to 16-gauge needle should be placed in the second or third intercostal space just superior to the rib in the midclavicular line until a chest tube can be placed.
6. Treat any tachyarrhythmia or bradyarrhythmia (see Section I, Chapter 60, Tachycardia, V, p 329, Section I, Chapter 8, Bradycardia, V, p 42, and Section I, Chapter 45, Irregular Pulse, V, p 241.

REFERENCES

Hollenberg SM, Kavinsky CJ, Parrillo JE: Cardiogenic shock. Ann Intern Med 1999;131:47.

Jansen RWMM, Lipsitz LA: Postprandial hypotension: Epidemiology, pathophysiology, and clinical management. Ann Intern Med 1995;122:286.

43. HYPOTHERMIA

I. Problem. You are called to the emergency room to see a patient with a temperature of 32.0°C (89.6°F).

II. Immediate Questions

A. Does the patient have any possible source of infection? Septic patients may be hypothermic. Look for evidence of pneumonia, urinary tract infection, or any other cause of bacteremia; one study found that 41% of patients admitted for hypothermia had a serious infection.

B. **Is there a history of other medical problems?** Hypothyroidism, hypoglycemia, hypopituitarism, and hypoadrenalism all may present with hypothermia. Alcohol also predisposes humans to environment-induced hypothermia.

C. **What is the clinical setting? Is there a history of exposure to cold weather or inadequate heating or clothing?** The very young and very old are susceptible to hypothermia as a result of environmental exposure.

D. **Is the patient taking any medications?** Barbiturates and phenothiazines impair hypothalamic thermoregulation. Alcohol is a vasodilator and CNS depressant, thus increasing the risk for hypothermia from environmental exposure. The use of insulin, thyroid medication, or steroids may also suggest an etiology.

III. Differential Diagnosis

A. **Sepsis.** Bacteremia must be ruled out.

B. **Environmental exposure.** Was the patient found outdoors or in an unheated building? Such patients frequently have concomitant alcoholism, drug addictions, and mental illnesses.

C. **Metabolic abnormalities**

1. **Myxedema.** Thermoderegulation resulting in hypothermia associated with hypothyroidism may have concomitant mental status changes including coma. There is often a precipitating event.
2. **Hypoglycemia.** This condition has many potential causes (see Section I, Chapter 37, Hypoglycemia, p 202). It may also be associated with overwhelming sepsis or depleted glycogen stores due to chronic alcohol consumption.
3. **Adrenal insufficiency.** May be acute or chronic. Often there is a history of steroid ingestion. May be secondary to metastatic carcinoma or idiopathic.
4. **Uremia.** Easily ruled out by checking BUN and creatinine.
5. **Hypopituitarism.** Can result in hypoadrenalism and hypothyroidism. Can also cause hypoglycemia.

D. **CNS dysfunction**

1. **Cerebrovascular accident.** Look for focal neurologic findings such as motor weakness or sensory deficit, unilateral hyperreflexia, or plantar extension with Babinski reflex.
2. **Head trauma.** A history and careful examination of head, eyes, ears, nose, and neck should reveal any recent injury.
3. **Spinal cord transection.** Paraplegia or quadriplegia on examination.
4. **Wernicke's encephalopathy.** This condition is characterized by a triad of ophthalmoplegia, mental status changes, and ataxia. It is

secondary to thiamine deficiency from decreased intake associated most often in the United States with chronic alcohol ingestion.

5. **Drug ingestion.** See II.D.
6. **Miscellaneous.** Other diagnoses to consider are generalized erythroderma, protein–calorie malnutrition, and anorexia nervosa.

IV. Database

A. Physical examination key points

1. **Vital signs.** Record the core temperature accurately with a rectal thermometer; make sure that it is a low-recording thermometer. Standard thermometers may not record temperatures lower than 34.4°C (93.8°F). Keep in mind that hypotension and bradycardia frequently occur in hypothermia.
2. **Skin.** Look for evidence of frostbite, diffuse erythroderma, burns, or insulin injection sites. Hyperpigmentation (especially in the creases of the palms) suggests primary adrenal insufficiency.
3. **Heart.** Heart sounds may be distant, slow, or absent.
4. **Lungs.** Respirations may be slow and shallow. Look for signs of pneumonia.
5. **Abdomen.** Ileus may occur with hypothermia.
6. **Neurologic exam.** Look for signs of head trauma. Check pupil reactivity; pupils are often sluggish and react slowly to light. Occasionally in this setting, pupils are nonreactive to light. Mental status may vary from mental slowing to confusion and coma. Check deep tendon reflexes, which may be absent with severe hypothermia. A slow relaxation phase points to hypothyroidism.

B. Laboratory data

1. **Complete blood count.** Hypothermia can cause hemoconcentration and leukocytosis. Leukocytosis or leukopenia with an increase in banded neutrophils suggests sepsis.
2. **Platelet count.** A low platelet count can occur with either secondary sequestration or disseminated intravascular coagulation (DIC) caused by either hypothermia or associated with sepsis. (See Section I, Chapter 61, Thrombocytopenia, p 333).
3. **Prothrombin time (PT), partial thromboplastin time (PTT).** Elevation of the PT and PTT is consistent with DIC, which can be a complication of hypothermia or associated with sepsis. (See Section I, Chapter 12, Coagulopathy, p 66).
4. **BUN and creatinine.** To rule out uremia. The BUN:creatinine ratio may be increased secondary to hemoconcentration.
5. **Glucose.** Hypoglycemia may be the cause of hypothermia or associated with underlying cause.
6. **Thyroxine (T_4) and thyroid-stimulating hormone (TSH).** You will need to rule out hypothyroidism. The T_4 can be low in the euthyroid sick state, but the TSH is usually normal.
7. **Cortrosyn stimulation test.** See Section II, ACTH Stimulation Test, p 345. This test is to rule out adrenal insufficiency since a

single cortisol level can be misleading. Also, be sure to check adrenal reserve in all patients with severe hypothyroidism.

8. **Arterial blood gases.** Correct pH and pCO_2 findings to allow for changes in body temperature. For each 1°C below 37°C (98.6°F), add 0.015 to the pH. To correct the pCO_2, subtract 4.4% for each 1°C below 37°C (98.6°F). Your clinical lab will make these corrections for you as long as the patient's temperature is known. The pO_2 should also be corrected; however, this function is a nonlinear equation. Refer to the Scott et al 1999 reference listed at the end of this chapter for the equation. A metabolic or respiratory acidosis may be present secondary to the hypothermia.
9. **Blood cultures.** Rule out sepsis.
10. **Serum and urine drug screen.** Rule out barbiturates or phenothiazines as possible causes.

C. **Radiologic and other studies**

1. **Chest x-ray.** Obtain to rule out pneumonia as a source of infection. Pneumonia is also the most common sequela of hypothermia during the recovery period.
2. **Electrocardiogram.** Hypothermia can promote myocardial irritability and cause conduction abnormalities. The ECG may show T-wave inversion and PR, QRS, and QT prolongation as well as the unique J wave (or *Osborn wave*), which closely follows the QRS complex. Continuous ECG monitoring is important with a temperature below 32°C (89.6°F) because of the risk of cardiac arrhythmias. Atrial fibrillation is common. Ventricular tachycardia and fibrillation occurs frequently at temperatures below 86.0°F (30°C).

V. Plan

A. General support

1. Make sure the patient is hemodynamically stable. If ventricular fibrillation occurs, cardiopulmonary resuscitation (see Section I, Chapter 9, Cardiopulmonary Arrest, V, p 46) should be instituted and continued until the core temperature rises. In this clinical setting, the statement "A patient is not dead until they are warm and dead" applies.
2. If you suspect hypothermia secondary to environmental exposure, place an intravenous line to replace fluids because chronic hypothermia leads to volume depletion. The IV fluids can be warmed to 43°C (109.4°F).
3. Other therapeutic measures depend on the clinical setting. If sepsis is a possibility, then begin antibiotics immediately.
4. Give IV steroids if you suspect Addison's disease; or IV thyroxine if you suspect possible myxedema coma.
5. Some clinicians advocate administration of 100 mg of thiamine IV, an ampoule (50 mL) of 50% dextrose solution (D50), and 2 mg of

naloxone (Narcan) to all comatose hypothermic patients. Narcotic overdose should be suspected with bradypnea and pin-point pupils. Empiric dextrose administration is controversial because the administration of 50% dextrose solution (D50) has been associated with poorer outcomes in patients with anoxic or ischemic coma. Some experts recommend intravenous dextrose only if an immediate finger-stick glucose is low.

B. Rewarming techniques

1. In cases of environmental exposure, remove the patient from the cold environment and use some insulating material such as blankets. Patients with mild hypothermia (body temperature, 32.2°C to 35°C) and no circulatory compromise can be treated with passive rewarming.
2. Patients with moderate (body temperature, 28°C to < 32.2°C) or severe hypothermia (temperature, < 28 °C) should be treated with active rewarming. Some aggressive rewarming techniques are controversial. Active *external* rewarming with an electric blanket may produce hypovolemic shock through peripheral vasodilation, or cause "afterdrop" in core temperature through movement of the cold blood to the body core. External rewarming may also worsen a metabolic acidosis.
3. Such concerns have led to the use of active *core* rewarming for patients with core temperatures below 32°C (89.6°F), especially in the setting of chronic hypothermia secondary to environmental exposure. Active core rewarming techniques include gastrointestinal rewarming, peritoneal dialysis, inhalation of warmed oxygen, hemodialysis, and use of cardiopulmonary-bypass circuit. Some clinicians favor the latter two techniques in severe accidental hypothermia due to environmental exposure. Gastrointestinal rewarming involves the instillation of warmed normal saline via nasogastric and rectal tubes, removal of the fluid, and repeating the process.

REFERENCES

Browning RG, Olson DW, Stueven HA et al: 50% dextrose: Antidote or toxin? Ann Emerg Med 1990;19:683.

Danzl DF, Pozos RS: Accidental hypothermia. N Engl J Med 1994;331:1756.

Lazar HL: The treatment of hypothermia. N Engl J Med 1997;337:1545.

Lewin S, Brettman LR, Holzman RS: Infections in hypothermic patients. Arch Intern Med 1981;141:920.

Reuler JB: Hypothermia: Pathophysiology, clinical settings and management. Ann Intern Med 1978;89:519.

Scott MG, Heusel JW, LeGrys VA et al: Electrolyte and blood gases. In: Burtis CA, Ashwood ER, eds. *Tietz Textbook of Clinical Chemistry.* 3rd ed. Saunders;1999:1056.

Walpoth BH, Walpoth-Aslan BN, Mattle HP et al: Outcome of survivors of accidental deep hypothermia and circulatory arrest treated with extracorporeal blood warming. N Engl J Med 1997;337:1500.

Weinberg AD: Hypothermia. Ann Emerg Med 1993;22:370.

44. INSOMNIA

I. **Problem.** A patient hospitalized for lower-extremity cellulitis complains of lying awake for hours at night.

II. **Immediate Questions**

A. **What is the patient's mental status?** Delirium and dementia can both present with sleep disturbance. Delirium frequently results in a reversal of the normal sleep/wake cycle. It is important to avoid treatment with sedatives/hypnotics as they may actually worsen the symptomatology. Because some causes of delirium are potentially life-threatening, aggressive evaluation of delirious patients is warranted. (See Section I, Chapter 13, Coma, Acute Mental Status Changes, p 72).

B. **Is the patient kept awake by pain?** Painful stimuli result in a state of increased arousal that interferes with sleep and escalates the cycle of sleep disturbance and pain. Common examples include rheumatoid arthritis, in which a worsening of morning stiffness is associated with sleep disturbance, and fibrositis, in which symptoms can be reproduced by disturbing delta sleep in normal subjects.

C. **What is the patient's daytime sleep pattern?** Certainly, a patient who sleeps for extended periods during the day will not be able to fall asleep readily at night. Sleep hygiene interventions may be helpful.

D. **Does the patient take hypnotic medications regularly?** What are his or her current medications? Virtually all hypnotic agents show a tolerance effect with chronic use and a disruption of the sleep patterns that can interfere with normal sleep. Abrupt withdrawal of these agents almost invariably results in sleep disturbance, often termed *rebound insomnia.* It is also important to remember that withdrawal from barbiturates can be associated with convulsions and death. Remember to ask specifically about over-the-counter preparations. In addition to self-administered preparations, many medications prescribed in the hospital can interfere with normal sleep; a thorough review of the patient's medication record is warranted.

E. **What are the patient's food and beverage habits?** Ingestion of stimulant-containing beverages (coffee, tea, some soft drinks) and foods (some cheeses) can interfere with sleep. Cigarette smoking and alcohol consumption both have deleterious effects on normal sleep patterns. Alcohol use and withdrawal are also associated with sleep disturbance and are frequently not reported.

F. **Does the patient have difficulty lying flat?** Most often this is related to a cardiopulmonary condition and is often associated with dyspnea.

G. **What is the patient's customary sleep pattern?** Many clues to the etiology of sleep disturbance can be derived from a careful history of the sleep/wake cycle, including duration of periods of arousal and associated symptoms. Prolonged sleep latency is frequently associated with chronic or situational anxiety. Early-morning awakening is often seen with major depression, but may also be related to alcohol use. Frequent awakening with urinary urgency may be secondary to prostatic hypertrophy with bladder outlet obstruction, hyperglycemia with polyuria, or mobilization of fluid in a patient with congestive failure or chronic venous stasis and insufficiency. Awakening after a period of sleep with shortness of breath requiring a prolonged upright posture before resumption of sleep would suggest left ventricular failure.

III. Differential Diagnosis

A. Medical causes

1. **Delirium.** Evaluate the patient for systemic illnesses, sepsis, and liver dysfunction; also consider drug toxicities.
2. **Pain.** Control of this symptom frequently relieves the sleep disturbance.
3. **Cardiac disorders.** Ventricular dysfunction, arrhythmias, and ischemia can cause sleep disturbances. Ask about orthopnea, paroxysmal nocturnal dyspnea, dyspnea on exertion, palpitations, pre-syncope, syncope, and angina.
4. **Respiratory disorders.** Sleep disturbance can be seen in asthma, chronic obstructive airway disease, cystic fibrosis, sarcoidosis, pneumonia, and sleep apnea. Sleep apnea is most frequently seen in patients who are morbidly obese. Central apnea syndrome is not necessarily related to body habitus. These patients are frequently unaware of their frequent arousals and instead complain of excessive daytime drowsiness.
5. **Periodic limb movements or restless leg syndrome.** These disorders should be considered in patients with evidence of kicking during sleep or an uncomfortable sensation in their legs interfering with sleep continuity.
6. **Hyperthyroidism.** Associated symptoms and signs include weight loss, hyperdefecation, heat intolerance, anxiety, tachycardia, and tremor.

B. Drugs/toxins

1. **Tolerance to sleep medications from chronic usage**
2. **Abrupt withdrawal of sedative/hypnotics or antidepressant medications**
3. **Alcohol abuse.** There may be secondary disruption of appropriate sleep patterns as a result of chronic consumption or sudden withdrawal.
4. **Tobacco use**
5. **Caffeine ingestion.** When inquiring about the patient's beverage consumption, keep in mind that many soft drinks contain caffeine.
6. **Stimulant use or abuse**

C. **Psychiatric causes**
   1. **Depressive illness.** Either bipolar or unipolar. Hallmarks are decreased sleep with no perception of sleep deficiency and early-morning awakening, respectively.
   2. **Anxiety disorders.** Generally manifested by a prolonged sleep latency.

D. **Situational causes.** Frequently related to hospitalization.
   1. **Noise.** The ICU environment and talkative or emotionally distressed roommates are cited as common offenders.
   2. **Frequent disruptions.** Nursing duties such as administration of medications, recording of vital signs, and hygienic activities often interrupt patients' sleep.
   3. **Anger.** The patient may be troubled by unexpressed anger over illness or toward staff or family.
   4. **Anxiety.** This is a short-term response, usually related to the patient's medical condition or disorienting environment.

IV. **Database.** The most important components of the database in evaluating insomnia are the patient's history and an evaluation of his or her mental status.

A. **Physical examination key points**
   1. **Cardiopulmonary exam.** Rales, elevated jugular venous pressure, displaced point of maximal impulse, S_3 gallop, and peripheral edema all suggest congestive heart failure.
   2. **Respiratory exam.** Wheezing suggests obstructive airway disease but can be seen with pulmonary edema.
   3. **Neurologic exam.** Conduct a mental status examination for evidence of anxiety, depression, delirium, and dementia.

B. **Laboratory data.** The cause of insomnia is very often determined without the use of laboratory tests.
   1. **Screening chemistries.** Include hepatic and renal function tests to evaluate for possible delirium.
   2. **Thyroid hormone levels.** If indicated by clinical presentation. (See III.A.6.)
   3. **Urine drug screen.** To be obtained in cases where drug use is strongly suspected but denied.

C. **Radiologic and other studies.** CXR is indicated if congestive heart failure or pneumonia is suspected. Rarely a sleep study (polysomnography) is needed.

V. **Plan.** It is most important to determine the medical, psychologic, or situational causes of the patient's sleeplessness. Most cases are secondary to a situational cause and do not represent a pathologic situation. In cases where there is no contraindication to their use, it is reasonable to include a sleeping medication to be taken as needed with admission orders. When a specific cause is determined, it should be remedied if possible rather than treating the sleeplessness symptomatically.

A. Nonmedical treatments. These measures are often as effective as medical treatment and lack side effects. They include minimizing disturbances, trying to maintain the patient's normal waking and sleeping times, eliminating roommate problems when possible, eliminating caffeine and tobacco use, and minimizing noise from monitors or other hospital equipment.

B. Symptomatic treatment

1. **Oral sleeping medication.** Choices include the benzodiazepines, benzodiazepine receptor agonists, chloral hydrate, and antihistamines. Barbiturates are not recommended.
   a. **Benzodiazepines.** These are most frequently used for short-term treatment of insomnia. Newer hypnotics such as estazolam (ProSom) 0.5–2.0 mg, zolpidem (Ambien) 5–10 mg, or zaleplon (Sonata) 5–10 mg PO nightly are effective; reports suggest less disturbance of rapid eye movement (REM) sleep and lower abuse potential than with older benzodiazepines. Other older, rapidly absorbed, short half-life agents such as triazolam (Halcion) 0.125–0.25 mg PO every night; or temazepam (Restoril) 15–30 mg PO and flurazepam (Dalmane) 15–30 mg PO every night can be used.
   b. **Chloral hydrate.** Available in both oral and rectal forms; the dose is 500–1000 mg by either route. Do not use in patients with hepatic or renal failure.
   c. **Antihistamines.** Be conscious of anticholinergic side effects, particularly in the elderly.
      i. **Diphenhydramine (Benadryl) 25–50 mg PO or IM.**
      ii. **Hydroxyzine (Vistaril) 25–50 mg PO or IM.**
   d. **Antidepressants.** Many have significant anticholinergic side effects and should be used with caution in the elderly. Also be aware of cardiac side effects.
      i. **Amitriptyline (Elavil).** Give 25–50 mg PO Q HS. Has significant anticholinergic side effects; most useful when chronic pain syndromes accompany sleep disturbance.
      ii. **Imipramine (Tofranil).** Give 75 mg PO Q HS. Requires the same precautions as with amitriptyline but is less useful in chronic pain.
      iii. **Desipramine (Norpramin).** Give 50 mg PO every night. May have fewer anticholinergic side effects.
      iv. **Trazodone (Desyrel).** Give 25–50 mg PO Q HS.
2. **Alternative therapies.** Valerian, kava, and others are not to be recommended due to inadequate research regarding their effectiveness. Melatonin, which has been extensively studied, has vasoconstrictive properties, and cardiovascular disease is a contraindication.

REFERENCES

Gillin JC, Byerley WF: The diagnosis and management of insomnia. N Engl J Med 1990;322:239.

Goodman LS, Limbird LE, Milonoff PB, eds: *Goodman & Gilman's The Pharmacological Basis of Therapeutics.* 9th ed. McGraw-Hill;1996.
Klink ME, Dodge R, Quan S: The relationship of sleep complaints to respiratory symptoms in a general population. Chest 1994;105:151.
Meyer TJ: Evaluation and management of insomnia. Hosp Pract Dec 15, 1998;75.

45. IRREGULAR PULSE

(See also Section I, Chapter 60, Tachycardia, p 323, and Section I, Chapter 8, Bradycardia, p 39).

I. **Problem.** A 77-year-old man with mental status changes is reported to have an irregular pulse.

II. **Immediate Questions**

A. **What is the patient's heart rate?** The heart rate, as well as the frequency of irregularity, can assist the physician in developing a differential diagnosis of the irregular heart rhythm. For example, an irregularly irregular rhythm with an apical pulse of 130 beats per minute (bpm) suggests atrial fibrillation.

B. **What are the patient's other vital signs?** Low systolic blood pressure (less than 90 mm Hg) would signal an urgent situation. (See Section I, Chapter 42, Hypotension (Shock), p 224).

C. **Has the patient been noted to have an irregular pulse before?** A previous history of "skipped heartbeats" suggests a chronic problem. The intermittent occurrence of isolated premature atrial contractions (PACs) or premature ventricular contractions (PVCs) may be chronic. This is a common benign condition associated with several medical problems or with the use of a variety of medications, and can be seen occasionally in otherwise healthy individuals.

D. **Is there any history of previous cardiac disease?** A history of mitral stenosis hints to atrial fibrillation related to left atrial enlargement, whereas a history of previous myocardial infarction (MI) or long-standing hypertension with left ventricular hypertrophy or dilated cardiomyopathy might suggest ventricular arrhythmias.

E. **What medication is the patient taking?** Ask specifically about medications (eg, digoxin, antiarrhythmic agents, diuretics, bronchodilators [especially theophylline], and tricyclic antidepressants). Digoxin can cause atrioventricular heart block with variable conduction. Diuretic-induced hypokalemia and hypomagnesemia as well as the use of antiarrhythmic drugs can cause both PACs and PVCs, which may be responsible for an irregular rhythm. Many asthma drugs and other stimulants to the heart can cause an irregular heartbeat.

III. **Differential Diagnosis**

A. **Premature contractions**

1. **Premature atrial contractions (PACs).** PACs can result from acute illnesses. Think of PACs in patients with a significant history

of tobacco, alcohol, or caffeine use. PACs may occasionally lead to sustained supraventricular tachycardia (SVT), but usually PACs do not require acute therapy in the absence of sustained supraventricular tachyarrhythmia.

2. **Premature ventricular contractions (PVCs).** The prevalence of benign isolated PVCs increases with age. PVCs are also seen with serious infections and illnesses; during acute myocardial ischemia; with stress; with use of many types of anesthetic drugs; and with excessive use of tobacco, alcohol, caffeine, or other cardiac stimulants. PVCs may also be seen with hypoxemia, metabolic or respiratory acidosis or alkalosis, hypokalemia, and hypomagnesemia. Patients with hypertrophic cardiomyopathy and mitral valve prolapse may have frequent multifocal nonsustained runs of ventricular ectopy that are considered risk factors for sudden cardiac death. The presence of isolated PVCs does not increase mortality in the absence of underlying organic heart disease, and therefore usually does not require any specific therapy.

B. **Sinus arrhythmia.** Sinus arrhythmia occurs in almost every age group and is usually a normal variant. Treatment is rarely indicated or required. Sustained tachyarrhythmias rarely occur in otherwise healthy patients with sinus arrhythmia. The P wave and QRS morphologies will appear normal. Think about medications and other external cardiac stimulants.

C. **Sinoatrial exit block.** This is defined by the absence of a normally timed P wave, resulting in a pause that is a multiple of the P-to-P interval. This rhythm can be seen with vagal nerve stimulation, during acute myocarditis or acute MI, or with fibrosis of the conduction system. It can be related to the use of several cardiac drugs such as quinidine, procainamide, and digitalis. Syncope is a rare outcome.

D. **Atrial fibrillation.** Defined as chaotic atrial depolarizations and a grossly irregular ventricular response. Atrial fibrillation can be seen in patients with apparently normal hearts; or in patients with rheumatic heart disease, acute myocardial ischemia/infarction, myocarditis, pericarditis, hypertrophic and dilated cardiomyopathies, hypertensive heart disease, acute alcohol intoxication, pulmonary embolism (PE), and thyrotoxicosis. The resting ventricular response is usually between 100–160 bpm. It may, however, be < 100 bpm in the presence of AV node disease or certain medications.

E. **Atrial flutter.** The pulse may be irregular if the atrioventricular node conduction varies; however, the pulse during atrial flutter is frequently rapid and usually regular. Atrial flutter is associated with the same diseases as atrial fibrillation.

F. **Second-degree atrioventricular block.** Both Mobitz type I (Wenckebach) and Mobitz type II second-degree heart block can bring about an irregular pulse if the atrial to ventricular conduction is variable. Second-degree heart block can be seen with acute MI, degenerative disease of the cardiac conduction system, viral myocarditis, acute rheumatic fever, and Lyme disease. Mobitz type I second-degree AV block can be seen during times of increased parasympathetic tone, such as with painful stimuli. In this circumstance, it does not indicate disease of the intracardiac conduction system.

IV. Database

A. Physical examination key points

1. **Vital signs.** Palpate the brachial or carotid pulses to determine the heart rate and assess the degree of cardiac irregularity. The brachial, carotid, and femoral artery pulses are preferred for palpation over more peripheral pulses. Be careful to avoid mistaking a heartbeat with a variable pulsation amplitude from an irregular cardiac rhythm. Variations in pulsation amplitude can be seen during severe pulmonary bronchospasm, during an extensive MI, with decompensated congestive heart failure, with acute aortic insufficiency, or with pericardial tamponade. Rapid action must be taken if hypotension is present. A fever may suggest an infection, which can have associated PVCs or PACs. Several specific infections (eg, acute rheumatic fever and acute Lyme disease) can cause atrioventricular node block.
2. **Heart.** Atrioventricular node block with an associated murmur might suggest acute rheumatic fever. An S_4 suggests acute MI. Several cardiac arrhythmias may be present with an acute MI, including PVCs and PACs, variable degrees of atrioventricular block, atrial fibrillation, and atrial flutter. If atrial fibrillation is present, listen for the diastolic rumble of mitral stenosis at the cardiac apex. It is best heard using the bell of the stethoscope, with the patient in the left lateral decubitus position.

B. Laboratory data

1. **Electrolytes.** Rule out hypokalemia. A low serum bicarbonate suggests metabolic acidosis.
2. **Arterial blood gases.** If PVCs are present, exclude hypoxemia and severe acidemia or alkalemia.
3. **Medications.** A recent serum digoxin level is imperative if the patient is taking this medication. Digitalis intoxication can cause PVCs, sinoatrial exit block, or second-degree heart block. Consider measuring serum levels of other medications, such as quinidine, procainamide, and theophylline. An elevated digoxin level can occur if the level is obtained while the drug is in the distribution phase (6–8 hr).

C. Electrocardiogram and rhythm strip

1. Be sure to include a long rhythm strip in order to catch the pattern of the responsible arrhythmia.
2. Identify all of the P waves that are present and note their timing and relationship to the QRS complexes. P waves are best seen in

leads I, II, aVR, aVF, and V1. You may need to examine several rhythm strips from different leads in order to correctly identify the cardiac rhythm.

3. Be certain to examine the ECG for evidence of myocardial ischemia; drug effects such as prolongation of the QT interval; and for the electrocardiographic changes of pulmonary embolism (S_1, Q_3, T_3, acute right bundle branch block, acute right-axis deviation), and for pericarditis (diffuse ST elevation with upward concavity, T wave inversion, and PR segment depression).

V. Plan. Most of the cardiac arrhythmias that result in a detectably irregular pulse do not need emergent therapy; however, they should be identified and predisposing conditions treated appropriately. Possible exceptions to this statement include the following:

A. Frequent or multifocal PVCs following a myocardial infarction or with impaired left ventricular function. Be sure to exclude predisposing conditions, such as hypokalemia, hypoxemia, hypomagnesemia, acidosis, alkalosis, and myocardial ischemia. Beta-blockers are the agents of choice because they are the only class of drugs proven to decrease the incidence of sudden cardiac death in postinfarction patients. Beta-blockers may cause or worsen congestive heart failure, particularly in patients with impaired left ventricular function. If treatment with an antiarrhythmic drug is considered, it is recommended that consultation with a cardiac electrophysiologist be obtained prior to starting the patient on any long-term antiarrhythmic drug therapy. This recommendation is based on the results of the Cardiac Arrhythmia Suppression Trial (CAST) study, which showed that the pro-arrhythmic side effects of some of these medications (eg, encainide, flecainide, moricizine) might increase rather than decrease the risk of sudden cardiac death.

B. Mobitz type II second-degree atrioventricular block. This condition frequently progresses to third-degree heart block; therefore, exclusion of reversible causes and placement of a temporary transvenous pacemaker should be considered.

C. Atrial fibrillation and flutter. See Section I, Chapter 60, Tachycardia, V, p 329.

REFERENCES

Cardiac Arrhythmia Suppression Trial (CAST) Investigators: Preliminary report: Effect of encainide and flecainide on mortality in a randomized trial of arrhythmia suppression after myocardial infarction. N Engl J Med 1989;321:406.

Falk RH: Atrial fibrillation. N Engl J Med 2001;344:1067.

Miller JM, Zipes DP: Management of the patient with cardiac arrhythmias. In: Braunwald E, Zipes DP, Libby P, eds. *Heart Disease: A Textbook of Cardiovascular Medicine.* 6th ed. Saunders;2001:700.

Wagner GS, ed: *Marriott's Practical Electrocardiography.* 9th ed. Williams & Wilkins;1994.

46. JAUNDICE

I. **Problem.** A 66-year-old woman is admitted because of icteric sclerae and abdominal pain.

II. **Immediate Questions**

A. **What are the patient's vital signs?** Fever and tachycardia with or without hypotension could indicate sepsis associated with ascending cholangitis. This is a medical emergency and requires immediate aggressive intervention.

B. **Does the patient have diabetes?** Diabetes is a significant risk factor for ascending cholangitis.

C. **Is there a history of alcoholism or chronic alcohol use?** Cirrhosis may be a source of jaundice.

D. **Is there a history of intravenous drug abuse, sexual promiscuity, homosexual activity, or exposure to hepatitis?** Viral hepatitis could be the source of the jaundice. A viral prodrome is often elicited.

E. **Is there associated abdominal pain?** A history of postprandial right upper quadrant or epigastric pain, especially with radiation to the back, may represent biliary colic. Abdominal pain can be also associated with cancer.

F. **Is there a history of previous biliary surgery?** Jaundice may occur as a result of a retained common duct stone or biliary stricture.

III. **Differential Diagnosis.** The differential diagnosis of jaundice can be classified as either surgical or medical.

A. **Acute biliary obstruction (surgical).** This category includes carcinoma and common bile duct stones. Biliary obstruction may lead to cholangitis and potentially life-threatening sepsis.

B. **Alcoholic liver disease (medical).** Alcoholic cirrhosis is usually seen after at least 10 years of heavy ethanol ingestion. Check for stigmata of chronic liver disease (palmar erythema, spider telangiectasias, gynecomastia, and testicular atrophy).

C. **Viral hepatitis (medical).** Consider with a history of IV drug abuse, exposure to persons with jaundice, sexual promiscuity, male homosexual activity, travel to endemic areas, or recent history of transfusion.

D. **Other causes of hepatitis (medical).** Autoimmune disorders or drugs such as isoniazid and halothane.

E. **Hemolysis (medical).** Rarely raises the bilirubin over 5 mg/dL. Look for an increased reticulocyte count and an increased indirect bilirubin.

F. **Primary biliary cirrhosis (medical).** Usually found in middle-aged women who present with jaundice, fatigue, and pruritus.

G. **Drugs (medical).** May cause hepatitis, cholestasis, or hemolysis. Phenothiazines and estrogens are common causes of cholestasis.

H. **Total parenteral nutrition (medical).** Associated with high carbohydrate loads. Usually from long-term TPN.

I. **Pregnancy (medical).** An unusual cause of jaundice, but can be life-threatening.

J. **Postoperative cholestasis (medical).** Diagnosis of exclusion.

K. **Sepsis (medical).** Diagnosis of exclusion.

IV. **Database.** An experienced clinician can make an accurate diagnosis with history, physical examination, and simple laboratory tests 85% of the time.

A. **Physical examination key points**

1. **Vital signs.** A fever with rigors may suggest ascending cholangitis.
2. **Skin.** Palmar erythema and telangiectasia point toward chronic liver disease. Look for needle marks or "tracks" suggestive of IV drug abuse.
3. **Breasts (in males).** Gynecomastia is consistent with chronic liver disease.
4. **Abdomen.** The physical exam should be centered on the abdomen. Look for hepatomegaly or palpable gallbladder (*Courvoisier's sign*), which may indicate malignant obstruction. The presence or absence of abdominal tenderness, particularly right upper quadrant tenderness, and *Murphy's sign* (tenderness in the right upper quadrant during inspiration with palpation) should be documented. Ascites may be present with cirrhosis.
5. **Rectum/genitourinary system.** A rectal exam should be done; look for occult blood. Testicular atrophy may be present with chronic liver disease.

B. **Laboratory data**

1. **Liver function studies.** Including transaminases (AST and ALT), bilirubin total and fractionated, alkaline phosphatase, and γ-glutamyl transpeptidase (GGT). There are two basic patterns in liver function tests, hepatocellular and hepatocanalicular. The hepatocellular pattern is characterized by AST and ALT 10 $\times$ the upper limits of normal with much smaller increases in alkaline phosphatase or GGT and bilirubin. Conversely, the hepatocanalicular pattern is suggested when the alkaline phosphatase or GGT is 5–10 times normal with relatively normal transaminases. Bilirubin is also more commonly elevated. Transaminases > 300 virtually never occur in alcoholic liver disease without the combined effect of some other toxin such as acetaminophen (Tylenol). Bilirubin levels > 20 are very suggestive of extrahepatic cholestasis. An elevated indirect bilirubin suggests hemoly-

sis; a total bilirubin secondary to hemolysis seldom exceeds 5 mg/dL.

2. **Amylase.** Significant elevations in amylase (> 10 times the upper limits of normal) are suggestive of biliary disease.
3. **Prothrombin time.** Elevation that corrects with vitamin K is caused by extrahepatic obstruction, while failure to correct is seen in fulminant hepatitis or cirrhosis.
4. **Hepatitis serology.** Hepatitis B surface antigen, hepatitis B IgM core antibody, hepatitis A IgM antibody, and hepatitis C antibody. (See Section II, Laboratory Diagnosis, Hepatitis Tests, pp 363–365).
5. **Other serology.** Antinuclear (ANA), antimitochondrial, and anti–smooth muscle antibodies may be helpful. The triad of antimitochondrial antibody, elevated alkaline phosphatase, and an elevated class M immunoglobulin is consistent with primary biliary cirrhosis. A high ANA titer suggests autoimmune hepatitis. High titers of anti–smooth muscle antibodies are seen in chronic active hepatitis.

C. Radiologic and other studies

1. **Ultrasound and computerized tomography.** First examination in patients with intermediate or low risk for extrahepatic biliary obstruction. Ultrasound and CT are good primarily for detecting dilated ducts, pancreatic masses, and stones in the gallbladder. Detection of stones in the common bile duct is uniformly poor with both of these tests.
2. **Endoscopic retrograde cholangiopancreatography (ERCP) and percutaneous transhepatic cholangiogram (PTC).** Tests of first choice for extrahepatic obstruction. Selection of ERCP or PTC is based on local expertise and the clinical situation. ERCP is recommended in patients with ascites, coagulation abnormalities, a previous history of failed percutaneous transhepatic cholangiography, a suspicion of sclerosing cholangitis, and a planned sphincterotomy. It is also the test of choice when carcinoma of the pancreas is suspected, because a biopsy can be done. Indications for PTC include patients with dilated ducts, previous gastric surgery with Billroth II anastomosis, a previous failed ERCP, or a mass involving the proximal bile duct.
3. **Liver biopsy.** Generally not useful in the diagnosis of jaundice. Occasionally reveals an unsuspected medical cause such as metastatic tumor. Liver biopsy is sometimes performed in the evaluation of alcoholic liver disease or viral hepatitis.
4. **Nuclear scan (HIDA).** This scan is generally of low utility in the diagnosis of jaundice. It is very helpful if acute cholecystitis is suspected.

V. Plan. The tempo of diagnostic evaluation is dictated by the severity of the patient's illness. If acute cholangitis is suspected, the evaluation must proceed emergently. Patients with signs of liver failure, specifically significant coagulopathy and hepatic encephalopathy, need ICU monitoring and aggressive supportive care.

A. Hepatocellular (medical) cholestasis

1. **Viral hepatitis.** Patients who are dehydrated or vomiting or have significant coagulopathy will need admission for treatment with IV fluids, vitamin K, and fresh-frozen plasma.
2. **Alcoholic liver disease.** Requires aggressive supportive care, entailing dietary restriction of protein, full evaluation of any coagulopathy (see Section I, Chapter 12, Coagulopathy, V, p 70), and treatment of associated electrolyte deficiencies that are often encountered in alcoholics (eg, hypokalemia, hypomagnesemia, and hypophosphatemia). Thiamine, folate, and multivitamins may be needed. In a patient with ascites, a paracentesis should be performed (see Section III, Chapter 11, Paracentesis). With ascites, prophylactic antibiotics are recommended to prevent peritonitis if the total protein in the ascitic fluid is < 1 g/dL or if the patient had a previous episode of spontaneous bacterial peritonitis. Norfloxacin 400 mg Q day; ciprofloxacin 750 mg week; or trimethoprim-sulfamethoxazole DS, one pill per day, 5 days per week should be given indefinitely.

B. Extrahepatic (surgical) cholestasis

1. If there is a strong clinical suspicion of extrahepatic obstruction, proceed at once with ERCP or PTC.
2. If extrahepatic obstruction is possible but not definite, obtain a biliary ultrasound or CT scan first. If obstruction is confirmed, then proceed with ERCP or surgery. If ascending cholangitis is suspected and confirmed by ultrasound or CT scan, begin antibiotics (ampicillin and gentamicin; or imipenem; or ticarcillin/clavulanate) and request immediate surgical consultation.

C. Hemolysis. Treat underlying cause.

REFERENCES

Frank BB: Clinical evaluation of jaundice. JAMA 1989;262:3031.

Kamath PS: Clinical approach to the patient with abnormal liver function tests. Mayo Clin Proc 1996;71:1089.

Lidofsky S, Scharschmidt BF: Jaundice. In: Feldman M, Scharschmidt BF, Sleisenger MH, eds. *Gastrointestinal and Liver Diseases: Pathophysiology/Diagnosis/Management.* 6th ed. Saunders;1998:220.

Moseley RH: Evaluation of abnormal liver function tests. Med Clin North Am 1996;80:887.

47. JOINT SWELLING

I. Problem. A 35-year-old woman is admitted with right knee swelling and pain.

II. Immediate Questions

A. **Is there a previous history of joint swelling?** A history of multiple joint involvement suggests an etiology resulting in polyarthritis rather than monarthritis. Remember, many diseases causing a polyarthritis can present initially as a monarthritis. The pattern of joint involvement may suggest the cause; for example, the first metatarsophalangeal (MTP) joint in gout, or metacarpophalangeal (MCP) and proximal interphalangeal (PIP) joints in rheumatoid arthritis. The history of onset, such as acute, chronic, or migratory, may be helpful in diagnosis.

B. **Is there a history of trauma?** Trauma to the joint would lead the clinician to consider fracture, ligamentous tear, loose body, or dislocation. A sport and occupational history is essential.

C. **Does the patient have any constitutional symptoms?** The presence of fever suggests septic arthritis, although infection must be considered in any case of monarticular arthritis even in the absence of fever. Malaise, fatigue, and weight loss suggest a systemic arthritis. Morning stiffness of significant duration (> 1 hour) suggests inflammatory arthritis.

D. **Are there any other systemic symptoms?** It is important to obtain a full rheumatic disease systems review. A photosensitive rash suggests systemic lupus erythematosus (SLE), whereas diarrhea may occur with inflammatory bowel disease (IBD) and associated reactive arthritis. A partial list of systemic symptoms would include rash, alopecia, Raynaud's phenomenon, oral or genital ulcers, urethritis or cervicitis, diarrhea, eye inflammation, sicca symptoms, weakness, and CNS disturbances.

E. **What is the patient's past medical and family history?** Inquire about recent febrile illnesses, tick bites, and other events, as the patient may not associate these symptoms with the onset of arthritis. A medication history may provide a clue to diagnosis (eg, hemarthrosis associated with warfarin therapy); or a positive family history may suggest arthritis associated with psoriasis, hemoglobinopathies, or coagulopathies.

III. Differential Diagnosis.

Arthritis is classified as being either monarticular or polyarticular. Subclassification is often based on the joint fluid analysis (see Section IV). Remember that an arthritis that is generally polyarticular can present as a monarticular arthritis.

A. **Monarticular arthritis**

1. **Infection.** May be bacterial, viral, fungal, or tuberculous.
2. **Trauma.** Etiologies include loose foreign bodies, fracture, plant thorn synovitis, and internal derangement.
3. **Hemarthrosis.** Causes include hemoglobinopathy, coagulopathy, anticoagulation therapy, and pigmented villonodular synovitis.

4. **Tumors.** Consider osteogenic sarcoma, metastatic tumor, synovial osteochondromatosis, and paraneoplastic syndromes.
5. **Crystals.** Types of crystal associated with arthritis include gout (first MTP involvement characteristic), pseudogout (may be secondary to hyperparathyroidism and hemochromatosis), and hydroxyapatite.
6. **Noninflammatory diseases.** These include avascular necrosis, which is often associated with a history of trauma, steroid use, alcohol use, or sickle cell anemia; osteoarthritis; endocrine disorders; amyloid; osteochondritis dissecans; and neuropathy.
7. **Inflammatory–connective tissue diseases.** Rheumatoid arthritis or Reiter's syndrome.

B. Polyarticular arthritis

1. **Infection or associated with infection**
   a. **Gonococcal infection.** Frequently associated with a migratory arthritis, tenosynovitis, and a pustular rash.
   b. **Lyme disease.** Associated with both an acute arthritis and a late chronic destructive arthritis.
   c. **Rheumatic fever.** Primarily lower-extremity large joints. In the adult, arthritis is rarely migratory.
   d. **AIDS.** Septic arthritis, Reiter's syndrome, and a lupus-like presentation with nondestructive polyarthritis, rash, pleuritis, and CNS symptoms all have been described.
   e. **Subacute bacterial endocarditis**
   f. **Chronic active hepatitis.** Chronic hepatitis B and C infections are associated with arthritis alone, or with polyarteritis nodosa or mixed essential cryoglobulinemia.
2. **Crystals.** For example, gout, pseudogout, and hydroxyapatite.
3. **Metabolic disorders.** Etiologies include hypothyroidism, acromegaly, hemochromatosis, ochronosis (alkaptonuria, associated degenerative arthritis sparing the small joints, pigmentation of the skin and sclera, and urine turning black with time or alkalinization), hemophilia, and hyperparathyroidism. Hyperparathyroidism and hemochromatosis are associated with pseudogout.
4. **Noninflammatory diseases**
   a. **Osteoarthritis.** Consider when distal interphalangeal (DIP) and carpal-metacarpal joints of hands are involved.
   b. **Intestinal bypass surgery**
5. **Spondyloarthropathies**
   a. **Associated with involvement of spine and/or sacroiliac joints.** Peripheral arthritis is often asymmetric.
   b. **Psoriatic arthritis** can involve joints in both arms or legs but the joints tend to be different, unlike rheumatoid arthritis, which involves the same joints on both sides of the body. Psoriatic arthritis, unlike rheumatoid arthritis, can affect the DIP joints.

6. **Inflammatory disease**
   a. **Juvenile rheumatoid arthritis (JRA).** Also called adult Still's disease. Fever, sore throat, and often systemic complaints (myalgias) are present. Rheumatoid factor (RF) is negative.
   b. **Rheumatoid arthritis.** A symmetric arthritis characteristically involves the MCP and PIP joints of the hands.
   c. **Systemic lupus erythematosus (SLE).** Resembles rheumatoid arthritis but is rarely an erosive arthritis.
   d. **Scleroderma.** Significant joint swelling is uncommon.
   e. **Polychondritis**
   f. **Mixed connective tissue disease.** Defined by a positive anti-ribonuclear protein (anti-RNP) antibody. Includes features of rheumatoid arthritis, scleroderma, polymyositis, and SLE.
   g. **Sarcoidosis.** An acute migratory arthritis frequently associated with tenosynovitis and erythema nodosum, and a chronic pauciarticular form involving the knees and ankles.
   h. **Vasculitis.** Leukocytoclastic vasculitis and larger vessel vasculitides such as Churg-Strauss syndrome, Wegener's granulomatosis, polyarteritis nodosa, and Behçet's syndrome can rarely present with arthritis.

IV. **Database**

A. **Physical examination key points.** Physical exam must be complete. Systemic disease must be ruled out as the cause of the arthritis; there can be no shortcuts.
   1. **Skin.** A rash may indicate the etiology. For evidence of psoriasis, frequently overlooked areas include under the hairline or rectum. Telangiectasia, nailfold infarcts, palmar erythema, and livedo reticularis suggest connective tissue disease or vasculitis. Nodules are seen in rheumatoid arthritis and gout. Bluish-black pigmentation suggests ochronosis.
   2. **Eyes.** Retinal abnormalities (hemorrhages) may suggest an infectious etiology such as subacute bacterial endocarditis. Scleral pigmentation may be seen with ochronosis.
   3. **Mouth.** Oral and nasal ulcers point to SLE or Behçet's syndrome.
   4. **Musculoskeletal system.** All major joints should be examined for range of motion, tenderness, deformity, and swelling. True swelling (arthritis) must be present rather than bone pain, muscle pain, or pain from bursitis, tendinitis, or torn ligaments or menisci.

B. **Laboratory data**
   1. **Complete blood count with differential.** To rule out infection and to identify anemia or thrombocytopenia if a systemic arthritis is considered.
   2. **Joint fluid analysis**
      a. Any initial presentation of arthritis should be evaluated with joint aspiration if possible. (See Section III, Chapter 3, Arthro-

centesis, p 392). Fluid should be sent for Gram's stain, as well as bacterial, acid-fast bacillus, and fungal cultures if indicated. You should also obtain a crystal exam, and cell count with differential. A WBC count of 0–300 is normal, 300–2000 is noninflammatory, 2000–75,000 indicates an inflammatory process, and > 100,000 indicates septic arthritis; however, cell counts from a bacterial source may be as low as 5000 WBC/mL. A differential count with a predominance of neutrophils suggests septic arthritis, whereas lymphocytosis suggests leukemia or tuberculosis. These values are only guidelines as there is considerable overlap in all of these diseases.

b. Gram's stain smears are positive in only 66% of subsequent culture-proven cases of septic arthritis. A negative result does not therefore exclude the possibility of infection. The monosodium urate crystals of gout are rod-shaped, negatively birefringent crystals (3–10 μm) seen within WBCs during active disease and often extend beyond the cell wall. The crystal is yellow when parallel to the slow ray of the compensator. Calcium pyrophosphate dihydrate (CPPD) crystals are rhomboid-shaped, positively birefringent crystals that are blue when parallel to the slow ray of the compensator. The crystal is usually contained within the WBC. Calcium hydroxyapatite crystals are small (< 1 μm), minimally birefringent, irregularly shaped cytoplasmic inclusions that appear under light microscopy as "shiny coins" when extracellular. Calcium hydroxyapatite crystals are more commonly associated with acute episodes of bursitis, tendinitis, or periarthritis seen in chronic renal failure patients or in older women with the progressive destructive arthritis of Milwaukee shoulder syndrome.

3. **Other cultures.** Cultures of urine and blood should be obtained if septic arthritis is considered. If gonorrhea is considered, obtain cervical/urethral, rectal, and pharyngeal specimens.
4. **Creatinine.** Often obtained because many drugs, especially nonsteroidal anti-inflammatory drugs (NSAIDs), used in treatment are contraindicated if creatinine is elevated.
5. **Urinalysis.** Proteinuria, red blood cells, and casts may indicate a systemic cause such as SLE.
6. **Rheumatic disease workup.** If a collagen vascular disease is suspected, obtain a Westergren erythrocyte sedimentation rate (ESR), C-reactive protein (CRP), antinuclear antibodies (ANA), and rheumatoid factor (RF). Tests for anti–double-stranded DNA (anti-DSDNA), extractable nuclear antigens (anti-RNP, anti-Smith, anti-SSA(Ro), anti-SSB(La), complement (CH50, C3, C4), and cryoglobulin are usually not obtained initially. Measurement of hepatitis B and C serologies or anti-neutrophil cytoplasmic antibody (ANCA) may be considered if the history is suggestive. A positive

C-ANCA is highly suggestive of Wegener's granulomatosis. HLA-B27 is rarely helpful.

C. **Radiologic and other studies.** Plain films of the involved joints are often helpful, especially if the arthritis is chronic. If normal, they can serve as a baseline as the arthritis progresses. Films of the hands and feet are particularly helpful when rheumatoid arthritis is considered.

V. **Plan.** Treatment is dependent on the type of arthritis diagnosed. An individual discussion of each type is beyond the scope of this book.

A. **Drug therapy.** Ensure from the patient's history and laboratory tests that there are no contraindications to the medication chosen. The patient must be informed of side effects. The most commonly prescribed medications (NSAIDs) are contraindicated in patients with elevated creatinine, a history of hypersensitivity reaction to aspirin or NSAIDs, platelet abnormalities, and possibly peptic ulcer disease. In the elderly, one must be aware of the CNS side effects. The selective COX-2 inhibitors (rofecoxib [Vioxx] and celecoxib [Celebrex]) are less likely to cause gastrointestinal toxicity. The COX-2 inhibitors, however, have the same renal toxicity as other NSAIDs. Avoid using celecoxib in patients with an allergy to sulfa drugs.

B. **Supportive measures.** Depending on the diagnosis, heat or ice therapy, specific exercises, splinting, and physical therapy may be indicated.

C. **Septic arthritis**

1. Daily drainage of joint fluid is absolutely necessary. If the joint is not easily drained, open drainage may be necessary. Gram's stain will help direct the initial choice of antibiotic pending cultures.
2. If gonococcal arthritis is suspected, ceftriaxone should be given. (See Section VII, p 604).
3. In nongonococcal bacterial arthritis, gram-positive cocci on Gram's stain should be treated with a penicillinase-resistant penicillin or vancomycin if methicillin-resistant *Staphylococcus aureus* is prevalent or if *Staphylococcus epidermidis* is suspected. An aminoglycoside and an antipseudomonal penicillin or third-generation cephalosporin would be used for gram-negative bacilli. If the Gram's strain is negative in a compromised host, use broad-spectrum coverage for both gram-positive and gram-negative organisms.

REFERENCES

Baker DG, Schumacher HR: Acute monarthritis. N Engl J Med 1993;329:1013.

Kelley WN, Harris ED, Ruddy S et al, eds: *Textbook of Rheumatology.* 6th ed. Saunders;1997.

48. LEUKOCYTOSIS

I. **Problem.** A 63-year-old woman is admitted for hypoxemia, bilateral pulmonary infiltrates, and fever. Broad-spectrum IV antibiotics are begun after appropriate cultures are obtained. Her white blood cell count (WBC) remains about 25,000–30,000/μL.

II. **Immediate Questions**

A. **What is the patient's current clinical status?** Elevated WBC counts are often associated with infection; look for associated fever, rigors, hypotension, or tachycardia.

B. **Have any intervening clinically relevant episodes of physical stress occurred since admission?** Hypotension and other signs of shock can certainly be associated with a leukocytosis. The use of mechanical ventilation or resuscitative measures can stimulate leukocytosis.

C. **Is there a history suggestive of prior underlying systemic illness?** Weight loss, prior sustained fevers, night sweats, chronic cough or dyspnea, hemoptysis, myalgias, and bone pain are all suggestive of chronic illnesses such as mycobacterial or fungal infections, connective tissue diseases, or possibly a neoplastic disorder. A history of new symptoms argues against a chronic or subacute illness.

D. **Are there any prior complete blood counts with which to compare this leukocyte count?** Again, the presence or absence of prior leukocytosis aids in the evaluation. Sustained leukocytosis over weeks or months strongly implies a chronic or subacute process, whether it be an infection such as an abscess or tuberculosis (TB), or a neoplasm.

E. **Is there evidence of infection that has not been addressed, such as intra-abdominal infection (abscess), genitourinary infection, or CNS infection?** Pulmonary infiltrates may represent adult respiratory distress syndrome (ARDS) occurring as a reaction to underlying sepsis, such as an abdominal infection. Acute infectious causes of leukocytosis must be excluded since they are so readily treatable.

F. **Is the patient currently on any medication such as granulocyte colony-stimulating factor (G-CSF), granulocyte-macrophage colony-stimulating factor (GM-CSF), or any other growth factors used to stimulate white cell production that are now commonly used in a variety of oncologic or hematologic conditions? Has the patient received one of these growth factors recently?** In addition, other medications such as vasopressors and glucocorticoids can cause demargination and subsequent leukocytosis. Lithium also causes a benign reversible leukocytosis.

G. **Does the patient have a history of an underlying hematologic disorder?** Symptoms such as paresthesias, cyanosis in response to changes in ambient temperature, and easy bruising or bleeding all are suggestive of a primary bone marrow pathology.

H. **Does the patient have a history of prior abdominal trauma or surgery or, specifically, splenectomy?** The postsplenectomy state is often associated with a baseline WBC count that is above normal. In addition, after splenectomy the patient is at greater risk of developing sepsis, especially from encapsulated organisms such as *Streptococcus pneumoniae* or *Haemophilus influenzae.*

III. **Differential Diagnosis.** There are numerous causes of leukocytosis. It is a normal response to many noxious emotional and physical stimuli. *Leukocytosis* is defined as a WBC count greater than 10,000/μL. A broad division of causes separates leukocytosis into acute and chronic.

A. **Acute**
1. **Acute bacterial infection.** Either localized or generalized (sepsis).
2. **Other infections.** Mycobacteria, fungi, certain viruses, rickettsiae, or even spirochetes.
3. **Trauma**
4. **Myocardial infarction (MI), pulmonary embolism/infarction, mesenteric ischemia/infarction, or peripheral vascular disease with ischemia**
5. **Vasculitis, antigen-antibody complexes, and complement activation**
6. **Physical stimuli.** Extremes of temperature, seizure activity, and intense pain are associated with increased WBC counts.
7. **Emotional stimuli.** Occasionally can trigger acute leukocytosis.
8. **Drugs.** Can often cause or contribute to leukocytosis, especially vasopressor agents, corticosteroids, lithium, G-CSF, and GM-CSF.

B. **Chronic**
1. **Persistent infections.** Often the same infection that caused the acute leukocytosis.
2. **Partially treated or occult infections.** Osteomyelitis, subacute bacterial endocarditis (SBE), and intra-abdominal abscess can often present as chronic leukocytosis.
3. **Mycobacterial or fungal infections.** These are notorious for promoting a sustained leukocytosis, often with little other clinical pathology at initial evaluation.
4. **Chronic inflammatory states.** Rheumatic fever, connective tissue disease such as systemic lupus erythematosus (SLE), thyroiditis, myositis, drug reactions, and pancreatitis can all chronically elevate the WBC count.
5. **Neoplastic processes.** Solid tumors and lymphoproliferative disorders can have an associated chronic leukocytosis.
6. **Primary hematologic disorders.** These include myeloproliferative disorders (eg, polycythemia vera), myelodysplasia, leukemias, chronic hemolysis, and asplenic states.

7. **Congenital disorders (including Down's syndrome).** May be associated in rare cases with chronic leukocytosis.
8. **Drugs.** These are less common causes. Potential offending agents include glucocorticoids and lithium.
9. **Overproduction of ACTH or thyroxine.** May cause chronic elevation of the baseline WBC count.

IV. Database

A. Physical examination key points

1. **Vital signs.** Be especially careful to check for the presence of fever or hypothermia, which suggests infection or sepsis. Fever can also indicate a neoplastic process, infarction of various tissues, or a connective tissue disorder. (See Section I, Chapter 22, Fever, p 127). Hypotension may occur with sepsis.
2. **General.** Look for evidence of acute distress or a chronic disease state (cachexia, digital clubbing, bitemporal wasting).
3. **Lymph nodes.** Check for palpable lymph nodes and note their character. Soft and tender nodes are most consistent with an infectious etiology. Rubbery and generalized nodes are most often seen with lymphoproliferative disorders such as lymphoma. Hard, fixed, and localized nodes suggest carcinoma.
4. **Skin/mucosa.** Petechiae or ecchymoses suggest sepsis with disseminated intravascular coagulation (DIC), primary bone marrow pathology with altered platelet number or function, and/or a clotting disorder or vasculitis.
5. **Lungs.** Inspiratory rales imply pneumonitis or pneumonia. Diminished breath sounds and dullness to percussion suggest a pleural effusion or abscess. A pleural rub may accompany infectious or malignant processes or other conditions such as thromboembolism and SLE.
6. **Heart.** Tachycardia is consistent with acute stress. The presence of a new murmur, particularly with fever, is suggestive of bacterial endocarditis. Look for evidence of volume overload, sometimes triggered by infection or occasionally associated with leukemias or myeloproliferative disorders.
7. **Abdomen.** Tenderness on rebound suggests an acute abdominal process such as perforation or infarction of a viscus.
8. **Genitourinary/gynecologic exam.** Flank, pelvic, or prostate tenderness is suggestive of acute infection.
9. **Neurologic exam.** Altered mental status, confusion, seizures, and focally abnormal deep tendon reflexes all can be seen in a variety of situations associated with leukocytosis, including meningitis (infectious or neoplastic), sepsis, leukemias, lymphomas, and solid malignancies.

B. Laboratory data

1. **Blood.** *Personally reviewing the peripheral blood smear is absolutely critical.* Look for a coexisting anemia, polycythemia, or

abnormal platelet count. Leukocytosis with a "left shift," Döhle bodies, and toxic granulation suggests an acute infection, whereas a normal differential pattern implies a nonbacterial cause. A lymphocytosis points to a viral illness, lymphoma, or leukemia. An increase in monocytes is often seen with carcinoma or TB. Eosinophilia suggests connective tissue disease, possible drug reaction, or possible parasitic infection. Promyelocytes, myelocytes, or an increase in basophils is consistent with myeloproliferative disorders (leukemias most commonly), although severe infections, toxic insults, and inflammation can result in the release of early myeloid forms. (However, blasts are not seen except in leukemias.)

2. **Liver function tests.** Can be elevated in acute hepatitis, sepsis, leukemia, lymphoma, or metastatic carcinoma.
3. **Electrolytes.** Acute infection (especially pneumonia) and chronic infection involving the lung (TB} or central nervous system (tuberculous or fungal meningitis) can cause the syndrome of inappropriate antidiuretic hormone (SIADH) release, resulting in hyponatremia.
4. **Arterial blood gases.** A metabolic gap acidosis can accompany sepsis, leukemia, or solid tumors.
5. **Cultures.** Blood, urine, cerebrospinal fluid, sputum, and other cultures are vital to rule in or exclude an infectious etiology.

C. Radiologic and other studies

1. **Chest x-ray.** Check CXR for evidence of acute pneumonic process, mass lesion, or a mediastinal abnormality.
2. **CT scan.** Can be used to localize an abscess, define the extent of any suspicious masses or adenopathy, and determine the presence or extent of organomegaly.
3. **Tumor markers.** Tests like terminal deoxynucleotidal transferase (TdT), leukocyte alkaline phosphatase (LAP), and vitamin B_{12} level, as well as tests for monoclonal antibodies to carcinomas, can be quite useful. Frequently with a sustained leukocytosis, the LAP score can be one of the most useful initial lab tests to distinguish between an infectious/inflammatory etiology and a myeloproliferative disorder. The LAP score is usually elevated in infectious processes, whereas it is classically low in chronic granulocytic myelogenous leukemia (CML) and variable in the other myeloproliferative disorders. The LAP score is also elevated in polycythemia vera.
4. **Bone marrow aspiration and biopsy.** May be required to exclude a primary marrow disorder, metastatic tumor, or chronic infections. Cytogenic studies can be performed to look specifically for myelodysplasia and for myeloproliferative disorders such as leukemias or lymphomas. At times, this is the only way to differentiate between a reactive bone marrow and chronic myelogenous leukemia.

V. Plan. The etiology of the increased WBC count, of course, guides therapy. When obvious acute stress (infection, trauma, and inflammation) is not present, chronic infections, inflammation, carcinoma, or primary marrow pathology must be considered. As mentioned, strict attention to history, clinical presentation, and physical examination together with personal review of the peripheral blood smear is absolutely vital for the initial evaluation of leukocytosis. The overlooked or inappropriately treated infection can be catastrophic. For specific treatment of the various etiologies of leukocytosis, refer to any general reference.

REFERENCES

Arnold SM, Patchell R, Lowy AM et al: Paraneoplastic syndrome. In: Devita VT, Hellman S, Rosenberg SA, eds. *Cancer: Principles and Practice of Oncology.* 6th ed. Lippincott Williams & Wilkins;2001:2511.

Curnutte JT, Coates TD: Leukocytosis and leukopenia. In: Hoffman R, Benz EJ, Shattil SJ et al, eds. *Hematology: Basic Principles and Practice.* 3rd ed. Churchill Livingstone;2000:720.

Dale DC: Neutropenia and neutrophilia. In: Beutler E, Lichtman MA, Coller BS et al, eds. *William's Hematology.* 6th ed. McGraw-Hill;2001:823.

49. LEUKOPENIA

I. Problem. A 39-year-old man with a history of schizophrenia is placed on clozapine. Two months later, he returns with complaints of fever and chills. He appears toxic, and the white blood count is 1000/μL.

II. Immediate Questions

A. What is the absolute neutrophil count (ANC)? *Neutropenia* is defined as an absolute neutrophil count < 1500/L (ANC = % of segmented and banded neutrophils × total WBC count divided by 100). At ANCs < 1000/L, the risk of infection begins to increase. Neutropenia can be mild (ANC 1000–1500), moderate (ANC 500–1000), or severe (ANC < 500). This definition of neutropenia holds true for most ages and ethnic groups, with a few exceptions (see II.J.).

B. Has the patient reported any fever, gastrointestinal complaints, or viral symptoms or any other signs of infection? Several viral (infectious hepatitis, mononucleosis, HIV) and bacterial (salmonella, bacillary dysentery) illnesses and rickettsial infections have been associated with neutropenia. Neutropenic patients also are susceptible to infections that can be life-threatening if left untreated; therefore, this should be investigated by a thorough review of symptoms and physical examination.

C. What is the patient's occupation? Has the patient been exposed to any chemicals? Farmers and gardeners may be exposed to insecticides (DDT, lindane, chlordane) that can cause leukopenia. A painter, dry cleaner, or chemist may be exposed to benzene.

D. **Has the patient received any antineoplastic drugs or radiation therapy?** Myelosuppression is often an expected result of chemotherapy. Radiation is a direct myelosuppressant.

E. **What are the patient's medications?** Several commonly used drugs have been documented to cause neutropenia, including semisynthetic penicillins, phenothiazines, sulfonamides, phenytoin, cimetidine, clozapine, captopril, and ranitidine.

F. **Has the patient noted any tea-colored urine?** Paroxysmal nocturnal hemoglobinuria (PNH) and hepatitis may be associated with aplastic anemia.

G. **Does the patient have a history of alcohol abuse or any history of cirrhosis?** Ethanol is a direct myelosuppressant and can cause leukopenia. Folate deficiency, which can occur in alcoholics, may also cause leukopenia. Hypersplenism and sequestration of WBCs as well as platelets is seen with cirrhosis.

H. **Is there any psychiatric history or history of anorexia nervosa?** Several medications (eg, phenothiazines) used in the treatment of psychiatric disorders can cause leukopenia. Anorexia nervosa and starvation can cause leukopenia; however, the mechanism is unknown.

I. **Does the patient have rheumatoid arthritis?** *Felty's syndrome* is the constellation of splenomegaly, neutropenia, and rheumatoid arthritis.

J. **What is the patient's ethnic background?** African Americans and Yemenite Jews may have a normal racial variant of leukopenia.

K. **What is the patient's sexual and drug history?** Patients with high-risk sexual behavior and IV drug users are at increased risk for HIV infection, which can cause leukopenia.

L. **Has the patient experienced recurrent, cyclic fevers?** Cyclic neutropenia is a rare form of neutropenia that has fluctuations of the neutrophil count at fairly regular 3-week intervals. The only clue may be unexplained recurrent fevers every 3 weeks.

III. **Differential Diagnosis.** The causes of neutropenia can be grouped in three broad categories: (1) *bone marrow failure* (defective neutrophil production or maturation); (2) accelerated neutrophil removal; and (3) neutrophil redistribution. This classification can be useful in directing the choice of laboratory studies and management.

A. **Inadequate bone marrow production**

1. **Leukemia (acute).** About 25% of acute cases of leukemia present with pancytopenia.
2. **Myelodysplastic syndromes.** The bone marrow is normally hypercellular or normocellular, but the WBCs fail to reach the circulation.
3. **Megaloblastic syndromes.** Both vitamin B_{12} and folate deficiencies can result in neutropenia. There is increased intramedullary destruction of blood cells.

4. **Marrow infiltration**
   a. **Metastatic cancer**
   b. **Granulomatous diseases**
5. **Drugs.** Benzene, alkylating agents (melphalan), vinca alkaloids (vincristine or vinblastine), doxorubicin (Adriamycin), and antimetabolites (methotrexate).
6. **Radiation.** A direct marrow toxin.
7. **Aplastic anemia**
8. **Cyclic neutropenia**
9. **Racial or familial neutropenia**
10. **Infections.** In cases of infectious mononucleosis, 20–30% of patients have moderate neutropenia. Other viral infections (HIV, hepatitis A or B) and bacterial illnesses may have a direct myelosuppressive effect.
11. **Starvation/anorexia nervosa**
12. **Paroxysmal nocturnal hemoglobinuria (PNH)**

B. **Accelerated removal/consumption**
   1. **Drug induced**
      a. **Immune.** Such as hydralazine (Apresoline), quinidine, quinine, cefoxitin (Mefoxin), and nafcillin.
      b. **Nonimmune.** Such as phenacetin, indomethacin (Indocin), phenytoin, chloramphenicol, cimetidine, ranitidine, and phenothiazines.
   2. **Hemodialysis and cardiovascular bypass.** Exposure of blood to a dialysis coil of cellophane or nylon fiber appears to activate the complement pathway. This increases neutrophil adhesion, causing neutrophils to sequester in pulmonary capillaries.
   3. **Felty's syndrome.** Neutropenia associated with seropositive rheumatoid arthritis and splenomegaly suggests this diagnosis.
   4. **Infection.** At times, the peripheral requirements for neutrophils during overwhelming sepsis can exhaust the marrow reserves. This is particularly true in the debilitated patient, such as a patient with chronic alcohol abuse.

C. **Redistribution of neutrophils**
   1. **Enhanced neutrophil margination.** Endotoxemia in gram-negative sepsis can give rise to rapid margination of neutrophils to the tissue.
   2. **Hypersplenism.** Refers to the clinical situation in which, in the presence of splenomegaly and a relatively normal bone marrow, there is a decrease of one or more cell lines in the peripheral blood because of sequestration in the spleen.

IV. Database

A. **Physical examination key points**
   1. **Vital signs.** Fever suggests infection. Hypotension may be a sign of sepsis.
   2. **Skin.** Petechiae are consistent with Rocky Mountain spotted fever or disseminated intravascular coagulation (DIC). Rash may be

seen in connective tissue diseases, or with certain bacterial infections such as *Neisseria gonorrhoeae* or *N meningitidis.*

3. **HEENT.** Temporal wasting and oral thrush may occur in acquired immunodeficiency syndrome (AIDS). Nuchal rigidity suggests meningitis.
4. **Lymph nodes.** Lymphadenopathy can be seen in both malignant and infectious processes, including HIV infection.
5. **Lungs.** Pneumonia with overwhelming sepsis may cause or be secondary to neutropenia. Inspiratory crackles, increased tactile and vocal fremitus, and egophony suggest pneumonia.
6. **Abdomen.** Hepatosplenomegaly can be a sign of malignancy (leukemia or lymphoma), infection, or hypersplenism.
7. **Joints.** Look for classic findings of rheumatoid arthritis, such as symmetric swelling of the proximal interphalangeal (PIP) and metacarpophalangeal (MCP) joints. Rheumatoid nodules on the extensor surface of the arms near the elbows are also a classic sign.

B. **Laboratory data**

1. **Complete blood count with differential.** Presence of anemia and thrombocytopenia along with leukopenia may suggest B_{12} or folate deficiency, aplastic anemia, PNH, ethanol abuse, or leukemia. The mean corpuscular volume (MCV) will be increased with B_{12} or folate deficiency.
2. **Blood and urine cultures.** If an infectious process is suspected.
3. **Liver function test and hepatitis serologies.** If hepatitis is suspected. An elevated lactate dehydrogenase level may suggest B_{12} deficiency or lymphoma.
4. **Peripheral blood smear.** Dysplastic, degranulated neutrophils with pseudo-Pelger-Huet anomaly (a bilobed neutrophil) may suggest a myelodysplastic syndrome. Toxic granulation and Döhle bodies suggest infection. Neutrophils with five and six lobes point toward B_{12} deficiency. Blasts are consistent with leukemia.
5. **Leukocyte alkaline phosphatase (LAP) score.** Is increased in certain infectious and inflammatory diseases and polycythemia vera. In contrast, it is decreased in chronic myelogenous leukemia.
6. **Rheumatoid factor and antinuclear antibodies (ANA).** Obtain these values if collagen vascular disease is suspected.
7. **Carotene (serum).** Elevated in anorexia nervosa and decreased in starvation.
8. **Vitamin B_{12} and folate levels.** To rule out megaloblastic anemia.
9. **Sucrose water test/Ham test.** Useful in making the diagnosis of PNH. The *sucrose water test* involves mixing the patient's RBCs in an isotonic solution of sucrose dissolved in water. The *Ham test* is performed by mixing the patient's RBCs with acidified serum. Both tests promote the binding of a small amount of complement to the surface. This results in hemolysis in PNH.

C. **Radiologic and other studies**
   1. **Chest x-ray.** To rule out pneumonia if suspected.
   2. **Sinus films, dental Panorex.** As indicated when looking for source of fever in a neutropenic patient.
   3. **Lumbar puncture.** Indicated when meningitis (acute or chronic) is suspected.
   4. **Bone marrow biopsy and aspiration.** See Section III, Chapter 5, Bone Marrow Aspiration and Biopsy, p . . . . This procedure can provide critical information about granulocyte aplasia, hypoplasia or dysplasia, infiltration of marrow, cellularity, and cellular maturation. A bone marrow biopsy and aspiration can be essential in diagnosing the cause of neutropenia.

V. **Plan.** The major consequence of neutropenia is vulnerability to infection. The usual clinical manifestations of infection are often absent because of the lack of granulocytes (neutrophils). Thus, pneumonia may be present without a significant infiltrate on CXR; meningitis may occur without pleocytosis or meningeal signs; and pyelonephritis may be present without pyuria. A heightened awareness for infection is extremely important in the neutropenic patient, because an untreated infection can be fatal.

A. **Emergent management**
   1. **Evidence of infection or fever with an ANC below 500/µL.** The patient should immediately be pancultured (body fluid cultures as indicated, such as blood and urine, etc), and broad-spectrum antibiotics should be initiated. The specific pathogens found are almost always pyogenic or enteric bacteria or certain fungi. These are usually endogenous to the patient and include staphylococci from skin and gram-negative organisms from the GI tract or urinary tract. In febrile neutropenic patients who were bacteremic, one study found that 46% of the isolated organisms were gram-positive (as high as 60–70% in one reference); 42% gram-negative; and 12% polymicrobial. Antibiotics should therefore cover both gram-positive and gram-negative bacteria with one drug (a broad-spectrum semisynthetic penicillin or cephalosporin, such as ceftazidime, imipenem, cefepime, or meropenem); or two drugs—an aminoglycoside (amikacin, gentamicin, or tobramycin) plus an antipseudomonal beta-lactam (ceftazidime, piperacillin, ticarcillin, or ticarcillin plus clavulanate). An aminoglycoside may be added to a one-drug regimen, depending on how toxic the patient appears. Vancomycin should be added if the patient is at high risk (serious catheter-related infections, significant mucosal damage from chemotherapy, use of prophylactic quinolone antibiotics, septic shock or cardiovascular compromise, colonization with penicillin- or cephalosporin-resistant *Streptococcus pneumoniae* or with methicillin-resistant *Staphylococcus aureus,* and positive blood cultures for gram-positive bacteria prior to determination of antibiotic susceptibility). An antifungal agent (amphotericin B)

should be added on days 5–7 if the absolute neutrophil count remains < 500/mm^3 and the patient remains febrile despite antibiotics. Neutropenia with infection is a medical emergency requiring immediate investigation and treatment.

2. **Identify any potential drugs or chemicals that may have induced the neutropenia; discontinue them.**
3. **Always wash your hands prior to touching the patient.** The patient should avoid exposure to fresh fruits or vegetables, flowers, live plants, and persons with active infections. Avoid rectal manipulation such as with digital examination or rectal temperature.

B. **Definitive care.** After the patient has had a complete history and physical exam, the etiology of the neutropenia can usually be placed in one of the three broad categories discussed earlier (see III.). Subsequent tests can be obtained to confirm a specific diagnosis. In general, regardless of the etiology, supportive care is indicated for most of these patients (ie, antibiotics for infections and blood products for associated severe anemia or thrombocytopenia).

1. **Bone marrow failure.** For drug-induced neutropenia, remove the offending agent and give supportive care until the counts return (generally within 1–2 weeks). Now available colony-stimulating factors (CSFs) can be used for drug-induced (ie, by chemotherapy) neutropenia to speed recovery. Specific guidelines have been established by the American Society of Clinical Oncology for the use of CSFs in cancer patients receiving chemotherapy for primary and secondary prophylaxis. In general, the CSFs are used as primary prevention with chemotherapeutic regimens that are significantly myelosuppressive to help decrease the incidence of febrile neutropenia. The CSFs are started approximately 24–72 hours after completion of the chemotherapy and are given until the ANC is over 10,000 following the neutrophil nadir. For secondary use (ie, in the febrile patient with neutropenia), the CSFs may be used if the patient has clinical features of deterioration such as pneumonia, sepsis, or fungal infections. They are usually continued until ANC is over 10,000. The usual dose is 5 μg/kg/d for G-CSF (filgrastim) and 250 μg/m^2/d of GM-CSF (sargramostim). The treatment for viral etiology or myelodysplastic syndromes is generally supportive care. The use of CSFs can be considered in myelodysplastic patients if patients are experiencing neutropenic infections.
2. **Consumption.** Treat bacterial infections as indicated. Immune-mediated consumption may require steroids. Felty's syndrome generally requires no specific treatment for the neutropenia unless the patient has recurrent infections. Then, splenectomy may be required.
3. **Redistribution.** Patients with hypersplenism are generally able to immobilize the sequestered neutrophils and thus fight off infection; subsequently, they do not require any specific therapy.

REFERENCES

American Society of Clinical Oncology: Update of recommendations for the use of hematopoietic colony-stimulating factors: Evidence-based, clinical practice guidelines. J Clin Oncol 1996;14:1957.

Bodey GP, Buckley M, Sathe YS et al: Quantitative relationships between circulating leukocytes and infection in patients with acute leukemia. Ann Intern Med 1966;64:328.

Elting LS, Rubenstein EB, Rolston KV et al: Outcomes of bacteremia in patients with cancer and neutropenia: Observations from two decades of epidemiological and clinical trials. Clin Infect Dis 1997;25:247.

Hughes WT, Armstrong D, Bodey GP et al: 1997 Guidelines for the use of antimicrobial agents in neutropenic patients and unexplained fever. Clin Infect Dis 1997;25:551.

Shoenfeld Y, Alkan ML, Asaly A et al Benign familial leukopenia and neutropenia in different ethnic groups. Eur J Haematol 1988;41:273.

50. NAUSEA & VOMITING

I. **Problem.** A 39-year-old man is admitted with diffuse abdominal pain and fever. Later that evening the patient has severe nausea and vomiting.

II. **Immediate Questions.** When you are evaluating nausea and vomiting, a careful history and a complete physical exam are important to rule out serious causes requiring prompt intervention, such as peritonitis or intracranial lesions.

A. **What are the patient's vital signs?** Fever suggests an inflammatory process such as gastroenteritis, peritonitis, or cholecystitis. Hypotension may be secondary to volume depletion or associated sepsis. Hypertension and bradycardia may reflect increased intracranial pressure.

B. **When do the nausea and vomiting occur? Are they related to meals?** Vomiting during or soon after a meal suggests psychogenic causes or may be seen with pyloric channel ulcer, pancreatitis, or biliary tract disease. If abdominal pain is relieved with vomiting, an ulcer becomes more likely. Vomiting an hour or more after a meal is more characteristic of gastric outlet obstruction, pancreatitis, or motility disorders, such as diabetic gastroparesis and postvagotomy. Nausea and vomiting early in the morning on arising are often associated with alcoholism, pregnancy, uremia, and increased intracranial pressure.

C. **What are the appearance and volume of the vomitus?** Large amounts of vomitus or secretions usually indicate partial or complete bowel obstruction, gastric atony, or, in rare cases, Zollinger-Ellison syndrome. Vomiting of undigested food suggests the presence of esophageal disorders, such as achalasia or a diverticulum, as well as gastric outlet obstruction. The presence of bile indicates a patent pyloric channel. A fecal smell suggests lower intestinal obstruction. Occasionally, this can be seen with bacterial overgrowth in the proximal small intestine or a fistula. Blood or coffee-ground–appearing material points to an upper GI bleed. Vomiting can also induce hematemesis secondary to a Mallory-Weiss tear. (See Section I, Chapter 27, Hematemesis, Melena, p 158).

D. **Does the patient consume alcohol? Does the patient take any nonsteroidal anti-inflammatory drugs (NSAIDs)?** Pancreatitis or acute gastritis can be caused by ethanol and result in nausea and vomiting. A NSAID such as ibuprofen (Motrin) may induce gastritis.

E. **Is there associated abdominal pain?** This can be seen with most abdominal causes of nausea and vomiting. The location of the abdominal pain will help in deciding the etiology of the nausea and vomiting. (See Section I, Chapter 1, Abdominal Pain, p 1).

III. **Differential Diagnosis.** Disorders that are associated with nausea and vomiting and require immediate attention can be grouped as follows:

A. **Intra-abdominal or thoracic etiology**

1. **Gastric outlet obstruction.** Occurs in patients with a history of peptic ulcer disease (PUD), prior abdominal surgery, or neoplasms.
2. **Small or large bowel obstruction.** May be caused by fibrous bands and adhesions (usually after surgery), primary or secondary metastatic neoplasms, impacted feces, strictures from active inflammatory bowel disease (IBD), intestinal parasites, gallstones, incarcerated hernia, or a volvulus.
3. **Pseudo-obstruction or functional (paralytic) ileus.** Results from failure of normal intestinal peristalsis. Causes include abdominal surgery; retroperitoneal or intra-abdominal hematomas; severe infections; renal disease; metabolic disturbances such as hypokalemia; or drugs, particularly anticholinergics.
4. **Peptic ulcer disease (PUD).** Results from local irritation or edema surrounding a pyloric channel ulcer, causing a mechanical obstruction.
5. **Pancreatitis.** Usually associated with abdominal pain that frequently (in $> 50\%$ of cases) radiates to the back. A CT scan is helpful in demonstrating inflammation and pseudocyst formation. Retroperitoneal abscess formation can complicate pancreatitis.
6. **Biliary colic.** From distension of smooth muscle in bile ducts secondary to stones, inflammation, or neoplasms.
7. **Intestinal ischemia.** From local vascular compromise or from reduced cardiac output. Guaiac-positive stools are common findings.
8. **Pyelonephritis or nephrolithiasis**
9. **Hepatitis.** May be either viral or drug-induced.
10. **Appendicitis.** Often associated with right lower quadrant pain, fever, and leukocytosis with a left shift.
11. **Diverticulitis.** Lower abdominal pain and fever are common.
12. **Perforated viscus.** Usually presents as an acute abdomen.
13. **Pelvic inflammatory disease (PID)**

14. **Acute myocardial infarction (MI).** MI, especially involving the inferior wall, can present with nausea and vomiting; chest pain may be absent.

B. **Intracranial etiology**
   1. **Tumor or mass lesions leading to increased intracranial pressure.** Consider an acute cerebral vascular accident, neoplasm, or subdural hematoma.
   2. **Bacterial and viral meningitis**
   3. **Migraine headache.** Usually a unilateral headache, with photophobia and previous history of similar headache. May have prodrome (eg, aura).
   4. **Labyrinthitis**

C. **Metabolic etiology**
   1. **Uremia.** Often associated with weight loss, lethargy, and intense pruritus.
   2. **Hepatic failure.** From a variety of causes including cirrhosis, hypoxic injury, and drug-induced states such as acetaminophen overdose.
   3. **Adrenal insufficiency.** Can occur in patients on chronic corticosteroid therapy that is suddenly discontinued or in such patients when stressed (surgery, serious infection) and the steroid dose is not increased. Associated symptoms include weakness, fatigue, hypotension, and abdominal pain.
   4. **Metabolic acidosis.** See Section I, Chapter 2, Acidosis, p 9.
   5. **Electrolyte abnormalities.** Hypercalcemia, hyperkalemia, and hypokalemia can cause nausea.
   6. **Hypothyroidism with decreased intestinal motility or thyroid storm.** Weight gain, constipation, mental status changes, and dry skin suggest hypothyroidism. Weight loss, hyperdefecation, moist skin, hyperthermia, and mental status changes as well as a precipitating event are consistent with thyroid storm.

D. **Miscellaneous etiology**
   1. **Drug-induced.** Major offenders are dopamine agonists such as L-dopa and bromocriptine (Parlodel), opiate analgesics such as morphine, digoxin (Lanoxin), and certain chemotherapy agents such as cisplatin (Platinol). Also consider alcohol, NSAIDs, and aspirin.
   2. **Acute gastroenteritis.** Common in the outpatient setting with "food poisoning" from bacterial endotoxins. Diarrhea is often present. (See Section I, Chapter 17, Diarrhea, p 97).
   3. **Pregnancy.** Especially during the first trimester.

IV. Database

A. **Physical examination key points**
   1. **Vital signs.** Hypotension may result from volume depletion or sepsis. Orthostatic blood pressure changes suggest volume depletion. An orthostatic decrease in blood pressure without an in-

crease in heart rate suggests autonomic neuropathy, which may accompany diabetes with gastroparesis. Fever points to an inflammatory component, possibly infection. Tachycardia can result from associated pain.

2. **HEENT.** Look for signs of head trauma that would indicate an intracranial process. Scleral icterus suggests hepatic failure/hepatitis. Papilledema is consistent with an intracranial process or a hypertensive emergency. An enlarged thyroid gland occurs with hypothyroidism or hyperthyroidism.
3. **Skin.** Check the patient's skin turgor and mucous membranes to estimate volume status. Check for jaundice. Hyperpigmentation may be caused by adrenal insufficiency (*Addison's disease*).
4. **Chest.** Inspiratory crackles secondary to atelectasis can be associated with any intra-abdominal process limiting deep inspiration because of pain. They may also suggest left ventricular dysfunction associated with MI.
5. **Abdomen.** See Section I, Chapter 1, Abdominal Pain, p 1.
6. **Rectum.** Check for fecal impaction, rectal masses, and occult blood. Tenderness on the right side is consistent with appendicitis. Blood can be secondary to diverticulitis, IBD, PUD, and gastritis; or may result from vomiting (Mallory-Weiss tear).
7. **Female genitalia.** Helpful in diagnosing PID. A discharge is often present.
8. **Neurologic exam**
   a. Mental status changes may signify central nervous system (CNS) lesions, encephalopathy, sepsis or severe infection, or significant electrolyte disturbances.
   b. Focal neurologic findings such as weakness, unilateral hyperreflexia, or a positive Babinski on one side suggest an intracranial process.
   c. Pain with flexion of the neck is consistent with meningeal inflammation secondary to either a subarachnoid bleed or meningitis. A positive *Kernig's sign* also indicates meningeal irritation; it is obtained by flexing the patient's hip and knee to a 90-degree angle. Attempts to extend the leg at the knee will result in hamstring pain and resistance to movement.

B. Laboratory data

1. **Electrolytes.** Severe vomiting may lead to various electrolyte disturbances, such as hypokalemia, hypochloremia, and metabolic alkalosis.
2. **Complete blood count with differential.** A leukocytosis with an increase in banded neutrophils suggests an infection. An elevated hematocrit can be associated with volume depletion. Anemia suggests chronic GI blood loss or massive acute bleeding.
3. **BUN and creatinine.** To rule out renal failure.
4. **Urinalysis.** Look for white blood cells and casts suggesting pyelonephritis. Red blood cells, especially with flank pain, point to nephrolithiasis.

5. **Liver function tests, transaminases (AST and ALT), total bilirubin, and alkaline phosphatase.** To rule out acute hepatitis and biliary tract obstruction.
6. **Amylase and lipase.** If pancreatitis is suspected.
7. **Arterial blood gases.** Needed to evaluate the presence of an acid–base disturbance as a cause or consequence of vomiting. Vomiting associated with an acid–base disturbance is almost always related to a serious underlying problem.
8. **Serum intact human chorionic gonadotropin (HCG) serum.** If pregnancy is suspected.

C. **Radiologic and other studies**

1. **Acute abdominal series (KUB).** Air-fluid levels are seen in obstruction; free air under the diaphragm indicates perforation. If the patient may be pregnant, defer KUB until the result of HCG test is known.
2. **Electrocardiogram.** Helpful in evaluating for acute MI. ST segment depression or elevation, T wave inversion, or Q waves suggest myocardial ischemia or infarction. An electrocardiogram should be done early in evaluating an acute abdomen with vomiting.
3. **Abdominal ultrasound or HIDA scan.** These may aid in the diagnosis of cholecystitis, biliary duct obstruction, or abscesses. Biliary colic cannot be ruled out with a normal ultrasound. A HIDA scan is used to assess cystic duct function rather than just patency.
4. **Endoscopy.** Important in the diagnosis of PUD or esophageal diverticula.
5. **Gastric emptying scan.** Useful in suspected gastroparesis, especially in patients with long-standing diabetes who have nausea and vomiting.

V. **Plan.** Treatment of the underlying etiology is essential in the management. A nasogastric tube should be used for decompression if obstruction is present. Separate treatment of each cause is beyond the scope of this section. Commonly used medications are listed here.

A. **Phenothiazines.** Most commonly used antiemetics. Principal mode of action is via depression of CNS dopamine receptors. Prochlorperazine (Compazine) 10 mg PO Q 4–6 hr or 25 mg PR; chlorpromazine (Thorazine) 25 mg PO Q 8 hr, and promethazine (Phenergan) 12.5–25 mg PO, PR, or IM Q 6–12 hr prn are effective agents. Extrapyramidal side effects can be treated with benztropine (Cogentin) 2 mg IV or diphenhydramine (Benadryl) 25 mg IV or IM Q 4–6 hr.

B. **Butyrophenones.** These agents also block CNS dopamine receptors. Give haloperidol (Haldol) 2 mg PO or IM Q 4–6 hr; or droperidol (Inapsine) 2–5 mg IV or IM Q 4–6 hr.

C. **Miscellaneous drugs**

1. **Ondansetron (Zofran).** A selective 5-HT_3 receptor antagonist, it is very effective prophylaxis for chemotherapy-induced and postoperative nausea and vomiting. The recommended adult oral dose

is 8 mg (10 mL of oral solution) bid. 5-HT_3 receptor antagonists are not effective in treating nausea and vomiting once such symptoms occur.

2. **Metoclopramide (Reglan), high-dose.** At a dose of 1–2 mg/kg Q 4–6 hr, this constitutes a useful and very effective adjunct with cancer chemotherapy to prevent nausea and vomiting. Effective for both prevention and treatment.
3. **Benztropine 2 mg PO or IV or diphenhydramine 25–50 mg PO or IM.** Should be given prophylactically to prevent extrapyramidal reactions with high doses of metoclopramide.

REFERENCE

Makau L, Feldman M: Nausea and vomiting. In: Feldman M, Scharschmidt BF, Sleisenger MH, eds. *Gastrointestinal and Liver Diseases: Pathophysiology/Diagnosis/Management.* 6th ed. Saunders;1998:117.

51. OLIGURIA/ANURIA

I. **Problem.** You are called because a 68-year-old man admitted with pyelonephritis and diabetes mellitus Type 2 has had only 100 cc of urine output over the last 8 hours.

II. **Immediate Questions.** A medical history and review of the patient's chart and hospital course are essential in evaluating and treating oliguria.

A. **Are there any serious or life-threatening conditions?** Oliguria may be associated with shock, hypotension, pulmonary edema, uremia, hyperkalemia, uncompensated metabolic acidosis, or other electrolyte disorders.

B. **Is the patient in distress? Does the patient appear ill? Is the patient hemodynamically stable?** Oliguria may be an early manifestation of impending shock.

C. **What are the patient's latest serum chemistries and BUN and creatinine levels?** An elevated creatinine suggests different etiologies compared to a normal or only slightly elevated creatinine, especially with an elevated BUN-to-creatinine ratio.

D. **What is the etiology of the oliguria?** Prompt identification of the underlying cause(s) is essential to prevent or attenuate renal injury.

E. **What is the urine output?** *Oliguria* is defined as a 24-hour urine output between 100 and 400 mL. As a general rule, the minimal acceptable urine output is 0.5–1.0 mL/kg/hr. *Anuria,* less than 100 mL/d of urine, may indicate complete urinary obstruction, a catastrophic renal vascular event, bilateral cortical necrosis, severe rapidly progressive glomerulonephritis, or severe allergic interstitial nephritis (AIN)—as may be seen with patients taking rifampin. A urine pattern of fluctuating decreased and increased urine output may indicate intermittent obstruction.

F. **Are there any underlying diseases that could result in oliguria and/or renal failure?** Congestive heart failure (CHF), cirrhosis, nephrotic syndrome, and third spacing of fluid (eg, pancreatitis) may decrease renal perfusion. Autoimmune disorders may affect the kidneys. Infections may cause renal failure through direct extension as well as through immune mechanisms. Diabetics, the elderly, and patients with preexisting renal insufficiency are at increased risk for acute renal failure (ARF).

G. **Does the patient have any symptoms or predisposing conditions that suggest hypovolemia?** Hypovolemia is a common cause of oliguria. Early diagnosis and prompt treatment are essential. Prolonged prerenal causes of oliguria may result in ischemic acute tubular necrosis (ATN). Diarrhea, vomiting, gastrointestinal (GI) bleeding, high fever, and low oral intake are examples. Positional dizziness suggests hypovolemia.

H. **Is there any previous history of symptoms to suggest bladder outlet obstruction from prostatic hypertrophy? Has the patient recently had a Foley catheter?** A history of hesitancy, difficulty initiating voiding, and dribbling suggests prostatic hypertrophy.

I. **Has the patient been exposed to any potentially nephrotoxic agents?** Aminoglycosides, amphotericin B, radiocontrast agents, and certain chemotherapeutic agents may cause ATN. Cyclosporine, tacrolimus, angiotensin-converting enzyme inhibitors, and nonsteroidal anti-inflammatory drugs (NSAIDs) may cause renal vasoconstriction. Intratubular obstruction from deposition of crystals from acyclovir, sulfonamides, and methotrexate may occur. Several medications have been associated with AIN.

J. **Is there a history of hematuria?** Rapidly progressive glomerulonephritis may be associated with hematuria. Hematuria is a common sign of nephrolithiasis and bladder or renal cell carcinoma.

K. **Is there any history of prolonged hypotension?** This may lead to ischemic ATN.

L. **Is there any history of abdominal, suprapubic, or flank pain?** Suggests nephrolithiasis, urinary tract obstruction, infection, or a renal vascular event.

M. **During the initial assessment, do the medications, IV fluids, and dietary orders need to be adjusted?** Renally cleared medications may need to have the dose or dosing interval adjusted. Potassium may need to be removed from intravenous fluids.

N. **Are any diagnostic procedures involving radiocontrast agents planned?** Radiocontrast dye will likely add further injury to the kidneys.

III. **Differential Diagnosis.** The differential diagnosis for acute oliguria and acute renal failure is identical and may be divided into prerenal, renal, and postrenal causes.

A. **Prerenal causes. Relating to renal hypoperfusion.**
   1. **Shock/hypovolemia**
      a. **Hemorrhage.** From GI bleeding or trauma, or as a postoperative complication.
      b. **Inadequate fluid administration.** Fever, diarrhea, vomiting, poor oral intake without adequate fluid administration.
      c. **Sepsis.** Causes decreased renal perfusion from a decreased systemic vascular resistance.
   2. **Apparent intravascular hypovolemia.** A relative decrease in the effective circulating volume.
      a. **"Third-space" losses.** Pancreatitis, major burns, and after major operations.
      b. **CHF**
      c. **Cirrhosis.** Hepatorenal syndrome may be associated.
      d. **Nephrotic syndrome**
   3. **Vascular**
      a. **Renal artery occlusion (acute or chronic)**
      b. **Aortic dissection**
      c. **Emboli (such as cholesterol)**

B. **Renal causes**
   1. **Acute tubular necrosis**
      a. **Ischemia.** Secondary to shock from any cause, including sepsis.
      b. **Toxins.** These may include medications (aminoglycosides, amphotericin B), contrast media, and heavy metals.
      c. **Transfusion reaction.** Causes intravascular hemolysis.
      d. **Myoglobinuria.** Secondary to rhabdomyolysis; often seen in alcoholics. Muscle tenderness, elevated creatine phosphokinase, and pigmented casts point to myoglobinuria.
   2. **Acute interstitial nephritis**
      a. **Drugs.** Beta-lactamase–resistant penicillins (eg, methicillin); also sulfonamides, fluoroquinolones, NSAIDs, and many others.
      b. **Hypercalcemia**
      c. **Uric acid.** Tumor lysis syndrome (chemotherapy for leukemia or lymphoma).
      d. **Infections.** Staphylococcal or streptococcal infections, Legionnaires' disease, toxoplasmosis, tuberculosis, and others.
   3. **Acute glomerular disease**
      a. **Malignant hypertension**
      b. **Emboli, thrombosis, disseminated intravascular coagulation (DIC)**
      c. **Rapidly progressive glomerulonephritis**
      d. **Systemic diseases.** Wegener's granulomatosis, Goodpasture's syndrome, thrombotic thrombocytopenic purpura, systemic lupus erythematosus (SLE), scleroderma.

C. Postrenal causes

1. **Urethral obstruction.** Prostatic hypertrophy, catheter obstruction. Prostatic carcinoma is an unusual cause of postrenal obstruction.
2. **Bilateral ureteral obstruction.** Most often as a result of carcinoma or retroperitoneal fibrosis. Common cause of death in cervical carcinoma.
3. **Intratubular obstruction.** Precipitation of crystals from medications such as acyclovir, sulfonamides, and methotrexate.

IV. Database

A. Physical examination key points. The physical examination may help determine the cause and/or identify possible complications of oliguria. Also, review oral and intravenous fluid input and urine output (and drains and number of stools) and daily weights to assess volume status.

1. **Vital signs**
   a. **Temperature.** Fever points to infection (possibly sepsis) or acute AIN.
   b. **Heart rate.** An irregularly irregular pulse is consistent with atrial fibrillation, a common cause of emboli.
   c. **Blood pressure**
      i. **Hypertension.** Malignant hypertension may cause acute renal failure. Volume overload from oliguria may cause hypertension. Also long-standing hypertension can be a cause of chronic renal insufficiency.
      ii. **Orthostatic changes.** Most importantly, assess the patient for orthostatic blood pressure and pulse changes (a decrease in systolic blood pressure of 10 mm Hg or an increase in heart rate by 20 bpm 1 minute after movement from supine to standing position). Orthostatic hypotension without a change in heart rate can be found in the elderly secondary to autonomic insufficiency or in patients on beta-blockers who are volume depleted. An imbalance in intake and output (I&O) can cause volume depletion resulting in orthostatic changes in heart rate and blood pressure. Weight loss can be seen with volume depletion.
      iii. **Pulsus paradoxus.** If uremic pericarditis is suspected, pulsus paradoxus may indicate impending tamponade.
2. **Skin.** Decreased tissue turgor, dry mucous membranes, and loss of axillary sweating may occur with volume depletion. The presence of purpura may indicate thrombotic thrombocytopenic purpura. A maculopapular rash may indicate an allergic drug eruption, which may be seen with AIN. Livedo reticularis may be seen with cholesterol emboli.

3. **HEENT.** On funduscopic examination look for exudates, hemorrhages, papilledema, Roth spots, and Hollenhorst plaques (cholesterol emboli).
4. **Neck.** Flat neck veins with the patient supine suggest volume depletion. There may be an increase in jugular venous pressure secondary to volume overload from oliguria/anuria. Failure of neck vein distension with inspiration (*Kussmaul's sign*) may be seen in pericardial tamponade.
5. **Pulmonary.** Rales suggest CHF, possibly from volume overload.
6. **Cardiac.** S_3 suggests CHF; a new-onset murmur may be seen in endocarditis.
7. **Abdomen.** Look for ascites or a distended bladder. A palpable enlarged bladder suggests bladder outlet obstruction. Bruits may indicate renal artery stenosis.
8. **Genitourinary system.** Examine males for an enlarged prostate. Remember bladder outlet obstruction can occur even when the gland feels normal in size. In females, rule out a pelvic mass.
9. **Extremities.** Assess perfusion by skin color and temperature.

B. **Laboratory data.** See Section II, Table 2–7, p 386, for urinary indices used in evaluating renal failure.

1. **Urinalysis**
   a. High specific gravity suggests volume depletion or recent dye administration.
   b. Protein (large amount) or red blood cell casts suggest glomerular disease.
   c. Significant hematuria points toward renal embolization or ureteral calculi. White blood cell casts suggest pyelonephritis or severe inflammation (AIN). Eosinophils are seen with AIN; frequent granular casts are consistent with ATN. Uric acid crystals may be seen in acute uric acid nephropathy.
2. **Serum chemistries.** Compare the blood urea nitrogen (BUN) and creatinine. If their ratio is > 20:1, a prerenal cause is likely, although obstruction may also cause a high ratio, as can GI bleeding and catabolic states. If the ratio is < 15:1 and the BUN and creatinine are elevated, a renal cause is likely. Note the presence of hyponatremia or hypernatremia, hyperkalemia, and a low bicarbonate, any of which may complicate acute renal insufficiency.
3. **Urine electrolytes and creatinine.** In the face of oliguria, a urinary sodium < 20 mmol/L suggests a prerenal cause; a urinary sodium > 20 mmol/L suggests renal causes. The fractional excretion of sodium (FE_{Na}) is calculated as [urinary sodium × serum creatinine/urine creatinine × serum sodium] × 100. A $FE_{Na} < 1$ suggests volume depletion; a $FE_{Na} > 1$ suggests renal causes. Acute urinary tract obstruction and dye nephrotoxicity may also reduce the FE_{Na} to < 1.

C. **Radiologic and other studies**

1. **KUB.** Helpful in assessing for obstructing renal calculi or for emphysematous pyelonephritis with diabetes.
2. **Ultrasound.** Renal ultrasound is useful in determining renal size, the presence of stones, and the presence of hydronephrosis. Hydronephrosis may be absent in early obstruction. Bedside bladder ultrasound may be useful in detecting bladder outlet obstruction.
3. **Radionucleotide renal scans.** Technetium-labeled diethylenetriaminepentacetate (DTPA) or mercaptoacetyltriglycine nuclear medicine studies can assess renal perfusion (thrombosis, infarction, or emboli) or renal function via renogram, and through the excretory phase they can assess for obstruction. Gallium scans may be positive in AIN.
4. **Central venous pressure line or pulmonary artery catheter.** For a more accurate assessment of volume status.
5. **Retrograde pyelogram (RPG).** If obstruction is suspected, an RPG can reveal the cause and specific location of the obstruction. Additionally, ureteral stent placement at the time of the procedure can relieve the obstruction.
6. **Renal biopsy.** Useful in renal failure of unknown cause or of prolonged duration. May diagnose rapidly progressive glomerulonephritis or vasculitis, or suspected interstitial disease of unknown etiology.
7. **Renal duplex Doppler.** May be useful in detecting renal artery disease, but is operator dependent.
8. **CT scan, intravenous pyelogram (IVP), arteriography.** Radiocontrast studies are best avoided in acute oliguria unless specifically indicated. Examples include renal and inferior vena cava venography in suspected renal vein thrombosis and arteriography in suspected polyarteritis nodosa.
9. **MRI.** Is useful in the diagnosis of renal vein thrombosis and avoids radiocontrast media.
10. **Chest x-ray.** May be useful to assess for pulmonary edema and heart size.
11. **ECG.** Should be obtained in patients with hyperkalemia.
12. **Echocardiogram.** Useful to assess for suspected pericardial effusion and left ventricular function.

D. **Other diagnostic/therapeutic maneuvers**

1. **Urinary catheter.** Initially, if a urinary catheter is in place, make sure the catheter is working by irrigating with 50 mL sterile normal saline (NS), using a catheter-tip syringe. The fluid should pass easily and the entire amount should be aspirated. (See Section I, Chapter 24, Foley Catheter Problems, p 141). If there is not a urinary catheter in place and obstruction is suspected, an in-and-out bladder catheterization should be performed. If a large postvoid

residual is obtained, the catheter should be left in place. If a patient has very little urinary output, an indwelling catheter should be avoided due to the risk of infection.

2. **Volume challenge.** It is appropriate in most cases of oliguria to administer a volume challenge of 500 cc of NS without potassium given over 30 minutes. With a fragile cardiorespiratory status or in the elderly, smaller boluses should be given and central venous catheters used to monitor volume status. Then adjust the IV rate accordingly.
3. **Diuretics.** The use of diuretics in an attempt to convert an oliguric ARF to a nonoliguric ARF has been advocated. It should be emphasized that a decrease in urine output should not automatically trigger a trial of diuretics. The patient's volume status needs to be carefully assessed and diuretics need to be avoided if the patient is volume-depleted. Indiscriminate use of diuretics may lead to further volume depletion and exacerbation of renal failure.

E. **Loop diuretics.** High doses of loop diuretics may be required to initiate a diuretic response with an intrinsic renal disease. One must be cautious of the adverse extrarenal effects of loop diuretics, such as ototoxicity. Large doses of bumetanide may be associated with severe myalgias. To help avoid such adverse effects, large doses of diuretic should be infused over approximately 30–60 minutes. Initial doses of furosemide (40–80 mg), bumetanide (1–2 mg), or torsemide (20–50 mg) can be tried. If urine output does not increase within 1 hour, the doses can be progressively doubled until maximal doses are achieved (furosemide 360–400 mg, bumetanide 8–10 mg, or torsemide 200 mg). If a diuresis is established, loop diuretics may be administered as needed. Volume status should be monitored carefully to avoid volume depletion. An alternative strategy is to administer a bolus of loop diuretic followed by a continuous infusion that may be titrated according to need. (For example, a bolus of 80–160 mg of furosemide can be followed by 20 mg/hr titrating up by 10 mg/hr every hour as needed to a maximum of 80 mg/hr; or a bolus of 1–2 mg of bumetanide can be followed by an infusion of 0.5 mg/hr titrating up by 0.5 mg/hr to a maximal dose of 2 mg/hr.)

F. **Thiazide diuretics.** May be used synergistically with loop diuretics. Metolazone 5–10 mg PO may be tried. An alternative is IV chlorothiazide 500 mg infused over 30 minutes.

G. **Mannitol.** May be used to help establish a diuresis in cases of rhabdomyolysis, hemolytic transfusion reactions, acute uric acid nephropathy, contrast-induced oliguria, and other toxic nephropathies. A dose of 12.5–25 g (50–100 mL of a 25% solution) IV may induce an osmotic diuresis. May cause hyponatremia or hypernatremia, hypokalemia, or volume overload.

H. Dopamine. Early in the course of ATN, dopamine in renal doses (0.5–3 µg/kg/min) used in conjunction with loop diuretics may increase urine output if loop diuretics alone failed. There is no evidence that dopamine alters the natural history of ATN.

V. Plan

A. Management of specific causes of oliguria/ARF

1. Prerenal

a. Monitor volume replacement. Give crystalloid to increase central venous pressure above 10 mm Hg or pulmonary capillary wedge pressure above 12–14 mm Hg. A hematocrit > 25–30% is adequate.

b. Follow hourly urine output. Give specific criteria, such as have the house officer called if urine output is < 0.5 mL/kg/hr. Remove potassium and magnesium from IV solutions. If hypokalemia or hypomagnesemia is present, replace judiciously, preferably by the oral route.

2. Postrenal

a. Bladder outlet obstruction. Manage acutely with a Foley catheter. There are several concerns with this therapy, including acute bladder decompression, postobstructive diuresis, and increased risk of infection. Rapid bladder decompression has been a concern in the past because of possibly triggering a vasovagal episode or bladder hemorrhage. However, studies have demonstrated that large changes in bladder pressure occur with the first 100–250 cc of urine output. Thus intermittent clamping of the catheter is probably unnecessary.

b. Postobstructive diuresis. Occasionally relief of obstruction is followed by a brisk diuresis. This is thought to be the result of volume overload and is physiologic. Volume depletion and electrolyte disturbances may occur. The usual therapy is IV maintenance fluids such as ½ normal saline or 0.45% NaCl at 75 mL/hr. Replacement of urine output with IV fluids milliliter per milliliter should be avoided.

c. Risk of infection. Intermittent, instead of continuous, bladder catheterization should be considered to reduce infection risk.

d. Ureteral obstruction. Ureteral obstruction requires urologic consultation. The consultation is emergent if an infection is suspected in the obstructed kidney (*pyonephrosis*).

3. Renal causes. Therapy of renal causes should be directed at the specific etiology. The most common cause of intrinsic renal failure in hospitalized patients is ATN.

A. Management of ATN. The therapy of ATN is supportive care (see V.B.1–4).

B. Management of oliguria/ARF. General measures include the following:

1. **Fluid management.** Fluid management needs to be individualized. In general, IV fluids should not contain potassium. Accurate records of fluid intake and output are essential. Serum electrolytes need to be followed carefully. If the patient has a metabolic acidosis with pH < 7.10, sodium bicarbonate should be added. Excessive hypotonic fluids may lead to hyponatremia.
2. **Nutrition.** Patients with ARF need a diet restricted in potassium, sodium, protein, and total fluids.
3. **Medications.** Review the patient's medications and stop all nephrotoxic drugs. Doses of renally excreted drugs should be adjusted.
4. **Hemodialysis or peritoneal dialysis.** Should be considered in the following circumstances: severe hypervolemia unresponsive to diuretics, intractable acidosis, severe hyperkalemia, pericarditis thought secondary to uremia, and severe uremic symptoms or encephalopathy.

REFERENCES

Cadnapaphornchai P, Alavalapti RK, McDonald FD: Differential diagnosis of acute renal failure. In: Jacobson HR, Striker GE, Klahr S, eds. *The Principles and Practice of Nephrology.* 2nd ed. Mosby;1995:555.

Klahr S, Miller SB: Current concepts: Acute oliguria. N Engl J Med 1998;338:671.

Post TW, Rose BD: Approach to the patient with renal disease including acute renal failure. In: Fletcher SW, Fletcher RH, Aronson MD, editors-in-chief. UpToDate [CD-ROM]. Version 8.2. Wellesley, MA;2000. www.uptodate.com

Rose BD: Optimal dosage of loop diuretics. In: Fletcher SW, Fletcher RH, Aronson MD, editors-in-chief. UpToDate [CD-ROM]. Version 8.2. Wellesley, MA;2000. www.uptodate.com.

Rose BD: Rate of decompression of an enlarged bladder. In: Fletcher SW, Fletcher RH, Aronson MD, editors-in-chief. UpToDate [CD-ROM]. Version 8.2. Wellesley, MA;2000. www.uptodate.com.

Rose BD: Urine output in urinary tract obstruction and postobstructive diuresis. In: Fletcher SW, Fletcher RH, Aronson MD, editors-in-chief. UpToDate [CD-ROM]. Version 8.2. Wellesley, MA;2000. www.uptodate.com

Thadhani R, Pascual M, Bonventre JV: Acute renal failure. N Engl J Med 1996;334:1448.

Toto RD: Approach to the patient with acute renal failure. In: Greenberg A, ed. *Primer on Kidney Diseases.* 2nd ed. Academic Press;1998:253.

52. OVERDOSES

I. **Problem.** You are called to the emergency room to evaluate a 38-year-old woman who was found unconscious by her husband, with an empty pill bottle lying on the floor near her.

II. **Immediate Questions**

A. **Is the patient conscious? What are the vital signs?** Assessing the patient's hemodynamic and respiratory status is the first priority in managing overdoses. Many overdose patients will require ventilatory and/or blood pressure support. Unconscious patients need to have rapid assessment of blood glucose and immediate treatment with thiamine. Naloxone should be considered with respiratory depression even before opiate toxicity is confirmed. Only in instances where the health care team is at risk of exposure—such as in certain cases of inhalation overdose or in cases of topical organophosphate exposure—should other interventions come first.

B. What is the agent responsible for the overdose? Although supportive measures are the primary concern in overdose management, discovering the causative agent can help predict possible toxicity and direct further care. A detailed history and physical exam should provide the clues necessary to answer this question. In cases where the patient is unreliable or has an altered mental status, an exhaustive investigation is necessary. Question the patient's family and friends, thoroughly search the patient's belongings and the site of the overdose, and contact the patient's physician or pharmacy to determine possible medications ingested. All packaging of medication or chemical ingested should be obtained and pill counts made. Remember that with intentional overdoses the likelihood is high that more than one substance was taken.

III. Differential Diagnosis. The possible causes of acute overdoses are numerous. One method of simplifying the classification of overdoses is to group toxins by their effects. Six toxic syndromes encompass most of the common agents causing overdoses. A small group of additional agents do not fit any of the categories and are considered separately. Remember, even though causes of overdoses are grouped by common effects, there are characteristics and toxicities unique to individual agents even within the same group.

A. Anticholinergic agents. The anticholinergics cause delirium, choreoathetosis, hypertension, tachypnea, tachycardia, and hyperthermia. Other characteristic signs include dry mouth, reduced bowel sounds, flushing of skin, dilated pupils, and urinary retention. Examples: tricyclic antidepressants (also commonly cause arrhythmias), antihistamines, phenothiazines, cyclobenzaprine, and belladonna alkaloids.

B. Sympathomimetic agents. These toxins cause hyperalert and delusional mental states. Hyperthermia, hypertension, tachypnea, and tachycardia are common. Other signs include tremor, dilated pupils, diaphoresis, hyperreflexia, and, on occasion, seizures. Examples: cocaine, amphetamines, methamphetamines, pseudoephedrine, and theophylline.

C. Sedatives/hypnotics/opiates. These agents cause CNS depression and, in extreme cases, coma. Vital signs show hypothermia, bradycardia, bradypnea, and hypotension. Reflexes are depressed and noncardiogenic pulmonary edema is common. Examples: opiates (morphine, oxycodone, heroin), benzodiazepines (diazepam, lorazepam, oxazepam, alprazolam), barbiturates and alcohols (ethanol, isopropyl alcohol, ethylene glycol).

D. Cholinergic agents. The mnemonic **SLUDGE** describes the symptoms of cholinergic overdose. **S**alivation, **S**weating, **L**acrimation, **U**rination, **D**iarrhea, **G**I hypermotility and cramping, and **E**mesis are the common findings. Confusion, coma, and seizures can also occur. Pupils are constricted, bradycardia is present, and the respiratory rate and blood pressure can be elevated or decreased. Examples: organophosphates, insecticides, and nicotine.

E. Serotonin agents. These chemicals cause hyperthermia, confusion, and agitation. Neuromuscular findings include hyperreflexia, myoclonus, and ataxia. Diaphoresis, shivering, and dilated pupils are also seen. Vital signs show hypertension, tachycardia, and tachypnea. Examples: serotonin reuptake inhibitors (SSRIs) (a type of antidepressant), including citalopram, fluoxetine, paroxetine, and sertraline, and dextromethorphan.

F. Hallucinogens. These agents cause hallucination, agitation, perceptual distortion, and paranoia. Pupils are usually dilated and nystagmus is common. Vital signs are all elevated. Examples: D-lysergic acid (LSD), phencyclidine (PCP), mescaline, and "designer" amphetamines.

G. Other agents. The following causes do not fit any specific classification.

1. **Acetaminophen.** The patient can initially be asymptomatic. Anorexia, nausea, emesis, diaphoresis, and lethargy are common. Primarily hepatotoxic.
2. **Salicylates.** Cause vertigo, nausea, emesis, noncardiac pulmonary edema, and acid–base disturbances (most commonly a combined metabolic gap acidosis and respiratory alkalosis).
3. **Insulin/oral hypoglycemics.** Cause hypoglycemia (see Section I, Chapter 37, Hypoglycemia, p 202). In the case of oral agents this can be long lasting.
4. **Carbon monoxide (CO).** Headache, nausea, confusion, dyspnea, syncope, and coma can occur. Suspect in cold weather, often from faulty heating or improper ventilation for exhaust from car or some other machine or heating device.
5. **Heavy metals.** Iron, mercury, lead.
6. **Digoxin.** Causes nausea, emesis, fatigue, yellow-green halos; and ventricular arrhythmias, atrioventricular block, and junctional tachycardia.
7. **Antihypertensives.** Beta-blockers, calcium channel blockers.
8. **Lithium.** Causes tremor, fasciculation, ataxia, sluggishness, nausea, emesis, and hypotension.

H. New drugs of abuse. Recently the following drugs have become popular and need to be considered in cases of overdose. They are predominantly used by adolescents and young adults and are associated with "raves."

1. **Ecstasy (3,4-methylenedioxymethamphetamine, or MDMA).** Increases serotonin, dopamine, and norepinephrine release in the CNS and prevents reuptake. Causes diaphoresis, mydriasis, tachycardia, hypertension, hallucinations, delirium, muscle spasms and rigidity, arrhythmias, and in severe cases can lead to death.

Shares many similar features to serotonin syndromes and sympathomimetic syndromes.

2. **Gamma hydroxybutyrate (GHB).** Increases dopaminergic activity in the CNS. Causes drowsiness, confusion, aggressive behavior, incontinence, ataxia, tremors, and seizures in some cases. Also can lead to bradycardia, respiratory depression, hypothermia, nausea, and vomiting. Gamma-butyrolactone (GBL) and 1,4-butanediol (1,4-BD) are GHB prodrugs that are converted after ingestion to GHB. They are found in several health and fitness products.
3. **Ketamine.** A PCP derivative that causes agitation, nystagmus, mydriasis, hallucinations, hypertonicity, delirium, and a floating sensation. It can cause seizures, tachycardia, hypertension, and palpitations.

IV. Database

A. Physical examination key points

1. **Vital signs.** Often the vital signs can be used to help determine the etiology of the overdose (eg, sinus tachycardia is commonly seen in tricyclic antidepressant overdoses, whereas bradycardia is seen with beta-blocker or cholinergic overdoses). Temperature should be checked because hyperthermia (cocaine) and hypothermia (alcohol) are common. For accuracy, respirations should be counted rather than estimated.
2. **Skin.** The entire body surface should be examined. Examination should include investigation for bruising or other trauma, pressure sores, and track marks suggesting injection drug usage. Flushing and erythema suggest an anticholinergic or CO overdose. Even though the cherry–red appearance of the skin and mucous membranes is classic for CO overdoses, cyanosis is more common. Pale diaphoretic skin is seen in overdoses of sympathomimetics and hallucinogens. Desquamation is found in heavy metal poisonings. Cyanosis suggests hypoxia.
3. **HEENT.** Look for evidence of head trauma, which can be concurrent with an overdose. A cervical collar should be applied if there is a question of trauma. Pupil size should be recorded accurately and may be one more clue in determining the cause of the overdose. Constricted pupils are seen with opiate, clonidine, and organophosphate overdoses, whereas dilated pupils are seen with cocaine, amphetamine, LSD, antihistamine, and tricyclic antidepressant overdoses. The oropharynx should also be evaluated to determine moistness of the mucous membranes, which can differentiate between cholinergic and anticholinergic poisonings, and for injection marks under the tongue, a sign of IV drug abuse. Breath odors can also provide useful information. Alcohols cause a fruity breath odor; salicylates, an odor similar to wintergreen; and arsenic or organophosphates, the smell of garlic.

4. **Lungs.** Look for evidence of aspiration, a common complication. Also check for pulmonary edema (a complication of overdoses with hydrocarbons, antihypertensives, heavy metals, and inhalants).
5. **Cardiovascular.** Look for peripheral and central cyanosis.
6. **Abdomen.** The abdomen should be auscultated for bowel sounds, which can be decreased or increased depending on the cause of the overdose. Look for organomegaly. Check for melena or hematochezia.
7. **Neurologic exam.** Assessment of the patient's mental status can provide invaluable evidence in determining the cause of the overdose. A depressed mental state suggests overdose with a sedative or alcohol. An agitated state would be more consistent with sympathomimetic agents and hallucinogens. A routine neurologic exam should be done to evaluate for trauma or intracranial injury. With mental status changes, the gag reflex should be assessed and if it is depressed or absent, intubation may be indicated.
8. **Musculoskeletal.** Lithium and sympathomimetics cause tremor and fasciculations. Alcohols, neuroleptics, and CO cause rigidity. Heavy metals can cause weakness. Tricyclic antidepressants and antiepileptics cause choreoathetotic movements.

B. Laboratory data

1. **Serum and urine drug screens.** Although these tests are commonly ordered and can be useful, it is important to remember the following: (1) they often take several hours to complete, which decreases their usefulness; (2) they test for only a limited number of agents, and even a positive result does not confirm that the discovered agent caused the symptoms; and (3) urine screens may be falsely negative if obtained too early. Although recommended for overdoses of unknown etiology, these tests need not be ordered when the causative agent can be determined by history and examination or in overdoses of minor severity.
2. **Tests for specific agents.** Tests for common causes of overdoses such as acetaminophen; salicylate; alcohols; iron, lead, and other metals; lithium; and digoxin can be easily obtained. They should be used any time overdose with the agent in question is suspected by history and physical examination. Tests for acetaminophen, salicylate, and alcohols are recommended in instances where the causative agent is unknown or in suicide attempts where ingestion of multiple substances is suspected.
3. **Glucose.** All overdose patients, especially those with altered mental status, should have serum glucose tested by finger-stick so that hypoglycemia can be discovered early and treated.
4. **Serum creatine kinase (CK) and urine myoglobin.** To rule out suspected rhabdomyolysis.
5. **Arterial blood gases.** Useful with respiratory compromise and inhalation exposure, and in cases where an acid–base disturbance is suspected.

6. **Serum electrolytes, liver function tests, blood urea nitrogen, and serum creatinine.** Mandatory in severe overdoses. In less severe cases, order based on suspected toxicity of a particular agent or on clinical judgment. The anion gap can be helpful in alcohol and salicylate overdoses where acid–base disturbances are common.
7. **Serum osmolarity.** The osmol gap can be helpful in diagnosing overdose with alcohols such as ethylene glycol and methanol.

C. **Radiologic and other studies**

1. **ECG.** An ECG can be helpful in managing an overdose patient. It is mandatory in evaluating an overdose of a drug known to affect the heart (tricyclic antidepressants, antihypertensives, and digoxin). Look for arrhythmias or prolonged QT, QRS, or PR intervals. A QRS interval > 0.10 seconds places the tricyclic antidepressant overdose patient at risk for arrhythmias and seizures.
2. **Chest x-ray.** To look for evidence of aspiration, acute respiratory distress syndrome, or noncardiogenic pulmonary edema.
3. **Abdominal x-ray.** Helpful with ingestions where the toxin is radiopaque. Examples of such substances include: **C**hlorinated hydrocarbons, **C**alcium salts, **C**rack vials, **H**eavy metals, **I**odinated compounds such as thyroxin, **P**sychotropics, **P**ackets of drugs, **E**nteric-coated tablets such as aspirin, **S**alicylates, **S**odium salts, and **S**ustained-release tablets. The mnemonic **CHIPES** may be useful. Abdominal films should also be done anytime intestinal obstruction is suspected.
4. **Head CT scan.** If there are mental status changes and the etiology is unclear, especially in cases where there is evidence of trauma along with a suspected overdose.
5. **Cervical x-rays.** With suspected neck trauma to rule out cervical fracture.

V. **Plan.** There are four components in the treatment of overdose: stabilization and support, decontamination, antidotes, and enhanced elimination. In unconscious patients, consider immediate assessment of blood glucose and treatment with dextrose 50%, 50 mL IV if hypoglycemic. Also, give thiamine 100 mg IV since the mental status changes associated with Wernicke's encephalopathy include coma and in an unconscious patient it is impossible to assess for ataxia or ophthalmoplegia. Furthermore, naloxone 0.4–2.0 mg should be administered, especially if respiratory rate is depressed, even before opiate toxicity is confirmed.

A. **Stabilization and support**

1. **ABCs (airway, breathing, and circulation).** Should be addressed first.
2. **Intubation.** See Section III, Chapter 7, Endotracheal Intubation, p 407. Intubation should be performed when hypoxia, hypercapnia, or respiratory distress is not easily reversible. It should also be done in any instance where there is airway compromise or risk of aspiration. Some patients with altered mental status and agitation may need to be sedated and intubated to prevent hyperthermia and rhabdomyolysis.

3. **Hypotension.** See Section I, Chapter 42, Hypotension (Shock), V, p 227. This should initially be managed with fluid resuscitation. Always use an isotonic fluid solution such as NS or LR. If no response to IV fluids, use vasopressor agents.
4. **Hypertension.** See Section I, Chapter 35, Hypertension, V, p 197. Agitated patients should be treated initially with sedatives such as lorazepam. If medication is necessary, nitroprusside or labetalol can be used. With hypertension from sympathomimetic drugs, beta-blockers should not be used.
5. **Arrhythmias.** See Section I, Chapter 9, Cardiopulmonary Arrest, V, p 46, Chapter 60, Tachycardia, V, p 329, and Chapter 8, Bradycardia, V, p 42. Ventricular arrhythmias with adequate blood pressure should be treated with lidocaine except in tricyclic antidepressant overdose, where $NaHCO_3$ should be used first. Atropine can be used for severe bradycardia; however, transcutaneous or transvenous pacing may be needed. In instances of torsades de pointes or ventricular tachycardia secondary to a prolonged QT interval, overdrive pacing should be considered. Magnesium can be used for polymorphic ventricular tachycardia, especially torsades de pointes.
6. **Monitoring.** Overdoses causing potential respiratory or hemodynamic compromise or cardiac arrhythmias such as tricyclic antidepressant overdose require intensive care monitoring. Patients with altered mental status also have better outcomes if monitored closely. Pulse oximetry should be used with respiratory compromise. Suicidal patients must be continuously observed.

B. Decontamination. Decontamination should be performed as rapidly as possible since the best outcomes have been associated with early treatment. The purpose of decontamination is to prevent further absorption of the toxic agent. The method of decontamination is determined by the type of exposure.

1. **Ingestion.** Methods of decontamination include induction of emesis, gastric lavage, activated charcoal, whole bowel irrigation, and surgical or endoscopic removal of the toxin. Best results are obtained if these are performed in the first hour after ingestion. Activated charcoal has been shown to be the most effective method, and is recommended in all cases of overdose ingestion except where contraindicated. The appropriate dose is 1 g/kg given orally or by NG tube. Doses of activated charcoal should be repeated as indicated for the specific substance ingested. Often water or sorbitol is given in conjunction with the activated charcoal. Activated charcoal binds ingested drugs, preventing absorption. Contraindications to use include bowel obstruction, ingestion of hydrocarbons, ingestion of acidic or alkali corrosives, ingestion of substances that do not bind to charcoal (such as lithium and metals such as iron), and any instances where aspiration is a risk. Charcoal can be given to patients with aspiration risk after intubation. In special cases consider other methods of decontamination, such as whole bowel irrigation or endoscopic removal of the toxin.

2. **Ocular.** Decontamination of eye exposures starts with saline irrigation for at least 15–20 minutes. Surface particulate matter can be removed with a cotton swab. Imbedded material should be removed by an ophthalmologist. Alkali corneal burns require immediate attention by an ophthalmologist.
3. **Topical.** Aggressive saline or water irrigation of the exposed area for at least 15 minutes is the best immediate method to prevent dermal absorption of toxic chemicals. Remove all contaminated clothing, and protect personnel from exposure. Exposure to several chemicals requires special treatment.

C. **Antidotes.** Many agents that are commonly associated with overdoses have antidotes that can prevent toxic injury or mortality. Listed below are commonly overdosed substances and the antidotes available. Antidotes should be used when the cause of the overdose is known and the possible toxicity is determined to be severe enough that the benefits of therapy outweigh the risks of the antidote. If you are unsure of how to manage an overdose or ingestion of a specific toxin, the local poison-control hotline can be extremely helpful.

1. **Opiates.** Naloxone 0.4–2.0 mg IV, IM, or SC. The diagnosis should be questioned if there is no response after repeated doses to a total dose of 10 mg.
2. **Tricyclic antidepressants.** Bicarbonate 1–2 mEq/kg IV push, then a sodium bicarbonate drip (two or three 50-cc ampoules of $NaHCO_3$ [50 mEq] added to 1 L of D5W) at 150–200 cc/hr. Follow the arterial pH and serum bicarbonate. Alkalinization reverses the cardiac conduction abnormalities.
3. **Benzodiazepines.** Flumazenil 0.2 mg, followed by increasing doses every minute until effect is seen, generally to a total dose of 3 mg. Duration of reversal is dependent on the benzodiazepine dose, the half-life of the drug taken, and the flumazenil dose. Administration of flumazenil to patients receiving a benzodiazepine for seizure control may precipitate seizures. Rapid access to a benzodiazepine (eg, IV lorazepam) is recommended. CNS effects of benzodiazepines may be reversed; however, respiratory support still may be required. Flumazenil is not recommended for use in multiple-drug overdoses. The drug may reverse the CNS effects of benzodiazepines, but it may precipitate seizures, arrhythmias, and withdrawal symptoms in patients who also ingested a tricyclic antidepressant. ECG findings suggesting a tricyclic antidepressant overdose are a relative contraindication to the use of flumazenil.
4. **Calcium channel blockers.** Calcium chloride 1 g IV over 5 minutes and repeated every 10–20 minutes for 3–4 additional doses. Glucagon can also be used (5–10 mg hourly) following a bolus of 50–150 mcg/kg.
5. **Beta-blockers.** Glucagon, 50–150 mcg/kg, then 5–10 mg hourly. Atropine 0.5–1 mg and repeated every 3–5 minutes up to 0.04 mg/kg may be used.
6. **Anticholinergics.** Physostigmine 1–2 mg IV over 5 minutes.

7. **Methanol and ethylene glycol.** Ethanol 10%, 10 mL/kg load, then 0.15 mL/kg/hr. The goal is a serum ethanol concentration of 100–120 mg/dL. Double this rate during dialysis. In ethylene glycol overdose, pyridoxine 100 mg IV and thiamine 100 mg should be given daily. An alternative therapy to ethanol is fomepizole (4-methylpyrazole), 15 mg/kg IV loading dose, followed by 10 mg/kg every 12 hours for 4 doses, then 15 mg/kg every 12 hours until levels fall to target range.
8. **Organophosphates and carbamates.** Atropine 2–5 mg IV, may repeat every 10–30 minutes to maintain full atropinization, noted by dried secretions and clearing of rales. Pralidoxime may be necessary.
9. **Digoxin.** Digoxin-specific antibody. Dose is based on digoxin level.
10. **Acetaminophen.** *N*-acetylcysteine (Mucomyst), 140 mg/kg initially, then 70 mg/kg/d every 4 hr for a total of 17 doses. Activated charcoal should be used initially; treatment with Mucomyst is based on acetaminophen blood levels. Serum blood levels should be drawn at least 4 hours after ingestion and the blood level plotted against time since ingestion. Using a standard acetaminophen toxicity nomogram, the risk for hepatotoxicity is classified as probable, possible, or no risk.
11. **Iron.** Deferoxamine 15 mg/kg/hr IV, total daily dose usually up to 6 g.
12. **Lead.** EDTA 50–75 mg/kg/d by deep IM injection or slow IV infusion in 3–6 divided doses for up to 5 days. Treatment course may be repeated.

D. Enhanced elimination

1. **Alkalinization of urine and forced diuresis.** Useful for renally excreted chemicals, especially weakly acidic substances. Examples include salicylates and phenobarbital. The goal is to infuse enough fluid and bicarbonate to increase urine output to > 3 mL/kg/hr and urine pH > 7.5.
2. **Hemodialysis.** Useful for clearing methanol, ethylene glycol, salicylates, lithium, and theophylline.
3. **Hemofiltration.** Useful in clearing aminoglycosides, vancomycin, and metal chelate complexes.

REFERENCES

Brent J, McMartin K, Phillips S et al: Fomepizole for the treatment of methanol poisoning. N Engl J Med 2001;344:424.

Burns M, Schwartzstein R: General approach to drug intoxications. In: Fletcher SW, Fletcher RH, Aronson MD, editors-in-chief. UpToDate [CD-ROM]. Version 8.2. Wellesley, MA;2000. www.uptodate.com

Ellenhorn MI, Schonwald S, Ordog G et al, eds: *Ellenhorn's Medical Toxicology.* 2nd ed. Williams & Wilkins;1997.

Graeme K: New drugs of abuse. Emerg Med Clin North Am 2000;18:625.

Kulig K: Initial management of ingestions of toxic substances. N Engl J Med 1992;326:1677.

Rosen P, editor-in-chief: *Emergency Medicine Concepts and Clinical Practice.* 4th ed. Mosby-Year Book;1998.

Toll LL, Hurlbut KM, eds: POISINDEX System. Englewood, CO: MICROMEDEX, Inc.;2001.

53. PACEMAKER TROUBLESHOOTING

I. Problem. A 44-year-old man was admitted to the CCU for an acute myocardial infarction (MI) complicated by third-degree heart block, and a pacemaker was inserted. The CCU nurse calls later to report seeing pacemaker spikes but no capture.

II. Immediate Questions

A. What is the patient's condition and what are his or her vital signs? Bradycardia with hypotension warrants immediate attention, as does the development of symptoms of hypoperfusion (confusion, pre-syncope or syncope, chest pain, and dyspnea).

B. What were the circumstances surrounding pacemaker insertion? Prophylactic insertion of a temporary pacemaker wire in the setting of an acute MI and Mobitz type II second-degree heart block carries a different set of implications than the development of third-degree heart block and hypotension. The latter situation may rapidly deteriorate to cardiac arrest, whereas the former may require no intervention other than close observation.

III. Differential Diagnosis. Most problems encountered with pacemakers are generally classified into one of two categories: failure to capture a pacing impulse, or failure to sense a cardiac depolarization. Temporary pacemaker output is programmed to be inhibited by cardiac depolarization.

A. Failure to capture. *Failure to capture* occurs when the temporary intravenous (or transcutaneous) pacemaker generates an impulse (as evidenced by a narrow, vertical pacemaker "spike"), but there is no evidence of ventricular depolarization. Keep in mind that a transvenous pacing wire placed appropriately in the apex of the right ventricle should produce a wide complex depolarization immediately after the pacemaker spike. A 12-lead ECG will reveal a superior axis (~ –90°) with a left bundle branch block morphology. See Figure 1–4 for an example of failure to capture. Failure to capture represents one of the most common problems encountered in temporary transvenous pacing.

1. Problems intrinsic to the pacemaker

a. Malposition of the catheter resulting in loss of contact between the catheter tip and the endocardium. This can occur when the patient is repositioned in bed. Malposition will result in raising the pacing threshold, and thus failure to capture.

b. Inappropriate lead placement

c. Inappropriate generator settings. Be sure that the heart rate and output settings have not been changed.

d. Malfunction of the generator. This is an uncommon reason; however, generators run on alkaline batteries, which sometimes fail. Be sure to check the generator battery regularly.

e. Fractured pacing electrode

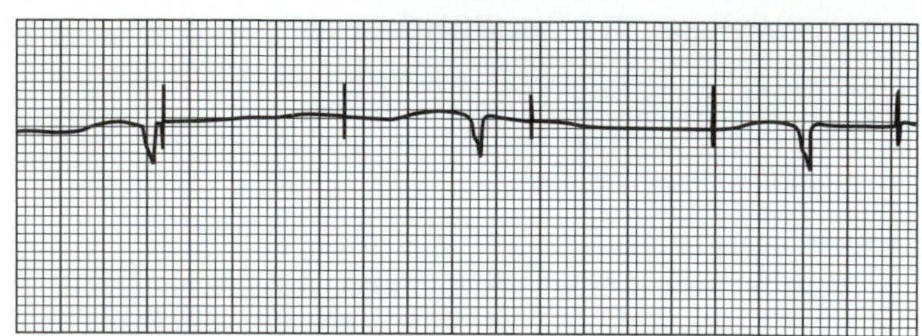

Figure 1–4. Failure to capture. The rhythm is a nodal rhythm at 40 beats per minute. The pacemaker spikes occur at 72 beats per minute. The pacemaker spikes are not associated with the ventricular depolarizations.

   f. **Poor connection between the electrodes and the generator**
2. **Local factors**
   a. **Profound hypoxemia**
   b. **Severe acidemia**
   c. **Marked hyperkalemia**
   d. **Fibrosis at the electrode**
   e. **Myocardial infarction** that includes the right ventricular apex
   f. **Myocardial edema at the catheter tip**
   g. **Drugs.** Type IIC antiarrhythmic agents (eg, flecainide, encainide) can raise the myocardial threshold for depolarization.

B. **Failure to sense.** *Failure to sense* occurs when the pacemaker fails to recognize a native depolarization and subsequently generates a pacemaker spike without being inhibited by the native depolarization. See Figure 1–5 for an example of failure to sense. Often, this inappropriate pacemaker spike will fall somewhere between the QRS complex and the T wave of the native depolarization, and a ventricu-

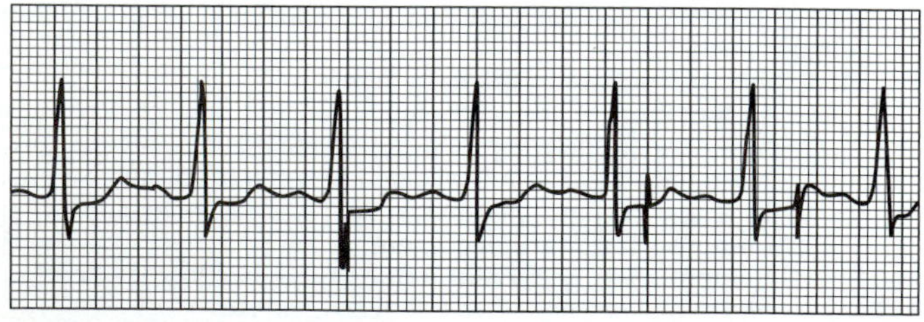

Figure 1–5. Failure to sense. A pacemaker spike is seen immediately after the 3rd, 4th, 5th, and 6th QRS complexes. The pacemaker should have been inhibited by the QRS complexes. (Photograph courtesy of Alberto Mazzoleni, MD.)

lar depolarization will *not* follow this pacemaker spike. This is because the pacemaker spike is occurring during the refractory period of the ventricle (the native depolarization was not sensed by the pacemaker). Failure to sense should not be interpreted as failure to capture, even though failure to capture often accompanies failure to sense, especially when the problem results from pacing electrode displacement and poor endocardial contact. In essence, the same circumstances that cause failure to capture can also cause failure to sense. If the timing of the pacemaker spike is on the T wave, sustained ventricular tachycardia can occur.

C. Other complications of transvenous pacemakers

1. **Oversensing of P waves and T waves**
2. **Myocardial perforation** with pericardial effusion and tamponade (rare)
3. **Ventricular ectopy**
4. **Tricuspid valve dysfunction**
5. **Line sepsis**
6. **Venous thrombosis**

IV. Database

A. Physical examination key points

1. **Vital signs.** Heart rate and blood pressure are essential to determine the need for immediate intervention.
2. **Cardiopulmonary examination.** An elevated jugular venous pressure, inspiratory rales at the bases, and an S_3 indicate congestive heart failure (CHF), possibly secondary to hypoperfusion. An elevated jugular venous pressure, new pericardial friction rub, and loss of a palpable apical impulse could indicate a pericardial effusion from myocardial perforation by the pacemaker wire.
3. **Neurologic exam.** A change in mental status or confusion may indicate hypoperfusion.

B. Laboratory data

1. **Portable chest x-ray.** To check placement of the catheter tip. Helpful if catheter displacement or myocardial perforation is a concern. In addition, comparison to post-insertion chest x-rays can be useful. Unfortunately, the most relevant information is obtained from the lateral projection, which often is not obtained after insertion and is often not feasible to obtain at the time of malfunction.
2. **Electrocardiogram and rhythm strip.** To rule out MI as a cause of the problem and to rule out myocardial ischemia as another indicator of hypoperfusion. Clues as to the current location of the catheter can be obtained from the surface ECG. For instance, a pacemaker in the right ventricular apex will result in a QRS configuration with a left bundle branch morphology. If a right bundle branch morphology is present, the clinician should suspect inter-

ventricular septum rupture and subsequent pacing from the left ventricle.

3. **Arterial blood gases.** To rule out acidemia or hypoxemia as a cause.
4. **Electrolytes.** To rule out hyperkalemia as a cause of the pacemaker's failure to sense or capture.

V. Plan

A. Electrode placement. If there has been any decline in the patient's condition or significant change in vital signs, ask the nurse to place anterior and posterior transcutaneous pacing electrodes in preparation for possible use until the transvenous pacing wire problem can be resolved. In addition, have the "crash cart" readily available in case of cardiopulmonary arrest.

B. Obtain back-up. There are few problems in internal medicine more anxiety-provoking than a dysfunctional pacemaker in a pacemaker-dependent patient. If a senior resident or cardiology fellow supervises you in the CCU, give him or her a call.

C. Inspect the generator and connections to the pacing wire. Care must be taken to avoid "short-circuiting" the system. Be sure you are wearing rubber gloves. Empiric replacement of a new generator "box" is generally preferred over attempts to replace batteries. In addition, replace the generator if something appears to be wrong with it. The pacing wire can be tested for electrode fracture by connecting the distal cathode to the V lead on the ECG machine, and then connecting the proximal anode to the V lead. If an ECG can be recorded from each electrode, the pacing wire has not fractured. When you cannot see a pacemaker spike, the problem usually lies with either the generator or the pacing wire. Pacemaker spikes are more easily seen with unipolar pacing (eg, the proximal anode is usually a subcutaneous wire). Also, a unipolar pacing configuration is more sensitive than a bipolar pacing configuration. Thus, changing from a bipolar to a unipolar configuration may help to restore both capture and sensing.

D. Adjust the pacemaker settings. Check the settings to be certain that the output, heart rate, and sensitivity settings are appropriate.

1. **Check the pacing threshold of the electrode.** First raise the pacing rate on the generator to a level at which the patient's rhythm is completely paced. Second, turn down the pacing output until pace beats no longer appear. This is the pacemaker's pacing threshold. Acceptable threshold values are usually < 2 mAmps. ***Caution:*** Be sure to raise the pacing output back to its original setting before leaving the patient's bedside.
2. **For failure to capture:** Increase the output until capture reappears. A high pacing threshold may be related to electrode displacement or other problems as listed above.

3. **For failure to sense:** Increase the sensitivity until it reliably detects and is inhibited by cardiac depolarization.

E. **Consider repositioning the catheter** if adjusting the pacemaker settings does not solve the problem. Pacemaker wires can be advanced and repositioned blindly by following the configuration of the ECG tracing recorded from the endocardium. *This should be done only by someone experienced in this technique.* It is much safer to use fluoroscopy, if available, or to rely temporarily on transcutaneous pacing until someone skilled in pacemaker insertion arrives. Many hospitals have fluoroscopy either available in a CCU procedure room or have portable fluoroscopy on a "C-arm." If either is available, repositioning of transvenous pacing electrodes under fluoroscopic visualization is advised.

REFERENCES

Emergency cardiac pacing. In: Cummins RO, ed. *Textbook of Advanced Cardiac Life Support.* American Heart Association;1994:5.

Narula OS: Clinical concepts of spontaneous and induced atrioventricular block. In: Mandel WJ, ed. *Cardiac Arrhythmias: Their Mechanisms, Diagnosis and Management.* Lippincott;1995:441.

Watanabe Y, Dreifus LS, Mazyalev T: Atrioventricular block: Basic concepts. In: Mandel WJ, ed. *Cardiac Arrhythmias: Their Mechanisms, Diagnosis and Management.* Lippincott;1995:417.

Wood M: Temporary cardiac pacing. In: Ellenbogen KA, Kay GN, Wilkoff BL, eds. *Clinical Cardiac Pacing.* Saunders;1995:687.

Wood M, Ellenbogen KA: Temporary cardiac pacing. In: Ellenbogen KA, ed. *Cardiac Pacing.* 2nd ed. Blackwell Science;1996:168.

54. PAIN MANAGEMENT

I. **Problem.** A 72-year-old man admitted for metastatic prostate cancer cannot sleep because of persistent back pain.

II. **Immediate Questions**

A. **Has the patient experienced this pain before?** The initial response is to assume that the pain results from metastatic disease; however, if the pain is of recent onset the patient will require a full evaluation to rule out other causes. For example, the pain may be from herpes zoster, acute pyelonephritis, renal colic, abdominal aortic aneurysm, or an epidural abscess.

B. **Is the patient currently receiving pain medication, and if so, what is the drug, dosage, and dosing interval?** If the patient has previously received narcotics, the pain may represent development of tolerance and therefore an inadequate dose of medication. Similarly, physicians frequently prescribe an inappropriately long interval between doses of narcotics.

III. **Differential Diagnosis.** The following discussion pertains chiefly to the management of pain in terminally ill cancer patients. The management of *chronic pain* (pain that has lasted longer than 3 months) is not discussed here. Pain in a patient with cancer may be caused by the malignancy itself, may occur as a complication of treatment, or may result from a psychological disorder.

A. Pain caused directly by tumors

1. **Tumor invasion of bone and pathologic fracture**
2. **Infiltration/compression of nerves**
3. **Obstruction of a hollow viscus**
4. **Expansion of a viscus or its capsule.** For example, liver metastases.
5. **Tissue ischemia after tumor invasion of lymphatics and blood vessels**
6. **Paraneoplastic syndromes.** Hypertrophic osteoarthropathy and neuropathy.

B. Iatrogenic causes of cancer pain

1. **Surgery.** Incisions; phantom limb pain.
2. **Chemotherapy.** May cause a variety of infectious, gastrointestinal, and neurologic causes of pain.
3. **Radiation.** Colitis, esophagitis.

C. Psychological pain. Anxiety, depression, and a feeling of loss of control are frequently associated with malignancy and may intensify the patient's perception of pain.

IV. Database

A. Physical examination key points

1. **Vital signs.** Tachycardia occurs with a variety of causes of acute pain and therefore is too nonspecific to suggest a specific etiology. Fever suggests an infectious etiology or acute venous thrombosis.
2. **Skin.** Chemotherapy and hematologic malignancies can predispose to herpes zoster infections; therefore, ascertain if the pain is in the distribution of a specific dermatome. Look for vesicles on an erythematous base that would suggest shingles. Pain may precede the development of the typical vesicular rash by 2–3 days.
3. **HEENT.** Papilledema would suggest increased intracranial pressure from cerebral metastases.
4. **Neck.** Nuchal rigidity could indicate infectious or carcinomatous meningitis causing back or neck pain.
5. **Chest.** In addition to auscultating the lungs for evidence of pneumonia, palpate the ribs and sternum for evidence of bone pain suggesting metastases.
6. **Abdomen.** In a patient with abdominal pain, examine for hepatomegaly, which could indicate liver metastases. Bowel obstruction could result from the underlying malignant process itself, or could occur as a result of decreased bowel motility from the administration of narcotics. A pulsatile epigastric mass would suggest an abdominal aortic aneurysm.

7. **Extremities.** Examine for evidence of bone pain, arthropathy, or deep venous thrombosis, which may occur with underlying malignancy.
8. **Neurologic exam.** In a patient complaining of headache, perform a careful neurologic exam looking for localizing findings that could indicate the presence of cerebral metastases. Stocking-glove distribution of pain may result from a peripheral neuropathy caused by underlying cancer or chemotherapeutic agents such as vincristine.

B. **Laboratory data**
   1. **Complete blood count.** Obtain if infection is suspected.
   2. **Alkaline phosphatase and serum calcium.** Order if bone metastases are suspected. Remember to correct the total calcium in the face of hypoalbuminemia or check an ionized calcium. See Section I, Chapter 36, Hypocalcemia, p 198.

3. **Alkaline phosphatase, γ-glutamyl transpeptidase (GGT), and transaminases (AST and ALT).** Obtain liver function tests if hepatic metastases are suspected.

C. **Radiologic and other studies.** Specific radiographs should be directed by findings from history and physical examination. Keep in mind that bone scintigraphy is more sensitive for bony metastases than plain films. Bone scintigraphy may be falsely negative if there is bone destruction without accompanying osteoblastic response, such as in multiple myeloma.

V. **Plan.** The following discussion pertains to the management of pain in a patient with malignancy, but the principles of pain management apply to patients with pain from other medical conditions as well. Fear of uncontrolled pain is one of the greatest concerns of a patient with malignancy. The physician should reassure the patient that every effort will be made to alleviate their pain. A frequent mistake made by physicians is reluctance to administer narcotics in a dosage sufficient to control pain for fear of subsequent addiction. This is an unfounded fear in treating patients with acute pain, especially those patients with pain related to malignancy. The great majority will *not* develop addiction or psychological dependence. Physical dependence and tolerance may occur after prolonged administration of narcotics. After the initial history and physical examination, and exclusion of potentially reversible causes of pain, the management of presumed cancer pain can proceed.

A. **Mild pain.** Non-narcotic analgesics may be tried initially.
   1. **Aspirin.** 650 mg PO Q 4 hr.
   2. **Acetaminophen (Tylenol).** Give 650–1000 mg PO Q 4 hr (up to a maximum of 4 g/d). Doses of 4 g/d can be toxic with liver disease or with a history of alcohol abuse.
   3. **Nonsteroidal anti-inflammatory drugs (NSAIDs)** such as ibuprofen (Motrin) 600 mg PO Q 6 hr or 800 mg PO Q 8 hr. Use cautiously

in patients with underlying renal insufficiency, congestive heart failure, or peptic ulcer disease. May be particularly effective as an adjunct with narcotics for pain from bone metastases.

B. **Moderate pain.** For patients whose pain persists despite the preceding measures, a weak narcotic-analgesic may be administered. Usually, these are administered in combination with either acetaminophen or aspirin, because the analgesic effect is greatly heightened by adding these agents.
   1. **Tylenol #3.** Acetaminophen 300 mg with codeine phosphate 30 mg PO Q 4 hr.
   2. **Percodan.** Aspirin 325 mg with oxycodone 5 mg PO Q 4 hr.
   3. **Percocet.** Acetaminophen 325 mg with oxycodone 5 mg PO Q 4 hr.

C. **Severe pain.** Although a variety of drugs may be used for more severe pain, morphine sulfate still remains the gold standard for management. It is important to emphasize that narcotics should be administered on a round-the-clock basis rather than on an as-needed basis. This provides a more sustained effect, reduces the overall narcotic requirement, and lessens overall patient suffering, since the goal is to circumvent the development of pain rather than to allow the patient to feel pain first and then request narcotics. Avoid the intramuscular route of administration because erratic absorption can occur, dose titration may be difficult, and onset of action may be delayed. Addition of a stool softener is essential to avoid constipation.
   1. **Morphine sulfate.** Oral dosing is the most convenient and least expensive means of administration. A reasonable starting dose for a patient not previously on narcotics would be 20 mg PO Q 4 hr. For patients previously taking a narcotic medication other than morphine, a narcotic conversion table could be used to estimate an appropriate starting dose. After initial titration with the immediate-release form of morphine, a longer-acting preparation such as MS Contin may be administered on an every-8-hour schedule. This preparation comes in 30- and 60-mg tablets. For patients unable to take morphine PO, consider use of transdermal fentanyl (Duragesic transdermal patch).
   2. **Demerol.** The use of this agent is discouraged in the management of acute pain because of its short half-life, requiring every-3-hour dosing. Use of Demerol may also result in accumulation of toxic metabolites that can cause CNS agitation and confusion, especially with renal insufficiency. Also, avoid use of this agent in patients taking monoamine oxidase inhibitors (can cause encephalopathy and death). Meperidine use should be limited to brief courses in otherwise healthy patients with prior adverse reactions to morphine.

D. **Adjunctive measures.** Most cancer patients (85–90%) obtain relief with one of the preceding regimens. For those with persistent pain, a variety of measures can be used.

1. **Spinal analgesia (epidural opioids)**
2. **Patient-controlled IV analgesia (PCA).** Allows patients to maintain control of their pain management. Intravenous opioids remain the standard of care for severe acute pain and should be used in patients in severe pain or unable to tolerate oral medication. A typical regimen provides loading doses of 3–5 mg of morphine sulfate every 5 minutes until pain is improved, then supplemental on-demand doses of 1 mg every 6 minutes can be provided. A basal continuous infusion of 0.5–1.0 mg/hr can be provided for nocturnal pain control.
3. **Corticosteroids.** Effective for neurologic compression syndromes due to tumor infiltration.
4. **Antidepressants.** Amitriptyline (Elavil) has some analgesic effect, especially for neuropathic pain. Depression can lower the pain threshold; therefore, do not ignore the importance of addressing the cognitive and emotional aspects of terminal malignancy.
5. **Anticonvulsants.** Both gabapentin and carbamazepine may be effective for neuropathic pain.

REFERENCES

Abramowicz M, ed: Drugs for pain. Med Lett Drugs Ther 2000;42:73.

Acute Pain Management Guideline Panel: *Acute Pain Management: Operative or Medical Procedures and Trauma.* Clinical Practice Guideline No. 1. US Dept of Health and Human Services, Public Health Service, Agency for Health Care Policy and Research;1992.

Ducharne J: Acute pain and pain control: State of the art. Ann Emerg Med 2000;35:592.

Martin JJ, Moore GP: Pearls, pitfalls, and updates for pain management. Emerg Med Clin North Am 1997;15:399.

55. POLYCYTHEMIA

I. **Problem.** A 65-year-old man is admitted because of chest pain; his hematocrit is 62%.

II. **Immediate Question. Are there any medical conditions that require the prompt institution of therapy directed at the elevated hematocrit?** Usually the finding of an elevated hematocrit is incidental, or it is discovered during the evaluation of a nonacute problem. You should determine that there is no evidence of decompensated congestive heart failure (CHF) and cardiac or cerebral ischemia that might benefit acutely from phlebotomy. Evidence of profound intravascular volume depletion requiring fluid replacement should be noted.

III. **Differential Diagnosis.** When you are confronted with an elevated hematocrit (> 50% for men, > 45% for women), you can simplify the differential diagnosis by separating polycythemia into three broad diagnostic categories.

A. **Relative polycythemia.** This condition is generally asymptomatic. Patients can, however, present with venous thrombosis, which can occur with severe volume depletion.

B. **Polycythemia vera.** Onset is usually insidious, often found on routine blood counts for other reasons. Polycythemia vera may present with major venous thrombosis or hemorrhage. Symptoms may include headache, dizziness, vertigo, tinnitus, diplopia, blurred vision, claudication, angina, symptoms of peptic ulcer disease (PUD), pruritus, mucosal bleeding, epistaxis, ecchymoses, symptoms of deep venous thrombosis, pulmonary embolism, or symptoms of cerebral vascular thrombosis. Polycythemia vera is usually a disease of middle and later years of life with a peak incidence in the sixth and seventh decades. There is a slight male predominance.

1. **The diagnosis is made by meeting three major criteria; or the first two major criteria and two minor criteria.**
   a. **Major criteria**
      - **Elevated red blood cell mass** (≥ 36 mL/kg in a male; ≥ 32 mL/kg in a female)
      - **Arterial oxygen saturation > than 92%**
      - **Splenomegaly**

   b. **Minor criteria**
      - **Platelet count > 400,000/mL**
      - **Elevated leukocyte alkaline phosphatase (LAP) score**
      - **Elevated vitamin B_{12}**
      - **Leukocytosis > 12,000/mL**

C. **Secondary polycythemia.** Classified by whether the polycythemia is physiologically appropriate (response to tissue hypoxia) or physiologically inappropriate (inappropriate stimulation or secretion of erythropoietin).

1. **Physiologically appropriate polycythemia**
   a. **High-altitude acclimatization**
   b. **Chronic obstructive pulmonary disease (COPD).** Caused by a pO_2 below 90% saturation. May occur as a result of desaturation at night or with exercise.
   c. **Cardiovascular disease (right-to-left shunts).** Most commonly as a result of congenital heart disease.
   d. **Alveolar hypoventilation.** Sleep apnea.
   e. **High-oxygen-affinity hemoglobins.** The patient may have a positive family history for this condition.
   f. **Congenital deficiency of 2,3-diphosphoglyceric acid**
   g. **Carboxyhemoglobinemia**
2. **Physiologically inappropriate polycythemia**
   a. **Renal vascular disease**
   b. **Hepatic tumors**
   c. **Uterine leiomyomas**
   d. **Cerebellar hemangioblastomas**

e. **Renal transplantation**
f. **Renal cell carcinoma**
g. **Ovarian carcinoma**
h. **Renal cysts.** Flank pain or hematuria may be present.
i. **Pheochromocytoma**

IV. Database

A. Physical examination key points

1. **Vital signs.** Hypertension is indicative of possible renal vascular disease or pheochromocytoma and may be present with polycythemia vera. Respiratory rate helps to assess presence of cardiac or pulmonary disease. Fever may indicate underlying systemic illness that may have caused volume depletion or be a sign of underlying malignancy.
2. **General appearance.** Plethora is not helpful in the distinction of polycythemia vera from secondary polycythemia. Clubbing should be noted as a sign of underlying pulmonary or cardiac disease. Cyanosis is usually an indicator of hypoxemia and might be more suggestive of a secondary polycythemia.
3. **HEENT.** Look for conjunctival injection and, on funduscopic exam, hemorrhages and engorged vessels. Congested mucous membranes are often present and are nonspecific. All these symptoms would be more in favor of polycythemia vera or secondary polycythemia.
4. **Heart.** The presence of any murmurs or an S_3 might either suggest a cardiac etiology or be a sign of cardiac dysfunction caused by polycythemia.
5. **Lungs.** Rales, barrel chest, or diminished breath sounds suggest COPD.
6. **Abdomen.** Hepatomegaly and abdominal masses suggest a secondary cause, whereas splenomegaly is one of the major criteria for diagnosing polycythemia vera.
7. **Extremities.** Clubbing, cyanosis, and edema point to secondary physiologically appropriate causes. Evidence of deep vein thrombosis may be a complication of polycythemia.
8. **Neurologic exam.** Look for evidence of focal findings consistent with cerebrovascular accident or tumor. Global findings consistent with hypoxic encephalopathy suggest a secondary cause of polycythemia.

B. Laboratory data.

If there are obvious clues from the history and/or physical exam, an extensive lab evaluation may not be indicated. For example, a patient with a history of vomiting and diarrhea, poor oral intake, and marked orthostasis and tachycardia with a hematocrit of 55% would be appropriately treated with fluid resuscitation and evaluation of the etiology of the volume loss. Unfortunately, the diagnosis is often not obvious and further evaluation is indicated.

1. **Hematocrit.** Generally, a hematocrit > 60% predicts a true increase in the RBC mass; hematocrits < 60% may result from either true or relative increases in the RBC mass.
2. **Platelet count.** A count > 400,000/μL suggests polycythemia vera.
3. **WBC count.** Leukocytosis > 12,000/μL suggests polycythemia vera.
4. **Arterial blood gases.** Oxygen saturation < 90% points to a physiologically appropriate secondary cause.
5. **LAP score.** An elevated LAP score is consistent with polycythemia vera.
6. **Vitamin B_{12}.** Elevated B_{12} or unbound B_{12} binding capacity is seen with polycythemia vera.
7. **p50 (Oxygen affinity of hemoglobin).** This test evaluates the presence of abnormal hemoglobins with high oxygen affinity.
8. **Carboxyhemoglobin level.** The presence of an elevated carboxyhemoglobin level points to a physiologically appropriate secondary cause.
9. **Erythropoietin level.** This value will be elevated with physiologically inappropriate causes (eg, hepatoma) as well as with physiologically appropriate causes.

C. Radiologic and other studies

1. **RBC mass.** A nuclear medicine study to distinguish between relative and true polycythemia. A normal RBC mass with a diminished or low normal plasma volume is characteristic of relative polycythemia. If this is found, no further evaluation of the elevated hematocrit is needed. An elevated RBC mass with a normal or increased plasma volume is found in true polycythemia. If this is the case, then further evaluation is indicated to determine if this represents a primary (polycythemia vera) or secondary polycythemia.
2. **Abdominal and pelvic CT scan.** To look for evidence of benign or malignant neoplasms of the liver, kidney, adrenals, and endometrium. Also look for splenomegaly.
3. **CT scan or MRI scan of the brain.** To rule out cerebellar tumor.
4. **Echocardiogram.** Look for right-to-left shunts. May also show left ventricular dysfunction, a possible complication of polycythemia.
5. **Pulmonary function studies.** May reveal severe obstructive lung disease.

V. Plan. Treatment depends on the type of polycythemia.

A. Relative polycythemia. This condition requires no therapeutic intervention directed specifically at reduction of the hematocrit, although the underlying disorder needs to be addressed (eg, volume depletion; or the impact of stress-related disorders such as obesity, hypertension, and nicotine addiction). Isovolemic phlebotomy can be used but has not been shown to affect morbidity or mortality.

B. True polycythemia of secondary cause

1. In physiologically appropriate secondary polycythemia, it may be difficult to determine if symptoms are due to the underlying dis-

ease or the elevated hematocrit. Remember that the elevated hematocrit is a physiologically important compensatory mechanism; you must prove that the erythrocytosis is detrimental prior to phlebotomy. In physiologically inappropriate polycythemia, therapy should be directed at the underlying cause.

2. **Therapeutic phlebotomy** is performed in physiologically appropriate polycythemia if the patient is clearly symptomatic from the elevated hematocrit. If phlebotomy is indicated, the goal should be to maintain the hematocrit between 50–60%. In patients with physiologically inappropriate polycythemia, phlebotomy is reasonable and can be done safely. The goal should be to maintain a hematocrit of 45%, especially if surgery is contemplated.
3. **Cytotoxic therapy** is contraindicated in any type of secondary polycythemia.

C. **Polycythemia vera.** Therapy is directed at overproduction of RBCs and frequently accompanying platelet disorders.

1. **Phlebotomy.** This procedure is quite effective in lowering the hematocrit. It is essentially free of complications as long as the patient is monitored for signs of hypovolemia during the phlebotomy and treated appropriately with crystalloid infusion should hypotension occur; or the volume should be replaced prophylactically if there is risk that a brief period of hypotension would be detrimental. An expected long-term complication with frequent phlebotomy is iron deficiency. It has been debated whether or not iron repletion should be undertaken in this setting, as this will increase the phlebotomy requirements. At least two reasons are commonly cited for iron replacement therapy.
   a. As RBCs become progressively more microcytic, there is an actual increase in the whole blood viscosity, which is the reason for doing therapeutic phlebotomy in the first place.
   b. There is a need for iron as a cofactor in many enzyme systems; the effects of iron depletion at this level are uncertain.
2. **Cytotoxic therapy.** In patients with a history of thrombotic or bleeding problems, phlebotomy may be inadequate therapy. These patients benefit from therapy with chemotherapeutic agents or radioactive phosphorus injections.
   a. **Hydroxyurea** has been shown to be effective, appearing to have minimal, if any, risk of induction of leukemia.
   b. **Alkylating agents** have been associated with an increased risk of secondary leukemias, especially in younger patients.
   c. **^{32}P** is also associated with an increased risk of secondary leukemias.
3. **Antiplatelet agents** such as aspirin and dipyridamole (Persantine) are inadequate therapy for polycythemia vera. However, patients with thrombocytosis unresponsive to hydroxyurea may benefit from either interferon or anagrelide (a platelet-aggregating agent).

4. **Recommendations for therapy by the Polycythemia Vera Study Group:**
   a. Most newly diagnosed patients should undergo phlebotomy to obtain symptomatic control of polycythemia. The rate and volume of phlebotomy are dictated by the patient's clinical condition. The goal is to reduce the hematocrit to the upper normal range (45%).
   b. The therapy chosen to manage disease long term should be influenced by the patient's age, whether or not there is a history of thrombosis and/or severe thrombocytosis. Patients younger than 50 years without thrombosis or severe thrombocytosis may be managed by phlebotomy alone. The risk of thrombosis increases with age; therefore, patients between 50 and 70 years of age may be managed with phlebotomy alone or with myelosuppressive therapy. Those older than 70 years and those with a history of thrombosis or severe thrombocytosis should receive myelosuppressive therapy. Hydroxyurea is the current myelosuppressive drug of choice.
   c. **Patients with other symptoms** such as pruritus, bone pain, and troublesome splenomegaly are best managed by a myelosuppressive agent.

REFERENCES

Berk PD et al: Therapeutic recommendations in polycythemia vera based on Polycythemia Vera Study Group Protocol. Semin Hematol 1986;23:132.

Gruppo Italiano Studio Policitemia: Polycythemia vera: The natural history of 1213 patients followed for 20 years. Ann Intern Med 1995;123:656.

Means RT: Polycythemia vera. In: Lee GR, Foerster J, Lukens F et al, eds. *Wintrobe's Clinical Hematology.* 10th ed. Lippincott Williams & Wilkins;1999:2374.

56. PRURITUS

I. **Problem.** A 25-year-old man is admitted for lethargy and a hematocrit of 21%. He also complains of severe generalized itching (*pruritus*).

II. **Immediate Questions**

A. **Is there an associated rash or other skin lesions?** In determining the etiology of pruritus, this is the initial question many experts use in helping establish a differential diagnosis. See III., Differential Diagnosis.

B. **Is the pruritus localized or generalized?** This is a very helpful question in determining the etiology.
   1. **Scalp.** Atopic dermatitis, folliculitis, pediculosis (*Pediculus capitis*), psoriasis, and seborrheic dermatitis.
   2. **Hands and arms.** Atopic dermatitis, contact dermatitis, dermatitis herpetiformis, eczema, and scabies (*Sarcoptes scabiei*).
   3. **Trunk.** Contact dermatitis, pediculosis (*Pediculus corporis*), pityriasis rosea, scabies, seborrheic dermatitis, tinea corporis, and urticaria.

4. **Groin.** *Candida albicans,* contact dermatitis, erythrasma, lichen planus, pediculosis (*Phthirus pubis*), scabies (*Sarcoptes scabiei*), and tinea cruris.
5. **Anus.** Contact dermatitis, *Enterobius vermicularis, Trichuris trichiura, Neisseria gonorrhoeae,* hemorrhoids, psoriasis, and tinea cruris.
6. **Legs.** Atopic dermatitis, dermatitis herpetiformis, eczema, lichen simplex, stasis dermatitis.
7. **Feet.** Contact dermatitis, erythrasma, and tinea pedis. An erythematous vesicular rash with intense pruritus may be seen at the point of entry of hookworm (*Necator americanus*).

C. **What is the duration of the symptoms?** A recent and sudden onset of pruritus is more often related to an exact cause such as a new medication or new laundry soap.

D. **Has the patient been exposed to any new medications, foods, clothing, detergents, or soaps?** These are common causes of pruritus in both the hospital and the ambulatory care setting.

E. **Are there any other symptoms?** Although uncommon, itching can be the first symptom of an anaphylactic reaction. See Section I, Chapter 4, Anaphylactic Reaction, p 24. You should inquire about dyspnea, swelling in and around the mouth, and wheezing. Dyspnea may point toward systemic mastocytosis or Löffler's syndrome (cough, fever as well as dyspnea, eosinophilia, and transient pulmonary infiltrates) associated with *Ascaris lumbricoides, N americanus,* and *Strongyloides stercoralis* infestation. Gastrointestinal symptoms may point to a parasitic infection, carcinoid, or systemic mastocytosis.

F. **Is there any history of any chronic medical conditions?** AIDS, uremia, cholestatic liver disease, hypothyroidism, hyperthyroidism, hyperparathyroidism, polycythemia vera, and multiple sclerosis are but a few of the chronic medical conditions associated with pruritus.

G. **Is there a history of travel or residence in the southeastern United States or an area endemic for parasitic infection?** Many parasitic infections may present with pruritus or have pruritus in addition to other symptoms such as diarrhea or weight loss or in addition to causing obstruction (intestinal and biliary), anemia, or malnutrition.

III. **Differential Diagnosis.** Clearly, most cases of pruritus seen in hospitalized patients are related to contact dermatitis or medications. One must rule out life-threatening conditions first, such as an anaphylactic reaction (see Section I, Chapter 4, Anaphylactic Reaction, p 24). Also, one must consider other causes of pruritus, including the causes associated with systemic medical conditions and skin disorders.

A. **Skin disorders.** Pruritus associated with visible skin lesions and conditions.

1. **Papulosquamous diseases.** Such as carcinoid, dermatomyositis, erythrasma (*Corynebacterium minutissimum*), fungal infections (tinea cruris, tinea corporis, tinea pedis, *C albicans*), lichen planus and lichen simplex, lymphoma (cutaneous T-cell), pityriasis rosea, psoriasis, parasitic infections (*A lumbricoides, N americanus, S stercoralis,* and *Trichinella*), seborrheic dermatitis. Carcinoid has associated flushing (especially the upper body) and wheals with central clearing.
2. **Bullous diseases.** Including bullous pemphigoid, dermatitis herpetiformis, pemphigus.
3. **Eczematous diseases.** Atopic dermatitis, contact dermatitis, eczema.
4. **Urticaria.** Can be from a variety of agents, heat or cold, local irritation such as insect bites, or as a systemic reaction to foods, intestinal parasites (including *Giardia lamblia*), systemic mastocytosis, or cancer.
5. **Allergic reactions**
   a. **Contact dermatitis.** Most often caused by soaps, detergents, adhesive tapes, antibacterial ointments (especially neomycin), or some other foreign material.
   b. **Urticaria.** In the hospital, often due to medications, such as analgesics, including narcotics (oral and epidural); antibiotics (penicillin and sulfonamides); aspirin; intravenous contrast; and thiazide diuretics. If a patient is allergic to aspirin, other nonsteroidal anti-inflammatory drugs (NSAIDs) may cause urticaria, and aspirin will likely exacerbate chronic urticaria.
6. **Infestation.** Pediculosis (lice) caused by *Pediculus capitis* (head louse), *P corporis* (body louse), and *Phthirus pubis* (pubic louse); scabies caused by *S scabiei.*
7. **Folliculitis.** *Pseudomonas aeruginosa* may cause "hot tub folliculitis," resulting in erythematous papules. "Hot tub folliculitis" also may be caused by *Staphylococcus aureus* often involving the scalp or extremities. Also *Pityrosporum* folliculitis presents with dome-shaped follicular papules and pustules.
8. **Fiberglass dermatitis.** Intense itching with macules and papules. Contact with fiberglass products such as insulation is likely.
9. **Xerosis (dry skin).** More common in the elderly and worse in the winter, colder climates, and dry humidity. Aggravated by hot water and multiple baths each day.
10. **Neurotic excoriations.** Seen in depression or obsessive-compulsive disorder.

B. **Systemic pruritus.** Can be caused by a variety of systemic conditions without an associated rash.
   1. **Liver disease.** Secondary to bile salts.
      a. **Primary biliary cirrhosis.** Often the earliest symptom is pruritus. Usually seen in middle-aged women.

   b. **Cholestasis of pregnancy.** Usually seen in the third trimester; pruritus is often the initial symptom. Fatigue is an accompanying symptom.
   c. **Biliary obstruction**
   d. **Hepatitis**
2. **Uremia.** Seen in many patients with chronic renal failure who receive hemodialysis; may be secondary to associated hyperparathyroidism.
3. **Metabolic.** Associated with hypothyroidism, hyperthyroidism, diabetes mellitus, hyperparathyroidism, and gout. Pruritus is infrequently the presenting symptom of diabetes mellitus.
4. **Hematologic**
   a. **Lymphoma.** Hodgkin's and non-Hodgkin's lymphomas, even though systemic symptoms are more likely seen with Hodgkin's lymphoma. Unlike other systemic symptoms (weight loss, fever, and night sweats), the absence or presence of pruritus does not affect prognosis.
   b. **Leukemia.** Various leukemias, including hairy cell leukemia, may have associated pruritus.
   c. **Multiple myeloma**
   d. **Polycythemia vera.** Caused by or aggravated by hot baths or showers. Pruritus is seen in about one-half of patients with polycythemia vera (see Section I, Chapter 55, Polycythemia, p 291).
   e. **Iron deficiency anemia.** Pruritus is seen with iron deficiency, with or without the anemia, and improves with repletion of iron stores.
   f. **Systemic mastocytosis.** A history of urticaria and other symptoms (fatigue, weight loss, and fever) is common. Other symptoms occurring less frequently include diarrhea, abdominal cramping, flushing, and headache. NSAIDs, penicillin, sulfa-containing medications, and morphine may precipitate symptoms. Papules (that may urticate) and macules that are hyperpigmented may be present.
5. **Malignancy.** Reported with breast, colon, gastric, lung, prostrate, thyroid, and uterine cancer.
6. **Parasitic infections.** Including *A lumbricoides, E vermicularis* (pinworm), *G lamblia, N americanus* (hookworm), *S stercoralis, Trichinella* (roundworm), and *T trichiura* (whipworm).
7. **Medications.** Pruritus secondary to medications will usually have an associated rash. The more common medications to cause pruritus without a rash are allopurinol, birth control pills, captopril, cephalosporins, cimetidine, clonidine, diuretics (decrease extracellular fluid and exacerbate xerosis), HMG-CoA reductase inhibitors, ketoconazole, narcotics, niacin, penicillin, phenothiazines, and phenytoin.

8. **Rheumatologic.** Sjögren's syndrome.
9. **Neurologic and psychiatric disorders.** Several neurologic and psychiatric conditions may have pruritus as a symptom, including cerebral lesions (infarction, abscess, tumor), Creutzfeldt-Jakob disease, multiple sclerosis, depression, and psychosis.

IV. Database

A. Physical examination key points

1. **Skin.** The skin is probably the single most helpful organ to examine in determining the cause of pruritus. Examine the entire patient, especially any areas of localized pruritus. Be sure to examine areas the patient cannot scratch (mid-upper back). What appears to be a rash may be excoriations secondary to scratching. Carefully record the distribution and appearance of the rash. Look for lice or nits (pediculosis) and mites, eggs, and burrows (scabies). Areas difficult to reach are usually spared and appear hypopigmented in neurotic excoriations. Look for fissuring, scaling, maceration in between the toes, or irregular, well-demarcated, red-brown macules with fine scales in the intertriginous areas (groin, axillae, buttocks, and underneath the breasts). Classically, in dermatomyositis a red to purple hue is present on the eyelids and extensor surfaces; violaceous flat papules are present over the knuckles.
2. **HEENT.** Stridor suggests a severe allergic reaction. Scleral icterus is seen with cholestasis, a common systemic cause of pruritus. Thyromegaly suggests hypothyroidism or hyperthyroidism as the cause of the pruritus.
3. **Chest.** Wheezing points toward an anaphylactic reaction as the cause.
4. **Abdomen.** Hepatomegaly points toward hepatitis, lymphoma, or some other malignancy or systemic mastocytosis. An enlarged spleen is seen with lymphomas, polycythemia vera, and systemic mastocytosis.
5. **Rectal exam.** Pinworms (*Enterobius vermicularis*) can be seen without magnification and may resemble a fiber or a piece of thread. Adhesive clear tape pressed against the perianal area in the early morning for several days is highly sensitive for detecting pinworms.
6. **Neurologic exam.** Check reflexes. A decrease (*fast return*) in the relaxation phase of the reflexes is seen in hyperthyroidism; an increase (*slow return*) in the relaxation phase of the reflexes is seen in hypothyroidism. Decreased proximal muscle strength is seen in dermatomyositis.
7. **Lymph nodes.** Lymphadenopathy suggests lymphoma, carcinoma, or systemic mastocytosis as the cause of pruritus.

B. Laboratory data

1. **Hemogram and differential.** An elevated hematocrit/hemoglobin, WBC count, and platelet count suggest polycythemia vera. A low

mean cell volume (MVC) and a low mean cellular hemoglobin (MCH) points toward iron deficiency anemia. A low hematocrit/hemoglobin, WBC count, and platelet count may be seen with lymphoma or carcinoma. Eosinophilia suggests an occult parasitic infection as the cause of the pruritus. An elevated WBC count (or decreased WBC count) with blasts, monoclonal lymphocytosis, or granulocytes at all stages of development suggests leukemia as the cause.

2. **Liver function tests.** Total bilirubin, alkaline phosphatase, γ-glutamyltransferase, and alanine aminotransferase (ALT) and aspartate aminotransferase (AST) should be obtained if the etiology is unclear, especially if a rash is not present.
3. **BUN and creatinine.** Uremia needs to be ruled out.
4. **Thyroid function tests.** Thyroid-stimulating hormone (TSH) will rule in or rule out hypothyroidism or hyperthyroidism.
5. **Glucose.** To rule out diabetes mellitus as the cause.
6. **Calcium.** To rule out hyperparathyroidism.
7. **Uric acid.** Especially if gout is considered; however, the diagnosis of gout is made by aspiration of joint fluid and examination of the fluid for crystals.
8. **Stool for ova and parasites.** Consider especially with gastrointestinal symptoms and eosinophilia.
9. **Other.** Specific tests such as serum and urine histamine (systemic mastocytosis) and 24-hour urine for 5-HIAA (carcinoid) may be helpful. An arterial blood gas test, leukocyte alkaline phosphatase (LAP) score, and vitamin B_{12} level will be helpful if polycythemia vera is considered (see Section I, Chapter 55, Polycythemia, p 291).

C. Radiologic and other studies

1. **Chest x-ray.** May reveal hilar adenopathy (lymphoma), a lung mass, or infiltrates (transient infiltrates seen with several parasitic infections).
2. **KOH (potassium hydroxide) preparation of skin scrapings.** Any rash suspected to be fungal in origin should be scraped with a #15 blade. Scrapings should fall on a microscopic slide recently wiped with an alcohol pad (will help keep the scrapings on the slide). Add one drop of KOH (10–20%), place a cover slip over the scrapings and KOH, and view under the microscope at magnifications of 10× and 40×. Heating the slide under an alcohol flame may facilitate the visualization of fungal elements.
3. **Wood's ultraviolet light.** Erythrasma will have a coral-red or pink color.
4. **Skin biopsy.** May be very helpful in establishing the diagnosis in systemic mastocytosis and various dermatologic conditions. The biopsy specimen should be sent for direct immunofluorescence if a primary blistering process is suspected (ie, bullous pemphigoid).

5. **Bone marrow biopsy.** May be needed if lymphoma, leukemia, multiple myeloma, or systematic mastocytosis is suspected.
6. **Red blood cell mass scan and spleen scan.** Helpful if polycythemia vera is considered.

V. Plan. Unless caused by a significant systemic disease or as an early sign of an anaphylactic reaction, pruritus usually does not require immediate treatment. However, pruritus may be a clue to a major illness. The patient's comfort during his or her hospitalization can greatly be enhanced by some simple measures until the underlying cause is established and specific therapy is instituted.

A. Specific causes

1. **Anaphylactic reaction.** See Section I, Chapter 4, Anaphylactic Reaction, V, p 26.
2. **Xerosis.** Patients should limit the amount of time in the bath or shower and the number of baths per week and use mild soaps. Immediately after bathing, they should apply an emollient. Patients should avoid any creams with an alcohol base. Humidifying the air and the use of petroleum and steroid ointment may also help.
3. **Uremia.** Cholestyramine, intravenous lidocaine, or ultraviolet B light may relieve the pruritus associated with uremia.
4. **Cholestasis.** Cholestyramine should be considered.
5. **Hematologic.** Aspirin, cyproheptadine, and ultraviolet B light are beneficial in treating pruritus secondary to polycythemia vera. Pruritus secondary to iron deficiency will resolve with iron replacement.
6. **Contact dermatitis.** Removal of the offending agent is essential. Topical steroids can be used for mild or very localized cases. Systemic steroids (prednisone 0.5–1.0 mg/kg/d for 2–3 days and then a tapering dose schedule) can be used in more severe and generalized cases.
7. **Eczematous dermatitis.** Prescribe emollients and steroid ointment.

B. Symptomatic treatment

1. **Antihistamines (H_1 blockers).** May provide relief. Nonsedating antihistamines (in the morning) such as cetirizine (Zyrtec), fexofenadine (Allegra), and loratadine (Claritin) may be less effective in relieving pruritus than other H_1 blockers. Patients should use the sedating antihistamines in the evening.
2. **Diphenhydramine (Benadryl).** Give 25–50 mg PO or IV Q 6–8 hr.
3. **Cyproheptadine (Periactin).** Give 4 mg PO Q 8 hr.
4. **Hydroxyzine (Atarax or Vistaril).** Give 25–50 mg Q 6–8 hr.
5. **Topical agents.** Camphor, menthol, phenol, and pramoxine are commonly used. Camphor, phenol, and pramoxine provide relief through local anesthetic effect. Menthol cools the skin. Other topical agents often used are Eucerin cream and Sarna lotion. Menthol and phenol are contained in Sarna lotion.

6. **Other.** Additional agents that have been shown to be effective are opiate antagonists (naloxone), doxepin (a tricyclic antidepressant with greater efficacy as an H_1 blocker than diphenhydramine or hydroxyzine), and capsaicin.

REFERENCES

Greco PJ, Ende J: Pruritus: A practical approach. J Gen Intern Med 1992;7:340.

Fleisher AB: Pruritus in the elderly. Adv Dermatol 1995;10:41.

Kantor GR, Lookingbill DP: Pruritus. In: Sams WM, Lynch PJ, eds. *Principles and Practice of Dermatology.* Churchill Livingstone;1990:861.

Yosipovitch G, David M: The diagnostic and therapeutic approach to idiopathic generalized pruritus. Int J Dermatol 1999;38:881.

57. PULMONARY ARTERY CATHETER PROBLEMS

(See also Section I, Chapter 10, Central Venous Line Problems, p 53, and Section III, Chapter 12, Pulmonary Artery Catheterization, p 421).

I. **Problem.** A 50-year-old man is admitted to the coronary care unit (CCU) with an anterior myocardial infarction (MI). A pulmonary artery (PA) catheter is placed. You are notified 24 hours later by the CCU nurse that he is having trouble interpreting the pressure tracings.

II. **Immediate Questions**

A. **What does the waveform look like?** The pulmonary artery waveform varies with inspiration and expiration and has a characteristic systolic/diastolic waveform. (See Figure 3–10, p 427; and Section III, Chapter 12, Pulmonary Artery Catheterization, p 421).

B. **Is there a waveform when the catheter is tapped?** The absence of a waveform or a "dampened" tracing suggests that the catheter is not patent; or that there are technical difficulties including transducer malfunction, cracked hub, loose connections, incorrect stopcock positions, too-tight skin sutures, and too-tight plastic sleeve diaphragms.

C. **Can the catheter be flushed? Can blood be withdrawn?** If the catheter cannot be flushed or blood withdrawn, the catheter may not be patent. The catheter may be kinked, or there may be a venous thrombus obstructing the catheter. (See Section I, Chapter 10, Central Venous Line Problems, p 53).

D. **Is the catheter in permanent wedge?** After a period of time within the patient's circulation, PA catheters tend to become softer and more pliable, and may migrate distally. With a decreasing pulmonary pressure, the same effect may occur as the pulmonary vascular bed shrinks relative to the catheter position. The catheter may end up wedged with its balloon deflated, a situation analogous to a pulmonary embolus. The catheter position must be corrected as soon as possible. Careful evaluation is needed to ensure that the problem is really a case of permanent wedge and not a kink or system malfunction. If all else fails to help distinguish the various causes of a flat tracing, wedge position can be confirmed with blood gas sampling, showing saturation in the arterial range, as opposed to the mixed venous range usually found when blood gases are sampled from the pulmonary artery position.

E. **Can a wedge tracing be obtained with the balloon inflated?** If not, the balloon may have ruptured or the catheter may have been partially removed. *Do not continue to inject air if the balloon has ruptured,* because the air is injected directly into the pulmonary artery.

F. **Are there any associated symptoms?** Chest pain may result from a PA catheter in permanent wedge, resulting in a pulmonary infarction. Hemoptysis can result from pulmonary infarction or from pulmonary artery rupture or erosion. This is usually associated with inflation of the balloon in a vessel smaller than the balloon, rupturing the pulmonary artery with entry of blood into the airways. Hemoptysis usually results and can sometimes be severe, but is rarely life-threatening. A fever may be secondary to catheter infection, catheter sepsis, or pulmonary infarction.

G. **What is the relative necessity of the pulmonary artery catheter?** If critical measurements are being made, such as hourly pulmonary artery wedge pressure readings, the situation is more serious than if the line has outlived its usefulness and can be removed.

III. **Differential Diagnosis.** Problems with PA catheters (Swan-Ganz) can be conveniently divided into problems occurring inside the patient and outside the patient.

A. **Outside the patient**

1. **Transducer error.** This type of error often results in a "dampened" or flattened tracing, and/or in an erratic nonlinear response to pressure changes. This has become an infrequent problem with the development of very reliable disposable transducers, but on occasion even these transducers can be defective or become damaged by rough handling or exposure to extreme conditions of light and heat. Bubbles within the transducer setup and any improper mounting will also result in a low-quality pressure tracing.
2. **Cables.** As with most electrical systems, particularly nondisposable systems, cables are a common source of problems. The best way to evaluate a cable is to simply use a different one, after first making sure that the transducer setup and its linear response are appropriate, that the system is properly zero-balanced, and that the monitor is set on the proper pressure scale for the measurements being made.
3. **Monitor-related problems.** Perhaps the most common monitor-related problems arise when the monitor is set on an improper scale or the transducer/monitor setup is not properly zero-balanced.

B. Inside the patient

1. **Catheter migration.** The catheter may have moved from its original insertion position, migrating either distally or proximally. Distal migration may result in a permanent wedge.
2. **Thrombosis.** A blood clot in the pressure-monitoring lumen may preclude good-quality pressure recordings.
3. **Kinks.** The most common sites for kinking are at the skin surface, under the clavicle, and at the proximal and distal ends of the sheath. Kinks are another cause of poor-quality tracings.
4. **Malfunctioning balloon.** If the catheter will not wedge, the balloon may have ruptured or the catheter may have migrated proximally. *Do not continue to inject air into the catheter system if a wedge tracing does not appear,* because a ruptured balloon may be the cause.

IV. Database

A. Physical examination key points

1. **General exam.** As in most technical areas of medicine, be sure that the information provided by your technology correlates with your clinical assessment.
2. **Vital signs.** The presence of fever suggests catheter infection or sepsis, especially if the catheter has been in place longer than 3 days.

B. Laboratory data

1. **Blood gases.** A blood gas sample obtained from the distal port of the catheter can be helpful in determining whether a PA catheter is in permanent wedge position. If the catheter is wedged, the oxygen saturation will approximate arterial oxygen saturation, whereas mixed venous saturation is found in pulmonary artery locations.
2. **Blood cultures.** Should be obtained in the presence of a fever or elevated WBC count with an increase in segmented and banded neutrophils.

C. Radiologic and other studies

1. **Chest x-ray.** A CXR is useful in determining whether the catheter is kinked or in the correct position. Permanent wedge may be suggested by a markedly distal location of the catheter tip. After injection with air, a deflated balloon also points to balloon rupture.
2. **Culture of PA catheter.** If catheter-related sepsis or infection is suspected, the PA catheter and the introducer sheath must be removed, and at least the subcutaneous portion of the introducer sheath should be sent for culture. It is unlikely that routinely culturing the PA catheter itself would yield additional useful information in most cases.

V. Plan. For replacement of a PA catheter, see Section III, Chapter 12, Pulmonary Artery Catheterization, p 421.

A. **Problems outside the patient.** If simple tapping on the catheter does not result in a waveform, the cause clearly resides outside the patient. Faulty line connections and stopcocks that are improperly set up, as well as transducer, cable, and monitor-related problems, should be addressed first.

B. **Problems inside the patient.** When a good waveform is obtained by tapping the catheter, the problem most likely resides within the patient.

1. **Permanent wedge.** This problem is reported much more frequently than actually exists. Often, a well-placed PA catheter is withdrawn when the position is fine.
   a. **System inspection.** Thoroughly inspect the PA catheter system before you attempt to move the catheter. The transducer should be evaluated for proper functioning. The system should be evaluated for leaks, loose connections, and similar mechanical problems, prior to any manipulation of the catheter.
   b. **CXR.** For PA catheter positioning and evaluation of the balloon. If the catheter is truly stuck in wedge, the CXR will show the catheter to be in the distal pulmonary circulation. Less commonly, the balloon will not deflate because the catheter is kinked.
   c. **Check the oxygen saturation.** As mentioned earlier, the oxygen saturation will be close to arterial when obtained from a truly wedged catheter.
   d. **Catheter withdrawal.** If the catheter is really wedged and the waveform cannot be returned to the expected waveform by manual aspiration or flushing of the catheter, withdraw the catheter centimeter by centimeter while flushing between each withdrawal using a pressure-bag flush system. During catheter withdrawal the balloon must be always completely deflated. When an appropriate waveform for pulmonary artery position returns, the balloon should be reinflated to be certain that the catheter will wedge when desired. With most properly placed PA catheters, the balloon needs to be inflated with only 1–1.5 mL of air to obtain the wedge tracing. Once the balloon is deflated, the original PA pressure waveform should return within 3–5 heartbeats.
2. **A balloon that will not wedge.** In most cases, the catheter has been pulled back too far, or the balloon is not functioning. The catheter should not be advanced unless a sterile sleeve protects the catheter portion lying outside the patient. If the balloon is malfunctioning, the catheter should be removed and a new one placed through the same introducer sheath if hemodynamic monitoring is still needed.
3. **Inaccurate or poorly reproducible cardiac outputs.**
   a. In cases of apparently inappropriate cardiac outputs, be sure that the constant on the cardiac output computer is correct for

the size/type of PA catheter used. The thermodilution technique is not accurate in patients with very low cardiac outputs (CO) or significant tricuspid regurgitation. Use the mixed venous oxygen saturation (should be below normal if CO is indeed low), and the Fick oxygen method to confirm the low CO. With the Fick method, the CO is calculated as the oxygen consumption ($\dot{V}O_2$) divided by the difference between arterial O_2 content (CaO_2) and venous O_2 content (CvO_2).

$$CO = VO_2 \div (CaO_2 - CvO_2)$$

The oxygen content of blood is calculated as the hemoglobin concentration (in grams per deciliter) × 1.36 (amount of O_2 in milliliters contained by 1 g of Hgb that is 100% saturated; values of 1.34 and 1.39 have also been used) × measured O_2 saturation (SaO_2 or SvO_2, as appropriate).

The amount of dissolved oxygen in the plasma is negligible and can be ignored. When a directly measured O_2 consumption is used, we call this the "direct Fick" method, but if an assumed normal O_2 consumption of 125 mL/min/m^2 is used instead, we call it "indirect Fick." ***Caution:*** Remember that to do these calculations correctly all volumes must be eventually expressed in the same units: mL, dL, or L.

b. If no cardiac output is obtained, the catheter may not be properly connected to the computer, or the wire connecting the thermistor to the computer may be fractured. Most computers will flash a code indicating that the catheter is at fault in this circumstance.

4. Pulmonary artery rupture or erosion. Treatment depends on the severity of the bleeding. It is prudent to remove the PA catheter; if it is crucial for managing the patient, it can be replaced. The new catheter should be directed toward the opposite lung. This procedure requires fluoroscopy. Careful attention to the adequacy of ventilation and blood pressure, serial CXRs, and a low threshold for requesting cardiothoracic surgery consultation are advisable in this situation. The complication of rupture or erosion can be avoided by always inflating the balloon slowly and carefully, and monitoring the pressure waveform so that the catheter is not overwedged or left in a "permanent" wedge position. For replacement of central venous catheters, see Section III, Chapter 6, Central Venous Catheterization, p 399.

REFERENCES

Davidson CJ, Bonow RO: Cardiac catheterization. In: Braunwald E, Zipes DP, Libby P, eds. *Heart Disease: A Textbook of Cardiovascular Medicine.* 6th ed. Saunders;2001:359.

Sprung CL, ed: *The Pulmonary Artery Catheter: Methodology and Clinical Applications.* 2nd ed. Crit Care Research Associates;1993.

58. SEIZURES

I. **Problem.** A 65-year-old man experiences a seizure-like episode the day after being admitted for a fractured hip.

II. **Immediate Questions**

A. **Did the patient have an epileptic seizure, or could something else have happened to explain this behavioral change?** The most common cause for a loss or alteration of consciousness is not an epileptic seizure. Disorders that may be confused with an epileptic seizure include syncope (orthostatic hypotension, arrhythmia, valvular heart disease), a transient ischemic attack, decorticate posturing from increased intracranial pressure, a sleep disorder (REM sleep disorder or somnambulism), a panic attack, neuroleptic malignant syndrome, or a psychogenic seizure. A detailed history from the patient and a reliable witness usually help to distinguish an epileptic seizure from another disorder.

B. **What type of epileptic seizure did the patient experience?** Seizures are classified depending on whether they are generalized or focal in onset (see Table 1–9, Classification by Seizure Type). Primary generalized seizures occur without warning and have nonlocalizing behavioral changes, whereas a warning, or aura, may precede partial seizures that exhibit localizing behavioral changes. Seizures that are localized in onset could be due to a focal, structural brain lesion.

C. **Was the seizure symptomatic or idiopathic?** Idiopathic seizures have no known cause and account for half of all cases; they often occur in younger patients who have a family history of idiopathic seizures. Symptomatic seizures indicate that the seizure is a symptom of another disorder that affects the central nervous system (CNS) (see III. Differential Diagnosis).

D. **Does the patient have a history of previous epileptic seizures?** If the patient was taking an anticonvulsant prior to admission, it may

TABLE I–9. CLASSIFICATION BY SEIZURE TYPE.

Primary generalized seizures
Primary generalized tonic-clonic seizures
Absence seizures
Myoclonic seizures
Tonic seizures
Clonic seizures
Atonic seizures
Partial seizures
Simple partial seizures
Complex partial seizures
Partial seizures evolving to 2° generalized seizures

have been discontinued, or other medications may have altered the absorption or metabolism of the anticonvulsant, leading to subtherapeutic anticonvulsant levels and breakthrough seizures. The most common cause for recurrent seizures is poor compliance. Other causes for uncontrolled seizures are the presence of severe CNS disease, an incorrect diagnosis of epileptic seizures, the wrong anticonvulsant for that type of seizure, or an anticonvulsant prescribed at a subtherapeutic dose.

E. **Does the patient have a history of alcohol or drug abuse?** Alcohol or drug withdrawal may trigger an epileptic seizure. Alcohol withdrawal seizures commonly occur 12–24 hours after cessation or reduction of alcohol intake in someone who drinks daily or binge drinks for 5 or more days. The seizures are usually self-limited, but sometimes status epilepticus occurs and should be treated similarly to other episodes of status. Additional causes for epileptic seizures such as meningitis, head injury, electrolyte abnormalities, and hypoglycemia should also be considered in alcohol and drug abuse.

III. **Differential Diagnosis.** An epileptic seizure is the result of abnormal electrical activity of the cerebral cortex and may result in loss of consciousness or confusion, abnormal motor activity, or sensory sensations. Generalized tonic-clonic seizures are typified by loss of consciousness with severe, tonic stiffening of muscles followed by clonic jerking. The entire episode usually lasts 2–3 minutes, after which the patient may sleep for several hours and later awaken confused. In adults, the first seizure is usually a partial seizure that secondarily becomes tonic-clonic.

A. **Head trauma.** Recent or remote head trauma that is sufficient to produce loss of consciousness or prolonged amnesia, a depressed skull fracture, dural tear, intracranial hemorrhage, or focal neurologic deficits is related to a high risk for epileptic seizures.

B. **Infections.** Bacterial, fungal, or viral meningitis or encephalitis; cerebral abscess; mycotic aneurysm; or parasitic infestation of cysticercosis, toxoplasmosis, or paragonimiasis may cause epileptic seizures.

C. **Stroke.** A common cause for epileptic seizures in the elderly. Cortical vein thrombosis is especially epileptogenic, but other vascular causes include subarachnoid hemorrhage, arteriovenous malformation, CNS vasculitis, hypertensive encephalopathy, or eclampsia.

D. **Carcinoma.** Epileptic seizures may be the presenting symptom of a primary or metastatic brain tumor. Common cancers that metastasize to the brain are lung, breast, kidney, gastrointestinal, and melanoma. Meningeal carcinomatosis, paraneoplastic disorders such as limbic encephalitis, and cancer-associated vascular disorders should be considered.

E. **Drugs.** Toxic or therapeutic doses of certain drugs may precipitate an epileptic seizure. They include psychotropics, isoniazid, high doses of penicillin, lidocaine, clozapine, theophylline, chemotherapeutic agents (etoposide, ifosfamide, and *cis*-platinum); and drugs of abuse such as amphetamines, cocaine, heroin, gamma hydroxybutyrate (GHB), and phencyclidine. Abrupt withdrawal of alcohol, benzodiazepines, or barbiturates also causes seizures. Certain medications such as bupropion and phenothiazines can decrease the seizure threshold.

F. **Neurodegenerative disorders.** Alzheimer's disease is associated with a high risk for seizures, which are usually myoclonic but can be generalized tonic-clonic seizures. Down's syndrome patients often develop Alzheimer's disease and may have epileptic seizures.

G. **Metabolic or toxic disorders.** Hypoglycemia, hyponatremia, hypocalcemia, hypomagnesemia, hypophosphatemia, uremia, severe alkalosis or acidosis, hepatic failure, and possibly hyperkalemia may precipitate epileptic seizures. Osmolar changes with hemodialysis for acute or chronic renal failure can cause seizures; multifocal myoclonus usually precedes the generalized seizures. Severe hypoxic encephalopathy following a cardiopulmonary arrest can cause myoclonic seizures. Toxins including methanol, ethylene glycol, or lead or carbon monoxide (CO) poisoning (with CO levels > 50%) can cause seizures.

H. **Nonepileptic psychogenic seizures.** Due to malingering or a conversion disorder, psychogenic seizures, or pseudoseizures, may be difficult to distinguish from an epileptic seizure. Prolonged complex movements, shaking side-to-side, pelvic thrusting, and failure to respond to therapeutic doses of anticonvulsants in a patient with a psychiatric history, no risk factors for epileptic seizures, and a normal exam without postictal confusion following the seizure are clues that it is a nonepileptic psychogenic seizure.

I. **Other causes.** Systemic lupus erythematosus, acute intermittent porphyria, Whipple's disease, sickle cell anemia, sarcoidosis involving the CNS, or neurofibromatosis in adulthood may have associated epileptic seizures. Porphyria as a cause should be considered if the seizure activity is exacerbated by standard anticonvulsants. Genetic disorders such as tuberous sclerosis, inherited inborn errors of amino acid metabolism (phenylketonuria), glycogen or lipid storage diseases, cerebral malformations, and prenatal or postnatal birth injuries usually present in childhood with epileptic seizures.

IV. Database

A. **Physical examination key points.** Although a detailed history and general physical examination are necessary for all patients who present with an epileptic seizure, key points include the following:

1. **Vital signs.** The blood pressure is often normal following a seizure, but hypotension in an elderly person may signal a recent myocardial infarction due to the profound muscular exertion ac-

companying a generalized tonic-clonic seizure. Hypertension may suggest a cause for the seizure, such as hypertensive encephalopathy, toxemia, or elevated blood pressure with a recent stroke.

2. **Skin.** Neurocutaneous syndromes including tuberous sclerosis, Sturge-Weber syndrome, ataxia-telangiectasia, von Hippel–Lindau syndrome, and neurofibromatosis would signify a cause for the epileptic seizure. Inspection of the skin for needle tracks might indicate illegal drug use, and a rash could suggest an underlying vasculitis or connective tissue disease. Enlarged lymph nodes could imply HIV or other infections, malignancy, sarcoidosis, or systemic lupus erythematosus.
3. **HEENT.** Presence of a deeply bitten and bleeding tongue is strongly associated with generalized tonic-clonic seizures and rarely if ever occurs in psychogenic seizures. Inspection of the skull for recent or remote head injuries, burr holes, or other deformities from craniotomies may be indicative of the cause. Intracranial hypertension from a tumor, infection, hemorrhage, or brain edema may be identified by funduscopy (papilledema). Measuring head circumference is important to detect microcephaly and the associated disorders, which can cause epileptic seizures. Meningismus, or nuchal rigidity, could signify a neck injury, meningitis, or a subarachnoid hemorrhage.
4. **Heart and lungs.** A cardiac dysrhythmia or valvular abnormality could suggest syncope rather than an epileptic seizure. Aspiration pneumonia or noncardiogenic pulmonary edema following generalized tonic-clonic seizures may lead to respiratory insufficiency.
5. **Genitourinary system and rectum.** Urinary or stool incontinence may occur with an epileptic seizure, though some patients with psychogenic seizures may be incontinent, too.
6. **Back and extremities.** Severe muscle contraction with generalized tonic-clonic seizures can cause vertebral body fractures in osteoporotic patients, whereas falls may cause fractures of long bones.

B. **Neurologic exam.** A detailed neurologic examination is necessary to identify the location of the lesion within the CNS, which may be the source of the epileptic seizure.

1. **Mental status.** Following an epileptic seizure, the patient may be confused for an hour or longer. The patient is usually alert and lucid immediately after a brief syncopal event or a psychogenic seizure.
2. **Cranial nerves.** An asymmetrical enlarged pupil could be an early sign of uncal herniation. Small pupils occur with metabolic disorders or narcotics; fixed and dilated pupils can accompany severe hypoxic encephalopathy or the use of drugs such as cocaine and atropine. Both upper and lower facial weakness on one side could suggest a basal skull fracture, but weakness limited to the

lower face on one side occurs with a contralateral brain stem lesion or cerebral hemisphere lesion. A visual field deficit may pinpoint a lesion in the occipital cortex.

3. **Motor and sensory.** Focal motor or sensory findings, asymmetrical reflexes, and presence of an abnormal Babinski reflex may occur subsequent to the epileptic seizure and aid in localizing the seizure focus. Transient hemiparesis following the seizure could represent a Todd's paralysis and point to a lesion or seizure focus in the contralateral motor cortex.

C. **Laboratory data**

1. **Serum glucose and electrolytes.** Rule out hypoglycemia, hypocalcemia, and hyponatremia or a hyperosmolar state due to hyperglycemia or hyponatremia. A high anion gap metabolic acidosis secondary to high lactate levels often occurs with a generalized tonic-clonic seizure, but can also be associated with methanol and ethylene glycol poisoning.
2. **Renal profile and creatine phosphokinase (CK).** Rule out acute or chronic renal failure. Rhabdomyolysis with myoglobinuria can complicate a generalized tonic-clonic seizure and precipitate acute renal failure.
3. **Drug screen.** Consider if the clinical history suggests the use of cocaine, amphetamines, phencyclidine, barbiturates, benzodiazepines, alcohol, methanol, or ethylene glycol.
4. **Levels of prescribed anticonvulsants.** Perform immediately to determine if the recent seizure is due to subtherapeutic levels secondary to poor compliance, prescribed subtherapeutic doses, or interference with absorption or metabolism of the anticonvulsant. If the level is within the therapeutic range, the dose can sometimes be increased. Or, if it is feared that increasing the dose will lead to drug toxicity, a new anticonvulsant may need to be started.
5. **Complete blood count with differential.** A high white blood cell count could indicate an underlying infection. However, following a generalized tonic-clonic seizure, a postictal leukocytosis sometimes occurs that can be distinguished from a leukemoid response to an infection by the presence of many mature granulocytes with few immature forms.
6. **Arterial blood gases.** To rule out hypoxemia or acidosis as a cause or complication of the epileptic seizure. Following a generalized tonic-clonic seizure, the patient hyperventilates to correct the metabolic and respiratory acidosis that occurred during the seizure. A severe alkalosis can also cause seizures.
7. **Other.** Consider obtaining prothrombin time and partial thromboplastin time if a lumbar puncture is anticipated. Sedimentation rate or antinuclear antibody should be obtained if the clinical findings suggest the presence of a vasculitis or lupus.

D. Radiologic and other studies

1. **CT or MRI brain scan.** A neuroimaging study should be performed on all patients who present with new-onset seizures and in whom no other cause for the seizure is apparent. A CT head scan is usually more convenient in the emergency situation, can be obtained quickly, and may provide good images when the patient is postictally confused and cannot lie quietly for very long. Heavy sedation or anesthesia is sometimes required to ensure a MRI brain scan does not show significant movement artifact in a restless and confused patient.
2. **Lumbar puncture.** See Section III, Chapter 10, Lumbar Puncture, p 412. It should be done immediately if meningitis, encephalitis, or meningeal carcinomatosis is suspected, or if there is clinical suspicion for a subarachnoid hemorrhage with a negative neuroimaging study. If immediately available, a neuroimaging study should precede the lumbar puncture, especially if there are focal neurologic findings or papilledema to suggest increased intracranial pressure.
3. **EEG.** Usually not necessary as an emergency procedure, but is helpful in classifying epileptic seizures. An interictal recording may demonstrate focal epileptiform activity consistent with a partial seizure disorder, whereas generalized epileptiform activity indicates a primary generalized seizure disorder. Though an interictal EEG recording is usually abnormal, a normal interictal EEG recording does not exclude the diagnosis. An immediate EEG is essential for monitoring patients in a pentobarbital coma for status epilepticus, or in a comatose patient with suspected subclinical epileptic seizures as a cause of the coma.
4. **Chest x-ray and ECG.** Helpful if aspiration pneumonia, noncardiogenic pulmonary edema, or an acute myocardial infarction is suspected as a complication of the epileptic seizure.

V. Plan. Support life functions with the ABCs (airway, breathing, and circulation) of cardiopulmonary resuscitation and protect the patient from self-inflicted injury during the seizure.

A. Emergency management. Place the patient in a lateral decubitus position with a suction device to prevent aspiration if vomiting occurs. Move objects away from the patient or place padding between the patient and the floor or other immovable items. Do not place objects in the patient's mouth or try to force the mouth open because these measures are unnecessary and may lead to injury to the patient or yourself.

B. Seizure control. See Section VII, Therapeutics, for a discussion of drugs listed here.

1. Most seizures are self-limited, will last no more than 2–3 minutes, and may not need immediate treatment until a detailed evaluation

is completed. *Status epilepticus* is recurrent seizures without complete recovery between seizures. Any seizure type can evolve into status epilepticus, but generalized tonic-clonic status epilepticus is a medical emergency requiring prompt treatment in order to prevent serious morbidity and mortality. In clinical practice, a generalized tonic-clonic seizure lasting more than 5–10 minutes or two generalized tonic-clonic seizures occurring in quick succession without the patient fully recovering between seizures should be treated as status epilepticus.

2. Immediately establish intravenous access and collect a serum specimen for laboratory tests. If hypoglycemia is a suspected cause, do not wait for the results of the laboratory tests. Promptly give 50 mL of 50% dextrose IV. If there is clinical suspicion for chronic alcohol abuse or other disorder associated with nutritional deprivation, give 50 mg thiamine IV with dextrose to prevent precipitation of Wernicke's encephalopathy.

3. For generalized tonic-clonic status epilepticus with the patient in an active seizure, give lorazepam 0.1 mg/kg at 1–2 mg/min IV, and repeat if necessary in 15 minutes (maximum dose 0.2 mg/kg or 5–10 mg total; doses > 0.2 mg/kg are usually unnecessary or ineffective). Diazepam may also be used at doses of 5–10 mg at 1–2 mg/min IV, and repeated if necessary in 15 minutes (maximum dose 20–40 mg). However, lorazepam may be preferred due to its longer effect. Both drugs may cause respiratory depression requiring intubation and ventilatory support.

4. If the patient is in status epilepticus but not in an active seizure, fosphenytoin can be given to prevent further seizures by loading intravenously with 15–20 mg phenytoin equivalents (PE)/kg at 100–150 mg PE/min. Phenytoin may also be used intravenously with a loading dose of 15–20 mg/kg but must be given at slower rates of ≤ 50 mg/min to avoid significant hypotension. Phenytoin extravasation can cause severe skin sloughing. Another option would be IV valproate at doses of 15 mg/kg. Phenobarbital with a loading dose of 10–20 mg/kg at 50–100 mg/min (maximum dose of 1.5–2 g) may be added if seizures recur with maximal doses of fosphenytoin.

5. If you are unable to immediately secure an IV access and the patient is in an active seizure, diazepam rectal gel may be given at a dose of 0.2 mg/kg (maximum 20 mg). Midazolam may be given IM at a dose of 0.07–0.08 mg/kg (approximately 5 mg), or fosphenytoin can be given IM at a dose of 15–20 mg/kg.

6. Generalized tonic-clonic status epilepticus refractory to the above measures may require general anesthesia with an agent such as pentobarbital. The loading dose is 15–20 mg/kg IV at 25–50 mg/min. Additional doses of 25–50 mg every 2–5 minutes may be given until burst suppression or adverse effects occur, then a maintenance dose of 1–2 mg/kg/hr. Continuous EEG monitoring is necessary to rule out subclinical status epilepticus. The patient must be intubated, and a central venous pressure monitor is required to monitor volume status. Dopamine or dobutamine drips may be necessary to treat hypotension due to the cardiac depressant effects of pentobarbital. Other options for refractory status include IV midazolam 0.2 mg/kg bolus, maintained at 0.75–10 mcg m/kg/min; or IV propofol 1–2 mg/kg bolus, maintained at 2–10 mg/kg/hr.

7. Not all isolated seizures need to be treated with an anticonvulsant. Epileptic seizures due to alcohol or drug withdrawal, drug abuse, severe sleep deprivation, or seizures associated with acute illness such as hypoglycemia do not need to be treated. If there is an associated history of brain injury, a structural lesion of the brain such as a tumor or arteriovenous malformation, or an abnormal EEG with epileptiform activity, or if the presentation with status epilepticus is at the onset, treatment with an anticonvulsant to prevent further seizures is recommended.

REFERENCES

Browne TR, Holmes GL: Epilepsy. N Engl J Med 2001;344:1145.

Delanty N, Vaughan CJ, French JA: Medical causes of seizures. Lancet 1998;352:383.

Leppik IE, ed: *Contemporary Diagnosis and Management of the Patient with Epilepsy.* 5th ed. Handbooks in Health Care;2000.

Lowenstein DH, Alldredge BK: Status epilepticus. N Engl J Med 1998;338:970.

Trescher WH, Lesser RP: The epilepsies. In: Bradley WG, Daroff RB, Fenichel GM et al, eds. *Neurology in Clinical Practice.* 3rd ed. Butterworth-Heinemann;2000:1745.

Wilder BJ, ed: Management of epilepsy: Consensus conference on current clinical practice. Neurology 1998;51(suppl 4):S1.

59. SYNCOPE

I. **Problem.** A patient admitted for palpitations and chest pain loses consciousness while being transported to the ICU.

II. **Immediate Questions**

Definition: *Syncope* is transient loss of consciousness with loss of postural tone. True syncope must be differentiated from dizziness, “spells,” or near syncope, which are not associated with loss of consciousness and are generally more benign.

A. **What was the patient’s activity and position immediately prior to the incident?** Syncope in the recumbent position is almost always due to Stokes-Adams attacks (high-grade atrioventricular block). Vasovagal syncope or fainting from orthostatic hypotension requires the patient to have been in the seated or upright position. Exertional syncope is frequently cardiac in origin. Other key activities to ask about include turning or twisting the head, coughing, getting up quickly, and micturition.

B. **Is the patient still unconscious?** Vasovagal syncope rarely lasts more than a few seconds and resolves with recumbency. Persistent unconsciousness suggests a cardiac or neurologic (brain stem stroke or seizure [see Section I, Chapter 58, Seizures, p 308]) cause.

C. **What were the vital signs during the episode? What are the vital signs now?** Vasovagal syncope is associated with bradycardia, but frequently a reflex tachycardia is noted after the episode. The blood pressure is usually normal after a vasovagal faint. Orthostatic changes in blood pressure and tachycardia are frequently evidence of volume depletion or blood loss as the cause. Neurologic causes are generally associated with a normal or elevated blood pressure. Cardiac syncope may occur when arrhythmias result in a pulse < 40 or > 180 bpm.

D. **Was there evidence of seizure activity?** Some clonic jerking of the limbs may occur with syncope, and in some rare instances, a brief tonic-clonic seizure may occur (*convulsive syncope*). Fecal and urinary incontinence are more typical of seizures than of other causes of syncope. Seizures that occur in the absence of typical postictal symptoms may suggest hypotension from an arrhythmia or vasovagal episode as a cause of the syncope.

E. **How quickly was consciousness regained? Was the patient immediately oriented?** Cardiac causes and vasovagal episodes are associated with a rapid return to full consciousness. Seizures are characterized by postictal confusion and headache.

F. **How did the patient feel immediately prior to the loss of consciousness?** Vasovagal episodes are normally preceded by a symptom complex consisting of sweating, lightheadedness, and abdominal queasiness. Seizures often have an *aura* (frequently recurring visual or olfactory sensations). Postural or exertional symptoms may be present in cardiac and orthostatic syncope; however, symptoms are often not present, or may only be associated with sensations of the room closing in or going dark. Dizziness and vertigo in association with syncope have been associated with increased psychiatric causes of syncope. However, dizziness may also be a sign of an arrhythmia.

G. **What medical conditions does the patient have?** Several medical conditions predispose to syncope. Diabetics are at risk for hypoglycemia as well as orthostasis secondary to autonomic dysfunction. A history of atherosclerotic vascular disease suggests arrhythmias as well as cerebrovascular events. Other important illnesses to ask about include a previous history of a seizure disorder, valvular disorders, presence of a pacemaker, migraines, and any history of head trauma.

H. **What medications is the patient receiving?** A variety of medications predispose to orthostatic hypotension, including diuretics, antihypertensives, and tricyclic antidepressants such as amitriptyline (Elavil).

Varying degrees of heart block can be induced by verapamil (Calan, Isoptin), diltiazem (Cardizem), digoxin (Lanoxin), and beta-blockers. Many Class I antiarrhythmics can also induce ventricular arrhythmias leading to syncope ("quinidine syncope"). Antianginals, analgesics, and CNS depressants have been associated with syncope.

III. Differential Diagnosis. In five population-based studies, the most common causes of syncope were vasovagal causes, heart disease and arrhythmias, orthostatic hypotension, and seizures. No diagnosis was found in 34% of patients. The cause of syncope may be placed into one of five categories.

A. Neural-mediated reflexes associated with vasodilatation or bradycardia

1. **Vasovagal syncope.** Also called neurocardiogenic syncope. It is by far the most common cause of syncope, and associated with the symptom complex previously described (see II.F.). Generally has a benign prognosis.
2. **Situational—sudden decrease in venous return**
   a. **Micturition syncope**
   b. **Cough syncope**
   c. **Valsalva maneuver.** Increases vagal tone.
   d. **Swallow syncope**
3. **Other**
   a. **Carotid sinus.** Associated with head turning or neck pressure
   b. **Glossopharyngeal neuralgia.** Intermittent tongue, larynx, or pharynx pain that can stimulate the vagus nerve, resulting in bradycardia.

B. Orthostatic hypotension

1. **Age-related physiologic changes**
2. **Volume depletion**
   a. **Dehydration**
   b. **Blood loss**
3. **Medications.** Diuretics, anti-hypertensives, and tricyclic antidepressants such as amitriptyline (Elavil)
4. **Autonomic insufficiency**
   a. **Shy-Drager syndrome.** Idiopathic autonomic dysfunction.
   b. **Diabetes.** Autonomic dysfunction with long-standing diabetes.
5. **Postprandial orthostasis in the elderly**

C. Psychiatric causes. Generally associated with frequent symptoms and lack of injury.

1. **Anxiety**
2. **Depression**
3. **Conversion disorder**

D. Neurologic causes

1. **Transient ischemic attack (TIA).** Most commonly vertebrobasilar area. Seldom will a cerebrovascular accident involving the an-

terior circulation result in syncope unless there is bilateral disruption of the reticular activating system.

2. **Migraines.** Basilar artery ("drop attacks")
3. **Seizures.** See Section I, Chapter 58, Seizures, p 308.
4. **Carotid sinus syndrome.** Presents as syncope caused by turning head to one side or having too tight a collar.
5. **Subclavian steal syndrome**
6. **Subarachnoid hemorrhage.** May present as brief syncope followed by severe headache.

E. **Cardiac syncope**
  1. **Organic heart disease**
     a. **Atrial myxoma.** Intermittent obstruction of a valve.
     b. **Aortic stenosis.** Associated with left ventricular outflow obstruction. Syncope is a marker for significant mortality.
     c. **Acute myocardial infarction with cardiogenic shock**
     d. **Primary pulmonary hypertension.** Caused by decreased pulmonary flow and left-sided return.
     e. **Idiopathic hypertrophic subaortic stenosis.** Same etiology as aortic stenosis.
     f. **Pulmonary embolism**
     g. **Aortic dissection**
     h. **Cardiac tamponade**
     i. **Pregnancy.** Aortocaval compression by an enlarged uterus.
  2. **Dysrhythmias**
     a. **Tachycardias.** See Section I, Chapter 60, Tachycardia, p 323.
        i. **Ventricular tachycardia**
        ii. **Paroxysmal atrial tachycardia**
        iii. **Atrial fibrillation with rapid ventricular response**
        iv. **Atrial flutter**
        v. **Wolff-Parkinson-White (WPW) syndrome.** Look for short PR interval and delta wave.
        vi. **Torsades de pointes**
     b. **Bradycardias.** See Section I, Chapter 8, Bradycardia, p 39.
        i. **Sinus bradycardia**
        ii. **Second- and third-degree atrioventricular block**
        iii. **Sinus node disease**
        iv. **Pacemaker syncope.** If the patient has a pacemaker, malfunction must be considered as a possible cause of syncope (see Section I, Chapter 53, Pacemaker Troubleshooting, p 283).

F. **Miscellaneous causes**
  1. **Hypoxemia**
  2. **Hyperventilation**
  3. **Hypoglycemia.** Often occurs in patients on insulin or oral hypoglycemics who miss a meal or receive the wrong dose.

G. **Unknown**

IV. Database. History and physical examination identifies approximately 45% of patients whose syncope has an identifiable cause.

A. Physical examination key points

1. **Vital signs (see II.C).** Vitals should be rechecked frequently during the evaluation.
2. **HEENT.** Look for evidence of trauma, and palpate for bony abnormalities. Look for subhyaloid hemorrhages as evidence of subarachnoid hemorrhage. Tongue or cheek lacerations suggest seizure activity. Meningitis and subarachnoid hemorrhage have associated neck stiffness. Carotid bruits suggest diffuse atherosclerosis.
3. **Chest.** Auscultate for crackles and wheezes that may accompany aspiration during the syncopal episode. Palpate for rib injury caused by a fall.
4. **Heart.** Assess rate and rhythm, data that are especially useful during or immediately after episode. Auscultate for new fourth heart sound (S_4), suggestive of acute myocardial infarction and murmur, listening for characteristic changes with position that would differentiate aortic stenosis and idiopathic hypertrophic subaortic stenosis from other systolic murmurs. Assess the jugular venous pulse as an indicator of volume status.
5. **Genitourinary system.** Look for evidence of urinary and/or fecal incontinence.
6. **Neurologic exam.** Slow resolution of mental status to normal points to a postictal state. Focal deficits suggest a cerebrovascular event. Persistent mental obtundation suggests hypoglycemia, hypoxemia, or other metabolic derangement.
7. **Reproduction of event.** Perform maneuvers intended to reproduce event. ***Caution:*** Do this only with appropriate monitoring and resuscitation equipment available (including venous access). Have the patient cough, turn her or his head, and hyperventilate; or perform carotid massage as appropriate.

B. Laboratory data. The American College of Physicians (ACP) suggests workup based on the following algorithm (Figure 1–6):

1. **Routine blood testing.** CBC, electrolytes, BUN, and glucose are not recommended in the ACP Syncope Guideline because they rarely led to diagnostically useful information. However, these tests are recommended to confirm an etiology suggested by history or physical exam.
2. **Electrocardiogram with a rhythm strip.** Look for tachyarrhythmias or bradyarrhythmias. A short PR interval and delta wave suggest Wolff-Parkinson-White syndrome. Also look for evidence of ischemia or myocardial damage and new conduction abnormalities. Approximately 5% of patients with syncope will have an identifiable cause on ECG. Despite the low yield, the ECG is risk-free and inexpensive, and abnormalities will guide further testing.

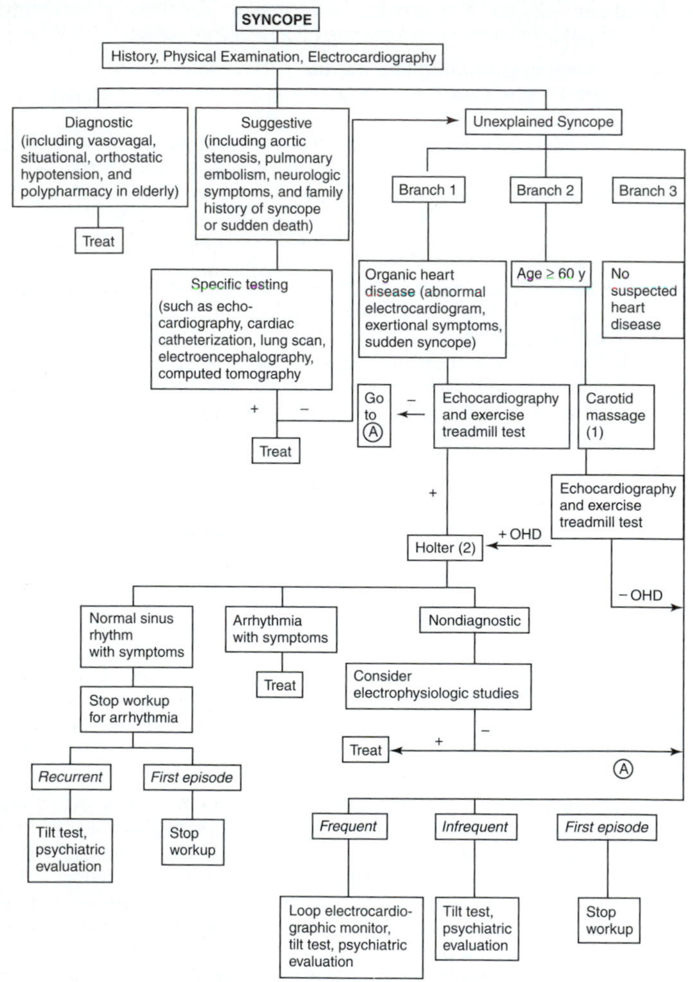

Figure 1–6. Algorithm for diagnosing syncope. (*Reprinted, with permission, from Linzer M, Yang EH, Estes M et al: Diagnosing syncope: Part I. Value of history, physical examination, and electrocardiography. Ann Intern Med 1997;126:989.*)

Footnotes to Figure I–6

(1) Cartoid massage can be performed in an office setting only in the absence of bruits, ventricular tachycardia, recent stroke, or myocardial infarction.
(2) Holter monitoring may be replaced by inpatient telemetry if there is a concern about arrhythmias.
OHD = Organic heart disease

Based on history, physical exam, and ECG, the remainder of the evaluation may be divided into one of three categories:

3. **Diagnostic** (ie, vasovagal, medication, orthostasis, situational). Treat the patient.
4. **Suggestive** (ie, aortic stenosis, neurologic symptoms, trauma, family history of sudden death). Perform specific testing such as echocardiography, CT scan, $\dot{V}\dot{Q}$ scan, or EEG. If workup is unrevealing then go to 5.
5. **Unexplained syncope**
   a. **Unexplained syncope with clinical organic heart disease or abnormal ECG**
      i. **Echocardiography.** Look for valvular lesion, thrombi, new wall motion abnormalities, or myxoma. Unsuspected findings are found in 5–10% of patients.
      ii. **Exercise testing.** With exertional symptoms, exercise testing may lead to a diagnosis of ischemia or an exercise-induced arrhythmia. Echocardiography should be performed first to exclude hypertrophic cardiomyopathy.
      iii. **24-hour Holter monitor.** Useful if an arrhythmia is suspected, particularly in patients with frequent attacks. An event recorder may be more useful if the attacks are infrequent and the evaluation is in the outpatient setting.
      iv. **Electrophysiologic (EP) testing.** Patients with normal hearts (ie, normal ECG and no evidence of underlying structural heart disease) should rarely undergo EP testing. EP studies will be most revealing with organic, structural, or conduction abnormalities.
      v. **Signal-averaged ECG.** In patients with coronary artery disease (CAD) and those in whom ventricular tachycardia is suspected, signal-averaged ECG has a high sensitivity and specificity for inducible tachycardia.
   b. **Unexplained syncope in the elderly (older than 60 years).** Carotid sinus massage may be performed if no bruits are present and there is no history of recent myocardial infarction, stroke, or ventricular tachycardia. It is advised to have intravenous access, cardiac monitoring, and atropine readily available prior to carotid sinus massage. If a cardioinhibitory response (asystole > 3 seconds) occurs, the patient may be treated with a pacemaker.

C. **Unexplained syncope with no CAD and no suspected CAD**
   1. **Long-term loop ECG.** A noninvasive event monitor will be most beneficial with frequent symptoms. The monitor constantly

records and is activated after an episode saving the last several minutes before and after an event.

2. **Head-up tilt-table.** Most helpful with a negative cardiac and arrhythmia evaluation. Passive tilt-table at 65 degrees for 45 minutes may be followed by the use of isoproterenol in patients who have a high pretest probability for neurally mediated syncope. The test is positive only if typical symptoms are reproduced.

V. **Plan.** This will be dictated by your initial impression based on the preceding evaluation. The causes of syncope range from a relatively benign vasovagal episode to life-threatening complete heart block. The treatment plan should reflect the severity of the underlying cause. Remember, injuries from a fall secondary to syncope can result in significant morbidity, especially in the elderly, so a thorough evaluation for injury should be performed.

A. **Vasovagal syncope**

1. Instruct the patient to assume a recumbent position at the onset of presyncopal symptoms. If unable to lie down, the patient should be seated with his or her head down.
2. The patient should be made aware of situations that bring on the episodes, such as prolonged standing, and should avoid these situations.
3. For patients with suspected recurrent neurocardiogenic syncope, consider head-up tilt-table testing to confirm diagnosis and direct further treatment (beta-blockers, disopyramide).

B. **Orthostatic hypotension**

1. Assess for signs of volume contraction and correct as indicated. Review medications to eliminate, if possible, those that could cause volume depletion or cause vasodilatation.
2. If gastrointestinal bleeding is diagnosed, see Section I, Chapter 27, Hematemesis, Melena, V, p 160, and/or Chapter 28, Hematochezia, V, p 165.
3. Instruct the patient to rise and change positions slowly, with adequate support available.

C. **Cardiac syncope**

1. Treat arrhythmias. See Section I, Chapter 8, Bradycardia, V, p. 42, Chapter 45, Irregular Pulse V, p. 241 and Chapter 60, Tachycardia, V, p. 329.
2. If an arrhythmia is suspected but cannot be confirmed with Holter monitoring, consider electrophysiologic testing, especially if ischemic heart disease is present.
3. If ischemia is suspected, treat as possible myocardial infarction, and institute a rule-out myocardial infarction protocol.

D. **Miscellaneous disorders**

1. **Carotid sinus syndrome (carotid sinus hypersensitivity).** Instruct the patient to avoid sudden turning of the head, tight collars, or vigorous rubbing with electric shavers.

2. **Micturition.** Instruct the patient to sit when voiding and to remain seated for several minutes after voiding.
3. **Cough and hyperventilation.** Informing the patient of the cause is frequently the only thing that can be done; however, if hyperventilation is due to anxiety, the anxiety should be addressed and treated appropriately.

REFERENCES

Kapoor WN: Evaluation and management of the patient with syncope. JAMA 1992;268:2553.

Linzer M, Yang EH, Estes M et al: Diagnosing syncope part 1: Value of history, physical examination, and electrocardiography. Ann Intern Med 1997;126:989.

Linzer M, Yang EH, Estes M et al: Diagnosing syncope part 2: Unexplained syncope. Ann Intern Med 1997;127:76.

60. TACHYCARDIA

I. **Problem.** You are asked to evaluate an 18-year-old woman with sudden onset of chest pain, palpitations, and dizziness. Cardiac monitoring reveals the presence of a rapid, regular, narrow-complex tachycardia at a rate of 180 beats per minute (bpm).

II. **Immediate Questions**

A. **What are the patient's other vital signs?** Hypotension accompanying a tachyarrhythmia requires immediate action. Tachypnea and tachycardia may be present with acute pulmonary embolism (PE); a severe pneumonia; an exacerbation of chronic obstructive pulmonary disease (COPD); or during the presentation of acute pulmonary edema. Tachycardia accompanied by a fever may suggest an infection or thyrotoxicosis. The presence of *pulsus paradoxus* (a variation in the systolic blood pressure of more than 10 mm Hg between tidal end inspiration and end expiration) suggests pericardial tamponade or an exacerbation of COPD.

B. **What has been the patient's heart rate previously?** A sudden change in heart rate may signify a change in cardiac rhythm, such as the sudden onset of atrial fibrillation.

C. **Does the patient have any symptoms related to the tachycardia?** Ask about dyspnea, chest pain, dizziness, syncope, agitation, or confusion.

D. **What medication is the patient currently taking?** Drugs that can cause tachyarrhythmias include diuretics, theophylline, sympathomimetic drugs, catecholamine infusions, digoxin, and thyroid supplements. Diuretics can lead to intravascular volume loss as well as hypokalemia and hypomagnesemia that can result in tachyarrhythmias. Theophylline, even in therapeutic doses, may cause sinus tachycardia; and in toxic doses (serum levels greater than 20 μg/mL) can lead to ventricular tachyarrhythmias.

III. Differential Diagnosis

A. **Sinus tachycardia.** This condition is defined as a sinus node controlled rhythm at a rate greater than 100 bpm. The extensive list of its causes includes varying states of emotion and pain; fever; anemia; hypoxemia; hemorrhage; infection; thyrotoxicosis; myocardial infarction; pneumothorax; pericarditis; use of drugs or medications that include caffeine, nicotine, and atropine; and ingestion or overdoses of amyl nitrite, quinidine, cocaine, antihistamines, decongestants, or tricyclic antidepressants. Sinus tachycardia is typically gradual in onset and termination. Vagal maneuvers and carotid sinus massage may slow the heart rate temporarily, but the tachycardia will return when these maneuvers are stopped. Sinus tachycardia rarely occurs in quiet patients at rates greater than 140 bpm. Fever can be expected to raise the sinus rate about 10 bpm for every degree above normal core body temperature.

B. **Supraventricular tachyarrhythmias (SVT).** When you are examining the ECG or rhythm strip of a suspected SVT for the first time, check the tracing for the following features:

1. **Regularity.** Atrial fibrillation, multifocal atrial tachycardia, and on occasion atrial flutter are irregular rhythms, whereas most other SVTs are regular.
2. **Baseline.** The *baseline* is that portion of the ECG between the end of the T wave and the beginning of either the P wave or the next QRS complex. If this section is flat, then the atria are either quiescent or fibrillating, or their activity is hidden in another section of the ECG.
3. **QRS complex.** SVTs generally have QRS complexes with axes and widths that are similar to those found during sinus rhythm, but not always. Wide QRS complexes can result from a rate-dependent bundle branch block, or antegrade conduction across an accessory atrioventricular pathway.
4. **P waves.** Determine if the P wave morphology and axis during the tachycardia is similar to or different from normal sinus rhythm. If different, then atrial activation is initiated somewhere other than the sinoatrial node.
5. **P wave–QRS complex relationship.** A constant timing relationship between P waves and the QRS complexes is found in most regular SVTs. Atrial flutter may demonstrate a variable relationship depending on the degree of AV conduction. The presence of atrioventricular dissociation would indicate a ventricular tachyarrhythmia.
6. After you examine the characteristics of a particular SVT, it is then helpful to classify the arrhythmia based on the mechanisms used to sustain it.
   a. **Atrial flutter.** Atrial flutter involves a reentry circuit localized entirely within the atrial myocardium. The atrial rate is typically

250–400 bpm. Coarse, saw-toothed "flutter waves" are usually visible in the inferior leads. The ventricular rate depends on conduction in the AV node and is usually 1:2 or 1:3 of the atrial rate. If AV conduction is rapid, and the atrial flutter waves are therefore hard to see, carotid sinus massage will transiently decrease AV node conduction and allow a better view of the baseline or the saw-toothed pattern of the ECG. Atrial flutter can be irregular or regular, depending on whether the conduction through the AV node is variable or constant. Atrial flutter can be seen with rheumatic heart disease or ischemic heart disease; with recent cardiac surgery, as part of the postpericardiotomy syndrome; in cardiomyopathy of various causes; and in atrial septal defect, acute PE, mitral or tricuspid valve disease, thyrotoxicosis, ethanol abuse, and pericarditis.

b. **Atrial fibrillation.** Atrial fibrillation is a rhythm that involves many disorganized atrial electrical circuits leading to chaotic atrial depolarizations. It is characterized by an atrial rate of 350–600 bpm. Distinct P waves are not visible. The ventricular rate is classically described as "irregularly irregular" and is controlled by the rate of conduction of the atrial impulses through the AV node. Ventricular rates are commonly 100–160 bpm in the untreated patient. Carotid sinus massage will temporarily decrease AV node conduction and slow the ventricular rate to allow the baseline to be better seen. Predisposing conditions are similar to those for atrial flutter.

c. **Automatic supraventricular tachycardias.** These tachycardias develop because of abnormally enhanced automaticity in the atrial myocardium or bundle of His.

   i. **Paroxysmal atrial tachycardia with block.** This tachycardia is usually related to digoxin toxicity and therefore occurs in patients with some type of organic heart disease. Enhanced automaticity in the atrial myocardium is the most likely mechanism. Hypokalemia may cause this arrhythmia. There is organized, visible atrial activity, although the P wave axis is different from normal P wave axis in sinus rhythm. The atrial rate is typically 180–240 bpm. Conduction of the rapid atrial discharges through the AV node is partially suppressed by digitalis, resulting in the intermittent AV block.

   ii. **Automatic atrioventricular junctional tachycardia.** The mechanism of this tachycardia is incompletely understood. It is generally attributed to increased automaticity of the pacemaker cells in the AV node. This tachycardia rarely occurs without underlying cardiac disease. It can be seen in digitalis intoxication, in acute inferior or posterior myocardial infarctions, following cardiac surgery, or with viral or rheumatic myocarditis. This arrhythmia is usually benign and self-limited. The QRS complex is usually narrow and resembles that of sinus rhythm. The rate rarely exceeds 130 bpm. Atrioventricular dissociation is commonly visible; P waves are visible between QRS complexes. This arrhythmia has a gradual onset and termination.

d. **Reentrant supraventricular tachycardia.** Reentry circuits are the most common mechanism sustaining regular SVTs. Reentry requires myocardium with differing degrees of refractoriness in order to maintain the electrical circuit. These reentry circuits are located within the AV node, the atrial myocardium, or the sinus node; or involve both the atria and ventricles in the case of accessory conduction pathways.

   i. **AV nodal reentry tachycardia.** This is the most common type of reentrant tachycardia, accounting for up to 30% of all SVTs. The reentry circuit usually consists of a slowly conducting antegrade AV nodal pathway and a rapidly conducting retrograde AV nodal pathway. This arrhythmia is characterized by the presence of normal QRS complexes at a regular rate between 150 and 250 bpm. P waves are usually not visible. The onset and termination of the tachycardia are usually abrupt. Carotid sinus massage or vagal maneuvers may result in the abrupt termination of the tachyarrhythmia.

   ii. **Atrioventricular reciprocating tachycardia.** This tachyarrhythmia, also known by the eponym Wolff-Parkinson-White syndrome, involves an accessory conduction pathway between the atria and the ventricles. The QRS complex is usually narrow during tachycardia because antegrade conduction moves through the AV node, and the accessory pathway is conducting the ventricular electrical activity retrograde to the atria. Heart rates may exceed 200 bpm. During sinus rhythm, a "delta" wave, representing ventricular pre-excitation, may be visible as a slurring of the upstroke of the QRS complex. This also results in an abnormally short PR interval (< 0.12 seconds). This tachyarrhythmia may account for up to 20% of all supraventricular tachycardias. P waves may be present inside the QRS complex, or in the QT interval. The P waves will have an abnormal axis reflective of the retrograde atrial depolarization.

e. **SVTs of uncertain mechanism.** *Multifocal atrial tachycardia* is an arrhythmia characterized by the presence of multiple foci of atrial depolarization, resulting in more than one P wave morphology. This arrhythmia is found most commonly with chronic pulmonary disease and pulmonary hypertension. The ventricular rhythm is usually irregular as a result of variable conduction through the AV node. The QRS complexes are generally normal. The ventricular rate can range from 100 to 140 bpm.

C. **Ventricular arrhythmias**

1. **Accelerated idioventricular rhythm (AIVR).** This is a rhythm of ventricular origin with a rate of 50–100 bpm. It can be seen with digitalis intoxication or acute myocardial infarction, as well as in otherwise healthy individuals. It is a common arrhythmia seen in patients given reperfusion therapy for acute myocardial infarction, where it is considered an indicator of successful coronary reperfusion. Most AIVRs are benign, except those associated with digitalis intoxication. Onset and termination are gradual. AIVRs do not usually result in hemodynamic collapse. The QRS complexes are wide, consistent with the ventricular origin of the arrhythmia. AIVRs can be recognized by the appearance of a monomorphic ventricular rhythm that appears to overtake a slower sinus rhythm; P waves and fusion beats are frequently visible. No specific therapy is necessary, unless digitalis intoxication is present. If hypotension does result from the AIVR, use of atropine to raise the sinus node rate will usually terminate this arrhythmia and restore hemodynamic stability.
2. **Ventricular tachycardia (VT).** These arrhythmias are characterized by a cardiac rhythm with wide QRS complexes and heart rates of 70–250 bpm. They usually compromise blood pressure and are a common cause of sudden cardiac death. Electrocardiographic criteria suggesting a ventricular arrhythmia, as opposed to a wide-complex supraventricular arrhythmia, include the following: (1) a QRS duration > 0.14 seconds; (2) the presence of fusion and capture beats; (3) identification of P waves in the baseline of the ECG, suggesting AV dissociation; and (4) a QRS morphology that appears similar to isolated premature ventricular contractions seen prior to the initiation of sustained VT. A *fusion beat* is a hybrid beat, in which a beat originating in the atrium fuses with one originating in the ventricle. Ventricular tachycardia is invariably associated with organic heart disease, especially coronary artery disease following myocardial infarction, and cardiomyopathies with impaired left ventricular function. The mechanism behind most ventricular tachyarrhythmias involves a reentry circuit located within the ventricular myocardium. There is usually an abnormality of impulse conduction, with a region of normally conducting myocardium located adjacent to a region of slowly conducting myocardium, frequently involving a section of scarred or fibrotic tissue. These areas of slow conduction are the myocardial substrate needed to maintain a reentry electrical circuit. This region of slowly conducting myocardium produces low-amplitude, high-frequency after-depolarizations that help to maintain the reentry circuit. These after-depolarizations are visible on signal-averaged electrocardiograms (SAECG).
3. **Ventricular fibrillation (VF).** This is the most common arrhythmia in cardiac arrest patients. Coronary artery disease is the major underlying etiology. Death is certain unless rapid and immediate

electrical defibrillation is instituted. If resuscitation efforts are successful, further investigation is indicated, as recurrence rates are as high as 30% during the first year. Invasive electrophysiologic studies are helpful in finding the patients who are at highest risk for recurrence of VT or VF; these studies have proven to be useful in guiding long-term therapy.

4. **Torsades de pointes.** This is a distinctive form of polymorphic ventricular tachycardia. This arrhythmia is uniquely characterized by a basic variation in the electrical polarity of the QRS complex, such that the QRS complexes appear to be twisting around an isoelectric baseline. Multiple leads may be necessary to accurately visualize the changes in the electrical polarity. The rate of the tachyarrhythmia can range from 150 to 280 bpm. Variation in the R–R interval is commonly seen. Spontaneous termination and recurrences are common. Torsades de pointes can occasionally progress to a sustained ventricular arrhythmia. The electrocardiographic abnormality that is the hallmark of this tachyarrhythmia is a prolonged corrected QT interval during sinus rhythm $>$ 0.50 seconds. This tachyarrhythmia is seen in quinidine and procainamide toxicity.

IV. Database

A. Physical examination key points

1. **Vital signs.** Hypotension requires rapid action. Palpation of carotid, brachial, or femoral pulses can give the examiner a rapid estimate of the adequacy of systolic pressure.
2. **Neck.** Distended jugular veins are present with acute decompensation of congestive heart failure, exacerbations of chronic pulmonary disease, pneumothorax, and pericardial tamponade. The presence of cannon "A" waves in the jugular venous pulsations suggests the presence of AV dissociation.
3. **Chest.** Rales and wheezes can be present in many of the associated cardiopulmonary diseases that predispose to tachyarrhythmias.
4. **Heart.** Listen in particular for S_3 or S_4 heart sounds or a murmur that might suggest mitral valve disease.
5. **Abdomen.** Localized or rebound tenderness pinpoint a source of infection as the cause of the tachyarrhythmia.
6. **Extremities.** Examine for signs of peripheral perfusion as an assessment of the adequacy of cardiac output.

B. Laboratory data

1. **Serum electrolytes.** Hypokalemia and hypomagnesemia can be responsible for sustained arrhythmias, particularly in patients taking digoxin. Both supraventricular and ventricular arrhythmias can result from potassium and magnesium deficiencies.
2. **Arterial blood gases.** Severe disturbances of acid–base status can be responsible for the initiation of tachyarrhythmias.

3. **Hemogram.** An elevated white blood cell count with a left shift suggests the presence of an infection.
4. **Thyroid function studies.** Check in order to exclude hyperthyroidism as a cause of an SVT.
5. **Serum drug levels.** In particular, digoxin, theophylline, and antiarrhythmic drug levels should be checked in patients with new onset of a sustained tachyarrhythmia.

C. **Electrocardiogram and rhythm strip.** A 12-lead ECG is the most important piece of diagnostic information in a patient with acute onset of sustained ventricular tachyarrhythmia. It should be obtained prior to initiating therapy as long as the patient's condition allows the extra time. Otherwise you will have to rely on a single-lead rhythm strip recorded from the cardiac monitor to direct therapy. Examine the ECG for the presence of visible P waves, fusion or capture beats, and their relationship to the QRS complexes, the rate and regularity of the rhythm, and the width of the QRS complexes. If a baseline ECG is available, look for prolongation of the QT interval.

V. **Plan.** A discussion of definitive or long-term therapy of tachyarrhythmias is not within the scope of this book. The reader is referred to the reference edited by Horowitz for an in-depth explanation of the use of antiarrhythmic medications, radiofrequency ablative procedures, automatic implantable cardioverter defibrillators, and anti-tachycardia pacemakers. The present discussion will deal primarily with the use of medications for acute treatment of sustained tachyarrhythmias.

A. **Treat any underlying predisposing conditions.** Correction of serum electrolyte imbalances is essential. Therefore, treatment with IV potassium and magnesium when appropriate may help prevent further episodes of sustained tachyarrhythmias related to these electrolyte disturbances. Administration of supplemental oxygen may be helpful in the hypoxic patient. If acute digitalis intoxication is responsible for the presence of a life-threatening recurrent tachyarrhythmia, consider treating the patient with digoxin immune Fab fragments (Digibind). The dose is based on the amount of digoxin acutely ingested or the serum digoxin concentration and body weight. See dosing charts provided with the drug.

B. **Synchronized electrical cardioversion.** If a tachyarrhythmia is responsible for causing an acute unstable episode of congestive heart failure, acute myocardial ischemia, or hemodynamic collapse, the quickest and most appropriate therapy for the termination of the tachyarrhythmia is synchronized electrical cardioversion. If the patient remains conscious during the tachycardia, it is appropriate to administer an intravenous sedative such as midazolam (Versed) prior to electrical cardioversion. Ventricular fibrillation may result if the electrical shock is not synchronized to the R wave in cases of

SVT and VT. Most SVTs can be terminated using 50–100 joules, and most ventricular tachyarrhythmias respond to 100–200 joules. ***Caution:*** Electrical cardioversion is contraindicated in cases of digitalis toxicity, and will not be helpful if used for sinus tachycardia.

C. **Carotid sinus massage.** This maneuver can be very helpful in establishing the diagnosis of many supraventricular tachycardias, and can result in the termination of some tachycardias, such as AV nodal reentry tachycardia. Carotid sinus massage or other maneuvers that raise vagal tone, like Valsalva's or Mueller's maneuver, should be tried first when you are treating an episode of SVT, as long as the patient's condition will allow the time. Vagal maneuvers should be repeated after each pharmacologic agent is administered until the arrhythmia stops. Carotid sinus massage should be done in a monitored setting because of the potential of inducing symptomatic bradycardia or sinus arrest in the case of hypersensitive carotid sinus syndrome.

D. **Medications**

1. **Adenosine (Adenocard).** The electrophysiologic effects of adenosine include a negative chronotropic action on the sinus node and a negative dromotropic effect on the AV node. Adenosine is helpful in the management of paroxysmal supraventricular tachycardias caused by a reentry circuit involving the AV node. Adenosine has also been used to diagnose the mechanism of a particular tachycardia, and occasionally to differentiate supraventricular tachycardias with aberrant conduction from VTs. Adenosine (6 mg) is administered as a rapid intravenous dose. The onset of action is 10–30 seconds, and its therapeutic effect lasts for only 60–90 seconds. If the initial dose does not terminate the tachycardia, a second bolus of 12 mg is given. Conduction over accessory atrioventricular pathways is not affected. Patients with unstable bronchial asthma should not receive intravenous adenosine. Patients with atrioventricular reciprocating tachycardias (Wolff-Parkinson-White syndrome) should be watched closely, as adenosine may induce atrial fibrillation, which could lead to acceleration of the tachyarrhythmia and subsequent cardiac arrest. Dipyridamole, cardiac glycosides, verapamil, and benzodiazepines can potentiate the electrophysiologic effects of adenosine. Therefore, the initial dose should be reduced for patients taking these medications. Aminophylline antagonizes the actions of adenosine, and therefore higher doses may be required.
2. **Amiodarone (Cordarone).** Indicated for VT, cardiac arrest (pulseless ventricular tachycardia or ventricular fibrillation), paroxysmal supraventricular tachycardia, atrial fibrillation, atrial flutter, and junctional tachycardia. The drug of choice by most experts for cardiac arrest due to pulseless ventricular tachycardia or ventricular fibrillation. The dose for arrhythmias other than cardiac arrest is 150 mg IV over 10 minutes, followed by 1 mg/min IV over 6

hours, then 0.5 mg/min. For cardiac arrest, the dose is 300 mg IV push; may follow with a second dose of 150 mg. Follow the initial bolus (es) with a continuous infusion as above. The maximum dose is 2.2 g over 24 hours. Dilute the bolus in 20–30 mL normal saline or 5% dextrose in water.

3. **Beta-blockers (propranolol, metoprolol, esmolol).** Beta-blockers are helpful in controlling a rapid heart rate with sinus tachycardia, atrial flutter and fibrillation, automatic atrial tachycardia, and SVTs associated with digitalis intoxication. Beta-blockers should be used with caution in impaired left ventricular function or COPD. The usual intravenous dose for propranolol (Inderal) is 1–3 mg (not to exceed 1 mg/min). May repeat if necessary in 2 minutes. No additional doses should be given in less than 4 hours. Metoprolol (Lopressor) 5–15 mg is given in divided doses (administered in doses of 5 mg given at about 2-minute intervals). Esmolol (Brevibloc) 500 μg/kg is given over 1 minute followed by a continuous infusion of 50 μg/kg/min.
4. **Digoxin (Lanoxin).** Digoxin is useful in the treatment of many supraventricular tachycardias in order to control the ventricular response. It is an established drug in the treatment of atrial fibrillation or flutter. An initial dose of 0.25–0.50 mg is given IV followed by additional doses of 0.25 mg every 4–6 hours (carefully assess clinical response and signs of toxicity prior to each additional dose), for a total loading dose of 1.0 mg. Daily maintenance doses of 0.125–0.25 mg are required to sustain adequate serum levels with normal renal function. If digoxin alone does not adequately control the ventricular rate of an SVT, addition of a calcium channel blocker such as verapamil or diltiazem may be helpful.
5. **Diltiazem (Cardizem, Dilacor).** Diltiazem comes in an injectable form for the acute management of new-onset atrial fibrillation or flutter, and the treatment of acute episodes of paroxysmal supraventricular tachycardia. The initial dose is 0.25 mg/kg IV administered over 2 minutes (maximum dose 20 mg), to be repeated 0.35 mg/kg in 15 minutes if needed. The patient can then be maintained on an IV infusion of 10 mg/hr, or started on oral maintenance doses of 60–90 mg given Q 6 hr. The dose can be changed to a long-acting preparation after 24 hours. Precautions are similar to those for verapamil.
6. **Lidocaine.** Lidocaine can be used for the treatment of ventricular tachyarrhythmias that are not associated with hemodynamic collapse; however, the evidence for the use of lidocaine is poor and methodologically weak. Amiodarone and procainamide are recommended before lidocaine for the initial treatment of hemodynamically stable wide-complex tachycardia. A loading dose of 1 mg/kg is given as an IV bolus followed by a continuous infusion of 1–4 mg/min. A second loading dose of 0.5 mg/kg is recommended and should be given 5–10 minutes after the initial bolus.

Lidocaine may also be helpful in arrhythmias associated with digoxin intoxication.

7. **Magnesium.** Indicated for polymorphic ventricular tachycardia (torsades de pointes) and suspected hypomagnesemia. The dose is 1–2 g IV over 15 minutes (for hypomagnesemia) and 2 g IV over 1–2 minutes followed by 0.5–1.0 g/hr (for torsades de pointes). Dilute the bolus in 50–100 mL of 5% dextrose in water.
8. **Procainamide (Pronestyl).** Procainamide can be used to convert ventricular tachyarrhythmias. A loading dose of 15–18 mg/kg is given IV at a rate of 25 mg/min, followed by a continuous infusion of 1–4 mg/min. Hypotension can develop during loading infusions if the drug is administered at rates in excess of 25 mg/min.
9. **Verapamil (Calan).** Verapamil IV will convert approximately 90% of episodes of AV nodal reentry tachycardia to sinus rhythm. It is also helpful in the acute management of atrial flutter and fibrillation. Give an initial bolus of 2.5–10 mg IV over 2 minutes, then start an oral maintenance dose of 80- to 120-mg tablets Q 8 hr. Verapamil is not the drug of choice for patients with congestive heart failure, poor left ventricular function, or acute myocardial infarction. It should *never* be used in the treatment of wide-complex tachyarrhythmias because it will frequently worsen the patient's condition.

   Special Note: Treatment of AV reciprocating tachyarrhythmias, or Wolff-Parkinson-White syndrome, should focus on drugs that prolong the refractory period of the accessory atrioventricular pathway or of the AV node. An acute-onset tachyarrhythmia suspicious for an accessory atrioventricular pathway (normal QRS width, regular R–R interval, rate around 200 bpm, and retrograde P waves visible in ST segment) can be approached with drugs that prolong conduction in the AV node, such as adenosine, verapamil, diltiazem, or beta-blockers, or with procainamide. Procainamide is the preferred drug of choice for initial management, as it will prolong the effective refractory period of the accessory bypass pathway and other involved myocardium, and has less chance of accelerating the rate of tachycardia. Procainamide's electrophysiologic properties make this drug an excellent choice for the initial pharmacologic therapy of AV reciprocating tachycardias. Digitalis may shorten the refractory period of the accessory pathway and accelerate ventricular response in some patients with AV reciprocating tachyarrhythmias.

REFERENCES

Falk RH: Atrial fibrillation. N Engl J Med 2001;344:1067.

Horowitz LN, ed: *Current Management of Arrhythmias.* Decker;1991.

Miller JM, Zipes DP: Management of patient with cardiac arrhythmias. In: Braunwald E, Zipes DP, Libby P, eds. *Heart Disease: A Textbook of Cardiovascular Medicine.* 6th ed. Saunders;2001:700.

Wagner GS, ed: *Marriott's Practical Electrocardiography.* 9th ed. Williams & Wilkins;1994.

Wellens HJJ, Bar FWH, Lie K: The value of the electrocardiogram in the differential diagnosis of tachycardia with widened QRS complex. Am J Med 1978;64:27.

61. THROMBOCYTOPENIA

I. Problem. You are called to see a 73-year-old patient admitted to the cardiology service with unstable angina. His admission laboratory data reveal a platelet count of 32,000/μL.

II. Immediate Questions

A. Is the patient bleeding? The risk of bleeding from trauma increases with a platelet count < 50,000/μL; the risk of spontaneous bleeding increases with a platelet count < 20,000/μL.

B. Is the count real? Rule out the phenomenon of platelet clumping. Review the peripheral smear if available. Recheck the platelet count using a different anticoagulant such as citrate or heparin. Clumping can occur in some patients using the more common anticoagulant, EDTA.

C. Is there an obvious cause? Recent chemotherapy or radiation can result in decreased production of platelets. Also, an enlarged spleen can result in sequestration of platelets.

D. Is there a past history of low platelet count? Does this appear to be an acute problem such as idiopathic thrombocytopenic purpura (ITP); or is there an underlying disorder contributing to the low platelet count, such as cirrhosis with hypersplenism, chronic ITP, or perhaps an inherited disorder such as Fanconi's syndrome or Wiskott-Aldrich syndrome?

E. Is the patient on any medicines that might cause thrombocytopenia? Drug-induced thrombocytopenia is one of the most common etiologies. Many drugs can cause thrombocytopenia. Quinidine and quinine together account for the largest number of cases. Other commonly associated drugs are ethanol, sulfonamides, heparin, gold, thiazide diuretics, cimetidine (Tagamet), and captopril (Capoten).

F. Is there a history of a preceding viral infection? A viral infection days to weeks before the onset of thrombocytopenia suggests a chronic form of ITP or acute interference with normal megakaryocyte maturation.

III. Differential Diagnosis. Quantitative platelet disorders can frequently be divided into two categories: decreased production; and peripheral destruction or sequestration.

A. Pseudothrombocytopenia. Thrombocytopenia may be artifactual, particularly when relying on an automated counter. Platelet autoagglutinins may cause clumping in the presence of EDTA or may cause adherence to neutrophils.

B. Decreased production

1. **Infiltrative processes.** Leukemias (acute or chronic), carcinoma, or lymphomas crowd out the normal marrow elements, resulting in a decreased number of megakaryocytes. Infection (granulomatous disease) such as tuberculosis can cause a similar picture.
2. **Myelodysplasia (preleukemic syndrome).** This condition frequently leads to morphologically abnormal megakaryocytes and results in low platelet levels.
3. **Drugs.** Virtually any drug can be associated with thrombocytopenia either by decreasing production or by an immune mechanism. Some known myelosuppressive drugs are particularly toxic to platelet production; for example, cytosine arabinoside (ARA-C), cyclophosphamide (Cytoxan), busulfan (Myleran), methotrexate (MTX), carboplatin (Paraplatin), and interferon. Thiazide diuretics have been associated with a decreased number of megakaryocytes leading to thrombocytopenia. Thiazides may also induce platelet-directed antibodies that can lead to peripheral destruction. Thrombocytopenia is common in chronic alcoholism. Ethanol has been shown to decrease the number of megakaryocytes.
4. **Radiation.** Ionizing radiation can affect all marrow elements, frequently megakaryocytes to a lesser extent. Patients who have had therapeutic radiation to large areas of marrow can have transient thrombocytopenia, and recovery to preradiation levels may not occur.
5. **Nutrition.** Malnutritional states, such as vitamin B_{12} and folate deficiency, and occasionally iron deficiency, can lead to depressed numbers of megakaryocytes.
6. **Virus infection.** Viral illnesses such as hepatitis B, rubella, and infectious mononucleosis may cause an acute interference with normal megakaryocyte maturation.
7. **Paroxysmal nocturnal hemoglobinuria.** Can be associated with insufficient platelet production. Episodic red-brown urine occurs most often with first morning urine. Associated thrombosis especially of the hepatic and mesenteric veins.

C. Peripheral destruction

1. **Immune-mediated disorders**
   a. **Idiopathic thrombocytopenic purpura (ITP).** ITP is an autoimmune disorder and a frequent cause of thrombocytopenia. The diagnosis can be made definitively if antiplatelet antibodies can be demonstrated; however, this test is not available in all clinical labs. There are two forms of ITP:
      i. **Chronic.** Usually seen in adults.
      ii. **Acute.** More frequently seen in children; often self-limiting.
   b. **Drugs.** May also cause immune destruction; quinidine is the best known. In addition to exerting a toxic effect on megakaryo-

cytes, quinidine may act as a hapten with antibody complex adhering to the platelet, followed by complement-mediated platelet destruction. Sulfa drugs work in a similar fashion.

c. **Systemic lupus erythematosus (SLE).** Can cause autoimmune thrombocytopenia.

d. **Human immunodeficiency virus (HIV).** An ITP-like syndrome has been associated with HIV. The thrombocytopenia is caused by an IgG antibody; platelet counts may fall below 10,000/μL. The incidence increases with the severity of the disease.

2. **Infection.** Direct platelet toxicity may occur from viruses, gram-positive organisms, or the lipopolysaccharides of gram-negative bacteria. Complement, immunoglobulins, and fibrinogen may also play a role. Disseminated intravascular coagulation (DIC), frequently caused by infection, can lead to a consumptive platelet loss. Thrombocytopenia may also be seen in the absence of DIC in septicemia, as with Rocky Mountain spotted fever and malaria.
3. **Snake bite.** Thrombocytopenia may be related to DIC or direct platelet destruction.
4. **Burns.** Thrombocytopenia may be secondary to sequestration within damaged tissue and can be further aggravated by concomitant sepsis.
5. **Glomerulonephritis.** Thrombocytopenia presumably secondary to immune-mediated mechanisms.
6. **Aortic valvular stenosis.** Occasional cause of thrombocytopenia. Presumed mechanism is direct platelet injury secondary to turbulent flow.
7. **Thrombotic thrombocytopenic purpura (TTP, Moschcowitz's syndrome).** This disease is a pentad of microangiopathic hemolytic anemia, thrombocytopenia, fluctuating neurologic findings, fever, and renal dysfunction.
8. **Direct toxins to platelets.** Heparin appears to cause a direct antiplatelet factor causing aggregation (Type II heparin-induced thrombocytopenia) and can induce aggregation in the absence of antibody (Type I heparin-induced thrombocytopenia). The incidence of heparin-induced thrombocytopenia is about 5%. Heparin-induced thrombocytopenia can occur with IV or SC delivery, and with bovine or porcine heparin, but is more common with bovine. This entity is infrequently associated with thromboembolism.

D. **Sequestration.** Normally, the spleen may contain 30% of the circulating platelet pool. When the spleen is enlarged and hypersplenism ensues, up to 90% of circulating platelets may be pooled within the spleen.

IV. Database

A. **Physical examination key points.** Look for evidence of bleeding and peripheral sequestration.

1. **Vital signs.** Fever requires consideration of infectious causes as well as TTP.
2. **Skin and mucous membranes.** Are there petechiae or purpura? The lower extremities frequently reveal petechiae when petechiae may not be easily seen elsewhere. Multiple bruises out of proportion to the degree of trauma may give further evidence of quantitative or qualitative platelet defects. Look for gingival hyperplasia or skin nodules, which suggest leukemia.
3. **Heart.** Severe aortic stenosis can cause thrombocytopenia. A new murmur may indicate bacterial endocarditis.
4. **Abdomen.** Splenomegaly may be associated with thrombocytopenia resulting from sequestration. Chronic alcoholics may have evidence of portal hypertension such as dilated abdominal and chest wall veins, ascites, and splenomegaly. Splenomegaly is also seen with lymphoproliferative and myeloproliferative disorders, as well as infectious causes (eg, infectious mononucleosis and endocarditis). The lack of splenomegaly is also important to note. The presence of palpable splenomegaly makes ITP much less likely.
5. **Neurologic exam.** Fluctuating neurologic findings are frequently seen in TTP.

B. Laboratory data

1. **Peripheral blood smear.** Extremely important to review to rule out pseudothrombocytopenia. Pseudothrombocytopenia can be confirmed by obtaining a normal platelet count from heparin-anticoagulated blood. Large platelets (megathrombocytes) are frequently seen with ITP and may indicate peripheral destruction. Morphology of red blood cells may indicate DIC or TTP with a microangiopathic picture. Look for blasts as a sign of acute leukemia. The presence of left-shifted granulocytes, nucleated red blood cells, and teardrops may indicate marrow infiltration. Left-shifted granulocytes and toxic granulation are consistent with a bacterial infection.
2. **Coagulation studies.** Elevated prothrombin time, partial thromboplastin time, and thrombin time may be seen with DIC and liver disease. They are normal in ITP and TTP. A bleeding time will always be abnormal in the face of a low platelet count and is never indicated in the evaluation for thrombocytopenia.
3. **Fibrinogen and D-dimers.** A decrease in fibrinogen and an increase in D-dimers are suggestive of DIC.
4. **Antinuclear antibodies (ANA).** To rule out collagen vascular disease as a cause.
5. **BUN and creatinine.** Renal failure can cause marrow suppression of megakaryocytes and may coexist with other causes such as sepsis, DIC, and TTP.
6. **Bone marrow.** See Section III, Chapter 5, Bone Marrow Aspiration & Biopsy, p 397. This is essential in the evaluation if there is

no obvious reason for thrombocytopenia. The presence of an adequate or increased number of megakaryocytes implies peripheral destruction. Marrow infiltration or primary marrow disease can be identified with a bone marrow aspirate and biopsy (often results in decreased megakaryocytes).

7. **Liver function tests.** Total bilirubin, alkaline phosphatase, and transaminases (AST and ALT) may support viral hepatitis, alcoholic liver disease, or sepsis from a biliary source as the cause.

C. Radiologic and other studies

1. **CT scan of the abdomen.** May demonstrate hepatosplenomegaly or lymphadenopathy in indicated situations.
2. **Liver/spleen scan.** Demonstrates splenomegaly in questionable cases, and also indicates hepatic dysfunction and findings consistent with portal hypertension.
3. **Platelet antibodies.** Much variability exists among the techniques for various assays. A negative antiplatelet antibody study does not rule out the presence of antiplatelet antibodies.

V. Plan

A. Bleeding. Initially, it is important to determine if there is life-threatening bleeding, in which case platelet transfusion is indicated. (See Section V, Blood Component Therapy, p 437). If there is no active bleeding and the thrombocytopenia is immunologic, platelet transfusions are to be avoided. In this situation, transfusions are frequently ineffective and may actually worsen the thrombocytopenia with further immunologic challenge.

B. Immune-mediated destruction. If this is suspected, all nonessential medicines should be stopped. Do not overlook heparin flush from catheters and Hep-Locks, as well as heparin-banded central venous catheters.

C. Treatment of underlying cause. Especially for leukemias, lymphomas, infections, and DIC.

D. ITP

1. **High-dose steroids (1–2 mg/kg prednisone) daily is the treatment for ITP.** IV immunoglobulins can also be used in steroid-unresponsive ITP or if steroids are contraindicated.
2. **Splenectomy** may be required in chronic ITP that is unresponsive to steroids or immunoglobulins. If the platelet count is consistently > 50,000/µL, close observation may be best, depending on the underlying medical condition(s).

E. TTP

1. **Plasmapheresis.** Considered standard treatment though the mechanism of action is unknown. May be related to removal of an offending agent or replacement of missing factor(s).
2. **High-dose prednisone.** Frequently used treatment; however, there is no proven benefit.

F. **Prophylactic platelet transfusion.** May be indicated with myeloproliferative disorders or bone marrow suppression from myelotoxic drugs. Frequently, transfusions are given for platelet counts < 20,000/μL. Three units per meter squared, or approximately six units, should give an adequate increment in most adults. Pheresed or single-donor platelets are often given to those who require repeated transfusion to decrease donor exposure and risk of developing antibodies. Repeated transfusion may cause alloimmunization, with resultant smaller increments after transfusion. Human leukocyte antigen–matched platelets will increase platelet survival, and are indicated in patients receiving multiple platelet transfusions who have a suboptimal response.

G. **Chemotherapy-related thrombocytopenia.** Oprelvekin (Neumega), a recombinant human interleukin-2, may be used for prevention of severe thrombocytopenia and decrease the need for platelet transfusion following myelosuppressive chemotherapy in nonmyeloid malignancies. The usual dose is 50 μg/kg SC every day and is initiated 6–24 hours after completion of chemotherapy and continued 14–21 days or until the postnadir platelet count is at least 50,000/μL. Discontinue at least 2 days before the next chemotherapy cycle.

REFERENCES

Beutler E: Platelet transfusions: The 20,000/microliter trigger. Blood 1993;81:1411.

George JN: Drug-induced thrombocytopenia: A systemic review of published case reports. Ann Intern Med 1998;129:886.

George JN, Rizvi MA: Thrombocytopenia. In: Beutler E, Lichtman MA, Coller BS et al, eds. *William's Hematology.* 6th ed. McGraw-Hill;2001:1495.

Rodgers G: Thrombocytopenia. In: Kjeldsberg C, ed. *Practical Diagnosis of Hematologic Disorders.* 3rd ed. ASCP Press;2000:739.

62. TRANSFUSION REACTION

(See also Section V, Blood Component Therapy, p 437).

I. **Problem.** During a transfusion of packed red blood cells (PRBCs), the patient's temperature rises to 38.5°C (101.3°F).

II. **Immediate Questions.** Fever is a common complication of transfusion and is a sign of transfusion reaction. Transfusion reactions are categorized into broad categories of noninfectious versus infectious complications and may be either mild febrile nonhemolytic transfusion reactions that are self-limited or severe life-threatening hemolytic reactions. Your initial assessment will be directed at differentiating among these.

A. **What are the patient's vital signs?** Presenting signs and symptoms of fever and chills, tachycardia, and tachypnea are nonspecific and will not allow you to differentiate reliably between a self-limited and a life-threatening transfusion reaction. Hypotension suggests a severe hemolytic transfusion reaction.

B. Does the patient have any complaints? Fever, frequently accompanied by shaking chills, may be the only clinical symptom of a febrile nonhemolytic transfusion reaction. However, severe acute hemolytic reactions are often accompanied by other symptoms, including nausea, vomiting, headache, and back pain. Often patients will experience bronchospasm and pulmonary edema.

C. Is there any evidence of generalized bleeding from mucosal membranes, previous venipuncture sites, or the present IV site? Diffuse bleeding would be consistent with disseminated intravascular coagulation (DIC); it suggests a severe, life-threatening hemolytic reaction.

D. Has the patient ever had a transfusion before? If so, has she or he ever reacted to blood products in the past? Patients who have prior histories of a transfusion are likely to have become alloimmunized to blood group antigens. Patients with a prior history of febrile reactions to transfusion likely have cytotoxic or agglutinating antibodies to HLA antigens present on granulocytes, lymphocytes, and platelets. Although these reactions are troublesome, they are typically self-limited.

E. Most important, does the name on the unit of packed cells match that on the patient's armband? Most fatal acute hemolytic transfusion reactions result from transfusion of ABO-incompatible blood. This is frequently the result of human error in patient or specimen identification occurring during situations of high stress.

III. Differential Diagnosis

A. Hemolytic transfusion reaction

1. **Severe sequelae from a hemolytic transfusion reaction.** Occur even when a small volume of incompatible blood is transfused. If there is concern that a patient may be experiencing a severe reaction, the transfusion must be stopped immediately. If the label on the transfusion unit of blood does not match that on the patient's armband, the blood bank should be notified immediately for assistance.
2. **Transfusion of ABO-incompatible blood results in intravascular hemolysis.** The naturally occurring anti-A or anti-B antibodies activate the classical complement pathway, resulting in membrane lysis and a liberation of free hemoglobin within the bloodstream. Fever, hypotension, shock, and renal failure may result.

B. Self-limiting febrile transfusion reaction. This reaction is not hemolytic. It often occurs in patients who have had numerous transfusions or in multiparous women. Although this type of reaction often results in interruption of the transfusion, if no further symptoms develop the transfusion may be restarted.

C. Transfusion of blood contaminated with microorganisms. This is an infrequent transfusion reaction. Blood contaminated by cold-growing organisms such as *Pseudomonas* should be considered.

D. Delayed hemolytic reaction. Should be suspected if a post-transfusion hemoglobin level cannot be maintained several days after the transfusion. Mild jaundice and fever with or without chills should alert the clinician to the possibility of a delayed hemolytic transfusion reaction. Many of these reactions are not detected because patients have been discharged from the hospital. The serologic findings of a delayed hemolytic transfusion reaction include a positive direct Coombs' test. The previously alloimmunized patient may not have had detectable antibody levels in his or her routine pretransfusion antibody screening study. However, after reexposure to the relevant antigen, an amnestic response to the transfused RBCs occurs. IgG antibody alone or IgG with complement may then be detected. A single antibody or multiple antibodies may be involved. The antibodies most often implicated are directed against Rh, Kidd, Duffy, or Kell antigens. Because the antibody titer may again drop to undetectable levels, a chart notation or Medic Alert card may prevent future reactions with known antibodies. Delayed hemolytic transfusion reactions are generally regarded as mild.

IV. Database

A. Physical examination key points

1. **Vital signs.** If the constellation of hypotension, fever, and tachycardia is present, the transfusion reaction must be considered to be a severe hemolytic reaction.
2. **Skin and mucous membranes.** Generalized bleeding may be part of a severe hemolytic reaction.
3. **Chest.** Wheezing or rales is consistent with a life-threatening reaction.

B. Laboratory data

1. **Hemogram.** May point to contaminated blood or show evidence of hemolysis.
2. **Prothrombin time, partial thromboplastin time, thrombin time, fibrinogen, and fibrin split products.** To rule out DIC.
3. **Peripheral smear.** Look for schistocytes as evidence for DIC.
4. **Urine for hemoglobinuria.** Supports the diagnosis of a severe transfusion reaction.
5. **Serum for free hemoglobin.** If positive, indicates hemolysis.
6. **Post-transfusion direct antiglobulin testing.** A negative study in the absence of serum-free hemoglobin supports that an acute hemolytic transfusion has not occurred.
7. **Gram's stain of remaining untransfused blood.** To rule out bacterial contamination of the unit.

V. **Plan.** The treatment plan depends on the type of reaction.

A. **Severe hemolytic reaction**

1. If a serious transfusion reaction is suspected, the transfusion should be stopped immediately.
2. **Supportive care** including IV fluids. The patient should be closely monitored for hypotension and decreasing urine output. If oliguria occurs, diuretics and mannitol may be required. A renal dose of dopamine (5 mcg/kg/min) may be considered as well. If physical signs and laboratory findings indicate DIC, administration of platelets and cryoprecipitate is recommended.

B. **Self-limiting febrile transfusion reactions.** The findings of isolated fever and chills with a previous history of a febrile reaction support the diagnosis of a self-limiting febrile transfusion reaction. Antihistamines and antipruritics may be administered. Meperidine (Demerol) may be used for patients experiencing severe shaking chills. After premedication, transfusion may be safely resumed. Steps to prevent this type of reaction in the future include decreasing the granulocytes in the transfused unit. Leukofiltration and premedication are indicated for future transfusions.

C. **Transfusion of blood contaminated with microorganisms.** If this is suspected, broad-spectrum antibiotics should be instituted.

REFERENCES

Andreu G, Dewailly J, Leberre C et al: Prevention of HLA immunization with leukocyte-poor packed red cells and platelet concentrates obtained by filtration. Blood 1988;72:964.

Brittingham TE, Chaplin H Jr: Febrile transfusion reaction caused sensitivity to donor leukocytes and platelets. JAMA 1957;165:819.

Brubaker DB: Clinical significance of white cell antibodies in febrile nonhemolytic transfusion reactions. Transfusion 1990;30:733.

Jeter EK, Spivey MA: Noninfectious complications of blood transfusion. Hematol Oncol Clin North Am 1995;9:187.

Sazama K: Reports of 355 transfusion associated deaths: 1976–1985. Transfusion 1990;30:583.

63. WHEEZING

I. **Problem.** You are asked to evaluate a patient recently admitted with chest pain who develops respiratory distress and wheezing.

II. **Immediate Questions**

A. **What are the vital signs?** A respiratory rate greater than 30/min may indicate the need for immediate treatment. Associated hypotension may suggest an anaphylactic reaction, an acute myocardial infarction (MI) with pulmonary edema, or a pulmonary embolism (PE). Fever may point to an underlying infection, PE, or MI.

B. **Were any diagnostic tests recently performed or medicines administered?** A beta-blocker may precipitate an acute attack of bronchospasm when given to a patient with stable or undiagnosed asthma. Wheezing after the administration of a drug such as penicillin or radiocontrast dye suggests an anaphylactic reaction.

C. **Why was the patient admitted?** Acute pulmonary edema may accompany an MI, and aspiration can result from gastric outlet obstruction secondary to a gastric ulcer.

D. **Is there a history of asthma?** Childhood asthma may reactivate at any age, given the right stimuli.

E. **Does the patient have any allergies to medications or other substances such as shellfish?** It is prudent to inquire about known allergies.

III. Differential Diagnosis

A. Diffuse wheezing

1. **Acute bronchospasm.** May be caused by asthma, exacerbation of chronic obstructive pulmonary disease (COPD), or an anaphylactic reaction.
2. **Aspiration.** May trigger bronchospasm from mucosal irritation or from impacted foreign bodies.
3. **Cardiogenic pulmonary edema.** The primary finding in "cardiac asthma" may be wheezing. Other findings of pulmonary edema should be present, and the chest x-ray will be diagnostic.
4. **Pulmonary embolism (PE).** Mediators may be released that cause not only hypoxemia but also transient bronchospasm.

B. Stridor (upper airway wheezing)

1. **Laryngospasm.** This may be part of an anaphylactic reaction or secondary to aspiration.
2. **Laryngeal or tracheal tumor.** A history of dysphagia, hoarseness, cough, or weight loss and anorexia may be present.
3. **Epiglottitis.** The patient is often unable to speak or to swallow secretions. The mouth is held open and there may be drooling. (Similar presentation may occur with Ludwig's angina or an abscess involving the floor of the mouth.)
4. **Foreign body aspiration**
5. **Vocal cord dysfunction.** Bilaterally paralyzed vocal cords may result in severe stridor and dyspnea. A subgroup of patients has recently been recognized to have "factitious asthma": they voluntarily adduct their vocal cords for psychogenic reasons.

C. Localized wheezing

1. **Tumors.** May obstruct one bronchus, leading to localized wheezing.
2. **Mucous plugging**
3. **Aspirated foreign body**

IV. Database

A. Physical examination key points. Localization of wheezing allows categorization, as outlined in the differential diagnosis (III.).

1. **Vital signs.** A fever may indicate an infectious etiology. A pulsus paradoxus greater than 16 mm Hg indicates severe respiratory distress. Hypotension requires immediate assessment and action.
2. **HEENT.** Check the mouth carefully. Examine the neck for angioedema—which may be precipitated by angiotensin-converting enzyme (ACE) inhibitors. Palpate the sternocleidomastoid muscles to assess accessory muscle use in obstructive lung diseases. Auscultate over the mouth and larynx in an effort to localize the wheezing.
3. **Chest.** Carefully auscultate for localized wheezing. Listen for bibasilar rales, which may be present in pulmonary edema. Rales, increased fremitus, and egophony suggest pneumonia.
4. **Heart.** Check carefully for evidence of an S_3 gallop or jugular venous distension, which points to cardiogenic pulmonary edema.
5. **Extremities.** Clubbing may indicate underlying lung cancer. Cyanosis indicates underlying hypoxemia. Edema may signify chronic congestive heart failure.
6. **Skin.** Urticaria suggests an acute allergic reaction. A malar rash points toward acute systemic lupus erythematosus, which can present with acute pneumonitis.

B. Laboratory data

1. **Arterial blood gases.** An elevated $PaCO_2$ indicates significant ventilatory failure. Hypoxemia is commonly present during bronchospasm because of $\dot{V}/\dot{Q}$ mismatch. It may worsen after beta-agonist aerosols.
2. **Complete blood count.** An increased white blood cell count may indicate an underlying infection; however, an increase in WBCs without a left shift can be seen with an acute MI or PE. Eosinophilia suggests an allergic or asthmatic etiology to the wheezing.

C. Radiologic and other studies

1. **Electrocardiogram.** An ECG may show an acute MI or ischemia. Occasionally it will be suggestive of a PE, showing an S wave in lead I, a Q wave in III, T wave inversion in lead III ($S_1Q_3T_3$), new right bundle branch block (RBBB), and right-axis shift. It may also show a change in rhythm.
2. **Chest radiograph.** A PE (with infarction) severe enough to cause wheezing may be evident on the chest film. Look for a pleural-based, wedge-shaped lesion (*Hampton's hump*) or localized oligemia of the pulmonary arteries. Kerley B lines, bilateral pleural effusions, vascular redistribution, and cardiomegaly may suggest congestive heart failure. Look for localized infiltrates or masses suggesting other causes.

V. Plan.

Treatment depends on the diagnosis. The preceding differential diagnoses and studies should enable you to form a tentative categorization on which to base initial therapy.

A. **Bronchospasm (asthma, COPD, allergic reaction)**
   1. **Methylprednisolone (Solu-Medrol).** Give 40–80 mg IV stat dose, then 40 mg Q 6 hr.
   2. **Nebulized albuterol.** Give 0.5 mL of 0.5% solution (2.5 mg) in 2.5 mL normal saline stat and Q 20 minutes for 3 doses, then Q 1–4 hours as needed. Alternatively, four puffs albuterol MDI via spacer device may be given Q 20 minutes up to 4 hours (12 doses), then Q 1–4 hours as needed.

B. **Stridor**
   1. **Methylprednisolone 40 mg IV stat dose**
   2. **Nebulized racemic epinephrine.** Give 0.5 mL in 3 mL normal saline.
   3. **Continuous positive airway pressure (CPAP).** Give 10–15 cm H_2O applied continuously; if ventilatory failure is suspected, consider bidirectional positive airway pressure (BiPAP) instead at 15/10 cm H_2O.
   4. **Intubation or tracheostomy.** If there is no response to the above measures.

C. **Pulmonary edema**
   1. **Furosemide (Lasix) 20–80 mg IV**
   2. **Nitroglycerin.** Give 0.4 mg sublingually, or paste ½ in. on skin, or nitroglycerin drip 10–20 mcg/min and increase by 5–10 mcg Q 10 minutes.
   3. **Afterload reduction.** Use agents such as intravenous nitroprusside (Nipride), or oral agents such as captopril (Capoten) or enalapril (Vasotec), or any other ACE inhibitor.
   4. **Intravenous morphine.** For venodilation and to relieve anxiety. Morphine may suppress respiratory drive and cause further respiratory compromise, necessitating intubation.
   5. **Oxygen.** Start with 100% O_2 by non-rebreather mask, as long as the patient is not a carbon dioxide retainer.
   6. **CPAP (10 cm) or BiPAP (12/8 cm).** Recently proven efficacious in acute pulmonary edema.

D. **Miscellaneous disorders.** Treatment varies with the disease. PE should be treated with anticoagulants (see Section I, Chapter 11, Chest Pain, V, p 63). Suspected tumors require additional tests such as bronchoscopy before reasonable treatment can be initiated.

REFERENCES

Aboussouan LS, Stoller JK: Diagnosis and management of upper airway obstruction. Clin Chest Med 1994;15:35.

Leatherman J: Life-threatening asthma. Clin Chest Med 1994;15:453.

NHLBI Expert Panel Report 2: *Guidelines for the Diagnosis and Management of Asthma.* NIH Publication # 97-4051; April 1997.

II. Laboratory Diagnosis

Notes: The ranges of normal values are given below each test, first in conventional units such as metric (eg, milligrams per liter), and then in international units if there is a difference. Reference ranges for each laboratory may vary from the values given; therefore, you should interpret the results of a patient's laboratory value in light of an individual facility's range.

■ ACID-FAST STAIN

Positive: *Mycobacterium* species (tuberculosis and atypical mycobacteria such as *M avium-intracellulare*), *Nocardia.*

■ ACTH (ADRENOCORTICOTROPIC HORMONE)

8 am: 20–100 pg/mL or 20–100 ng/L; midnight value: ~ 50% of am value.

Increased: Addison's disease; ectopic ACTH production (small cell carcinoma, pancreatic islet cell tumors, thymic tumors, renal cell carcinoma).

Decreased: Adrenal adenoma or carcinoma, nodular adrenal hyperplasia, pituitary insufficiency.

■ ACTH STIMULATION TEST

Used to help diagnose adrenal insufficiency. Cosyntropin (Cortrosyn), an ACTH analogue, is given at a dose of 0.25 mg IM or IV. Collect blood at times 0, 30, and 60 minutes for cortisol.

Normal response: Basal cortisol of at least 5 μg/dL, an increase of at least 7 μg/dL, and a final cortisol of 16 μg/dL at 30 minutes or 18 μg/dL at 60 minutes.

Subnormal/abnormal response: Addison's disease (primary adrenal insufficiency) and secondary adrenal insufficiency: Secondary insufficiency is caused by pituitary insufficiency or suppression by exogenous steroids. An ACTH level and pituitary stimulation tests can be used to differentiate primary from secondary adrenal insufficiency.

■ ALBUMIN, SERUM

3.5–5.0 g/dL or 35–50 g/L.

Decreased: Malnutrition, nephrotic syndrome, cystic fibrosis, multiple myeloma, Hodgkin's disease, leukemia, protein-losing enteropathies, chronic glomerulonephritis, cirrhosis, inflammatory bowel disease, collagen-vascular diseases, hyperthyroidism.

■ ALBUMIN, URINE

Normal = < 30 mg/d.

Microalbuminuria 30–300 mg/d (a sign of early renal damage in diabetes mellitus; presence helps identify patients at risk for renal failure, neuropathy, retinopathy, and coronary artery disease. Renal function may be preserved with the use of an angiotensin-converting enzyme [ACE] inhibitor). Microalbuminuria can be detected by determining the albumin to creatinine ratio by obtaining a spot urine for albumin and creatinine. Normal is < 30 μg of albumin per milligram of creatinine, and microalbuminuria is defined as 30–300 μg of albumin per milligram of creatinine.

Note: Microalbuminuria can be seen with prolonged exercise, hematuria, fever, or prolonged upright posture.

Nephrotic proteinuria > 3.5 gm/d.

■ ALDOSTERONE

Serum—supine: 3–10 g/dL or 0.083–0.28 nmol/L early am, normal sodium intake; upright: 5–30 g/dL or 0.138–0.83 nmol/L.

Urinary—2–16 μg/24 hr or 5.4–44.3 nmol/d.

Increased: Hyperaldosteronism (primary or secondary). Should confirm after oral or IV salt loading.

Decreased: Adrenal insufficiency.

■ ALKALINE PHOSPHATASE

Adult 20–70 U/L.

A γ-glutamyltransferase (GGT) is often useful to differentiate whether an elevated alkaline phosphatase has its origin from bone or liver. A normal GGT suggests bone origin.

Increased: Increased calcium deposition in bone (hyperparathyroidism), Paget's disease, osteoblastic bone tumors, osteomalacia, pregnancy, childhood, liver disease, and hyperthyroidism.

Decreased: Malnutrition, excess vitamin D ingestion.

■ ALPHA-FETOPROTEIN (AFP)

< 30 ng/mL or < 30 μg/L

Increased: Hepatoma, testicular tumor (embryonal carcinoma, malignant teratoma), spina bifida (in mother's serum).

■ ALT (ALANINE AMINOTRANSFERASE) (SGPT: SERUM GLUTAMIC-PYRUVIC TRANSFERASE)

8–20 U/L.

Increased: Liver disease–liver metastases, biliary obstruction, liver congestion, hepatitis (ALT is more elevated than AST in viral hepatitis; AST is more elevated than ALT in alcoholic hepatitis).

■ AMMONIA

Arterial: 15–45 μg/dL or 11–32 μmol N/L.

Increased: Hepatic encephalopathy, Reye's syndrome.

■ AMYLASE

25–125 U/L.

Increased: Acute pancreatitis, pancreatic duct obstruction (stones, stricture, tumor, sphincter of Oddi spasm), alcohol ingestion, mumps, parotiditis, renal disease, macroamylasemia, cholecystitis, peptic ulcers, intestinal obstruction, mesenteric thrombosis, after surgery (upper abdominal), ovarian cancer, ruptured ectopic pregnancy, and diabetic ketoacidosis.

Decreased: Pancreatic destruction (pancreatitis, cystic fibrosis), liver disease (hepatitis, cirrhosis).

■ ANION GAP

8–12 mmol/L.

Note: The anion gap is a calculated estimate of unmeasured anions and is used to help differentiate the cause of metabolic acidosis.

$$\text{Anion gap} = (Na^+) - (Cl^- + HCO_3^-)$$

Increased (High): (> 12 mmol/L): Lactic acidosis, ketoacidosis (diabetic, alcoholic, starvation); uremia; toxins (salicylates, methanol, ethylene glycol, paraldehyde). In addition, dehydration, alkalosis, use of certain penicillins (carbenicillin), and salts of strong acids such as sodium citrate (used as a preservative in packed red blood cells) can cause a mild increase in the anion gap.

Decreased (Low): (< 8 mmol/L): Seen with bromide ingestion, hypercalcemia, hypermagnesemia, multiple myeloma, and hypoalbuminemia.

■ ANTICARDIOLIPIN ANTIBODIES

See Antiphospholipid Antibodies, p 349.

■ ANTI-NEUTROPHIL CYTOPLASMIC ANTIBODIES (ANCAS)

Negative = < 10 EV/mL.
Equivocal = 10–20 EV/mL.

Positive = > 20 EV/mL.

Antibodies to cytoplasmic components of neutrophils, seen in vasculitides. Two types:

1. **C-ANCA (Cytoplasmic-staining ANCA).** Present in ~ 90% of patients with generalized Wegener's granulomatosis; also seen in rapidly progressive glomerulonephritis and a type of polyarteritis nodosa (microscopic). May be used to follow disease activity; also especially useful in distinguishing active disease from an infectious complication. C-ANCA is not present in other collagen-vascular diseases.
2. **P-ANCA (Perinuclear-staining ANCA).** Seen in a variety of collagen-vascular diseases such as limited Wegener's granulomatosis, polyarteritis nodosa, Goodpasture's syndrome, and other vasculitides; and also seen in several types of glomerulonephritides.

■ ANTINUCLEAR ANTIBODIES (ANA)

Negative: A useful screening test in patients with symptoms suggesting collagen-vascular disease, especially if titer is > 1:160.

Positive: Systemic lupus erythematosus (SLE), drug-induced lupus (procainamide, hydralazine, isoniazid, etc), scleroderma, mixed connective tissue disease (MCTD), rheumatoid arthritis, polymyositis, juvenile rheumatoid arthritis (JRA) (5–20%). Low titers are also seen in non-collagen-vascular disease.

Specific Immunofluorescent ANA Patterns

1. ANA Patterns
   - **Homogenous:** Nonspecific, from antibodies to deoxyribonucleoproteins (DNP) and native double-stranded deoxyribonucleic acid (DNA). Seen in SLE and a variety of other diseases. Antihistone is consistent with drug-induced lupus.
   - **Speckled:** Pattern seen in many connective tissue disorders. From antibodies to extractable nuclear antigens (ENA) including antiribonucleoproteins (anti-RNP), anti-Sm, anti-PM-1, and anti-SS. Anti-RNP is positive in MCTD and SLE. Anti-Sm is found in SLE. Anti-SS-A and anti-SS-B are seen in Sjögren's syndrome and subacute cutaneous lupus. The speckled pattern is also seen with scleroderma.
   - **Peripheral RIM Pattern:** From antibodies to native double-stranded DNA and DNP. Seen in SLE.
   - **Nucleolar Pattern:** From antibodies to nucleolar ribonucleic acid (RNA). Positive in Sjögren's syndrome and scleroderma.
2. Other Autoantibodies
   - **Antimitochondrial:** Primary biliary cirrhosis.
   - **Anti-Smooth Muscle:** Low titers are seen in a variety of illnesses; high titers (> 1:100) are suggestive of chronic active hepatitis.
   - **Antimicrosomal:** Hashimoto's thyroiditis.

■ ANTIPHOSPHOLIPID ANTIBODIES

Note: There are two basic categories of antiphospholipid antibody—anticardiolipin and lupus anticoagulant. Both are associated with recurrent arterial or venous thrombosis or fetal demise.

Anticardiolipin antibody. Two forms: IgG, IgM.
IgG normal < 23u.
IgM normal < 11u.

Lupus anticoagulant
Negative = normal.
Positive = presence.
Should be suspected with an isolated elevated partial thromboplastin time (PTT) with no other likely cause.

■ AST (ASPARTATE AMINOTRANSFERASE) (SGOT: SERUM GLUTAMIC-OXALOACETIC TRANSFERASE)

8–20 U/L.
Generally parallels changes in ALT in liver disease.

Increased: Liver disease, acute myocardial infarction, Reye's syndrome, muscle trauma and injection, pancreatitis, intestinal injury or surgery, factitious increase (erythromycin, opiates), burns, brain damage.

Decreased: Beri-beri, diabetes mellitus with ketoacidosis, liver disease.

■ B_{12} (VITAMIN B_{12})

140–700 pg/mL or 189–516 pmol/L.

Increased: Leukemia, polycythemia vera.

Decreased: Pernicious anemia, bacterial overgrowth, dietary deficiency (rare—humans normally have 2–3 years of stores), malabsorption, pregnancy.

■ BASE EXCESS/DEFICIT

See Table 2–1, p 350. A decrease in base (bicarbonate) is termed *base deficit;* an increase in base is termed *base excess.*

Excess: Metabolic alkalosis (see Section I, Chapter 3, Alkalosis, p 18), respiratory acidosis (see Section I, Chapter 2, Acidosis, p 9).

Deficit: Metabolic acidosis (see Section I, Chapter 2, Acidosis, p 9), respiratory alkalosis (see Section I, Chapter 3, Alkalosis, p 18).

TABLE 2–1. NORMAL BLOOD GAS VALUES.[1]

Measurement	Arterial	Mixed Venous[2]	Venous
pH (range)	7.40 (7.36–7.44)	7.36 (7.31–7.41)	7.36 7.31–7.41)
pO_2 (decreases with age)	80–100 mm Hg	35–40 mm Hg	30–50 mm Hg
pCO_2	36–44 mm Hg	41–51 mm Hg	40–52 mm Hg
O_2 saturation (decreases with age)	>95%	60–80%	60–80%
HCO_3^-	22–26 mmol/L	22–26 mmol/L	22–29 mmol/L
Base difference (deficit/excess)	–2 to +2	–2 to +2	–2 to +2

[1]*Modified and reproduced with permission from Gomella LG, ed.* Clinician's Pocket Reference. *9th ed. McGraw-Hill; 2002.*
[2]From right atrium.

■ BENCE–JONES PROTEINS—URINE

Negative: Normal.

Positive: Multiple myeloma, idiopathic Bence–Jones proteinuria.

■ BICARBONATE (SERUM HCO_3^-)

22–29 mmol/L.

See Tables 2–1 and 2–2. Also see Carbon Dioxide, Arterial, p 353, for pCO_2 values.

Increased: Metabolic alkalosis, compensation for respiratory acidosis. See Section I, Chapter 2, Acidosis, p 9; and Section I, Chapter 3, Alkalosis, p 18.

TABLE 2–2. ACID–BASE DISORDERS WITH APPROPRIATE COMPENSATION.

	Changes in Normal Values		
Disorder	pH	HCO_3^-	pCO_2
Metabolic acidosis	↓	↓↓	↓
Metabolic alkalosis	↑	↑↑	↑
Acute respiratory acidosis	↓	slight↑	↑↑
Chronic respiratory acidosis	slight↓	↑	↑↑
Acute respiratory alkalosis	↑	slight↓	↓↓
Chronic respiratory alkalosis	slight↑	↓	↓↓

Decreased: Metabolic acidosis, compensation for respiratory alkalosis. See Section I, Chapter 2, Acidosis, p 9; and Section I, Chapter 3, Alkalosis, p 18.

■ BILIRUBIN

Total: < 0.2–1.0 mg/dL or 3.4–17.1 μmol/L;

Direct: < 0.2 mg/dL or < 3.4 μmol/L;

Indirect: < 0.8 mg/dL or < 13.7 μmol/L.

Increased Total: Hepatic damage (hepatitis, toxins, cirrhosis), biliary obstruction (gallstone or tumor), hemolysis, fasting.

Increased Direct (Conjugated): Biliary obstruction (gallstone, tumor, stricture), drug-induced cholestasis, Dubin-Johnson syndrome, and Rotor's syndrome.

Increased Indirect (Unconjugated): Hemolytic anemia (transfusion reaction, sickle cell, collagen-vascular disease), Gilbert's disease, Crigler-Najjar syndrome.

■ BLEEDING TIME

Duke, Ivy: < 6 min; Template: < 10 min.

Increased: Thrombocytopenia, thrombocytopenic purpura, von Willebrand's disease, defective platelet function (aspirin, nonsteroidal anti-inflammatory drugs, uremia).

■ BLOOD GAS, ARTERIAL

See Tables 2–1 and 2–2, p 350. For acid–base disorders, see Section I, Chapter 2, Acidosis, p 9; and Chapter 3, Alkalosis, p 18.

■ BLOOD GAS, VENOUS

See Table 2–1, p 350. **Note:** There is little difference between arterial and venous pH and bicarbonate (except with congestive heart failure and shock); therefore, the venous blood gas may be occasionally used to assess acid–base status, but venous oxygen levels are significantly lower than arterial levels.

■ BLOOD UREA NITROGEN (BUN)

7–18 mg/dL or 1.2–3.0 mmol urea/L.

Increased: Renal failure, prerenal azotemia (decreased renal perfusion secondary to congestive heart failure, shock, volume depletion), postrenal obstruction, gastrointestinal bleeding, hypercatabolic states.

Decreased: Starvation, malnutrition, liver failure (hepatitis, drugs), pregnancy, infancy, nephrotic syndrome, overhydration.

■ BLOOD UREA NITROGEN/CREATININE RATIO

Between 10 and 20:1.

Elevated Ratio **(> 20:1):** Congestive heart failure, dehydration, gastrointestinal bleeding, increased protein intake, drugs such as tetracycline and steroids. Infection (sepsis), high fevers, burns, cachexia.

Decreased Ratio: **(< 10:1):** Acute tubular necrosis, low-protein diet, starvation, malnutrition, liver disease, syndrome of inappropriate antidiuretic hormone, pregnancy, and rhabdomyolysis.

Note: The ratio may not be appropriate if the patient is in diabetic ketoacidosis or receiving drugs such as cephalosporin.

The ratio can be altered by interferences in the chemical methods used to measure the creatinine or the BUN, resulting in spurious results. The presence of Ketones may seriously elevate the serum creatinine level. Drugs such as cephalosporins, ascorbic acid and barbiturates may also interfere with the serum creatinine measurement.

■ CALCITONIN

< 100 pg/mL or < 100 g/L.

Increased: Medullary carcinoma of the thyroid, pregnancy, chronic renal insufficiency, Zollinger-Ellison syndrome, pernicious anemia.

■ CALCIUM, SERUM

8.4–10.2 mg/dL (4.2–5.1 mEq/L) or 2.10–2.55 mmol/L;

Ionized: 4.5–4.9 mg/dL (2.2–2.5 mEq/L) or 1.1–1.2 mmol/L.

Note: To interpret a total calcium value, you must know the albumin level. If the albumin is not within normal limits, a corrected calcium can be roughly calculated with the following formula. Values for ionized calcium need no special correction.

$$\text{Corrected total Ca} = 0.8\,(\text{normal albumin} - \text{measured albumin}) + \text{reported Ca}$$

Increased: See Section I, Chapter 31, Hypercalcemia, p 175.

Decreased: See Section I, Chapter 36, Hypocalcemia, p 198.

■ CALCIUM, URINE

Average calcium diet: 100–300 mg per 24-hour urine.

Increased: Hyperparathyroidism, hyperthyroidism, hypervitaminosis D, distal renal tubular acidosis (type I), sarcoidosis, immobilization, osteolytic lesions (bony metastasis, multiple myeloma), Paget's disease, glucocorticoid excess (either endogenous or exogenous), furosemide.

Decreased: Thiazide diuretics, hypothyroidism, renal failure, steatorrhea, rickets, osteomalacia.

■ CARBON DIOXIDE, ARTERIAL (PCO_2)

36–44 mm Hg. See Tables 2–1 and 2–2, p 350.

Increased: Respiratory acidosis, compensation for metabolic alkalosis. See Section I, Chapter 2, Acidosis, p 9; and Chapter 3, Alkalosis, p 18.

Decreased: Respiratory alkalosis, compensation for metabolic acidosis. See Section I, Chapter 2, Acidosis, p 9; and Chapter 3, Alkalosis, p 18.

■ CARBOXYHEMOGLOBIN

Nonsmoker: < 2%.
Smoker: < 6%.
Toxic: > 15%.

Increased: Smoking, smoke inhalation; exposure to automobile exhaust, faulty heating units with inadequate ventilation.

■ CARCINOEMBRYONIC ANTIGEN (CEA)

Nonsmoker: < 3.0 g/mL or < 3.0 μg/L;
Smoker: < 5.0 g/mL or < 5.0 μg/L.

Increased: Carcinoma (colon, pancreas, lung, stomach), smokers, nonneoplastic liver disease, Crohn's disease, and ulcerative colitis. Test used predominantly to monitor patients for recurrence of carcinoma, especially after colon carcinoma resection.

■ CATECHOLAMINES, FRACTIONATED

Note: Values are variable and depend on the lab and method of assay used. Normal levels listed in Table 2–3 are based on high-performance liquid chromatography technique.

Increased: Pheochromocytoma, neural crest tumors (neuroblastoma). In extra-adrenal pheochromocytoma, norepinephrine may be markedly elevated compared with epinephrine.

TABLE 2–3. FRACTIONATED CATECHOLAMINES.

Catecholamine	Plasma (Supine)	Urine
Norepinephrine	70–750 pg/mL 414–4435 pmol/L	14–80 μg/24-hr 82.7–473 nmol/d
Epinephrine	0–100 pg/mL 0–100 pg/mL	0.5–20 μg/24-hr 2.73–109 nmol/d
Dopamine	<30 pg/mL <196 pmol/L	65–400 μg/24-hr 424–2612 nmol/d

■ CATECHOLAMINES, URINE, UNCONJUGATED

> 15 years old: < 100 μg/24 hr.
Measures free (unconjugated) epinephrine, norepinephrine, and dopamine.

Increased: Pheochromocytoma, neural crest tumors (neuroblastoma).

■ CBC (COMPLETE BLOOD COUNT, HEMOGRAM)

Note: For normal values, see Table 2–4. For differential, see specific tests.

TABLE 2–4. NORMAL CBC VALUES—ADULTS.[1]

WBC	4800–10,800 cells/μL
RBCs	M: 4.7–6.1 × 10^6 cells/μL F: 4.2–5.4 × 10^6 cells/μL
Hemoglobin	M: 14–18 g/dL F:12–16 g/dL
Hematocrit	M: 40–54% F: 37–47%
MCV	M: 80–94 fL F: 81–99 fL
MCH	27–31 pg
MCHC (%)	33–37%
RDW	11.5–14.5
Platelets	150,000–450,000/μL
■ Differential	
Segmented neutrophils	41–71%
Banded (stab) neutrophils	5–10%
Lymphocytes	24–44%
Monocytes	3–7%
Eosinophils	1–3%
Basophils	0–1%

[1]Refer to hospital reference values. *Modified and reproduced with permission from Gomella LG, ed.* Clinician's Pocket Reference. *9th ed. McGraw-Hill; 2002.*

■ CHLORIDE, SERUM

98–106 mEq/L.

Increased: Metabolic nongap acidosis such as diarrhea, renal tubular acidosis, mineralocorticoid deficiency, hyperalimentation, medications (acetazolamide, ammonium chloride).

Decreased: Vomiting, diabetes mellitus with ketoacidosis, mineralocorticoid excess, renal disease with sodium loss.

■ CHLORIDE, URINE

110–250 mmol per 24-hour urine.

See Urinary Electrolytes, p 385.

■ CHOLESTEROL (TOTAL)

140–240 mg/dL or 3.63–6.22 mmol/L.

Desired level: < 200 mg/dL or 5.18 mmol/L.

Increased: Primary hypercholesterolemia (types IIA, IIB, III), elevated triglycerides (types I, IV, V), biliary obstruction, nephrosis, hypothyroidism, diabetes mellitus, pregnancy.

Decreased: Chronic liver disease, hyperthyroidism, malnutrition (cancer, starvation), myeloproliferative disorders, steroid therapy, lipoproteinemias.

High-Density Lipoprotein (HDL) Cholesterol

Fasting male: 40–60 mg/dL or 0.78–1.81 mmol/L.

Fasting female: 40–60 mg/dL or 0.78–2.07 mmol/L.

Note: HDL highly correlates with the development of coronary artery disease; a decreased HDL (< 35 mg/dL) leads to an increased risk, and an increased HDL (> 65 mg/dL) is associated with a decreased risk.

Increased: Estrogen (females), exercise, ethanol.

Decreased: Male gender, beta-blockers, anabolic steroids, uremia, obesity, diabetes, liver disease, Tangier's disease.

Low-Density Lipoprotein (LDL) Cholesterol

Desired: < 130–160 mg/dL or 3.36–4.14 mmol/L. In the presence of coronary artery disease or diabetes mellitus, desired LDL is < 100 mg/dL or 2.58 mmol/L.

Increased: Excess dietary saturated fats, myocardial infarction, hyperlipoproteinemia, biliary cirrhosis, endocrine disease (diabetes, hypothyroidism).

Decreased: Malabsorption, severe liver disease, abetalipoproteinemia.

Triglycerides

See Triglycerides, p 381.

■ COLD AGGLUTININS

Normal = < 1:32.

Increased: *Mycoplasma* pneumonia; viral infections (especially mononucleosis, measles, mumps); cirrhosis; some parasitic infections.

■ COMPLEMENT C3

80–155 mg/dL or 800–1550 ng/L;
> 60 years: 80–170 mg/dL or 80–1700 ng/L.
Note: Normal values may vary greatly depending on the assay used.

Increased: Rheumatic fever, neoplasms (gastrointestinal, prostate, others).

Decreased: Systemic lupus erythematosus, glomerulonephritis (poststreptococcal and membranoproliferative), vasculitis, severe hepatic failure.

Variable: Rheumatoid arthritis.

■ COMPLEMENT C4

20–50 mg/dL or 200–500 ng/L.

Increased: Neoplasia (gastrointestinal, lung, others).

Decreased: Systemic lupus erythematosus, chronic active hepatitis, cirrhosis, glomerulonephritis, hereditary angioedema.

Variable: Rheumatoid arthritis.

■ COMPLEMENT CH50 (TOTAL)

33–61 mg/mL or 330–610 ng/L. Tests for complement deficiency in the classical pathway.

Increased: Acute-phase reactants (eg, tissue injury, infections).

Decreased: Hereditary complement deficiencies, any cause of deficiency of individual complement components. See Complement C3, and Complement C4.

■ COOMBS' TEST, DIRECT

Uses patient's erythrocytes; tests for the presence of antibody or complement on the patient's red blood cells.

Positive: Autoimmune hemolytic anemia (leukemia, lymphoma, collagen-vascular diseases, eg, systemic lupus erythematosus); hemolytic transfusion reaction; sensitization to some drugs (methyldopa, levodopa, penicillins, cephalosporins).

■ COOMBS' TEST, INDIRECT

More useful for red blood cell typing. Uses serum that contains antibody from the patient.

Positive: Isoimmunization from previous transfusion, incompatible blood as a result of improper cross-matching.

■ CORTISOL

Serum—8 am: 5.0–23.0 µg/dL or 138–635 nmol/L; 4 pm: 3.0–15.0 µg/dL or 83–414 nmol/L.

Urine (24-hour): 10–100 µg/d or 27.6–276 nmol/d.

Increased: Adrenal adenoma, adrenal carcinoma, Cushing's disease, non-pituitary ACTH-producing tumor, steroid therapy, oral contraceptives.

Decreased: Primary adrenal insufficiency (Addison's disease), Waterhouse-Friderichsen syndrome, ACTH deficiency.

■ CORTROSYN STIMULATION TEST

See ACTH Stimulation Test, p 345.

■ COUNTERIMMUNOELECTROPHORESIS (CIE)

Normal = negative.

CIE is an immunologic technique that allows rapid identification of infectious organisms from body fluids, including serum, urine, cerebrospinal fluid, and others. Organisms that can be identified include *Neisseria meningitidis, Streptococcus pneumoniae, Haemophilus influenzae,* and group B streptococcus.

■ C-PEPTIDE

Fasting: ≤ 4.0 g/mL or ≤ 4.0 µg/L;
male > 60 years: 1.5–5.0 g/mL or 1.5–5.0 µg/L;
female: 1.4–5.5 g/mL or 1.4–5.5 µg/L.

Decreased: Diabetes (insulin-dependent diabetes mellitus), insulin administration, hypoglycemia.

Increased: Insulinoma. Test is useful to differentiate insulinoma from surreptitious use of insulin as a cause of hypoglycemia.

■ C-REACTIVE PROTEIN (CRP)

Normal: < 8 mg/L.

An acute-phase reactant with a relatively short half-life.

Increased: Infections (increase in bacterial infections > increase in viral infections); tissue injury or necrosis (acute myocardial infarction, malignant disease [especially lung, breast, and gastrointestinal] and organ rejection following transplantation); and inflammatory disorders (rheumatoid arthritis, systemic lupus erythematosus, inflammatory bowel disease, and vasculitides).

■ CREATINE PHOSPHOKINASE (CK)

25–145 mU/mL or 25–145 U/L.

Increased: Cardiac muscle (acute myocardial infarction, myocarditis, defibrillation); skeletal muscle (intramuscular injection, hypothyroidism, rhabdomyolysis, polymyositis, muscular dystrophy); cerebral infarction.

CK isoenzymes MM, MB, BB: MB (normal < 6%) increased in acute myocardial infarction (increases in 4–8 hours, peaks at 24 hours), cardiac surgery; BB not useful.

■ CREATININE CLEARANCE

Male: 100–135 mL/min or 0.963–1.300 mL/s/m^2.

Female: 85–125 mL/min or 0.819–1.204 mL/s/m^2.

A concurrent serum creatinine and a 24-hour urine creatinine are needed. A shorter time interval can be used and corrected for in the formula. A quick formula for estimation is also found in Table 7–18, Aminoglycoside Dosing, p 614.

$$\text{Creatinine clearance} = \frac{(\text{urine creatinine} \times \text{total urine volume})}{(\text{plasma creatinine} \times \text{time in minutes})}$$

To verify if the urine sample is a complete 24-hour collection, determine if the sample contains at least 14–26 mg/kg/24 hr or 124–230 mmol/kg/d creatinine for adult males; or 11–20 mg/kg/24 hr or 97–177 mmol/kg/d for adult females. This test is not a requirement.

Decreased: A decreased creatinine clearance results in an increase in serum creatinine, usually secondary to renal insufficiency. Clearance normally decreases with age. See Creatinine, Serum, Increased, p 359.

Increased: Pregnancy, prediabetic renal failure.

■ CREATININE, SERUM

Male: 0.7–1.3 mg/dL.
Female: 0.6–1.1 mg/dL.

Increased: Renal failure (prerenal, renal, or postrenal), acromegaly, ingestion of roasted meat, large body mass. Falsely elevated with ketones and certain cephalosporins, depending on assay.

■ CREATININE, URINE

Male total creatinine: 14–26 mg/kg/24 hr or 124–230 μmol/kg/d.
Female: 11–20 mg/kg/24 hr or 97–177 μmol/kg/d. See Creatinine Clearance, p 358.

■ CRYOCRIT

≤ 0.4%. (Negative if qualitative.) Cryocrit, a quantitative measure, is preferred over the qualitative method. It should be collected in nonanticoagulated tubes and transported at body temperature. Positive samples can be analyzed for immunoglobulin class, and light-chain type on request.

> 0.4%. (Positive if qualitative.) *Monoclonal*—Multiple myeloma, Waldenström's macroglobulinemia, lymphoma, chronic lymphocytic leukemia.

Mixed polyclonal or mixed monoclonal—Infectious diseases (viral, bacterial, parasitic) such as subacute bacterial endocarditis or malaria, systemic lupus erythematosus, rheumatoid arthritis, essential cryoglobulinemia, lymphoproliferative diseases, sarcoidosis, chronic liver disease (cirrhosis).

■ DEXAMETHASONE SUPPRESSION TEST

Used in the differential diagnosis of Cushing's syndrome.

Overnight Dexamethasone Suppression Test

In the rapid version of this test, the patient takes dexamethasone 1 mg PO at 11 pm; a fasting 8 am plasma cortisol is obtained. Normally, the cortisol level should be < 5 μg/dL or < 138 nmol/L. A value > 5 μg/dL or > 138 nmol/L suggests the diagnosis of Cushing's syndrome; however, suppression may not occur with obesity, alcoholism, or depression. In these patients, the best screening test is a 24-hour urine for free cortisol.

Low-Dose Dexamethasone Suppression Test

After collection of baseline serum cortisol and 24-hour urine free cortisol levels, dexamethasone 0.5 mg PO is administered Q 6 hr for eight doses. Serum cortisol and 24-hour urine for free cortisol are repeated on the second day. Failure to suppress to a serum cortisol of < 5 μg/dL (138 nmol/L) and a urine free cortisol < 30 μg/dL (82 nmol/L) confirms the diagnosis of Cushing's syndrome.

High-Dose Dexamethasone Suppression Test

If the low-dose test is positive, dexamethasone 2 mg PO Q 6 hr for eight doses is administered. A fall in urinary free cortisol to 50% of the baseline value occurs in patients with Cushing's disease, but not in patients with adrenal tumors or ectopic ACTH production.

■ ERYTHROPOIETIN (EPO)

Normal = 5–30 mU/mL.

There is an inverse relationship between erythropoietin and hematocrit.

Decreased or normal levels: Myelodysplastic syndrome, polycythemia vera, chronic renal disease, early pregnancy, and in preterm infants.

Increased: AZT-treated HIV infection, normocytic anemia, and microcytic anemia.

RIA measurement detects erythropoietin in both the active and inactive forms while the mouse bioassay assesses functional hormones.

■ ETHANOL LEVEL

See Drug Levels, Table 7–16, p 613.

■ FERRITIN

Male: 15–200 ng/mL or 15–220 μg/L.

Female: 12–150 ng/mL or 12–150 μg/L.

Decreased: Iron deficiency, severe liver disease.

Increased: Hemochromatosis, hemosiderosis, sideroblastic anemia, any inflammatory process (acute-phase reactant).

■ FIBRIN DEGRADATION PRODUCTS (FDP)

< 10 μg/mL.

Increased: Any thromboembolic condition (deep venous thrombosis, myocardial infarction, pulmonary embolus); disseminated intravascular coagulation; hepatic dysfunction.

■ FIBRINOGEN

150–450 mg/dL or 150–450 g/L.

Decreased: Congenital; disseminated intravascular coagulation (sepsis, amniotic fluid embolism, abruptio placentae, prostatic or cardiac surgery); burns; neoplastic and hematologic malignancies; acute severe bleeding; snake bite.

Increased: Inflammatory processes (acute-phase reactant).

■ FOLATE RED BLOOD CELL

160–640 ng or 360–1450 nmol/mL RBC.

More sensitive for detecting folate deficiency from malnourishment if the patient has started proper nutrition before the serum folate is measured (even one well-balanced hospital meal).

Increased: See Folic Acid (Serum Folate).

Decreased: See Folic Acid.

■ FOLIC ACID (SERUM FOLATE)

2–14 ng/mL or 4.5–31.7 nmol/L.

Increased: Folic acid administration.

Decreased: Malnutrition, malabsorption, massive cellular growth (cancer), hemolytic anemia, pregnancy.

■ FTA-ABS (FLUORESCENT TREPONEMAL ANTIBODY ABSORBED)

Nonreactive.

Positive: Syphilis (test of choice to confirm diagnosis). May be negative in early primary syphilis; may remain positive after adequate treatment.

■ FUNGAL SEROLOGIES

Negative (< 1:8). Complement-fixation fungal antibody screen that usually detects antibodies to *Histoplasma, Blastomyces, Aspergillus,* and *Coccidioides.*

■ GAMMA-GLUTAMYLTRANSFERASE (GGT)

Male: 9–50 U/L.

Female: 8–40 U/L. Generally parallels changes in serum alkaline phosphatase and 5′-nucleotidase in liver disease.

Increased: Liver disease (hepatitis, cirrhosis, obstructive jaundice); pancreatitis.

■ GASTRIN

Male: < 100 pg/mL or < 100 ng/L.
Female: < 75 pg/mL or < 100 ng/L.

Increased: Zollinger-Ellison syndrome, pyloric stenosis, pernicious anemia, atrophic gastritis, ulcerative colitis, renal insufficiency, steroid and calcium administration.

■ GLUCOSE

Fasting: 70–105 mg/dL or 3.89–5.83 nmol/L.
2 hours postprandial: 70–120 mg/dL or 3.89–6.67 mmol/L.

Increased: See Section I, Chapter 32, Hyperglycemia, p 180.

Decreased: See Section I, Chapter 37, Hypoglycemia, p 202.

■ GLYCOHEMOGLOBIN (HEMOGLOBIN A_{1C})

4.0–6.0%.

Increased: Poorly controlled diabetes mellitus.

■ GRAM'S STAIN

Rapid Technique

Spread a thin layer of specimen onto glass slide and allow to dry. Fix with heat. Apply Gentian violet (15–20 seconds); follow with iodine (15–20 seconds), then alcohol (just a few seconds until effluent is barely decolorized). Rinse with water and counterstain with safranin (15–20 seconds). Examine under oil immersion lens: gram-positive bacteria are dark blue and gram-negatives are red.

Gram-Positive Cocci: *Staphylococcus, Streptococcus, Enterococcus, Micrococcus, Peptococcus* (anaerobic), and *Peptostreptococcus* (anaerobic) species.

Gram-Positive Rods: *Clostridium* (anaerobic), *Corynebacterium, Listeria,* and *Bacillus.*

Gram-Negative Cocci: *Neisseria, Branhamella, Moraxella, Acinetobacter* species.

Gram-Negative Coccoid Rods: *Haemophilus, Pasteurella, Brucella, Francisella, Yersinia,* and *Bordetella* species.

Gram-Negative Straight Rods: *Acinetobacter (Mima, Herellea), Aeromonas, Bacteroides* (anaerobic), *Campylobacter* (comma-shaped) species, *Eikenella, Enterobacter, Escherichia, Fusobacterium* (anaerobic), *Helicobacter, Klebsiella, Legionella* (small, pleomorphic; weakly staining), *Proteus, Providencia, Pseudomonas, Salmonella, Serratia, Shigella, Vibrio, Yersinia.*

■ HAPTOGLOBIN

26–185 mg/mL.

Increased: Obstructive liver disease; any inflammatory process.

Decreased: Hemolysis (eg, transfusion reaction); severe liver disease.

■ *HELICOBACTER* ANTIBODIES

Normal = negative.

Serological test to detect antibodies to *Helicobacter pylori* in patients with peptic ulcer disease. High titers of IgG to *Helicobacter* are indicative of *H pylori* infection (sensitivity > 95% and specificity > 95%). More sensitive than biopsy for detecting presence of *H pylori.* It may take 6 months or longer for antibodies to decline appreciably after treatment.

■ HEMATOCRIT

See Table 2–4, p 354, for normal values.

Increased: See Section I, Chapter 55, Polycythemia, p 291.

Decreased: See Section I, Chapter 5, Anemia, p 27.

■ HEMOGLOBIN

See Table 2–4, p 354, for normal values.

Increased: See Section I, Chapter 55, Polycythemia, p 291.

Decreased: See Section I, Chapter 5, Anemia, p 27.

■ HEPATITIS TESTS

See Table 2–5, p 364.

- **HBsAg:** Hepatitis B surface antigen (formerly Australia antigen). Indicates either chronic or acute infection with hepatitis B. Used by blood banks to screen donors.

TABLE 2–5. HEPATITIS PANEL TESTING.

Profile Name	Tests	Purpose
■ Screening		
Admission: High-risk patients (homosexuals, IV drug users, dialysis patients)	HBsAg Anti-HCV	To screen for chronic or active infection.
All pregnant women	HBsAg	To screen for chronic or active infection.
Percutaneous inoculation	HBsAg Anti-HCV	Test serum of patient (if known) for possible infectivity. Start Hep B vaccination if health care worker not previously immunized.
	Anti-HBs	Determine if vaccinated health care worker is immune and protected.
Pre-HBV vaccine in high-risk patients	HBsAg Anti-HBc	To determine if an individual is infected or already has antibodies and is immune.
■ Diagnosis		
Differential diagnosis of acute hepatitis	Anti-HAV IgM HBsAg Anti-HBc IgM Anti-HCV	To differentiate between hepatitis A, hepatitis B, and hepatitis C (Anti-HCV may take 4–8 weeks to become positive)
Differential diagnosis of chronic hepatitis (Abnormal Liver Function Tests [LFTs])	HBsAg Anti-HCV (and RIBA or HCV RNA if Anti-HCV is positive)	To rule out chronic hepatitis B or C as a cause of chronically elevated LFTs.
■ Monitoring		
Chronic hepatitis B	LFTs HBsAg HBeAg/Anti-HBe Anti-HDV IgM α-fetoprotein HBV DNA	To test for activity, late seroconversion, or disease latency in known hepatitis B carrier, superinfection with HDV, development of hepatoma, or resolution of infection after therapy or spontaneously.
Chronic hepatitis C	LFTs HCV RNA α-fetoprotein	To test for activity of hepatitis likelihood of response to interferon, or development of hepatoma
Postvaccination screening	Anti-HBs	To ensure immunity after vaccination
Sexual contact	HBsAg	To monitor sexual partners with acute or chronic hepatitis B

- **Total Anti-HBc:** IgG and IgM antibody to hepatitis B core antigen. Confirms either previous exposure to hepatitis B virus (HBV) or ongoing infection. Used by blood banks to screen donors.
- **Anti-HBc IgM:** IgM antibody to hepatitis B core antigen. Early and best indicator of acute infection with hepatitis B.
- **HBeAg:** Hepatitis B_e antigen. When present, indicates high degree of infectiousness. Order *only* when evaluating a patient with *chronic* HBV infection.
- **Anti-HBe:** Antibody to hepatitis B_e antigen. Order with HbeAg. Presence is associated with resolution of active inflammation; but often means virus is integrated into host DNA, especially if host remains HBsAg positive.
- **Anti-HBs:** Antibody to hepatitis B surface antigen. Typically indicates immunity associated with clinical recovery from an HBV infection or previous immunization with hepatitis B vaccine. Order *only* to assess effectiveness of vaccine.
- **HBV-DNA:** Detects presence of viral DNA in serum (pg/mL) quantitatively to confirm infection and assess therapy. Very expensive assay.
- **Anti-HAV:** Total antibody to hepatitis A virus. Confirms previous exposure to hepatitis A virus.
- **Anti-HAV IgM:** IgM antibody to hepatitis A virus. Indicates recent acute infection with hepatitis A virus.
- **Anti-HDV:** Total antibody to delta-agent hepatitis. Confirms previous exposure. Order *only* in patients with known chronic HBV infection.
- **Anti-HDV IgM:** IgM antibody to delta-agent hepatitis. Indicates recent infection. Order *only* in patients with known chronic HBV infection.
- **Anti-HCV:** Antibody against hepatitis C (formerly known as non-A non-B hepatitis). Order to evaluate both acute and chronic hepatitis. Has a low false-positive rate. Used by blood banks to screen donors.
- **Anti-HCV RIBA:** Measures antibody to 4 separate HCV antigens. Used to confirm positive anti-HCV test.
- **HCV-RNA:** Detects presence of virus by either sensitive RT-PCR or quantitatively by branched DNA. Confirms infection or response to therapy. Very expensive assay.

■ 5-HIAA (5-HYDROXYINDOLEACETIC ACID)

2–8 mg or 10.4–41.6 μmol/24-hr urine collection. 5-HIAA is a serotonin metabolite.

Increased: Carcinoid tumors; certain foods (banana, pineapple, tomato).

■ *HISTOPLASMA CAPSULATUM* ANTIGEN, URINE

< 1.0 units/mL

Elevated in disseminated histoplasmosis, less commonly elevated in localized pulmonary *Histoplasma* infections. The most sensitive and rapid diagnostic test available for disseminated histoplasmosis in AIDS patients.

After amphotericin B treatment, levels fall to low or nondetectable range. If measurement increases, it is an indication of relapse.

■ HOMOCYSTEINE

5–18 mmol/mL.

Increased: Arteriosclerotic vascular disease, deep venous thrombosis, pregnancy complicated by neural tube defects.
Increases with aging, smoking, and many drugs.

■ HUMAN CHORIONIC GONADOTROPIN, SERUM (HCG BETA SUBUNIT)

< 3.0 mIU/mL;
7–10 days postconception: > 3 mIU/mL; 30 days: 100–5000 mIU/mL;
10 weeks: 50,000–140,000 mIU/mL; > 16 weeks: 10,000–50,000 mIU/mL; thereafter: levels slowly decline.

Increased: Pregnancy, testicular tumors, trophoblastic disease (hydatidiform mole, choriocarcinoma levels usually > 100,000 mIU/mL).

■ HUMAN IMMUNODEFICIENCY VIRUS (HIV) ANTIBODY TEST

Negative: Used in the diagnosis of acquired immunodeficiency syndrome (AIDS) and HIV infection, and to screen blood for use in transfusion. May be negative in early HIV infection.

ELISA (Enzyme-Linked Immunosorbent Assay)

Used to detect HIV antibody. A positive test is usually repeated and then confirmed by Western blot analysis.

Positive: AIDS, asymptomatic HIV infection, false-positive test.

Western Blot

The technique used as the reference procedure for confirming the presence or absence of HIV antibody, usually after a positive HIV antibody by ELISA determination.

Positive: AIDS, asymptomatic HIV infection.
Note: Polymerase chain reaction is becoming a useful tool for detection of the HIV virus. It will be especially useful in very early infection, when antibody may not be present.

■ INTERNATIONAL NORMALIZED RATIO (INR)

See also Prothrombin Time, p 376.

Normal = 1.0.

The INR is used to standardize prothrombin results in patients taking anticoagulants.

- **INR 2–3:** Therapeutic range for most indications, including atrial fibrillation, deep venous thrombosis, pulmonary embolus, and transient ischemic attacks.
- **INR 3.0–4.0:** Prevention of arterial thromboembolism with mechanical valves. This range may also be required in hypercoagulable states, or in recurrent arterial or venous thromboembolic disease.

■ IRON

Males: 65–175 μg/dL or 11.64–31.33 μmol/L.

Females: 50–170 μg/dL or 8.95–30.43 μmol/L.

Increased: Hemochromatosis, hemosiderosis caused by excessive iron intake, excess destruction or decreased production of erythrocytes, liver necrosis.

Decreased: Iron deficiency anemia, nephrosis (loss of iron-binding proteins), anemia of chronic disease.

■ IRON BINDING CAPACITY, TOTAL (TIBC)

250–450 μg/dL or 44.75–80.55 μmol/L.

The normal iron/TIBC ratio is 20–50%; < 15% is characteristic of iron deficiency anemia. An increased ratio is seen with hemochromatosis.

Increased: Acute and chronic blood loss, iron deficiency anemia, hepatitis, oral contraceptives.

Decreased: Anemia of chronic disease, cirrhosis, nephrosis, hemochromatosis.

■ 17-KETOGENIC STEROIDS (17-KGS)

Males: 5–23 mg or 17–80 μmol/24-hr urine;

Females: 3–15 mg or 10–52 μmol/24-hr urine.

Increased: Adrenal hyperplasia.

Decreased: Panhypopituitarism, Addison's disease, acute steroid withdrawal.

■ 17-KETOSTEROIDS (17-KS)

Males: 9–22 mg or 31–76 μmol/24-hr urine;

Females: 6–15 mg or 21–52 μmol/24-hr urine.

Increased: Cushing's syndrome, 11- and 21-hydroxylase deficiency, severe stress, exogenous steroids, excess ACTH or androgens.

Decreased: Addison's disease, anorexia nervosa, panhypopituitarism.

■ KOH PREP

Negative: Normal.

Positive: Superficial mycoses (*Candida, Trichophyton, Microsporum, Epidermophyton, Keratinomyces*).

■ LACTATE DEHYDROGENASE (LDH)

45–100 U/L.

Increased: Acute myocardial infarction, cardiac surgery, hepatitis, pernicious anemia, malignant tumors, pulmonary embolus, hemolysis, renal infarction.

■ LACTIC ACID (LACTATE)

4.5–19.8 mg/dL or 0.5–2.2 mmol/L.

Increased: In hypoxia, hemorrhage, circulatory collapse, sepsis, cirrhosis, with exercise.

■ LEUKOCYTE ALKALINE PHOSPHATASE SCORE (LAP SCORE)

70–140.

Increased: Leukemoid reaction, Hodgkin's disease, polycythemia vera, myeloproliferative disorders, pregnancy, liver disease, acute inflammation.

Decreased: Chronic myelogenous leukemia, pernicious anemia, paroxysmal nocturnal hemoglobinuria, nephrotic syndrome.

■ LIGASE CHAIN REACTION FOR *NEISSERIA GONORRHOEAE* AND *CHLAMYDIA TRACHOMATIS* FOR URINE

Normal: Not detected.

This is a useful screening test for infections by these agents in populations where there is high prevalence. The patient should not have voided 2 hours prior to providing specimen.

■ LIPASE

Variable depending on the method; 10–150 U/L by turbidimetric method.

Increased: Acute pancreatitis; pancreatic duct obstruction (stone, stricture, tumor, drug-induced spasm); fat emboli. Usually normal in mumps.

■ LUPUS ANTICOAGULANT

See Antiphospholipid Antibodies, p 349.

■ LYMPHOCYTES, TOTAL

1800–3000/mL.

Used to assess nutritional status. Calculated by multiplying the white blood cell count by the percentage of lymphocytes: < 900, severe; 900–1400, moderate; 1400–1800, minimal nutritional deficit. Lymphopenia is also seen with certain viral infections, including HIV.

■ MAGNESIUM

1.6–2.4 mg/dL or 0.80–1.20 mmol/L.

Increased: Renal failure, hypothyroidism, magnesium-containing antacids, Addison's disease, severe dehydration.

Decreased: See Section I, Chapter 39, Hypomagnesemia, p 210.

■ MAGNESIUM, URINE

6.0–10.0 mEq/d or 3.00–5.00 mmol/d.

Increased: Hypermagnesemia, diuretics, hypercalcemia, metabolic acidosis, hypophosphatemia.

Decreased: Hypomagnesemia, hypocalcemia, hypoparathyroidism, metabolic alkalosis.

■ METANEPHRINES, URINE

Total: < 1.0 mg or 0.574 mmol/24-hr urine;

Fractionated metanephrines-normetanephrines: < 0.9 mg or 0.517 mmol/24-hr urine;

Fractionated metanephrines: < 0.4 mg or 0.230 mg/24-hr urine.

Increased: Pheochromocytoma, neural crest tumors (neuroblastoma), false-positives with drugs (phenobarbital, hydrocortisone, others).

■ MONOSPOT

Negative: Normal.

Positive: Mononucleosis.

■ MYOGLOBIN, URINE

Qualitative negative.

Positive: Disorders affecting skeletal muscle (crush injury, rhabdomyolysis, electrical burns, delirium tremens, surgery), acute myocardial infarction.

■ 5′-NUCLEOTIDASE

2–15 U/L.

Increased: Obstructive liver disease.

■ OSMOLALITY, SERUM

275–295 mOsm/kg.

A rough estimation of osmolality is [2(Na) + BUN/2.8 + glucose/18]). The calculation will not be accurate if foreign substances that increase the osmolality (eg, mannitol) are present. If foreign substances are suspected, osmolality should be measured directly.

Increased: Hyperglycemia; alcohol or ethylene glycol ingestion; increased sodium resulting from water loss (diabetes insipidus, hypercalcemia, diuresis); mannitol.

Decreased: Low serum sodium, diuretics, Addison's disease, hypothyroidism, syndrome of inappropriate antidiuretic hormone (SIADH), iatrogenic causes (poor fluid balance).

■ OSMOLALITY, URINE

Spot 50–1400 mOsm/kg; > 850 mOsm/kg after 12 hours of fluid restriction.

The loss of the ability to concentrate urine, especially during fluid restriction, is an early indicator of impaired renal function.

■ OXYGEN, ARTERIAL (PO_2)

See Table 2–1, p 350; see also Section VI, Ventilator Management, p 450.

Decreased:

- **Ventilation-perfusion ($\dot{V}/\dot{Q}$) abnormalities:** COPD, asthma, atelectasis, pneumonia, pulmonary embolus, adult respiratory distress syndrome, pneumothorax, cystic fibrosis, obstructed airway.
- **Alveolar hypoventilation:** Skeletal abnormalities, neuromuscular disorders, Pickwickian syndrome.
- **Decreased pulmonary diffusing capacity:** Pneumoconiosis, pulmonary edema, pulmonary fibrosis.
- **Right-to-left shunt:** Congenital heart disease (tetralogy of Fallot, transposition, others).

■ PARATHYROID HORMONE (PTH)

Normal based on relationship to serum calcium, usually provided on the lab report. Also, reference values will vary depending on the laboratory and whether N-terminal, C-terminal, or midmolecule is measured.

PTH midmolecule: 0.29–0.85 ng/mL or 29–85 pmol/L with calcium 8.4–10.2 mg/dL or 2.1–2.55 mmol/L.

Increased: Primary hyperparathyroidism, secondary hyperparathyroidism (hypocalcemic states such as chronic renal failure, others).

Decreased: Hypercalcemia not resulting from hyperparathyroidism and hypoparathyroidism.

■ PARTIAL THROMBOPLASTIN TIME (PTT)

27–38 seconds.

Prolonged: Heparin and any defect in the intrinsic clotting mechanism, such as severe liver disease or disseminated intravascular coagulation (includes factors I, II, V, VIII, IX, X, XI, and XII); prolonged use of a tourniquet before drawing a blood sample; hemophilia A and B; lupus anticoagulant; liver disease. Also, elevated in the presence of lupus anticoagulant. See Section I, Chapter 12, Coagulopathy, p 66.

■ pH, ARTERIAL

See Tables 2–1 and 2–2, p 350.

Increased: Metabolic and respiratory alkalosis. See Section I, Chapter 3, Alkalosis, p 18.

Decreased: Metabolic and respiratory acidosis. See Section I, Chapter 2, Acidosis, p 9.

■ PHOSPHORUS

2.7–4.5 mg/dL or 0.87–1.45 mmol/L.

Increased: Hypoparathyroidism, pseudohypoparathyroidism, excess vitamin D, secondary hypoparathyroidism, acute and chronic renal failure, acromegaly, tumor lysis (lymphoma or leukemia treated with chemotherapy), alkalosis, factitious increase (hemolysis of specimen).

Decreased: See Section I, Chapter 41, Hypophosphatemia, p 220.

■ PLASMINOGEN

7–17 mg/dL.

Plasminogen activity: 75–140%.

Decreased: Uncommon cause of inherited thrombosis, primary and secondary fibrinolysis, liver disease, after fibrinolytic therapy.

■ PLATELETS

See Table 2–4, p 354.

Platelet counts may be normal in number, but abnormal in function (eg, aspirin therapy); platelet function with a normal platelet count can be assessed by measuring bleeding time.

Increased: Primary thrombocytosis (idiopathic myelofibrosis, agnogenic myeloid metaplasia, polycythemia vera, primary thrombocythemia, chronic myelogenous leukemia). Secondary thrombocytosis (collagen-vascular diseases, chronic infection [osteomyelitis, tuberculosis], sarcoidosis, hemolytic anemia, iron deficiency anemia, recovery from B_{12} deficiency or iron deficiency or heavy ethanol ingestion, solid tumors and lymphomas; after surgery, especially postsplenectomy; response to drugs such as epinephrine, or withdrawal of myelosuppressive drugs).

Decreased: See Section I, Chapter 61, Thrombocytopenia, p 333.

■ POTASSIUM, SERUM

3.5–5.1 mmol/L.

Increased: See Section I, Chapter 33, Hyperkalemia, p 186.

Decreased: See Section I, Chapter 38, Hypokalemia, p 206.

■ POTASSIUM, URINE

25–125 mmol/24-hr urine; varies with diet. See Urinary Electrolytes, p 385.

■ PROLACTIN

Females: 1–25 ng/mL.
Males: 1–20 ng/mL.

Increased: Pregnancy, nursing after pregnancy, prolactinoma, hypothalamic tumors, sarcoidosis or granulomatous disease of the hypothalamus, hypothyroidism, renal failure, Addison's disease, phenothiazines, butyrophenones (eg, haloperidol [Haldol]).

Decreased: Sheehan's syndrome.

■ PROSTATE-SPECIFIC ANTIGEN (PSA)

< 4 ng/dL.

Most useful as a measure of response to therapy for prostate cancer. Also used for screening for prostate carcinoma. Values > 8.0 ng/dL are associated with carcinoma at the 90% confidence level.

Increased: Prostate cancer, some cases of benign prostatic hypertrophy, prostatic infarction, post ejaculation (returns to normal level in 48 hours), vigorous exercise (returns to normal in 48–72 hours).

Decreased: Total prostatectomy, response to therapy for prostatic carcinoma.

■ PROTEIN ELECTROPHORESIS, SERUM AND URINE (SERUM PROTEIN ELECTROPHORESIS [SPEP]; URINE PROTEIN ELECTROPHORESIS [UPEP])

Quantitative analysis of the serum proteins is often used in the evaluation of hypoglobulinemia, macroglobulinemia, α_1-antitrypsin deficiency, collagen disease, liver disease, myeloma, and occasionally in nutritional assessment. Serum electrophoresis yields five different bands (see Figure 2–1, p 374; and Table 2–6, p 375). If a monoclonal gammopathy or a low globulin fraction is detected, quantitative immunoglobulins should be checked.

Urine protein electrophoresis can be used to evaluate proteinuria and can detect Bence–Jones (light-chain) protein that is associated with myeloma, Waldenström's macroglobulinemia, and Fanconi's syndrome.

■ PROTEIN, SERUM

6.0–7.8 g/dL or 60–78 g/L.

Increased: Multiple myeloma, Waldenström's macroglobulinemia, benign monoclonal gammopathy, lymphoma, sarcoidosis, chronic inflammatory disease.

Decreased: Any cause of decreased albumin or any cause of hypogammaglobulinemia such as common variable hypogammaglobulinemia.

■ PROTEIN, URINE

See also Albumin, Urine, p 346.

< 100 mg/24-hr urine;
Spot: < 10 mg/dL (< 20 mg/dL if early-morning collection);
Dipstick: negative.

Increased: Nephrotic syndrome, glomerulonephritis, lupus nephritis, amyloidosis, renal vein thrombosis, severe congestive heart failure, multiple

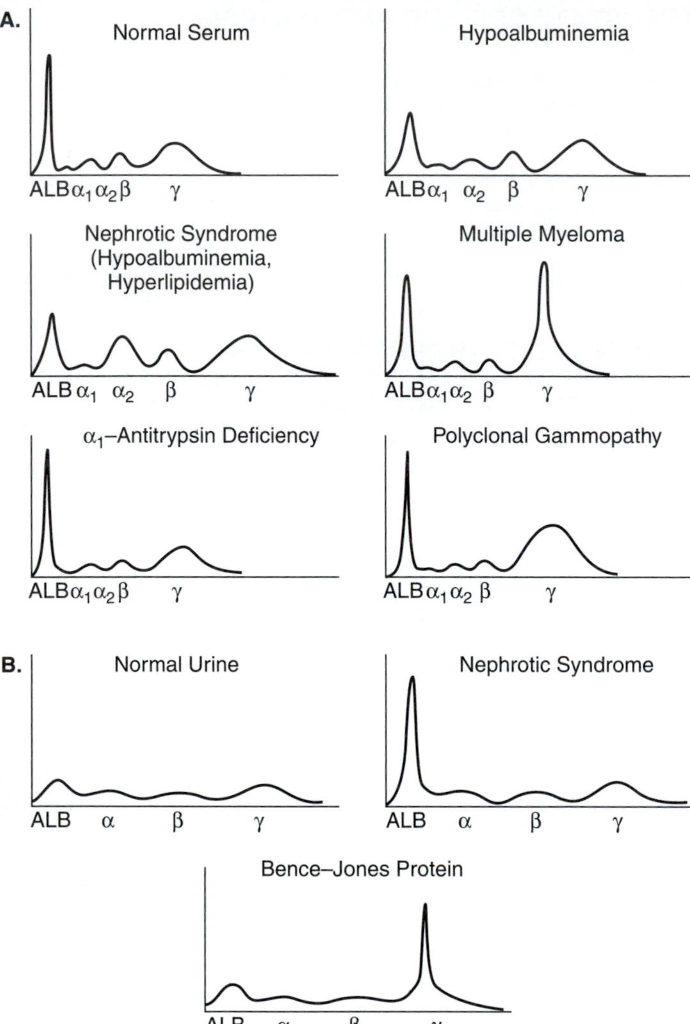

Figure 2–1. Protein electrophoresis patterns. Examples of (**A**) serum and (**B**) urine protein electrophoresis patterns.

TABLE 2–6. NORMAL SERUM PROTEIN COMPONENTS AND FRACTIONS AS DETERMINED BY ELECTROPHORESIS ALONG WITH ASSOCIATED CONDITIONS.[1]

Protein Fraction	Percentage of Total Protein	Constituents	Increased	Decreased
Albumin	52–68	Albumin	Dehydration (only known cause)	Nephrosis, malnutrition, chronic liver disease
α_1-Globulin	2.4–4.4	Thyroxine-binding globulin, antitrypsin, lipoproteins, glycoprotein, transcortin	Inflammation, neoplasia	Nephrosis, α_1-antitrypsin deficiency (emphysema-related)
α_2-Globulin	6.1–10.1	Haptoglobin, glycoprotein, macroglobulin, ceruloplasmin	Inflammation, infection, neoplasia, cirrhosis	Severe liver disease, acute hemolytic anemia
β-Globulin	3.5–14.5	Transferrin, glycoprotein, lipoprotein	Cirrhosis, obstructive jaundice	Nephrosis
γ-Globulins (immunoglobulins)	10–21	IgA, IgG, IgM, IgD, IgE	Infections, collagen-vascular diseases, leukemia, myeloma	Agammaglobulinemia, hypogammaglobulinemia, nephrosis

[1] *Reproduced with permission from Gomella LG, ed.* Clinician's Pocket Reference. *9th ed.: McGraw-Hill; 2002.*

myeloma, pre-eclampsia, postural proteinuria, polycystic kidney disease, diabetic nephropathy, radiation nephritis, malignant hypertension.

False-positive: Gross hematuria, very concentrated urine, Pyridium, very alkaline urine.

■ PROTEIN C, PLASMA

Normal = 60–130%.

Decreased: Hypercoagulable states resulting in recurrent venous thrombosis; chronic liver disease; disseminated intravascular coagulation (DIC); postoperatively; neoplastic disease and autosomal recessive deficiency.

■ PROTEIN S, PLASMA

Normal = 60–140%.

Decreased: See Protein C, Plasma. Protein S is a cofactor of protein C; should be ordered along with protein C.

■ PROTHROMBIN TIME (PT)

See International Normalized Ratio (INR), p 366.
11.5–13.5 seconds.
Evaluates extrinsic clotting mechanism (factors I, II, V, VII, and X).

Prolonged: Drugs such as sodium warfarin (Coumadin), decreased vitamin K, fat malabsorption, liver disease, prolonged use of a tourniquet before drawing a blood sample, disseminated intravascular coagulation (DIC), lupus anticoagulant (usually selectively increased PTT). See Section I, Chapter 12, Coagulopathy, p 66.

■ QUANTITATIVE IMMUNOGLOBULINS

IgG: 650–1500 mg/dL or 6.5–15 g/L;
IgM: 40–345 mg/dL or 0.4–3.45 g/L;
IgA: 76–390 mg/dL or 0.76–3.90 g/L;
IgE: 0–380 IU/mL or KIU/L;
IgD: 0–8 mg/dL or 0–80 mg/L.

Increased: Multiple myeloma (myeloma immunoglobulin increased, other immunoglobulins decreased), Waldenström's macroglobulinemia (IgM increased, others decreased), lymphoma, carcinoma, bacterial and viral infections, liver disease, sarcoidosis, amyloidosis, myeloproliferative disorders.

Decreased: Hereditary immunodeficiency, leukemia, lymphoma, nephrotic syndrome, protein-losing enteropathy, malnutrition.

■ RAPID PLASMA REAGIN (RPR)

See VDRL, p 387.

■ RED BLOOD CELL COUNT (RBC)

See Table 2–4, p 354. Also see Hematocrit, p 363.

■ RED BLOOD CELL INDICES

See Table 2–4, p 354.

MCV (Mean Cell Volume)

Increased: Megaloblastic anemia (B_{12}, folate deficiency), reticulocytosis, chronic liver disease, alcoholism, hypothyroidism, aplastic anemia.

Decreased: Iron deficiency, sideroblastic anemia, thalassemia, some cases of lead poisoning, hereditary spherocytosis.

MCH (Mean Cellular Hemoglobin)

Increased: Macrocytosis (megaloblastic anemias, high reticulocyte counts).

Decreased: Microcytosis (iron deficiency).

MCHC (Mean Cellular Hemoglobin Concentration)

Increased: Severe and prolonged dehydration; spherocytosis.

Decreased: Iron deficiency anemia, overhydration, thalassemia, sideroblastic anemia.

RDW (Red Cell Distribution Width)

Measure of the degree of homogenicity of RBC size.

Increased: An increase in the RDW suggests two different populations of RBCs, such as a combination of a macrocytic and microcytic anemia or recovery from iron deficiency anemia (microcytosis plus reticulocytosis).

■ RED BLOOD CELL MORPHOLOGY

Poikilocytosis: Irregular RBC shape (sickle, burr).

Anisocytosis: Irregular RBC size (microcytes, macrocytes).

Basophilic stippling: Lead, heavy metal poisoning, thalassemia.

Howell-Jolly bodies: Seen after a splenectomy and in some severe anemias.

Sickling: Sickle cell disease and trait.

Nucleated RBCs: Severe bone marrow stress (hemorrhage, hemolysis), marrow replacement by tumor, extramedullary hematopoiesis.

Target cells: Thalassemia, hemoglobinopathies (sickle cell disease), obstructive jaundice, any hypochromic anemia, after splenectomy.

Spherocytes: Hereditary spherocytosis, immune or microangiopathic hemolysis.

Helmet cells (schistocytes): Microangiopathic hemolysis, hemolytic transfusion reaction, other hemolytic anemias.

Burr cells (acanthocytes): Severe liver disease; high levels of bile, fatty acids, or toxins.

Polychromasia: Appearance of a bluish-gray RBC on routine Wright's stain suggests reticulocytes.

■ RETICULOCYTE COUNT

0.5–1.5%.

If the patient's hematocrit is abnormal, a corrected reticulocyte count should be calculated as follows:

$$\text{Corrected reticulocyte count} = \%\ \text{reticulocytes} \times \frac{\text{patient's hematocrit}}{45\%}$$

Increased: Hemolysis, acute hemorrhage, therapeutic response to treatment for iron, vitamin B_{12}, or folate deficiency.

Decreased: Infiltration of bone marrow by carcinoma, lymphoma, or leukemia, marrow aplasia, chronic infections such as osteomyelitis, toxins, drugs (> 100 reported), many anemias.

■ RHEUMATOID FACTOR (RA LATEX TEST)

< 15 IU by microscan kit or < 1:40.

Increased: Rheumatoid arthritis, systemic lupus erythematosus, Sjögren's syndrome, scleroderma, dermatomyositis, polymyositis, syphilis, chronic inflammation, subacute bacterial endocarditis, hepatitis, sarcoidosis, interstitial pulmonary fibrosis.

■ SEDIMENTATION RATE (ESR)

- **Wintrobe Scale:** Males: 0–9 mm/hr;

Females: 0–20 mm/hr.

- **ZETA Scale:** 40–54%, normal; 55–59%, mildly elevated; 60–64%, moderately elevated; > 65%, markedly elevated.
- **Westergren Scale:** Males < 50 years: 15 mm/hr; males > 50 years: 20 mm/hr;
- Females < 50 years, 25 mm/hr; females > 50 years: 30 mm/hr.

- This is a very nonspecific test. The ZETA method is not affected by anemia. The Westergren scale remains the preferred method.

Increased: Infection, inflammation, rheumatic fever, endocarditis, neoplasm, acute myocardial infarction.

■ SGGT (SERUM GAMMA-GLUTAMYLTRANSFERASE)

See Gamma-Glutamyltransferase (GGT), p 361.

■ SGOT (SERUM GLUTAMIC-OXALOACETIC TRANSFERASE) OR AST (SERUM ASPARTATE AMINOTRANSFERASE)

See AST, p 349.

■ SGPT (SERUM GLUTAMIC-PYRUVIC TRANSFERASE) OR ALT (SERUM ALANINE AMINOTRANSFERASE)

See ALT, p 346.

■ SODIUM, SERUM

136–145 mmol/L.

Increased: See Section I, Chapter 34, Hypernatremia, p 190.

Decreased: See Section I, Chapter 40, Hyponatremia, p 214.

■ SODIUM, URINE

40–210 mmol/24-hr urine. See Urinary Electrolytes, p 385.

■ STOOL FOR OCCULT BLOOD (HEMOCCULT TEST)

Negative: Normal.

Positive: Swallowed blood; ingestion of red meat; any gastrointestinal tract lesion (ulcer, carcinoma, polyp); large doses of vitamin C (> 500 mg/d). See also Section I, Chapter 28, Hematochezia, p 162; and Chapter 27, Hematemesis, Melena, p 158.

■ STOOL FOR WBC

Occasional WBCs, usually PMNs.

Increased: *Shigella, Salmonella,* enteropathogenic *Escherichia coli,* pseudomembranous colitis (*Clostridium difficile*), ulcerative colitis.

■ T_3 (TRIIODOTHYRONINE) RADIOIMMUNOASSAY

120–195 ng/dL or 1.85–3.00 nmol/L.

Increased: Hyperthyroidism; T_3 thyrotoxicosis; exogenous T_4; any cause of increased thyroid-binding globulin such as oral estrogens, pregnancy, or hepatitis.

Decreased: Hypothyroidism, euthyroid sick state, any cause of decreased thyroid-binding globulin (eg, malnutrition).

■ T_3 RU (RESIN UPTAKE)

24–34%.

Increased: Hyperthyroidism; medications (phenytoin, anabolic steroids, corticosteroids, heparin, aspirin, others); nephrotic syndrome.

Decreased: Hypothyroidism, pregnancy, medications (estrogens, iodine, propylthiouracil, others).

■ T_4 TOTAL (THYROXINE)

5–12 µg/dL or 65–155 nmol/L.
Males: 5–10 µg/dL: 5–10 µg/dL or 65–129 nmol.
Females: 5.5–10.5 µg/dL or 71–135 nmol/L.

Increased: Hyperthyroidism; exogenous thyroid hormone; any cause of increased thyroid-binding globulin (eg, estrogens, pregnancy, or hepatitis); euthyroid sick state.

Decreased: Hypothyroidism, euthyroid sick state, any cause of decreased thyroid-binding globulin (eg, malnutrition).

■ THROMBIN TIME

10–14 seconds.

Increased: Heparin, disseminated intravascular coagulation, elevated fibrin degradation products, fibrinogen deficiency, congenitally abnormal fibrinogen molecules. See Section I, Chapter 12, Coagulopathy, p 66.

■ THYROGLOBULIN

0–60 ng/mL or < 60 µg/L.
Used primarily to detect recurrence of nonmedullary thyroid carcinoma after resection.

Increased: Differentiated thyroid carcinomas (papillary, follicular), thyroid adenoma, Graves' disease, toxic goiter, nontoxic goiter, thyroiditis.

Decreased: Hypothyroidism, testosterone, steroids, phenytoin.

■ THYROID-BINDING GLOBULIN (TBG)

1.5–3.4 mg/dL or 15–34 mg/L.

Increased: Hypothyroidism, pregnancy, medications (oral contraceptives, estrogens), hepatitis, acute porphyria, familial.

Decreased: Hyperthyroidism, medications (androgens, anabolic steroids, corticosteroids, phenytoin), nephrotic syndrome, severe illness, liver failure, malnutrition.

■ THYROID-STIMULATING HORMONE (TSH)

0.7–5.3 mU/mL.

Newer sensitive assays are excellent screening tests for hyperthyroidism as well as hypothyroidism; they allow you to distinguish between a low normal and a decreased TSH.

Increased: Hypothyroidism.

Decreased: Hyperthyroidism. Fewer than 1% of cases of hypothyroidism are from pituitary or hypothalamic disease resulting in a decreased TSH.

■ TRANSFERRIN

220–400 mg/dL or 2.20–4.00 g/L.

Increased: Acute and chronic blood loss, iron deficiency anemia, hepatitis, oral contraceptives.

Decreased: Anemia of chronic disease, cirrhosis, malnutrition nephrosis, hemochromatosis.

■ TRIGLYCERIDES

Males: 40–160 mg/dL or 0.45–1.81 mmol/L.

Females: 35–135 mg/dL or 0.40–1.53 mmol/L; may vary with age.

Increased: Hyperlipoproteinemias (types I, IIb, III, IV, V), hypothyroidism, liver diseases, diabetes mellitus, alcoholism, pancreatitis, acute myocardial infarction, nephrotic syndrome.

Decreased: Malnutrition, congenital abetalipoproteinemia.

TROPONIN I

< 0.6 ng/mL or < .6 μg/L.

Increased: In myocardial injury levels > 1.5 ng/mL (1.5 μg/L) is consistent with myocardial infarction. Sensitivity is similar to CK-MB but more specific. Does not tend to be elevated with skeletal muscle injury nor chronic renal disease as much as the CK-MB. False-positives can be seen in clotted specimens and in the presence of heterophil antibodies. Elevated within 4–8 hours of myocardial injury with peak at 12–16 hours, but remains elevated for 5–9 days.

TROPONIN T

< 0.1 ng/mL or < .1 μg/L.

Increased: In myocardial injury but also in muscle disease such as muscular dystrophy. Not as valuable in assessing acute myocardial injury though it parallels troponin I. Its importance may be in risk stratification of cardiac patients (determining those patients with unstable angina who are more likely to have a cardiac-related death).

TRYPTASE

5.6–13.5 μg/L.

Increased: Diseases of mast cell activation such as anaphylaxis or mastocytosis.

Released in a slower manner than histamine and more stable so that it can be detected for a longer period of time than histamine. In anaphylaxis, histamine peaks in 5 minutes and returns to normal in less than 1 hour. Tryptase peaks in 1–2 hours and returns to normal after a few hours.

URIC ACID

Males: 4.5–8.2 mg/dL or 0.27–0.48 mmol/L.

Females: 3.0–6.5 mg/dL or 0.18–0.38 mmol/L.

Increased: Gout; renal failure; destruction of massive amounts of nucleoproteins (tumor lysis after chemotherapy, leukemia or lymphoma); toxemia of pregnancy; drugs (especially diuretics); hypothyroidism; polycystic kidney disease; parathyroid diseases.

Decreased: Uricosuric drugs (salicylates, probenecid, allopurinol), Wilson's disease, Fanconi's syndrome, pregnancy.

URINALYSIS, ROUTINE

Appearance

- **Normal:** Yellow, clear, straw-colored
- **Pink/red:** Blood, hemoglobin, myoglobin, food coloring, beets

- **Orange:** Pyridium, rifampin, bile pigments
- **Brown/black:** Myoglobin, bile pigments, melanin, cascara bark, iron, nitrofurantoin, metronidazole, sickle cell crisis
- **Blue:** Methylene blue, *Pseudomonas* urinary tract infection (rare), hereditary tryptophan metabolic disorders
- **Cloudy:** Urinary tract infection (pyuria), blood, myoglobin, chyluria, mucus (normal in ileal loop specimens), phosphate salts (normal in alkaline urine), urates (normal in acidic urine), hyperoxaluria
- **Foamy:** Proteinuria, bile salts

pH

(4.6–8.0)

Acidic: High-protein diet; methenamine mandelate; acidosis; ketoacidosis (starvation, diabetic); diarrhea; dehydration.

Basic: Urinary tract infection, involving *Proteus;* renal tubular acidosis; diet (high vegetable, milk, immediately postprandial); sodium bicarbonate or acetazolamide therapy; vomiting; metabolic alkalosis; chronic renal failure.

Specific Gravity

Normal: 1.001–1.035.

Increased: Volume depletion, congestive heart failure (CHF), adrenal insufficiency, diabetes mellitus, syndrome of inappropriate antidiuretic hormone (SIADH), increased proteins (nephrosis). If markedly increased (1.040–1.050), suspect artifact, excretion of radiographic contrast medium, or some other osmotic agent.

Decreased: Diabetes insipidus, pyelonephritis, glomerulonephritis, water load with normal renal function.

Bilirubin

Negative dipstick.

Positive: Obstructive jaundice, hepatitis, cirrhosis, CHF with hepatic congestion, congenital hyperbilirubinemia (Dubin-Johnson syndrome).

Blood (Hemoglobin)

Negative dipstick.

Positive: Hematuria (See Section I, Chapter 29, Hematuria, p 166); free hemoglobin (from trauma, transfusion reaction, or lysis of red blood cells); or myoglobin (crush injury, burn, or tissue ischemia).

Glucose

Negative dipstick.

Positive: Diabetes mellitus; other endocrine disorders (pheochromocytoma, hyperthyroidism, Cushing's syndrome, hyperadrenalism); stress states (sepsis, burns); pancreatitis; renal tubular disease; medications (corticosteroids, thiazides, birth control pills); false-positive with vitamin C ingestion.

Ketones

Negative dipstick.

Positive: Starvation, high-fat diet, alcoholic and diabetic ketoacidosis, vomiting, diarrhea, hyperthyroidism, pregnancy, febrile states.

Leukocyte Esterase

Negative dipstick.

Positive: Infection (test detects 5 or more WBC/HPF or lysed WBCs).

Microscopy

Note: Many laboratories will no longer perform urine microscopy on a routine basis when the dipstick is negative and the gross appearance is normal.

- **RBCs:** (Normal: 0–3/HPF.) Trauma, urinary tract infection, prostatic hypertrophy, genitourinary tuberculosis, nephrolithiasis, malignant and benign tumors, glomerulonephritis.
- **WBCs:** (Normal: 0–4/HPF.) Infection anywhere in the urinary tract, genitourinary tuberculosis, renal tumors, acute glomerulonephritis, radiation damage, interstitial nephritis (analgesic abuse). (Glitter cells represent WBCs lysed in hypotonic solution.)
- **Epithelial cells:** (Normal: occasional.) Acute tubular necrosis, necrotizing papillitis.
- **Parasites:** (Normal: none.) *Trichomonas vaginalis, Schistosoma haematobium.*
- **Yeast:** (Normal: none.) *Candida albicans* (especially in diabetics and immunosuppressed patients, or if a vaginal infection is present).
- **Spermatozoa:** (Normal: after intercourse or nocturnal emission.)
- **Crystals:** Normal:

Acid urine: Calcium oxalate (small square crystals with a central cross), uric acid.

Alkaline urine: Calcium carbonate, triple phosphate (resemble coffin lids).

Abnormal: Cystine, sulfonamide, leucine, tyrosine, cholesterol, or excessive amounts of the crystals noted earlier.

- **Contaminants:** Cotton threads, hair, wood fibers, amorphous substances (all usually unimportant).

- **Mucus:** (Normal: small amounts.) Large amounts suggest urethral disease. Ileal loop urine normally has large amounts.
- **Hyaline cast:** (Normal: occasional.) Benign hypertension, nephrotic syndrome.
- **RBC cast:** (Normal: none.) Acute glomerulonephritis, lupus nephritis, subacute bacterial endocarditis, Goodpasture's disease, vasculitis, malignant hypertension.
- **WBC cast:** (Normal: none.) Pyelonephritis or interstitial nephritis.
- **Epithelial cast:** (Normal: occasional.) Tubular damage, nephrotoxin, viral infections.
- **Granular cast:** (Normal: none.) Results from breakdown of cellular casts, leads to waxy casts.
- **Waxy cast:** (Normal: none.) End stage of a granular cast; evidence of severe chronic renal disease, amyloidosis.
- **Fatty cast:** (Normal: none.) Nephrotic syndrome, diabetes mellitus, damaged renal tubular epithelial cells.
- **Broad cast:** (Normal: none.) Chronic renal disease.

Nitrite

Negative dipstick.

Positive: Bacterial infection (a negative test does not rule out infection).

Protein

See also Albumin, Urine, p 346.
Negative dipstick.

Positive: See Protein, Urine, p 373.

Reducing Substance

Negative dipstick.

Positive: Glucose, fructose, galactose.

False-positives: Vitamin C, antibiotics.

Urobilinogen

Negative dipstick.

Positive: Bile duct obstruction, suppression of gut flora with antibiotics.

■ URINARY ELECTROLYTES

These "spot urines" are of limited value because of large variations in daily fluid and salt intake. Results are usually indeterminate if a diuretic has been given. Sodium is most useful in the differentiation of volume depletion, oliguria, or hyponatremia. Chloride is useful in the diagnosis and treatment of metabolic alkalosis. Urinary potassium levels are often used in the evaluation of hypokalemia.

- **Chloride < 10 mmol/L:** Chloride-sensitive metabolic alkalosis. See Section I, Chapter 3, Alkalosis, p 18.
- **Chloride > 20 mmol/L:** Chloride-resistant metabolic alkalosis. See Section I, Chapter 3, Alkalosis, p 18.
- **Potassium < 10 mmol/L:** Hypokalemia, from extrarenal losses.
- **Potassium > 10 mmol/L:** Renal potassium wasting (diuretics, brisk urinary output).
- **Sodium < 20 mmol/L:** Volume depletion, hyponatremic states, prerenal azotemia (CHF, shock, others), hepatorenal syndrome, edematous states.
- **Sodium > 40 mmol/L:** Acute tubular necrosis, adrenal insufficiency, renal salt wasting, syndrome of inappropriate antidiuretic hormone (SIADH).
- **Sodium > 20–40 mmol/L:** Indeterminate.

■ URINARY INDICES

See Table 2–7. These indices are used in determining the etiology of oliguria. See Section I, Chapter 51, Oliguria/Anuria, p 266.

■ VANILLYLMANDELIC ACID (VMA), URINE

2–7 mg/dL or 10.1–35.4 mmol/d.

VMA is urinary metabolite of both epinephrine and norepinephrine.

TABLE 2–7. URINARY INDICES IN ACUTE RENAL FAILURE ACCOMPANIED BY OLIGURIA: DIFFERENTIAL DIAGNOSIS OF OLIGURIA.[1]

Index	Prerenal	Renal (ATN)
Urine osmolality	> 500	< 350
Urinary sodium	< 10–20	> 30–40
Urine/serum creatinine	> 40	< 20
Fractional excreted sodium[2]	< 1	> 1
Renal failure index[3]	< 1	> 1

[1]*Modified and reproduced with permission from Gomella LG, ed.* Clinician's Pocket Reference. *9th ed. McGraw-Hill; 2002.*

[2] $\text{Fractional excreted sodium} = \dfrac{(\text{urine / serum sodium})}{(\text{urine / serum creatinine})} \times 100.$

[3] $\text{Renal failure index} = \dfrac{(\text{urine sodium} \times \text{serum creatinine})}{(\text{urine creatinine})}$

Increased: Pheochromocytoma; neural crest tumors (neuroblastoma, ganglioneuroma). False-positive with methyldopa, chocolate, vanilla, others.

■ VDRL TEST (VENEREAL DISEASE RESEARCH LABORATORY) OR RAPID PLASMA REAGIN (RPR)

Normal: Nonreactive.

Good for screening syphilis. Almost always positive in secondary syphilis, but frequently becomes negative in late syphilis. Also, in some patients with HIV infection, the VDRL can be negative in primary and secondary syphilis.

Positive (reactive): Syphilis, systemic lupus erythematosus, pregnancy and drug addiction. If reactive, confirm with FTA-ABS (false-positives may occur with bacterial or viral illnesses).

■ WHITE BLOOD CELL COUNT

See Table 2–3, p . . . .

Increased: See Section I, Chapter 48, Leukocytosis, p 251.

Decreased: See Section I, Chapter 49, Leukopenia, p 255.

■ WHITE BLOOD CELL DIFFERENTIAL

See Table 2–4, p 354. Many hospitals are now performing differentials on automated machines. The newer automated differentials can differentiate neutrophils, lymphocytes, monocytes, eosinophils, and basophils. A manual differential must be done to differentiate segmented and banded neutrophils.

Neutrophils

40–70% segmented neutrophils, 5–10% banded neutrophils.

Increased: Exercise, pain, stress, infection, burns, drugs, thyrotoxicosis, steroids, malignancy, chronic inflammatory disease (vasculitis, collagen-vascular disease, colitis), lithium, epinephrine, asplenia, idiopathic.

Decreased: Congenital, immune-mediated, drug-induced, infectious (viral, rickettsial, parasitic).

Lymphocytes

Normal: 24–44%.

Increased: Measles; German measles (rubeola); mumps, whooping cough (*Bordetella pertussis*); smallpox; chickenpox (Varicella); influenza; viral hepatitis; infectious mononucleosis (Epstein-Barr virus); virtually any viral infection; acute and chronic lymphocytic leukemias.

Decreased: Following stress, burns, trauma; normal finding in 22% of population; uremia; some viral infections (including HIV).

Lymphocytes, Atypical

Normal: 0–3%.

> 20%: Infectious mononucleosis (Epstein-Barr virus), cytomegalovirus infection, viral hepatitis, toxoplasmosis.

3–20%: Viral infections (mumps, rubeola, Varicella), rickettsial infections, tuberculosis.

Monocytes

Normal: 3–7%.

Increased: Subacute bacterial endocarditis, brucellosis (*Brucella*), typhoid fever (*Salmonella typhi*), kala-azar (visceral leishmaniasis), trypanosomiasis (*Trypanosoma*), rickettsial infection, ulcerative colitis, sarcoidosis, Hodgkin's disease, monocytic leukemias, collagen-vascular diseases.

Decreased: Myelodysplasia, aplastic anemia, hairy cell leukemia, cyclic neutropenia, thermal injuries, collagen-vascular diseases.

Eosinophils

Normal: 0–3%.

Increased: Allergies, parasites, skin diseases, malignancy, drugs, asthma, Addison's disease, collagen-vascular diseases. (A handy mnemonic is **NAACP: N**eoplasm, **A**llergy, **A**ddison's disease, **C**ollagen-vascular diseases, **P**arasites).

Decreased: After steroids; ACTH; after stress (infection, trauma, burns); Cushing's syndrome.

Basophils

Normal: 0–1%.

Increased: Chronic myeloid leukemia; rarely, in recovery from infection and from hypothyroidism.

Decreased: Acute rheumatic fever, lobar pneumonia, after steroid therapy, thyrotoxicosis, stress.

■ WHITE BLOOD CELL MORPHOLOGY

- **Auer rod:** Acute myelogenous leukemias.
- **Döhle bodies:** Severe infection, burns, malignancy, pregnancy.
- **Hypersegmentation:** Megaloblastic anemias, iron deficiency, myeloproliferative disorders, drug induced.
- **Toxic granulation:** Severe illness (sepsis, burns, high temperature).

■ ZINC

60–130 μg/dL or 9–20 μmol/L.

Increased: Atherosclerosis, coronary artery disease.

Decreased: Inadequate dietary intake (parenteral nutrition, alcoholism); malabsorption; increased needs such as pregnancy or wound healing; acrodermatitis enteropathica.

REFERENCES

Burtis CA, Ashwood ER: *Tietz's Textbook of Clinical Chemistry.* 3rd ed. Saunders;1999.

Coudrey L: The troponins. Arch Intern Med 1998;158:1173.

Jurado R, Mattix H: The decreased serum urea nitrogen-creatinine ratio. Arch Intern Med 1998;115:2509.

Pettijohn TL, Doyle T, Spiekerman AM et al: Usefulness of positive troponin-T and negative creatine kinase levels in identifying high-risk patients with unstable angina pectoris. Am J Cardiol 1997;80:510.

Tchetgen M-B, Song JT, Strawderman M et al: Ejaculation increases the serum prostate-specific antigen concentration. Urology 1996;47:511.

III. Procedures

1. ARTERIAL LINE PLACEMENT

(See also Section I, Chapter 6, Arterial Line Problems, p 34).

Indications: Frequent sampling of arterial blood; hemodynamic monitoring when continuous blood pressure readings are needed, such as in a patient with malignant hypertension or a patient in shock, where indirect cuff pressures may be inaccurate.

Contraindications: Poor collateral circulation. Avoid the femoral artery if severe aortoiliac atherosclerosis is present. Coagulopathy is a relative contraindication. See Section I, Chapter 12, Coagulopathy, p 66.

Materials: 20-gauge (or smaller) 1.5- to 2-in. catheter-over-needle assembly (Angiocath), arterial line setup per ICU routine (transducer, tubing, and pressure bag with heparinized saline), armboard, sterile dressing, lidocaine.

Procedure

1. The radial artery is most frequently used; this approach is described here. Other sites, in decreasing order of preference, are the dorsalis pedis, femoral, brachial, and axillary arteries. Axillary arteries are infrequently used; catheters in these arteries should be placed by an intensivist or anesthesiologist.
2. Verify the patency of the collateral circulation between the radial and ulnar arteries using the **Allen test.** See Section III, Chapter 2, Arterial Puncture, p 391.
3. Place the extremity on an armboard with a roll of gauze behind the wrist to hyperextend the joint. Prep with povidone-iodine and drape with sterile towels. The operator should wear gloves and a mask.
4. Raise a very small skin wheal at the puncture site with 1% lidocaine using a 25-gauge needle. Carefully palpate the artery and choose the puncture site where it appears most superficial.
5. While palpating the path of the artery with your nondominant hand, advance the 20-gauge catheter-over-needle assembly into the artery at a 30-degree angle to the skin with the needle bevel up. Once a "flash" of blood is seen in the hub, hold the needle steady and advance the entire unit 1–2 mm so that the needle and catheter are in the artery. Advance the catheter over the needle into the artery. Remove the needle while briefly occluding the artery with manual pressure and connect the pressure tubing.
6. Suture in place with 3-0 silk and apply a sterile dressing.
7. Splint the dorsum of the wrist to limit mobility and provide catheter stability.

8. Kits are available with a needle and guide wire that allow the Seldinger technique to be used, which is especially useful for femoral artery cannulation.
9. Arterial lines should be replaced using a different site every 4 days to decrease risk of infection.

Complications: Thrombosis, hematoma, arterial embolism, arterial spasm, infection, hemorrhage, pseudoaneurysm formation.

2. ARTERIAL PUNCTURE

Indications: Blood gas determination; need for arterial blood in certain chemistry determinations.

Contraindications: Systemic fibrinolytic states, such as following thrombolytic therapy, are relative contraindications to arterial puncture.

Materials: Blood gas sampling kit *or* 3- to 5-mL syringe, 23- to 25-gauge needle (20–22 gauge for femoral artery), 1 mL heparin (1000 U/mL), alcohol or povidone/iodine swabs, and a cup of ice.

Procedure

1. Use a heparinized syringe for blood gas and a nonheparinized syringe for chemistry determinations. Obtain a blood gas kit (contains a preheparinized syringe), or a small syringe (3–5 mL) with a small-gauge needle (23–25 gauge for radial artery, 20–22 gauge is acceptable for femoral artery). Heparinize the syringe (if not preheparinized), by drawing up about 0.5–1 mL of heparin, pulling the plunger all the way back, and discarding the heparin.
2. Arteries, in the order of preference, are radial, femoral, and brachial. If using the radial artery, perform the **Allen test** to verify collateral flow from the ulnar artery. Have the patient make a tight fist. Occlude both the radial and ulnar arteries at the wrist and have the patient make a fist and release several times. Then have the patient open her or his hand. The hand should appear pale. While maintaining pressure on the radial artery, release the ulnar artery. If the ulnar-brachial arterial arch is patent, the entire hand should flush red within 10 seconds. If the Allen test is positive (the radial distribution will remain white beyond 10 seconds), the artery should not be used.
3. Hyperextension of the wrist joint or elbow will often bring the radial and brachial arteries closer to the surface.
4. If you are using the femoral artery, the mnemonic **NAVEL** will aid in locating the important structures in the groin. Palpate the femoral artery just two fingerbreadths below the inguinal ligament. From lateral to medial, the structures are **n**erve, **a**rtery, **v**ein, **e**mpty space, **l**ymphatic. You may wish to inject 1% lidocaine subcutaneously for anesthesia. Palpate the artery proximally and distally with two fingers, or trap the artery between two fingers placed on either side of the vessel.

5. Prep the area with either a povidone-iodine solution or an alcohol swab. Hold the syringe like a pencil with the needle bevel up and enter the skin at a 60- to 90-degree angle. Maintain slight negative pressure on the syringe.
6. Obtain blood on the downstroke or on slow withdrawal. Aspirate very slowly. A good arterial sample should require only minimal backpressure. If a glass or blood-gas syringe is used, the barrel will usually rise spontaneously. You should obtain 2–3 mL.
7. If the vessel cannot be located, redirect the needle without taking it out of the skin.
8. Withdraw the needle quickly and apply *firm* pressure at the site for at least 5–10 minutes, even if the sample was not obtained, to avoid a hematoma.
9. If the sample is for a blood gas, expel any air from the syringe, mix the contents thoroughly by twirling the syringe between your fingers, and make the syringe airtight with a cap. Place the syringe on ice before the sample is taken to the laboratory.

Complications: Localized bleeding; thrombosis of the artery, which may lead to arterial insufficiency; infection.

3. ARTHROCENTESIS (DIAGNOSTIC & THERAPEUTIC)

Indications

Diagnostic. Arthrocentesis is helpful in the diagnosis of new-onset arthritis, and to rule out infection in acute or chronic unremitting joint effusion.

Therapeutic. The procedure is used to instill steroids and maintain drainage of septic arthritis.

Contraindications: None. Care must be taken, however, not to cause excessive trauma if a coagulopathy or thrombocytopenia is present or if the patient is taking anticoagulant medications.

Materials: Betadine, alcohol swabs, sterile gloves, 1% lidocaine or ethyl chloride spray, an 18- or 20-gauge needle (a smaller-gauge needle if aspirating finger or toe joints), a large syringe (size depends on the amount of fluid present), a 3-mL syringe with a 25-gauge needle, and two heparinized tubes for cell count and crystal examination.

Discuss with your microbiology laboratory staff their preference for transporting fluid for bacterial, fungal, and acid-fast bacillus (AFB) cultures, and Gram's stain. A Thayer-Martin plate is needed if you suspect *Neisseria gonorrhoeae* (GC). A small syringe containing a long-acting corticosteroid such as Depo-Medrol or triamcinolone is optional for therapeutic arthrocentesis.

Procedure

General

1. Obtain consent. Describe the procedure and complications.

2. Determine the optimal site for aspiration and mark with indelible ink. Alternatively, make an indentation in the skin with the retracted tip of a ballpoint pen.
3. Wear gloves (universal precautions) to protect yourself against hepatitis and HIV. When aspiration is to be followed by corticosteroid injection, maintaining a sterile field with sterile implements minimizes the risk of infection to the patient.
4. Clean the area with Betadine, and dry and wipe over the aspiration site with alcohol. Betadine can render cultures negative. Let the alcohol dry before beginning the procedure.
5. Anesthetize the area with lidocaine using a 25-gauge needle, taking care not to inject the solution into the joint space. Lidocaine is bactericidal. Avoid preparations containing epinephrine, especially in a digit. Alternatively, spray the area with ethyl chloride just prior to needle aspiration.
6. Insert the aspirating needle, applying a small amount of vacuum to the syringe. Remove as much fluid as possible, repositioning the syringe if necessary.
7. If a corticosteroid is to be injected, remove the aspirating syringe from the needle, which is still in the joint space. It is helpful to ensure that the syringe can easily be removed from the needle before undertaking Step 6. Attach the syringe containing the corticosteroid, pull back on the plunger to ensure that the needle is not in a vein, and inject contents. ***Caution:*** *Never inject steroids when there is a possibility that the joint is infected.* Remove the needle and syringe, and apply pressure to the area. Generally, the equivalent of 40 mg of methylprednisolone is injected into large joints such as the knee and 20 mg into medium-sized joints such as the ankle or wrist. Preparations of intra-articular steroids are equivalent in potency. Injections of 0.5 cc into the knee or shoulder and 0.25 cc into the ankle or wrist are recommended dosages.
8. Joint fluid is sent for cell count and differential, crystal exam, Gram's stain, and cultures for bacteria, fungi, and AFB as indicated. See Section I, Chapter 47, Joint Swelling, p 245.

Arthrocentesis of the Knee

1. The knee should be fully extended with the patient supine. Wait until the patient's quadriceps muscle has relaxed, because its contraction plants the patella against the femur, making aspiration painful.
2. Insert the needle posterior to the lateral portion of the patella into the patellar-femoral groove. Direct the advancing needle slightly posteriorly and superiorly. (See Figure 3–1.)

Arthrocentesis of the Wrist. The easiest site for aspiration lies between the navicular bone and radius on the dorsal wrist.

1. Locate the distal radius between the tendons of the extensor pollicis longus and the extensor carpi radialis longus of the second finger. This site is just ulnar to the anatomic snuff box.

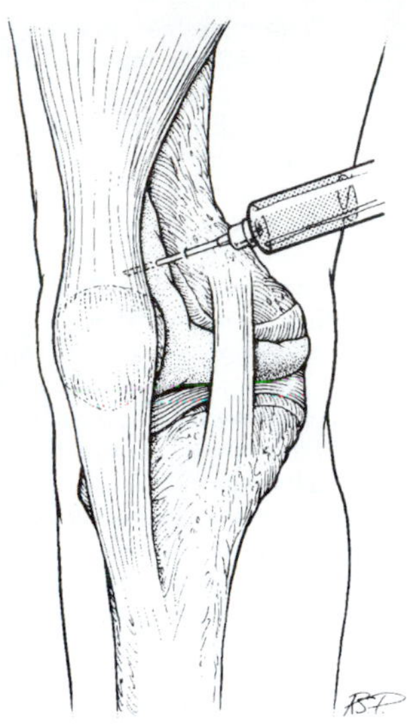

Figure 3–1. Arthrocentesis of the knee.

2. Direct the needle perpendicular to the mark. (See Figure 3–2.)

Arthrocentesis of the Ankle

1. The most accessible site lies between the tibia and the talus. The angle of the foot to leg is positioned at 90 degrees. Make a mark lateral and anterior to the medial malleolus and medial and posterior to the tibialis anterior tendon. Direct the advancing needle posteriorly toward the heel.
2. The subtalar ankle joint does not communicate with the ankle joint and is difficult to aspirate even by an expert. Keep in mind that "ankle pain" may originate in the subtalar joint rather than in the ankle. (See Figure 3–3.)

Complications: Infection, bleeding, pain. Postinjection flare-ups of joint pain and swelling can occur after steroid injection and can persist up to 48 hours. This complication is thought to be a crystal-induced synovitis resulting from the crystalline suspension used in long-acting steroids.

4. BLADDER CATHETERIZATION

(See also Section I, Chapter 24, Foley Catheter Problems, p 141).

Indications: Relieve urinary retention; collect an uncontaminated urine sample; monitor urinary output; perform bladder tests (cystogram, cystometrogram, determine postvoid residual urine quantity).

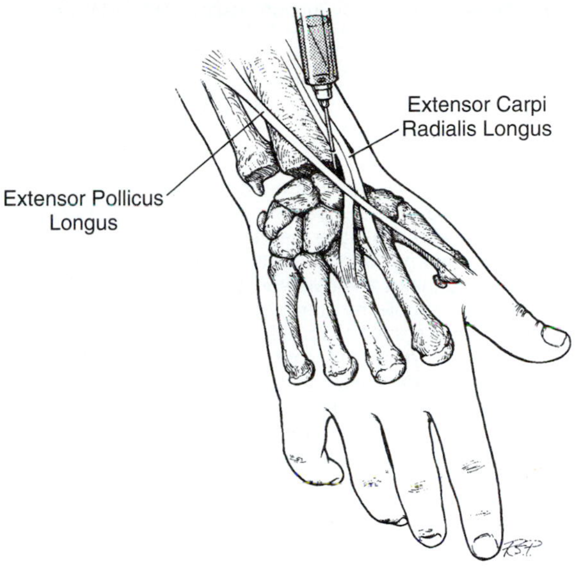

Figure 3–2. Arthrocentesis of the wrist.

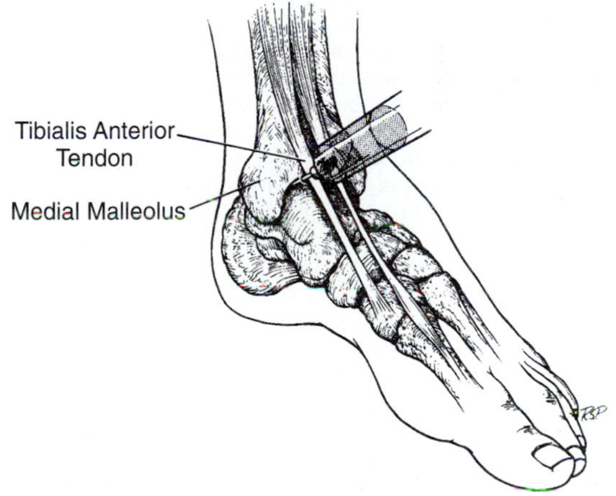

Figure 3–3. Arthrocentesis of the ankle.

Contraindications: Urethral disruption associated with pelvic fracture, acute prostatitis (relative).

Materials: Prepackaged Foley catheter tray (may need to add a catheter), catheter of choice (16- to 20-French Foley in adults).

Procedure

1. Have the patient in a well-lit area in a supine position. With females, knees should be flexed, hips internally rotated, and heels placed together to adequately expose the meatus.
2. Open the kit and put on the gloves. Prepare all the materials before you attempt to insert the catheter. Open the prep solution and soak the cotton balls; apply the sterile drapes.
3. Inflate and deflate the balloon of the Foley catheter with 5–10 mL of sterile water to ensure proper functioning. Coat the end of the catheter with lubricant jelly.
4. In females, use one gloved hand to prep the urethral meatus in a pubis-toward-anus direction; hold the labia apart with the other gloved hand. With uncircumcised males, retract the foreskin to prep the glans; use a gloved hand to hold the penis still.
5. The hand used to hold the penis or labia should not touch the catheter while you are inserting it. You can use disposable forceps in the kit to insert the catheter, or use the forceps to prep; you can then insert the catheter with your gloved hand.
6. In males, stretch the penis upward perpendicular to the body to eliminate any folds in the urethra that might create a false passage. Use *gentle* pressure to slowly advance the catheter. Any significant resistance that is encountered may represent a stricture and requires urologic consultation. In males with benign prostatic hypertrophy (BPH), a Coude-tip catheter may facilitate passage. Other means to facilitate catheter passage are ensuring that the penis is well stretched; and instilling 30–50 mL of sterile surgical lubricant into the urethra with a catheter-tipped syringe.
7. In both males and females, insert the catheter to the hilt of the drainage end. Compress the penis toward the pubis. These maneuvers ensure that the balloon will be inflated in the bladder and not in the urethra. Inflate the balloon with 5–10 mL of sterile water. After inflation, pull the catheter back so that the balloon will come to rest against the bladder neck. There should be good urine return when the catheter is in place. ***Caution:*** *Any male who is uncircumcised should have the foreskin repositioned to prevent massive edema of the glans after the catheter is inserted.*
8. If no urine returns, attempt to irrigate with 25–50 mL of sterile saline via a catheter-tipped syringe. ***Note:*** *A catheter that will not irrigate is in the urethra, not the bladder.*
9. Catheters in females can be taped to the leg. In males, the catheter should be taped to the abdominal wall to decrease urethral stricture formation (avoids catheter damage to urethra at penoscrotal junction).

Complications: Infection, bleeding, false passage.

5. BONE MARROW ASPIRATION & BIOPSY

Indications: Evaluation of anemia, thrombocytopenia, leukopenia, leukocytosis, thrombocytosis, malignancy primary to the marrow (leukemia, myeloma) or metastatic to the marrow (lung cancer, breast cancer); evaluation of iron stores; evaluation for possible disseminated infection (tuberculosis, fungal disease).

Contraindications: Infection near the puncture site. Relative contraindications include severe coagulopathy or thrombocytopenia uncorrected by transfusion of cryoprecipitate, fresh-frozen plasma, or platelets.

Materials: Commercial kits containing all necessary materials are presently available. If you do not have such a kit, you will need the following items: bone marrow biopsy needle (Jamshidi, Westerman, or similar type); sterile gloves and surgical drapes; iodine prep solution and alcohol; 22- and 26-gauge needles; at least two 10–mL syringes; 1% lidocaine solution; No. 11 scalpel blade, 4 × 4 gauze pads; and several microscope slides for staining.

Procedure

1. You must explain the procedure in detail to the patient or legally responsible individual and obtain an informed consent.
2. Local anesthesia is usually all that is required; however, it is reasonable to premedicate extremely anxious patients with an anxiolytic or sedative such as diazepam (Valium) or lorazepam (Ativan), or with an analgesic.
3. Bone marrow can be obtained from numerous sites, the most common being the posterior and anterior iliac crests and the sternum. The posterior iliac crest is the safest and is the method described here. The patient may be positioned on either the abdomen or on the side opposite the biopsy site.
4. Identify the posterior iliac crest with palpation and mark the desired biopsy site with indelible ink.
5. Use sterile gloves and follow strict aseptic technique for the remainder of the procedure.
6. Prep the biopsy site with sterile iodine solution and allow the skin to dry. Then wipe the site free of iodine with sterile alcohol. Next, cover the surrounding areas with surgical drapes.
7. Using a 26-gauge needle, administer 1% lidocaine solution subcutaneously to raise a skin wheal. Then, with the 22-gauge needle, infiltrate the deeper tissues with lidocaine until you reach the periosteum. At this point, you should advance the needle just through the periosteum and infiltrate lidocaine subperiosteally. An area approximately 2 cm in diameter should be infiltrated, using repeated periosteal punctures.

8. Once local anesthesia has been obtained, use a No. 11 scalpel blade to make a 2- to 3-mm skin incision over the biopsy site.
9. Insert the bone marrow biopsy needle through the skin incision; then advance it with a rotating motion that alternates between clockwise and counterclockwise rotation and gentle pressure until you reach the periosteum. Once the needle is firmly seated on the periosteum, advance it through the outer table of bone into the marrow cavity with the same rotating motion and gentle pressure. Generally, a slight change in the resistance to needle advancement signals entry into the marrow cavity. At this point, you should advance the needle 2–3 mm.
10. Remove the stylet from the biopsy needle and attach a 10-mL syringe to the hub of the biopsy needle. Withdraw the plunger on the syringe briskly and aspirate 1–2 mL of marrow into the syringe. The patient may experience severe, instantaneous pain. Slow withdrawal of the plunger or collection of more than 1–2 mL of marrow with each aspiration will result in excessive contamination of the specimen with peripheral blood.
11. The marrow aspiration specimen can be used to prepare coverslips for viewing under the microscope, and for special studies such as cytogenetics and cell markers or for culture. Repeat aspirations may be required to obtain enough marrow to perform all of the preceding tests. Also note that certain studies may require heparin or EDTA for collection. You should contact the appropriate laboratory prior to the procedure to be sure that you collect the specimens in the appropriate solution.
12. If a biopsy specimen is to be obtained, replace the stylet and withdraw the needle. Reinsert the needle at a slightly different angle and location, still within the area of periosteum previously anesthetized. Once you have reentered the marrow cavity, remove the stylet again. Advance the needle 5–10 mm using the same alternating rotating motion with gentle pressure. Withdraw the needle several millimeters (but not outside of the marrow cavity) and redirect it at a slightly different angle; then advance it again. Repeat this maneuver several times. About 2 or 3 cm of core material should enter the needle. Rotate the needle rapidly on its long axis in a clockwise and then counterclockwise direction. This will sever the biopsy specimen from the marrow cavity. Withdraw the needle completely without replacing the stylet. Some operators prefer to hold their thumb over the open end of the needle to create a negative pressure in the needle as it is withdrawn. This may help to prevent loss of the core biopsy specimen.
13. Remove the core biopsy specimen from the needle by inserting a probe (provided with the biopsy needle) into the distal end of the needle and then gently pushing the specimen the full length of the needle and finally out the hub end. The direction is important, as an attempt to push the specimen out the distal end may damage the biopsy specimen. Most biopsy needles are tapered at the distal end, presumably allowing the specimen to expand inside the needle and to prevent specimen loss when the needle is withdrawn from the patient.

14. The core biopsy specimen is usually collected in formalin solution. Again, plans for special studies should be made prior to the procedure to allow for any special handling of the biopsy material.
15. Observe the biopsy site for excess bleeding and apply local pressure for several minutes. Clean the area thoroughly with alcohol and apply an adhesive strip or gauze patch. Instruct the patient to assume a supine position, and place a pressure pack between the bed or table and the biopsy site for 10–15 minutes. This is not an absolute requirement unless there is an underlying coagulopathy or thrombocytopenia, but this will decrease local hematoma formation. Patients with an underlying tendency to bleed should maintain pressure for 20–25 minutes. A patient who is stable at this point may resume normal activities.

Complications: Local bleeding and hematoma, pain, possible infection.

6. CENTRAL VENOUS CATHETERIZATION

(See also Section I, Chapter 10, Central Venous Line Problems, p 53).

Indications: Administration of fluids and medications when peripheral administration is impossible, inappropriate, or unreliable; hemodynamic monitoring; transvenous pacemaker placement.

Contraindications: A coagulopathy dictates the use of the femoral or median basilic vein approach to avoid bleeding complications.

Materials: Generally, two approaches are used to place central venous lines. One of these involves puncturing the vein with a relatively small needle through which a thin guide wire is placed in the vein. After the needle has been withdrawn, the intravascular appliance—or a sheath through which a smaller catheter will be placed—is introduced into the vein over the guide wire. The other technique involves puncturing the vein with a larger-bore needle through which the intravascular catheter will fit. There are commercially available disposable trays that provide all necessary needles, wires, sheaths, dilators, suture materials, and topical anesthetics. Some hospitals insist that these materials be assembled when central line placement becomes necessary. If needles, guide wires, and sheaths are collected from different places, it is very important to make sure that the needle will accept the guide wire, that the sheath and dilator will pass over the guide wire, and that the appliance to be passed through the sheath will indeed fit the inside lumen of the sheath. Supplies should include the following items:

1. Small needle (16-18 gauge)
2. Guide wire
3. 5- to 10-mL syringe
4. Scalpel

5. Intravascular appliance (triple-lumen catheter or a sheath through which a Swan-Ganz pulmonary artery catheter could be placed)
6. Heparinized flush solution: 1 mL of 1:100 U heparin in 10 mL of normal saline (to be used to fill all lumens prior to placement, to prevent clotting of the catheter during placement)
7. Lidocaine 1% with or without epinephrine
8. Povidone-iodine (Betadine) prep solution
9. Alcohol pads
10. Sterile towels
11. 4 × 4 gauze sponges
12. 21-gauge needle to draw up the lidocaine.

Also, sterile procedure is highly recommended (mask, sterile gown, and gloves).

Note: If the catheter is introduced through a large-bore needle, an appropriately sized large-bore needle is required (12-14 gauge); a smaller needle and guide wire are not required. There seems to be little rationale for placement of a single-lumen catheter when multiple lumens can be installed for potential use at virtually the same risk. For these reasons, the ensuing discussion focuses on the over-the-guide-wire technique and placement of either a triple-lumen catheter or a sheath through which a smaller catheter will eventually be placed.

Right Internal Jugular Vein Approach

Actually, three different sites are described and used in accessing the right internal jugular vein: (1) anterior (medial to the sternocleidomastoid muscle belly); (2) middle (between the two heads of the sternocleidomastoid muscle belly); and (3) posterior (lateral to the sternocleidomastoid muscle belly). The middle approach is most commonly used and has the advantage of well-defined landmarks.

Procedure

1. Sterilize the site with povidone-iodine and drape with sterile towels.
2. Administer local anesthesia with lidocaine in the area to be explored.
3. Place the patient in Trendelenburg (head down) position.
4. Use a small-bore thin-walled needle with syringe attached to locate the internal jugular vein. It may be helpful to have a small amount of anesthetic (1% lidocaine) in the syringe to inject during exploration for the vein, if the patient notes some discomfort. Some operators find the vein with a long 21-gauge needle, leave the needle in place off the syringe, and pass the 19-gauge needle directly behind it, following the same course to the deep vein puncture site.
5. The internal diameter of the needle used to locate the internal jugular vein should be large enough to accommodate the passage of the guide wire. Some operators prefer a “micro-puncture” kit, which utilizes a smaller puncture needle, followed by a smaller-diameter guide wire, followed by a small-caliber dilator. The dilator actually then allows pas-

sage of the same guide wire usually passed via a 19-gauge needle. Less trauma is felt to occur due to the smaller puncture needle.

6. Percutaneous entry should be made at the apex of the triangle formed by the two heads of the sternocleidomastoid muscle and the clavicle.
7. The needle should be directed slightly laterally toward the ipsilateral breast and kept as superficial as possible.
8. Often a notch can be palpated on the posterior surface of the clavicle. This actually can help locate the vein in the lateral/medial plane, as the vein lies deep to this shallow notch.
9. Successful puncture of the vein is usually accomplished at a depth of needle insertion of 2–4 cm, and is heralded by sudden aspiration of nonpulsatile venous blood.
10. After the needle is detached from the syringe, the guide wire should pass with ease all the way to the right atrium. Once the wire is passed, remove the needle.
11. Leave enough wire outside the patient to accommodate the length of the intravascular catheter, sheath, etc, **with an adequate amount to allow control over the distal end of the guide wire at all times.**
12. Nick the skin with a No. 11 scalpel blade just adjacent to the guide wire.
13. The catheter or sheath should be introduced over the guide wire while the depth of the guide wire is kept relatively constant, to avoid irritation of the right atrium or ventricle and possible ventricular ectopy.
14. When the sheath or catheter is placed over the guide wire, the proximal end of the guide wire should be held until the catheter or sheath completely passes over the distal end of the guide wire.
15. Then the distal end of the guide wire is controlled while the catheter or sheath is advanced through the incised skin and into the vein.
16. Once the catheter or sheath is in place, the guide wire is removed.
17. An occlusive sterile dressing should be applied.
18. A chest x-ray should be obtained to verify position of the line as well as to identify complications such as a pneumothorax.

Complications

1. Relatively safe, with a low risk of pneumothorax.
2. It is likely that errant attempts at internal jugular puncture will end up in the mediastinum. It is possible to perforate endotracheal tube cuffs by this approach. This is usually not a subtle event and generally requires prompt replacement of the now-faulty endotracheal tube before safe deep line placement can proceed.
3. The other procedural miscue is inadvertent puncture of the carotid artery. This commonly occurs if the needle is inserted medial to where it should be on the middle approach; it is also common with the anterior approach. With arterial puncture, the syringe fills without negative pressure because of arterial pressure, and bright red blood pulsates from the needle after the syringe is removed. The needle should be removed and manual pressure applied for 10–15 minutes to ensure adequate hemostasis.

4. A chest x-ray should always be obtained after the procedure to check for positioning of the catheter and to rule out pneumothorax.

Advantages: Central venous access from this site allows virtually every potential use of the deep line, including hemodynamic assessment (both central venous pressure and pulmonary artery measurements are easily done); temporary pacemaker placement; endomyocardial biopsy; as well as administration of fluids, drugs, and parenteral nutrition.

Disadvantages

1. The major disadvantage of this site is patient discomfort. The site is difficult to dress, and is uncomfortable for patients who have the capacity to turn their heads.
2. The risk of infectious contamination for this line is intermediate between that for femoral lines and that for subclavian lines, and is probably related to the difficulty in keeping the site occlusively dressed. Reports from centers in Europe have shown a markedly reduced incidence of catheter infection by including at least an 8-cm subcutaneous tunnel from the percutaneous venipuncture site to the skin exit site of the catheter. The procedure is more demanding by virtue of having to construct the tunnel, not described here.

Left Internal Jugular Vein Approach

The left internal jugular vein is not commonly used for central line placement. Better options exist and should be exhausted before resorting to this approach.

Procedure: Similar to right internal jugular vein approach.

Complications: In addition to the usual procedural complications common to central lines, this approach has some unique complications.

1. There are case reports of inadvertent left brachiocephalic vein and superior vena cava puncture with intravascular wires, catheters, and sheaths.
2. Laceration of the thoracic duct.

Advantages: None over right internal jugular vein approach.

Disadvantages: See Complications for Right Internal Jugular Vein Approach. Laceration of the thoracic duct and puncture of the left brachiocephalic vein and superior vena cava are also possible.

Subclavian Approach (Left or Right)

Procedure

1. A small rolled-up towel placed between the shoulder blades facilitates this approach.

2. Place the patient in Trendelenburg position (15–30°).
3. Use sterile preparation and appropriate draping.
4. Anesthetize the skin with local anesthetic.
5. Percutaneous entry is then made caudal to the mid-clavicle and directed toward the suprasternal notch.
6. The needle is "marched" down the clavicle, keeping near the clavicle, to avoid the pleura.
7. A small amount of topical anesthetic in the syringe can be used to anesthetize periosteal surfaces while the vein is located, but hopefully only one puncture will be needed.
8. The guide wire should fit inside the lumen of the needle used to find the vein. As with internal jugular cannulation, some operators prefer the "micro puncture" approach. Some interventional radiologists use Doppler flow to mark the course of the subclavian vein, and some radiologists have contrast injected through an arm vein under fluoroscopy to help direct the puncture. These techniques are either not available for bedside use, or have not been associated with benefit in trials evaluating patient safety.
9. Direct the needle under the clavicle, above the first rib and toward the suprasternal notch. (See Figure 3–4.)
10. Apply constant negative pressure while the needle is advanced.
11. Successful entry is marked by free flow of nonpulsatile venous blood.

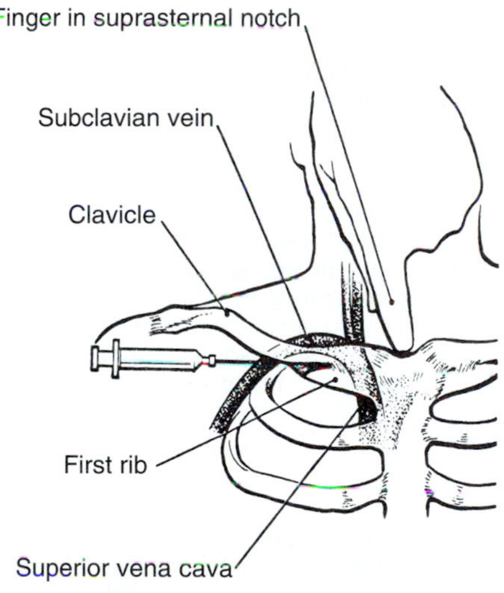

Figure 3–4. Technique for catheterization of the subclavian vein. (Reproduced, with permission, from Gomella LG, ed. *Clinician's Pocket Reference.* 9th ed. McGraw-Hill;2002.

12. The patient's head should be directed to face the operator while the guide wire is inserted. This facilitates guide wire placement down the superior vena cava as opposed to up the internal jugular vein.
13. Remove the syringe.
14. Advance the guide wire through the needle.
15. The guide wire should slide easily through the needle, essentially to the hub of the needle.
16. If there is resistance to passage of the guide wire, it is important to reattach the syringe and reposition the needle so that the blood flows freely.
17. If the resistance is more distal than the tip of the needle, the guide wire is likely coursing cephalad at the internal jugular vein (an awake patient may remark that the ipsilateral ear hurts). Another pass of the guide wire with the entry needle pulled back slightly is appropriate. Placing the guide wire in the internal jugular vein from the subclavian approach accomplishes nothing. The catheter placed over the guide wire will also end up in the internal jugular vein.
18. Once the guide wire is passed, remove the needle.
19. Follow steps 11 through 18 for placement via the right internal jugular vein approach.

Complications

1. Arterial puncture is usually obvious, because bright red blood spurts from the needle when the syringe is detached or the syringe spontaneously fills without negative pressure. The needle is then withdrawn and manual pressure applied to stop arterial bleeding. Significant bleeding deep to the clavicle may occur and is heavily dependent on the patient's coagulation system and the size of the puncture. This underscores the importance of knowing the patient's coagulation profile before making the decision on which approach to use for central line placement.
2. Pneumothorax can be detected when a sudden gush of air is aspirated instead of blood. A postprocedure chest x-ray should always be done to rule out pneumothorax and check for line placement. A pneumothorax requires chest tube placement in virtually all cases, especially when the patient is being supported on a ventilator. The left-sided approach is associated with higher risk for pneumothorax because of the higher dome of the left pleura compared with the right.
3. Hemothorax.
4. Air embolus.

Advantages

1. The left subclavian approach affords a gentle, sweeping curve to the apex of the right ventricle, and is the preferred entry site for placement of a temporary transvenous pacemaker without fluoroscopic assistance.

2. Hemodynamic measurements are often easier to record from the left subclavian approach.
3. From the left subclavian vein approach, the catheter does not have to negotiate an acute angle, as is commonly the case at the junction of the right subclavian with the right brachiocephalic vein en route to the superior vena cava. This is also a common site for kinking of the deep line.
4. Lowest risk of infection of various central line sites.

Disadvantages: Risk of pneumothorax.

Femoral Vein Approach

The femoral line is an option probably underutilized in critical care settings.

Procedure

1. Place the patient in the supine position.
2. Use sterile preparation and appropriate draping. Administer local anesthesia in the area to be explored.
3. Palpate the femoral artery.
4. Guard the artery with the fingers of one hand.
5. Explore for the vein just medial to the operator's fingers with a needle and syringe.
6. It may be helpful to have a small amount of anesthetic in the syringe to inject with exploration.
7. The needle is directed cephalad at about a 30-degree angle and should be inserted below the femoral crease.
8. Puncture is heralded by the return of venous, nonpulsatile blood on application of negative pressure to the syringe.
9. Advance the guide wire through the needle.
10. The guide wire should pass with ease into the vein to a depth at which the distal tip of the guide wire is always under the operator's control. The operator should maintain control of the guide wire at its entry point through the skin while passing the sheath/dilator or catheter over the distal end of the wire.
11. Remove the needle once the guide wire has advanced into the femoral vein.
12. If the catheter is 6-French or larger, a skin incision with a scalpel blade is generally needed. The catheter can then be advanced along with the guide wire in unison into the femoral vein. **Be sure always to control the distal end of the guide wire.**
13. Follow steps 14 through 17 for the right internal jugular vein approach.

Complications

1. The femoral deep line has the highest incidence of contamination and sepsis. If an occlusive dressing can remain in place and remain free

from contamination, this is a safe option. Recent randomized series from centers in Europe testify to the benefit of a 10-cm-long subcutaneous tunnel between the vein puncture site to the skin exit site of the catheter. A fourfold decrease in catheter-related infections was noted. The procedure is still done at bedside but is more involved in that the tunneling subcutaneously must be added to the percutaneous venipuncture.

2. Deep venous thrombosis (DVT) has occurred from femoral vein catheterization as well as with other sites. The risk for DVT increases if the catheter remains in place for prolonged periods.

Advantages

1. The procedure is safe, in that arterial and venous sites are compressible. This route or the median basilic vein approach is preferred in the presence of a coagulopathy or severe lung disease.
2. It is impossible to cause pneumothorax from this site.
3. Placement can be accomplished without interrupting cardiopulmonary resuscitation.
4. This site can be used to place a variety of intravascular appliances, including temporary pacemakers, pulmonary artery catheters (expertise with fluoroscopy is needed), and triple-lumen catheters.

Disadvantages

1. This approach has the highest rate of infection.
2. Fluoroscopy is required for placement of pulmonary artery catheters or transvenous pacemakers.

Median Basilic Vein Approach

It is possible in some patients, particularly men with well-developed upper extremities, to place an 8-French-sized introducer into the median basilic vein. The median basilic vein is directed medially at the antecubital fossa. The cephalic vein should be avoided. It runs laterally at the antecubital fossa and should not be relied on to pass a deep line because the line will commonly hang up at the origin of the axillary vein. Passage to the central circulation may occur via the cephalic vein, but should be tested using a long, thin guide wire and fluoroscopy before this approach is counted on for central access.

Procedure

1. Use sterile preparation with appropriate draping.
2. Administer local anesthesia with lidocaine.
3. Place an Intracath needle into the vein through which the guide wire will pass. Alternatively, the "micro-puncture" technique described above is also applicable for use in the upper extremities as well.
4. Advance the guide wire through the Intracath/intermediate dilator.

5. Once the guide wire has passed into the median vein, remove the Intracath/intermediate dilator.
6. Incise the skin with a No. 11 scalpel. Advance the sheath/dilator system or triple-lumen catheter over the wire and into the vein **while controlling either the proximal or distal end of the guide wire at all times.**
7. Follow steps 14 through 17 for the right internal jugular vein approach.

Complications: Thrombophlebitis (line should be removed in 48–72 hours).

Advantages

1. Noncompressible bleeding is avoided. This route or the femoral route is preferred in the presence of coagulopathy or severe lung disease.
2. No risk of pneumothorax.

Disadvantages

1. Cannot be used in all patients.
2. Fluoroscopy is required for placement of pulmonary artery catheters or temporary pacemakers.
3. Uncomfortable and immobilizing.

REFERENCES

Maki DG, Stolz SM, Wheeler S et al: Prevention of central venous catheter-related bloodstream infection by use of an antiseptic-impregnated catheter. Ann Intern Med 1997;127:257.

Raad I, Darouiche R, Dupuis J et al: Central venous catheters coated with minocycline and rifampin for the prevention of catheter-related colonization and bloodstream infections. Ann Intern Med 1997;127:267.

Timsit J-F, Bruneel F, Cheval C et al: Use of tunneled femoral catheters to prevent catheter-related infection. Ann Intern Med 1999;130:729.

Timsit J-F, Sebille V, Farkas J-C et al: Effect of subcutaneous tunneling on internal jugular catheter-related sepsis in critically ill patients. JAMA 1996;276:1416.

7. ENDOTRACHEAL INTUBATION

(See also Section VI, Ventilator Management, p 442).

Indications: These include cardiac arrest, acute hypoxemic respiratory failure, ventilatory failure, and the poorly responsive patient at risk for aspiration. Also needed to ensure a patent airway in the presence of neurologic or mechanical impairment and provide pulmonary toilet in the presence of overwhelming secretions or massive hemoptysis.

Contraindications: (Relative) massive maxillofacial trauma, fractured larynx, suspected cervical spinal cord injury. Nasotracheal intubation is contraindicated in suspected basilar skull fractures. Fiberoptic intubation or tracheostomy may be indicated in these instances.

Materials: Endotracheal tube (ETT), usually 7.0–9.0 mm internal diameter for most adults; laryngoscope handle and blade (No. 3 straight or curved); 10-mL syringe; adhesive tape; suction equipment; lubricant; malleable stylet (optional); gloves; protective eye wear; oximeter and end tidal CO_2 monitoring (if available).

Procedure: Orotracheal intubation is most commonly used and is described here.

1. If the patient is hypoxic or apneic, use a bag and mask with 100% oxygen prior to and during the intubation procedure. The risk of hypoxemia during intubation can be minimized by preoxygenation with 100% oxygen at high flow rates for 3–4 minutes and by avoiding prolonged periods without ventilation. Monitor O_2 saturation throughout the procedure if possible.
2. Prepare the equipment. Extend the laryngoscope blade to 90 degrees to verify that the light is working. Inflate the cuff to ensure competency. Apply a water-soluble lubricant to the tube. Enlist a respiratory therapist to maintain oxygenation and assist in airway control during the procedure.
3. Position the patient. This is likely the most important component of the procedure. Place folded towels under the patient's head to achieve the "sniffing position" (neck flexed and head slightly extended). Adjust the bed to a comfortable height. Remove the headboard and lock the wheels.
4. Intravenous sedation may be required in patients who are agitated, uncooperative, or combative. Consider using midazolam 1–2 mg IV every 5 minutes, fentanyl 25–50 mg IV, or etomidate 0.3 mg/kg IV.
5. Open the mouth by placing the thumb and index finger of the right hand on the lower and upper incisors, respectively, and spreading the thumb and finger with a scissorlike motion.
6. Grip the laryngoscope with the left hand. Insert the extended blade into the right side of the mouth. Use the blade to push the tongue to the left while keeping the tongue anterior to the blade. Advance carefully toward the midline until the epiglottis is seen. (See Figure 3–5.)
7. Pass the straight (Miller) laryngoscope blade posterior and inferior to the epiglottis. When using the curved (MacIntosh) blade, pass it anterior and superior to the epiglottis. Thrust the left arm upward at a 45-degree angle from the horizontal and visualize the vocal cords or the arytenoid cartilage. Avoid using the maxillary teeth as a fulcrum by keeping the wrist rigid and lifting only with the arm and shoulder. If the cords are not visualized, the straight blade may have progressed too posterior and inferior into the esophagus. In that case, slowly retract the laryngoscope while watching for the cords to appear. With either type of blade, application of cricoid pressure by an assistant may be a useful adjunct while attempting cord visualization.
8. While maintaining visualization of the cords, grasp the ETT in the right hand, pass it into the right corner of the mouth, and advance the cuff

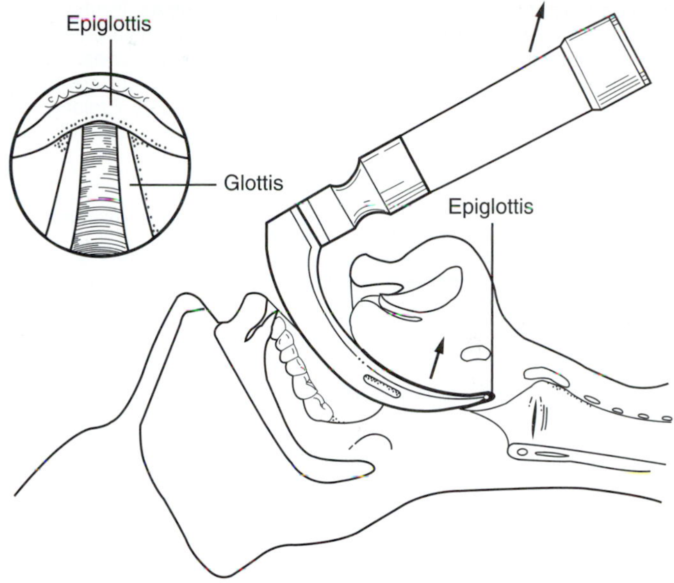

Figure 3–5. Endotracheal intubation. Advance blade to groove between base of tongue and epiglottis. (Reproduced, with permission, from Vander Salm TJ, ed. *Atlas of Bedside Procedures.* 2nd ed. Little, Brown;1988:21.)

beyond the cords. With more difficult intubations, a malleable stylet can be used to direct the tube. In average-sized individuals, the incisors should be at the 23-cm mark for males and 21-cm mark for females.

9. Gently inflate the cuff with air until an adequate seal is obtained (about 5 mL). Auscultate over the epigastrium (with ventilation, loud gurgling over the epigastrium suggests a gastric intubation), then auscultate over the left and right anterior and mid-axillary chest. If the left side lacks breath sounds, a right mainstem bronchus intubation is likely. In that case, deflate the cuff, retract the ETT 1–2 cm, reinflate the cuff, and reassess breath sounds. End-tidal CO_2 monitoring will confirm tracheal intubation. Confirm the positioning with a stat chest x-ray. The end of the endotracheal tube should be 3–4 cm superior to the carina.
10. Secure tube position with tape. Record the cm mark at the incisors. Insert an oropharyngeal airway to prevent the patient from biting the ETT.

Complications: Oropharyngeal trauma, aspiration, improper tube positioning (esophageal or right mainstem bronchus intubation). Complications associated with a prolonged intubation attempt include cardiac arrest, seizures, and gastric distension. Right mainstem bronchus intubation has adverse consequences including pneumothorax and left lung atelectasis. Prolonged intubation (greater than 10–14 days) can lead to tracheal stenosis.

REFERENCES

Einarsson O, Rochester CL, Rosenbaum SH: Airway management in respiratory emergencies. Clin Chest Med 1994;15:13.

Kaur S, Heard SO: Airway management and endotracheal intubation. In: Irwin RS, Rippe JM, Cerra FB et al, eds. *Procedures and Techniques in Intensive Care Medicine.* 2nd ed. Lippincott Williams & Wilkins;1999:3.

Pingleton SK: Management of complications of acute respiratory failure. In: Bone RC, ed. *Pulmonary and Critical Care Medicine.* 6th ed. Mosby;1998:R11-6.

8. GASTROINTESTINAL TUBES

Indications: Gastrointestinal (GI) decompression (paralytic ileus, obstruction, postoperatively); lavage of the stomach for GI bleeding or drug overdose; prevention of aspiration in obtunded patient (you should protect the airway by endotracheal intubation first); feeding a patient who is unable to swallow.

Contraindications: Nasal fractures, basilar skull fracture.

Materials: Gastrointestinal tube of choice, lubricant jelly, catheter tip syringe, glass of water with straw, stethoscope.

1. **Nasogastric tubes**
   a. **Levine:** Single-lumen tube that must be placed on intermittent suction to evacuate gastric contents.
   b. **Salem sump:** The best tube for continuous suction. The Salem sump is a double-lumen tube, with the smaller tube acting as an air intake vent. Use 14- to 18-French size in adults.
   c. **Ewald:** Large (18–36 French) single-lumen tube, especially suited for gastric lavage of drug overdoses; more often inserted by the orogastric route.
2. **Feeding tubes.** Although any small-bore nasogastric tube can be used as a feeding tube, certain weighted tubes are designed to pass into the duodenum and decrease the risk of aspiration of gastric contents.
   a. **Dobbhoff, Entriflex, Keogh:** These have a weighted mercury tip with stylet.
   b. **Vivonex:** Tungsten-tipped.
3. **Sengstaken-Blakemore tube:** A triple-lumen tube used exclusively for tamponade of esophageal varices to control bleeding. One lumen is for aspiration, one is for the gastric balloon, and the third is for the esophageal balloon.

Procedure

1. Inform the patient of the nature of the procedure and encourage the patient to cooperate. Choose the nasal passage that appears most patent by occluding one nostril and having the patient sniff.
2. Lubricate the distal 3–4 inches of the tube with a water-soluble jelly (K-Y Jelly or viscous 2% lidocaine) and insert the tube gently along the floor of the nasal passageway. Maintain gentle pressure that will allow the tube to pass into the nasopharynx. Running the tube under warm water prior to lubrication makes it more pliable and may help facilitate its placement. Flexing the head also helps facilitate passage of the tube.
3. When the patient can feel the tube in the back of the throat, ask him or her to swallow small amounts of water through a straw as you advance the tube 2–3 inches at a time.
4. To be sure that the tube is in the stomach, aspirate gastric contents or blow air into the tube and listen over the stomach with your stethoscope for a "pop" or "gurgle."
5. Attach sump tubes (Salem sump) to "continuous low wall suction" and the single-lumen tube (Levine) to "intermittent suction."
6. Feeding tubes are more difficult to insert because they are more flexible. You can use a stylet or guide wire, or attach the smaller tube to a larger, stiffer tube by wedging both into a gelatin capsule. Pass the tube in the usual fashion and allow it to remain in the stomach for 10–15 minutes. After this time, the capsule will dissolve and the larger tube can be removed.
7. **Always** verify the position of feeding tubes by chest x-ray before beginning feedings.
8. Tape the tube securely in place but do not allow it to apply pressure to the nasal ala. Patients have been disfigured by ischemic necrosis of the nose caused by a poorly positioned tube.

Complications: Inadvertent passage into the trachea; coiling of the tube in the mouth or pharynx; bleeding from the nose, pharynx, or stomach; and sinusitis.

9. INTRAVENOUS TECHNIQUES

Indications: To establish intravenous access for the administration of fluids, blood, or medications.

Materials: Intravenous fluid, connecting tubing, tourniquet, alcohol swab, intravenous cannulas (a catheter over a needle, such as Intracath, Angiocath, and Jelco or a butterfly needle), antiseptic ointment, dressing, and tape. You will find it helpful to rip the tape into strips and to flush the air out of the tubing with the intravenous fluid before you begin the procedure.

Procedure

1. An upper, nondominant extremity is the site of choice for an IV. Choose a distal vein so that if the vein is damaged, you can reposition

the IV more proximally. Avoid veins that cross joint spaces. Also avoid the leg, as there is a high incidence of superficial thrombophlebitis. If no extremity vein can be found, try the external jugular vein. If all these fail, the only alternative is a central line or a cutdown.

2. Apply a tourniquet above the proposed IV site. Techniques to help expose difficult-to-locate veins include (1) wrapping the extremity in a warm towel; (2) leaving the arm in a dependent position for a few minutes after the tourniquet is applied; or (3) using a blood pressure cuff as a tourniquet, inflated so that the arterial flow is still maintained. Carefully clean the site with an alcohol or povidone-iodine swab. If a large-bore IV is to be used (16 or 14 French), local anesthesia with 1% lidocaine may be helpful.
3. Stabilize the vein distally with the thumb of your free hand. Using the catheter-over-needle assembly (Intracath or Angiocath), enter the skin alongside the vein first, and then stick the vein along the side at about a 20-degree angle. Once the vein is punctured, blood should appear in the "flash" chamber. Advance 4–5 mm to be sure that BOTH the needle AND the tip of the catheter have entered the vein. Carefully withdraw the needle as you advance the catheter into the vein. (See Figure 3–6.) *Never withdraw the catheter over the needle because this procedure can shear off the plastic tip and cause a catheter embolus.* Apply pressure with your thumb over the vein just proximal to the site, to prevent significant blood loss while you connect the IV line to the catheter.
4. Observe the site with the IV fluid running for signs of induration or swelling that indicate improper placement or damage to the vein.
5. Tape the IV securely in place; apply a drop of povidone-iodine or antibiotic ointment and a sterile dressing at the puncture site over the needle. Ideally, the dressing should be changed every 24–48 hours to help reduce infections. Armboards are also useful to help maintain an IV site, especially near a joint.
6. If the veins are deep and difficult to locate, a small 3- to 5-mL syringe can be mounted on the catheter assembly. Proper position inside the vein is determined by aspiration of blood.
7. If venous access is limited, a "butterfly" needle can be used (see Figure 3–7); or the external jugular vein may be considered as an alternative site.
8. All intravenous lines should be changed every 72 hours to decrease the risk of infection.

Complications: Thrombophlebitis; localized infection or sepsis.

10. LUMBAR PUNCTURE

Indications: For the diagnosis of central nervous system (CNS) infection, post infectious, or inflammatory disorders; intracranial pressure disorders (eg, pseudotumor cerebri, intracranial hypertension, or hypotension); meningeal

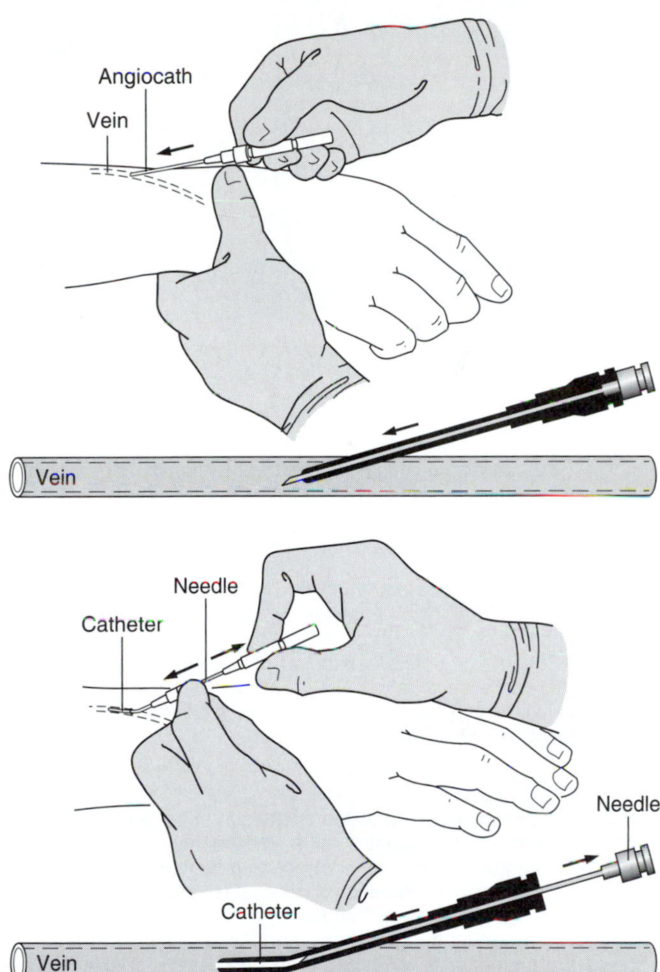

Figure 3–6. To insert a catheter-over-needle assembly into a vein, stabilize the skin and vein with gentle traction. Enter the vein and advance the catheter while holding the needle steady; then remove the needle. (Reproduced, with permission, from Gomella LG, ed. *Clinician's Pocket Reference.* 9th ed. McGraw-Hill;2002.)

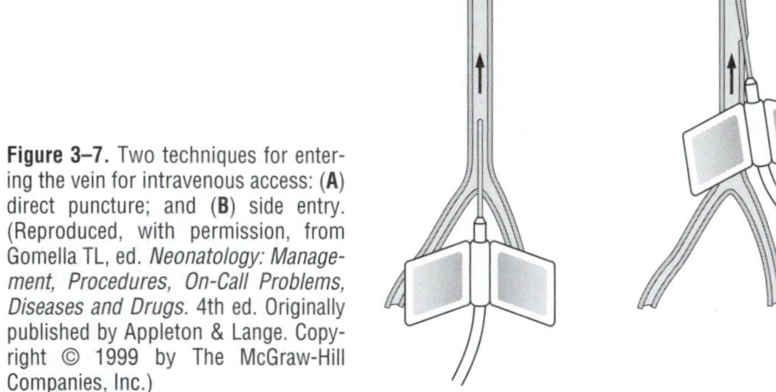

Figure 3–7. Two techniques for entering the vein for intravenous access: (**A**) direct puncture; and (**B**) side entry. (Reproduced, with permission, from Gomella TL, ed. *Neonatology: Management, Procedures, On-Call Problems, Diseases and Drugs.* 4th ed. Originally published by Appleton & Lange. Copyright © 1999 by The McGraw-Hill Companies, Inc.)

carcinomatosis; subarachnoid hemorrhage; or demyelinating disorders. Lumbar puncture (LP) may also be necessary for the injection of diagnostic or therapeutic agents (contrast media, antibiotics, or chemotherapy).

Contraindications: Evidence of infection near the planned puncture site or bleeding disorder. The presence of papilledema or a focal neurologic deficit is a contraindication unless neuroimaging can rule out a mass lesion, obstruction or displacement of the ventricles, or midline shift. If the patient is on heparin, the heparin should be discontinued for 4–6 hours prior to the lumbar puncture. Patients on coumadin should not undergo lumbar puncture if the international normalized ratio (INR) > 1.3 or until anticoagulation has been reversed with fresh-frozen plasma and/or vitamin K. An elective LP should be delayed if myelography is anticipated.

Procedure

1. Prior to the procedure, a detailed evaluation of the patient and careful consideration of the potential risks and benefits must be made. A neuroimaging procedure should precede a lumbar puncture if the patient has evidence of increased intracranial pressure (papilledema, focal neurologic findings, or headache).
2. The most important detail in the performance of a successful LP is to place the patient in a comfortable and accessible position. A lateral decubitus position with the back close to the edge of the bed or table and with the neck, back, knees, and hips maximally flexed to facilitate an open, clear approach to the vertebral interspaces is most effective. The hips and shoulders must be absolutely perpendicular to the bed. Padding placed between the iliac crest and inferior costal margin helps prevent sagging and keeps the spinal column straight and par-

allel with the bed. A pillow between the legs prevents the pelvis from rotating forward out of the perpendicular plane with the bed. It is often useful for an assistant to keep the patient in the optimal position. Alternatively, the LP may be performed with the patient sitting, leaning forward over the backrest of the chair or bed stand. However, in this position, accurate interpretation of the opening and closing pressures and comparison to standard pressures (which can only be done with the patient in a lateral decubitus position) are impossible.

3. The spinal needle should be inserted through the L_4–L_5 or L_5–S_1 interspace. An imaginary line drawn across the top of the iliac crests usually crosses the spine at about the L_4 vertebral body. Marking the skin overlying the L_4–L_5 interspace with an indentation of your fingernail is helpful in finding the spot later once the patient is prepped and draped.
4. Open the LP kit and put on sterile gloves. Prep the area with povidone-iodine solution in a circular fashion starting in the center and gradually working outward. Repeat this step two more times. Next, drape the patient.
5. Anesthetize the overlying skin by raising a small wheal using a 25-gauge needle and 1% lidocaine. Avoid injecting too much solution, as this may cause undue swelling of the tissues and obscure palpable landmarks. With a 1½-inch 22-gauge needle, infiltrate deeper tissues with 1% lidocaine.
6. Inspect the spinal needle, stylet, manometer, 3-way stopcock, and collection tubes for defects. Loosen the caps of the collection tubes and make certain that they are properly marked and that you are familiar with the sequence in which they will be used to collect serial specimens of cerebrospinal fluid (CSF).
7. Using a 20- or 22-gauge spinal needle with a well-fitting stylet, insert the needle into the subcutaneous tissues. Having the beveled tip parallel to the long axis of the spine minimizes injury to the longitudinal dural fibers and reduces the chances of a post-spinal headache. Guide the needle just caudal to the L_4 spinous process, keeping the needle parallel to the floor and mostly perpendicular to the spine but directed slightly cephalad, targeting the tip of the needle toward the umbilicus. Keep pressure on the hub of the stylet to avoid having it displaced from the needle. One useful technique to help avoid misdirecting the needle is to hold the needle between the index fingers of both hands with the thumbs holding the hub of the needle and stylet while guiding the needle into the subarachnoid space (see Figure 3–8).
8. Continue to advance the needle slowly until a "give" or "pop" is felt, indicating that the tip has passed the resistance of the longitudinal ligament and has entered the subarachnoid space. Remove the stylet and check for CSF flow. Replacing the stylet and rotating the needle 90–180 degrees may facilitate flow if it is absent or slow. If this fails,

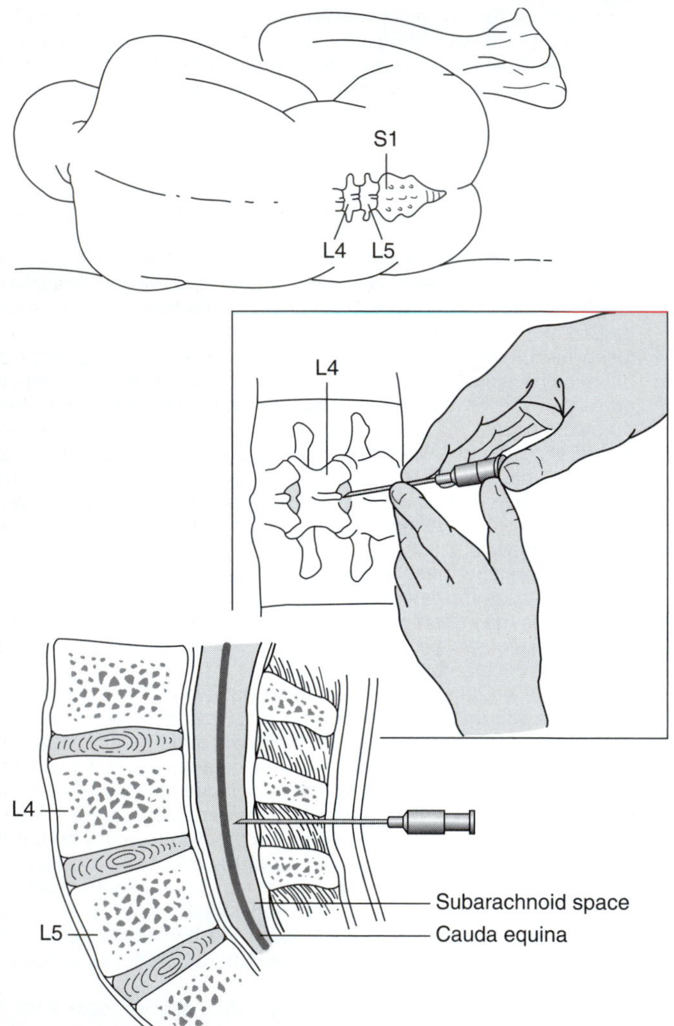

Figure 3–8. When you are performing a lumbar puncture, place the patient in the lateral decubitus position and locate the L4–L5 interspace. Control the spinal needle with two hands and enter the subarachnoid space. (Reproduced, with permission, from Gomella LG, ed. *Clinician's Pocket Reference.* 9th ed. McGraw-Hill; 2002.

replace the stylet and advance the needle a few millimeters, stopping each time to remove the stylet and check for CSF flow. Pressing on the abdomen or having the patient undergo a Valsalva maneuver can improve flow when very low CSF pressure is encountered. Never advance the needle without first replacing the stylet. The hollow barrel of the needle may become occluded with epidermis, which can be introduced into the subarachnoid space, leading to an epidermoid tumor later.

9. If you are unsuccessful at the L_4–L_5 interspace, attempt the procedure one interspace above or below this location.

10. Once the subarachnoid space is penetrated and CSF flow is obtained, attach the stopcock with the manometer and carefully measure the opening pressure. Be careful because unintentional movements during manipulation of the stopcock or manometer may displace the needle. Some LP trays contain a short piece of flexible tubing that can be attached between the needle hub and stopcock, which dampens these movements and makes displacement of the needle less likely. Normal opening CSF pressure with the patient lying comfortably in a lateral decubitus position is 70–180 mm H_2O, but may be as high as 250 mm H_2O in the severely obese patient. Straining may falsely elevate the CSF pressure, as will positive pressure devices attached to mechanical ventilators. An elevated pressure may be due to cerebral edema, mass lesions, and infectious or noninfectious CNS inflammatory disorders. Hyperventilation, chronic CSF leak, or subarachnoid block from a spinal tumor or meningitis can lower the CSF pressure. However, a low pressure more often occurs due to incomplete needle penetration of the subarachnoid space, a needle that is too small (25 gauge), or other faulty technique.

11. Collect the CSF in four serially labeled containers. The quantity depends on the tests to be performed, plus a small extra amount for additional tests thought of later. Usually 20 mL is adequate, but repeating an LP because insufficient fluid was collected should rarely occur. The collection tubes should be numbered in the order they were collected, and taken immediately to the laboratory for processing. It is often helpful to specify what laboratory studies are to be obtained from each tube; an example would be as follows:
    - Tube 1 for cell count and differential
    - Tube 2 for glucose and protein
    - Tube 3 for bacterial culture and Gram's stain
    - Tube 4 for cell count and differential

Although there may be an advantage to requesting fungal and AFB smears and cultures, or cytology from the last tube collected, special studies may be obtained from any of the other tubes. Other studies include VDRL, counterimmune electrophoresis (CIE) or latex agglutination for common bacterial antigens, multiple sclerosis profile, angiotensin-converting enzyme, viral cultures, etc.

Blood in the CSF may be due to a traumatic LP or subarachnoid hemorrhage (SAH). Clues that help to differentiate a traumatic LP from a SAH include visual clearing of the blood from one tube to the next, higher RBC count in the first tube than the last, the proportion of WBC count to RBC count similar to that of peripheral blood, the proportion of protein to RBC count the same as that of peripheral blood, centrifuged CSF showing a clear supernatant, and opening pressure that is normal. A SAH that has been present for at least 2–4 hours shows the supernatant to be pigmented or xanthochromic, there is no visual clearing of the blood from one tube to the next, the RBC count is about the same from one tube to the last, and the proportion of WBC count or protein to the RBC count may be higher than found in the peripheral blood. The opening pressure with SAH may be elevated or normal.

12. Withdraw the needle and place a sterile dressing over the puncture site. Instruct the patient to remain flat in bed for 12–24 hours and avoid straining, which may help to prevent a post-LP headache. Table 3–1, p 419, demonstrates typical CSF results for various disorders.
13. Carefully document the procedure in the patient's medical record, being sure to include opening and closing pressures, amount of CSF removed and its general appearance, the patient's position for the procedure, the vertebral interspace that was punctured, and any complications that were encountered.

Complications: The most common complication is a post-LP headache, which is improved by recumbency and aggravated by an upright position. It may occur within 1–2 days, or as long as a week after the procedure. Using a needle smaller than 22-gauge may reduce the risk, but resistance of a very small gauge needle to CSF flow prolongs the procedure and may falsely lower the measured pressures. A persistent post-LP headache that does not respond to strict bed rest may need treatment with a blood patch by an anesthesiologist. Other complications from an LP procedure include brain herniation, meningitis, trauma to nerve roots, cranial subdural hematoma, spinal subdural or epidural hematoma, diplopia, transient hearing loss, and, rarely, implantation of an epidermoid tumor.

REFERENCES

Fishman RA, ed: *Cerebrospinal Fluid in Diseases of the Nervous System.* 2nd ed. Saunders;1992.

Lumbar puncture and the examination of the cerebrospinal fluid. In: Haerer AF, ed. DeJong's *The Neurologic Examination.* 5th ed. Lippincott;1992:755.

11. PARACENTESIS

Indications: Determination of the cause of ascites; ruling out bacterial peritonitis; therapeutic removal of fluid in patients with tense ascites for symptomatic relief (early satiety, abdominal discomfort, dyspnea).

TABLE 3–1. DIFFERENTIAL DIAGNOSIS OF CEREBROSPINAL FLUID.[1]

Condition	Color	Opening Pressure (mm H_2O)	Protein (mg/100 mL)	Glucose (mg/100 mL)	Cells (per mL)
Adult (normal)	Clear	70–180	15–45	45–80	0–5 lymphs
Bacterial meningitis	Cloudy	Increased	50–1500	Decreased, may be < 20	25–10,000 polys
Granulomatous (TB, fungal)	Clear or cloudy	Increased	Increased, usually < 500	Decreased, may be 20–40	10–500 lymphs
Viral	Clear or slightly cloudy	Normal, or slightly increased	Normal, or slightly increased	Normal	10–500 lymphs (polys early)

[1]*Modified and reproduced with permission from Gomella LG, ed.* Clinician's Pocket Reference. *9th ed. McGraw-Hill; 2002.*
WBC = white blood cell; RBC = red blood cell; lymphs = lymphocytes; polys = polymorphonuclear leukocytes; TB = tuberculosis.

Contraindications: Coagulopathy (consider platelet transfusion if platelet count < 50,000 or fresh-frozen plasma if international normalized ratio [INR] > 1.5); multiple prior abdominal operations; uncooperative patient.

Materials: Minor procedure tray; Angiocath or Jelco assembly (18- to 20-gauge with a 1½-in. needle); 20- to 60-mL syringe; sterile specimen containers.

Procedure

1. Obtain informed consent. The patient's bladder needs to be empty. Some physicians prefer to place the patient in the lateral decubitus position so that the bowel floats upward away from the needle.
2. If there is any doubt about the presence of ascites, confirmation should be made by abdominal ultrasound. If the amount of ascites is small, ultrasound can be used to help locate the fluid during the procedure.
3. The entry site is usually the midline, 3–4 cm below the umbilicus. Avoid old surgical scars since bowel may adhere to the abdominal wall. Alternatively, you can locate an entry site in the left or right lower quadrant 4–5 cm above and medial to the anterior superior iliac spine (lateral to the rectus sheath).
4. Prep the patient's skin with povidone-iodine solution and apply sterile drapes. Raise a skin wheal with 1% lidocaine over the proposed entry site.
5. With the Angiocath mounted on the syringe, advance the needle into the anesthetized area carefully while gently aspirating. You will meet some resistance as you enter the fascia. When you get free return of fluid, leave the catheter in place, remove the needle, reattach the syringe, and aspirate. Sometimes it is necessary to reposition the catheter because of abutting omentum or bowel wall.
6. Aspirate the amount of fluid needed for tests (30–50 mL). Bedside inoculation of blood culture bottles with ascitic fluid increases the sensitivity of cultures. For a therapeutic tap, a 16- to 18-gauge steel needle can be connected to vacuum bottles with phlebotomy tubing. Large-volume paracentesis (5–10 L) can be safely performed in patients with tense ascites if the fluid is removed over 60–90 minutes.
7. Remove the needle quickly, apply a sterile 4 × 4 gauze, and apply pressure to the site with tape.
8. Depending on the clinical picture, send samples for albumin, total protein, glucose, lactate dehydrogenase, amylase, cell count and differential, Gram's stain, bacterial culture, acid-fast bacillus and fungal smears, and cultures and cytology. See Table 3–2 (p 421) for differential diagnosis of the fluid obtained.

Complications: Peritonitis; perforated bowel; intra-abdominal hemorrhage; perforated bladder, abdominal wall hematoma, and abdominal wall abscess.

TABLE 3–2. TESTING OF ASCITIC FLUID.

1) Albumin Gradient
   $ALB_{serum} - ALB_{ascites} = X$
   if X > 1.1g/dL, then portal hypertension
   If X < 1.1 g/dL, then not from portal hypertension
2) Total Protein < 1.0 g/dL, high risk for spontaneous bacterial peritonitis
3) Cell Count—absolute neutrophil count > 250/μL, presume infected
4) Bacterial Culture: Blood culture bottles 85% sensitivity
   Routine cultures 50% sensitivity
5) Bacterial Peritonitis—Spontaneous versus secondary
   Secondary: A) polymicrobial; B) total protein > 1.0 g/dL; C) LDH > normal serum value; D) glucose < 50 mg/dL
6) Food Fibers: Found in most cases of perforated viscus.
7) Cytology: Bizarre cells with large nuclei may represent reactive mesothelial cells and *not* a malignancy. Malignant cells suggest tumor.

REFERENCES

Marx JA: Peritoneal procedures. In: Roberts JR, Hedges JR, eds. *Clinical Procedures in Emergency Medicine.* 3rd ed. Saunders;1998:733.

Runyon BA: Care of patients with ascites. N Engl J Med 1994;330:337.

Runyon BA, Montano AA, Akriviadis EA et al: The serum-ascites albumin gradient is superior to the exudate-transudate concept in the differential diagnosis of ascites. Ann Intern Med 1992;117:215.

12. PULMONARY ARTERY CATHETERIZATION

(See also Section I, Chapter 57, Pulmonary Artery Catheter Problems, p 303).

Introduction: Controversy about the "value" of pulmonary artery catheters, or PACs (also called Swan-Ganz catheters), has been going on for over a decade, probably starting with Dr. Robin's editorials in 1985 and 1987 and nearly reaching the level of public hysteria with the publication of the article by Dr. Connors et al in 1996 (see references at the end of this chapter). The PAC is only a diagnostic tool, with no intrinsic therapeutic value. Thus, its ability to have a favorable impact on outcome in the clinical setting is entirely dependent on three basic conditions being met:

1. The PAC can provide, with a reasonable degree of safety, specific diagnostic information that is not otherwise readily available, and this information is germane to the management of the patient.
2. The physicians using this device know how to use it safely and how to obtain accurate information from it.
3. The therapy chosen in response to the diagnostic data obtained from the PAC is appropriate and timely for the specific clinical problem being addressed.

Published evidence has clearly suggested that many physicians and nurses who routinely use PACs are less than proficient in their use (Iberti et al 1990, 1994). Also, there is growing concern that management of shock and hemodynamic compromise may be done in a suboptimal manner by physicians without appropriate critical care expertise. Reynolds and colleagues (1988) at a single hospital showed that after going to full-time critical care physicians, there was a nearly 20% increase in the rate of PAC use for managing septic shock, accompanied by a 17% decrease in mortality and an 11% shift in overall ICU costs from nonsurvivors to survivors. Similarly, Knaus and colleagues (1982) reported that for critically ill patients with severe gastrointestinal illnesses (eg, acute gastrointestinal bleeding, pancreatitis), mortality in American ICUs was statistically significantly better than in comparable French ICUs, and that US physicians used PACs in these patients much more often than did their French counterparts. In both of these studies, claiming that the improved results were due to the increased rate of PAC use would be as misleading as it would be to blame the PAC for the lack of improvement or worse outcome associated with its use that was found in some retrospective observational studies (Robin 1987; Connors et al 1996).

The issues of when and by whom should a PAC be used, and also of whether similar diagnostic information could be better obtained in the ICU by other means (eg, "continuous" echocardiography or bioimpedance studies), remain legitimate areas of research. Likewise, studying different therapeutic approaches for a specific type of hemodynamic derangement also remains a high priority. In any case, only experienced personnel should use PACs. Similarly, proper PAC use requires clearly defined diagnostic and/or therapeutic goals that can be achieved using the data obtained from this device.

Indications: Pulmonary artery catheterization is generally undertaken in acutely ill patients *as a diagnostic intervention* when a question exists regarding the patient's volume status, cardiac output, or peripheral vascular resistance. Some specific examples include (1) establishing the cause of hypotension or shock when this is not immediately apparent; (2) differentiating between congestive heart failure, acute respiratory distress syndrome (ARDS), or pneumonia as the etiology of pulmonary infiltrates; (3) determining whether poor urine output is due to volume depletion, acute renal failure, or poor forward cardiac output; and (4) determining whether a patient with acute myocardial infarction and tachycardia has volume depletion, pain, anxiety, or left ventricular failure. Table 3–3 outlines the various types of PAC data in different types of shock. Please note that critically ill patients often have more than one disease process going on simultaneously, and hemodynamic data may become somewhat confusing without careful correlation with the whole clinical context and all other available data.

Contraindications: If a PAC is needed to manage a patient in a critical care setting, there are no absolute contraindications. For patients who are candidates for or who have received thrombolytic therapy, jugular and sub-

TABLE 3–3. PULMONARY ARTERY CATHETER: DIAGNOSIS OF SHOCK.

Type of Shock	Central Venous Pressure (CVP)	Pulmonary Artery Pressure (PAP)	Pulmonary Wedge Pressure (PWP)	Cardiac Output (CO)	Systemic Vascular Resistance (SVR)	Mixed Venous Oxygen Saturation (SvO_2)
Oligemic[1]	↓	Normal to ↓	↓↓↓	↓	↑	↓
Cardiac[2]	↑	↑	↑	↓↓↓	↑	↓
Distributive or "low SVR"[3]	Often ↓, may be normal or even ↑	Usually normal, may be ↓ or ↑	Usually ↓, may be normal or even ↑	Usually ↑, may become ↓	↓↓↓	Usually ↓, rarely can be normal or even ↑[4]
Obstructive, extra-cardiac[5]	Usually ↑	Usually ↑	Can be ↑ (eg, in tamponade), or ↓ (eg, with thromboembolism)	↓↓↓	↑	↓

[1]Oligemic shock refers to intravascular volume depletion, whether caused by true blood loss, by water loss (diarrhea, sweating, fever, burns, etc), or by venodilation and massive third-spacing (eg, SIRS or sepsis).
[2]Cardiac (or cardiogenic) shock can be subdivided into myopathic and valvular causes.
[3]Septic shock is the classic model of distributive (low SVR) shock, but this group includes other entities: anaphylaxis, toxic shock, drug-induced (eg, IL-2 given for bladder cancer therapy), and neurogenic. In all these scenarios, increased venous capacitance (venodilation) and/or massive third-spacing often initially add a hypovolemic picture, while specifically in sepsis myocardial depression may add a feature of myocardial failure. Thus the increased CO "classically" described in distributive shock is dependent on adequate fluid resuscitation, and may not be seen at all in septic patients with profound myocardial depression.
[4]Although oxygen uptake by the tissues is impaired in sepsis, in the presence of shock this results in an above-normal SvO_2 only in very rare instances. Initially the SvO_2 is usually below 60% (reflecting the decreased O_2 delivery to the tissues at a time when O_2 requirements are increased), even if maybe not as low as it would have been with normal peripheral extraction of O_2.
[5]The main examples of extracardiac obstructive shock are tamponade (where pressures tend to "equalize"), tension pneumothorax, and massive pulmonary thromboembolism.

clavian approaches should be avoided. As with all indwelling catheters that involve frequent manipulation, maintaining strict sterile conditions at all times, particularly at the time of placement, is essential to avoid infections. There are no convincing data showing that routine site changes at 3- or 4-day intervals are clearly beneficial and cost-effective, but of course, like all indwelling catheters, the PAC should be removed immediately as soon as it is no longer needed.

Materials: In most institutions, a single brand of a flow-directed balloon-tipped PAC is available. Use an insertion kit that provides the catheter as well as a sheath and the various syringes, needles, preparation material, local anesthetic, and other items that will be used to insert the catheter.

The PAC has four or five ports: air inflation or balloon port, thermistor, distal port, right atrial or proximal port, and (in some) a port for fluid or medication administration. (See Figure 3–9). The air inflation port is used to inflate the balloon to facilitate passage of the catheter from the right cardiac chambers to the

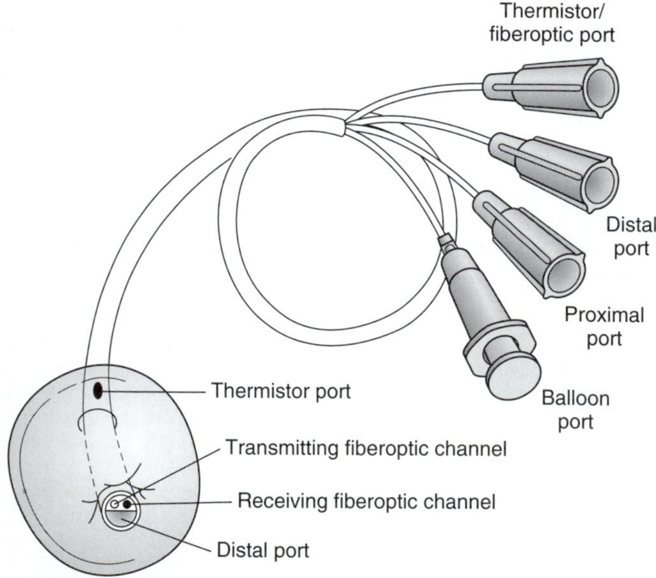

Figure 3–9. An example of a pulmonary artery catheter. This one features an oximetric measuring feature. (Reproduced, with permission, from Gomella LG, ed. *Clinician's Pocket Reference.* 9th ed. McGraw-Hill; 2002.

pulmonary artery. The thermistor can be used to measure cardiac outputs by thermal dilution when connected to a cardiac output computer. The distal port is used to measure pulmonary artery pressure and pulmonary capillary wedge pressure (PCWP) with the catheter in the pulmonary artery. The right atrial port is used to administer fluids, to measure right atrial pressure, or to inject fluid to measure cardiac output in conjunction with the thermistor and the cardiac output computer. (See Figure 3–9.) The catheter is often marked so that the clinician can determine how far the distal tip lies from the entry site. This information may help in catheter placement without fluoroscopy.

Procedure

1. The patient's informed consent is usually required.
2. Choose the site of operation; prep and drape the area. The choice of site is dictated by patient variables and operator experience. The easiest sites to place a PAC without fluoroscopic guidance are the right internal jugular vein and the left subclavian vein. In a patient receiving thrombolytic therapy, femoral and median basilic veins are preferable routes when/if it is felt that placement of the PAC cannot be safely delayed for a few hours (the preferred option).
3. **Always** use a strict sterile approach with a properly large sterile field, and wear gown, gloves, and mask.
4. Prepare the PAC by flushing the lumens with heparinized saline solution (1 mL of 1:100 U heparin in 10 mL of normal saline). Check the balloon function, and tap the catheter to be sure that a waveform is generated. You should set the pressure transducer level to the middle of the patient's chest.
5. Cannulate the central vein. (See Section III, Chapter 6, Central Venous Catheterization, p 399, for details.) In general, *never* push a guide wire when there is resistance; *always* keep one hand on the guide wire, either proximal or distal to the dilator, needle, etc.
6. Once the sheath is in place, you can advance the prepared catheter into the sheath. Once it has been advanced approximately 15 cm, the balloon will have cleared the tip of the sheath. You can then gently inflate the balloon with about 1.0–1.5 cm^3 of air. The maximum amount of air for use with smaller catheters (5 French) is ≤ 1.0 cm^3. If there is resistance to full inflation, check to see that the balloon has cleared the sheath or that it is not in an extravascular location (with an x-ray, or with fluoroscopy if available).
7. Once the balloon is inflated, advance the catheter to the level of the right atrium under the guidance of the pressure waveform and the electrocardiogram. Monitor the waveform and electrocardiogram at all times while advancing the balloon catheter. Remember to always advance the catheter with the balloon inflated and withdraw it with the balloon deflated. PACs usually come with a preformed curve on the tip. You should insert the catheter with its tip pointing anteriorly and to the left. Positioning in the right atrium is probably best determined by

watching for the characteristic waveform. The right atrium is generally located approximately 20 cm from the right internal jugular or subclavian vein insertion sites and approximately 25–30 cm from the left subclavian vein insertion site. The catheter should be advanced steadily. An abrupt change in the pressure tracing will occur as the catheter enters the right ventricle. There is generally little ectopy on entry into the right ventricle; however, as you advance the catheter into the right ventricular outflow tract, premature ventricular contractions (PVCs) may occur. Keep advancing the catheter until the ectopy disappears and the pulmonary artery tracing is obtained. If this does not occur, deflate the balloon, withdraw the catheter, and try again with the balloon inflated after slightly rotating the catheter. The PCWP will then be obtained by advancing the catheter another 10–15 cm. The catheter's final position should be such that the PCWP is obtained with full balloon inflation and the pulmonary artery pressure (PAP) tracing is present with the balloon deflated. In the "ideal position," transition from PAP to PCWP (and vice versa) will occur within three or fewer heartbeats. ***Caution:*** *Never* withdraw the catheter with the balloon inflated. See Figure 3–10, p 427, for normal waveforms. See Table 3–4, p 428, for normal PAC measurements.

8. Suture the catheter in place and dress the site according to your institution's practice. A chest x-ray should be obtained to document the catheter's present position as well as to rule out a pneumothorax or other complication from central venous catheterization.

9. Common problems: Catheter placement is much more difficult if severe pulmonary artery hypertension is present. If there is significant cardiac enlargement, particularly dilation of the right heart structures, the catheter may have a propensity to coil and get lost in its path to the right ventricular outflow tract. Fluoroscopy may be required to get the catheter into the correct position; moreover, it will hold this position poorly. Placement of the catheter in the pulmonary artery may also be difficult in the setting of a low cardiac output because the balloon-tipped catheter is dependent on blood flow to carry it through the right heart chambers.

10. Cardiac output can be measured by thermal dilution. First, connect the thermistor port of the PAC to a cardiac output computer into which the correct catheter's constant and the proper volume and temperature of the injectate have been entered. After this is done, rapidly inject fluid (usually 10 mL of normal saline at room temperature) through the right atrial port. If feasible, it is preferred to time the injection to occur at the same point of the respiratory cycle in all trials, usually at the end of inspiration. The computer will display the cardiac output. Repeat this procedure **at least** two more times. The variability of serial thermodilution cardiac output measurements should not exceed 20%, and usually is 15% or less. For normal cardiac output and index, consult Table 3–4, p 428.

11. You can often differentiate various clinical entities by measuring the blood pressure, PCWP, and cardiac output, and calculating the sys-

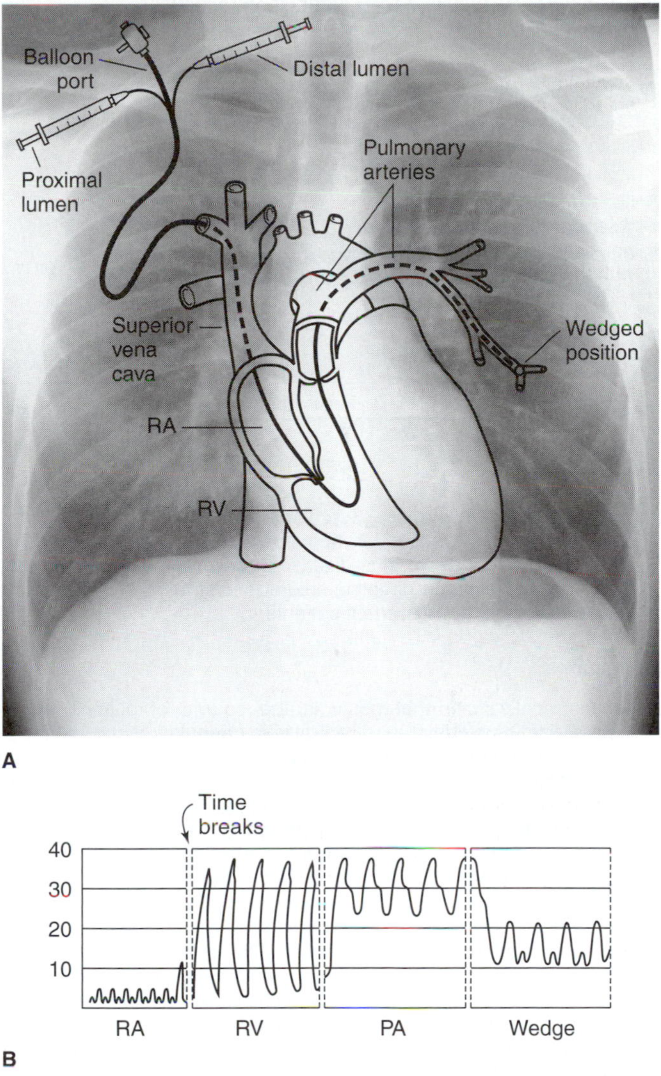

A

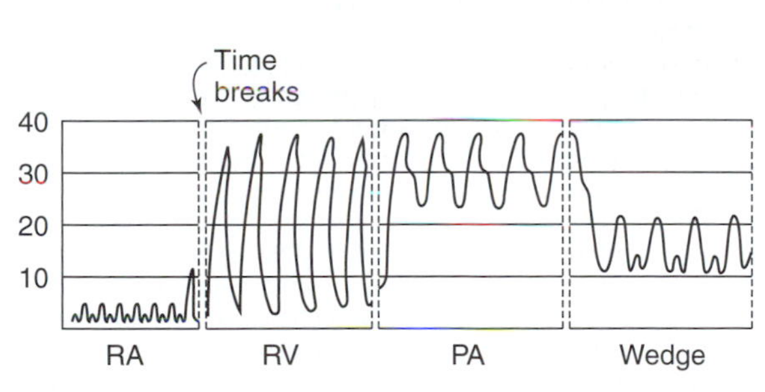

B

Figure 3–10. (**A**) Positioning and (**B**) pressure waveforms seen as the pulmonary artery catheter is advanced. (Reproduced, with permission, from Stillman RM, ed. *Surgery Diagnosis & Therapy.* Originally published by Appleton & Lange. Copyright © 1989 by The McGraw-Hill Companies, Inc.)

TABLE 3–4. NORMAL PULMONARY ARTERY CATHETER MEASUREMENTS.

Parameter	Range
Right artery pressure (RAP)	1–7 mm Hg
Right ventricular systolic pressure	15–25 mm Hg
Right ventricular diastolic pressure	0–8 mm Hg
Pulmonary artery systolic pressure	15–25 mm Hg
Pulmonary artery diastolic pressure	8–15 mm Hg
Pulmonary artery mean pressure	10–20 mm Hg
Pulmonary capillary wedge pressure (PCWP) (wedge)	6–12 mm Hg
Cardiac output (CO)	3.5–5.5 L/min
Cardiac index (CI)	2.8–3.2 L/min/m^2
Mixed venous O_2 saturation	> 60%
Systemic vascular resistance (SVR)	900–1200 dynes/sec/cm^5

$$SVR = \frac{\text{(mean arterial pressure} - \text{central venous pressure (or RAP)}}{\text{CO}} \times 80$$

temic vascular resistance. (See Table 3–3, p 423). Abnormalities in various pressures obtained from pulmonary artery catheterization can often help diagnose various disease states (see Table 3–5, p 429), and may be helpful in directing fluid administration and inotropic and vasopressor therapy in certain patients.

Complications

1. Most complications that occur in the course of pulmonary artery catheterization are related to central vein cannulation and include arterial puncture and pneumothorax, as well as inadvertent placement of the catheter outside the vascular tree, most often in the pleural space.
2. Arrhythmias are another common complication. The most common of these are transient PVCs that occur when the catheter is advanced into the right ventricular outflow tract. If a patient with a PAC suddenly develops frequent PVCs, displacement of the catheter should be suspected. Sustained ventricular tachycardia (VT) and ventricular fibrillation (VF) are both very rare occurrences.
3. Transient right bundle branch block (RBBB) occurs occasionally as the catheter passes through the right ventricular outflow tract. In a patient with preexisting left bundle branch block, this can result in complete heart block. In this setting, some form of backup pacing should be readily available. Complete heart block has been reported but is a rare occurrence.
4. Significant pulmonary infarcts and pulmonary artery rupture are potentially very serious but infrequent complications of PACs caused by “per-

TABLE 3–5. DIFFERENTIAL DIAGNOSIS OF COMMON PULMONARY ARTERY CATHETER READINGS.[1]

Low right atrial pressure	Volume depletion
High right atrial pressure	Volume overload; congestive heart failure; cardiogenic shock; increased pulmonary vascular resistance (hypoxia, ventilator effect of PEEP, pulmonary disease, primary pulmonary hypertension)
Low right ventricular pressure	Volume depletion
High right ventricular pressure	Volume overload; congestive heart failure; cardiogenic shock; increased pulmonary vascular resistance (hypoxia, ventilator effect of PEEP, pulmonary disease, primary pulmonary hypertension)
High pulmonary artery pressure	Congestive heart failure; increased pulmonary vascular resistance (hypoxia, ventilator effect of PEEP, pulmonary disease, primary pulmonary hypertension); cardiac tamponade
Low wedge pressure	Volume depletion
High wedge pressure	Cardiogenic shock, left ventricular failure, ventricular septal defect, mitral regurgitation and stenosis, severe hypertension, volume overload, cardiac tamponade

[1] *Modified and reproduced with permission from Gomella LG, Lefor AT. eds.* Surgery On Call Reference. *3rd ed.: McGraw-Hill; 2001.*
PEEP = Positive end-expiratory pressure

manent" wedge or peripheral placement of the catheter. Fortunately, these complications can be easily avoided with careful monitoring of the wave tracing to make sure that the PAC is not continuously or intermittently showing "spontaneous" PCWP position or "wedge."

5. Most complications and problems related to PACs tend to increase with the length of time that the catheter is left in place. Particularly relevant among them is the high risk of bacteremia and even subacute bacterial endocarditis that is seen in severely ill patients with chronic catheter placement. Thus, in the setting of unexplained fever the PAC and introducer sheath should always be removed and cultured. It is essential to always culture the introducer sheath, but whether the PAC itself should also be routinely cultured is not well established. A new catheter and sheath can be placed at a different site if use of a PAC is still indicated.

REFERENCES

Connors AF, Speroff T, Dawson NV et al: The effectiveness of right heart catheterization in the initial care of critically ill patients. JAMA 1996;276:889.

Iberti TJ, Daily EK, Leibowitz AB et al: Assessment of critical care nurses' knowledge of the pulmonary artery catheter. Crit Care Med 1994;22:1674.

Iberti TJ, Fisher EP, Leibowitz AB et al: A multicenter study of physician's knowledge of the pulmonary artery catheter. JAMA 1990;264:2928.

Knaus WA, LeGall JR, Wagner DP et al: A comparison of intensive care in the USA and France. Lancet 1982;2:642.

Reynolds HN, Haupt MT, Thill-Baharozian MC et al: Impact of critical care physician staffing on patients with septic shock in a university hospital medical intensive care unit. JAMA 1988;260:3446.

Robin ED: The cult of the Swan-Ganz catheter: Overuse and abuse of pulmonary flow catheters. Ann Intern Med 1985;103:445.

Robin ED: Death by pulmonary artery flow-directed catheter: Time for a moratorium? Chest 1987;92:721.

13. SKIN BIOPSY

Indications: To confirm or establish a diagnosis of any skin lesion or eruption.

Contraindications: Any skin lesion that is suspected to be a melanoma should be referred to a dermatologist or surgeon for an excisional biopsy. Punch biopsies are contraindicated in this setting as they do not provide adequate tissue for the measurement of tumor thickness. A platelet count less than 10,000/mm^3 is a relative contraindication.

Materials: A skin punch between 2 and 5 mm; 3 mL buffered lidocaine 1% with epinephrine; 3-mL syringe; 30-gauge needle; gloves; 4×4 gauze pads; alcohol pad; pair of curved iris scissors and fine-tooth forceps; a specimen bottle containing 10% formalin; 4-0 or 5-0 nonabsorbable suture; skin-marking pen.

Procedure

1. If more than one lesion is present, it is important to choose a representative site. For patients with vesiculobullous disease or suspected vasculitis, an early intact lesion not older than 24–48 hours is preferable. For bullous or vesicular lesions, biopsy the edge of the blister or include the entire lesion if possible. For eruptions involving the trunk and extremities, choose a well-developed lesion on the trunk, avoiding a biopsy of the lower leg when possible.
2. Note the orientation of the resting skin tension lines. Wipe the area to be biopsied with the alcohol pad. Mark the area with a skin-marking pen. Apply gloves. Inject the lidocaine slowly, infiltrating an area slightly larger than the biopsy site.
3. Immobilize the skin with one hand, pulling the skin perpendicular to the resting skin tension lines. With the other hand, hold the skin punch vertical to the skin surface and apply firm pressure. Rotate the punch alternating between clockwise and counterclockwise rotation while continuing to apply firm pressure. As the punch enters the subcutaneous fat, resistance will lessen. Remove the punch. The core of tissue can be elevated slightly by applying downward pressure on either side of the biopsy site. The tissue can then be snipped at the level of the subcutaneous fat with the scissors. If the tissue cannot be elevated, the core can be speared using the 30-gauge needle and lifted outward, allowing it to be snipped with the scissors.
4. The biopsy specimen should be immediately placed in the specimen container. If a primary blistering process (ie, bullous pemphigoid) is

suspected, the specimen should be sent for direct immunofluorescence as well as hematoxylin & eosin staining. A 3- to 4-mm biopsy should be performed from perilesional nonbullous skin. The specimen being sent for direct immunofluorescence should be sent in a separate container in Michel's solution.

5. Hemostasis is achieved by applying pressure with the gauze pads.
6. Defects from 2-mm punches generally do not require suture placement. Punch defects larger than 2 mm should be closed with one or two sutures, placed perpendicular to skin tension lines to minimize the appearance of scarring.
7. Lubricant jelly (Vaseline) and an appropriately sized bandage should be applied. The dressing can be removed the following day, but the wound should be kept moist with Vaseline until completely healed.
8. Sutures can be removed as early as 3 days postprocedure from the face and 7–10 days from other areas.

Complications: Infection (unusual); hemorrhage (usually controlled with pressure, rare even in patients taking warfarin or aspirin); scarring and keloid formation.

REFERENCES

Robinson J, LeBoit P: Biopsy techniques: Description and proper use. In: Arndt KA, ed. *Cutaneous Medicine and Surgery.* Saunders;1996:120.

Zachary C: Surgical therapy. In: Sams WM, Lynch PJ, ed. *Principles and Practice of Dermatology.* Churchill Livingstone;1990:63.

14. THORACENTESIS

Indications: Diagnosis of pleural effusion; therapeutic removal of pleural fluid; instillation of sclerosing compounds to obliterate the pleural space.

Contraindications: Pneumothorax, hemothorax, or respiratory impairment on the contralateral side; coagulopathy (relative); a patient receiving positive pressure ventilation (relative).

Materials: Prepackaged thoracentesis kit; or minor procedure tray plus 20- to 60-mL syringe, 20- or 22-gauge 1.5-in. needle, three-way stopcock, specimen containers, 500- or 1000-cc vacuum bottles, hemostat.

Procedure

1. It takes at least 300 mL of fluid to visualize a pleural effusion on a standard posteroanterior chest x-ray.
2. Discuss the procedure with the patient and obtain informed consent. Teach the patient the Valsalva maneuver; or make sure the patient can hum (to increase intrathoracic pressure at a later point in the procedure).
3. The usual site for a thoracentesis is the posterolateral back 5–10 cm lateral to the spine. Percuss out the fluid level, or use the chest x-ray and count ribs. Enter just above the rib to avoid the neurovascular bundle

that traverses below the rib. Do not attempt thoracentesis below the eighth intercostal space in order to avoid injury to the spleen or liver. For high-risk patients or small effusions (less than 1 cm on a lateral decubitus radiograph), consider using ultrasound guidance.

4. Prep the area with povidone-iodine and drape. The patient should be sitting up comfortably; leaning too far forward causes the effusion to move anteriorly away from the thoracentesis site. The bed stand is helpful in order to keep the patient upright and leaning slightly forward.
5. Make a skin wheal over the proposed site with a 25-gauge needle and lidocaine. Change to a 22-gauge 1½-in. needle, and infiltrate up and over the rib; try to anesthetize the deeper structures and the pleura. During this time, you should be aspirating. (See Figure 3–11.) Once fluid returns, note the depth of the needle and mark it with a hemostat. This gives you the approximate depth before you enter the pleural space. Remove the needle.
6. Measure the 16- to 18-gauge thoracentesis needle with a hemostat to the same depth as the first needle, and attach to a 50-cc syringe with a three-way stopcock. Open the stopcock to the syringe. Penetrate through the anesthetized area with the thoracentesis needle entering over the top of the rib to avoid the neuromuscular bundle that runs below the rib. (See Figure 3–11.) After advancing to the depth premeasured by the hemostat, aspirate the amount of fluid needed. For a large-volume therapeutic thoracentesis, a catheter-thru-needle kit can be used. After entering the pleural space, the catheter is advanced through the needle, which is then removed. One end of the drainage tubing is attached to the catheter, the other to a needle, which in turn

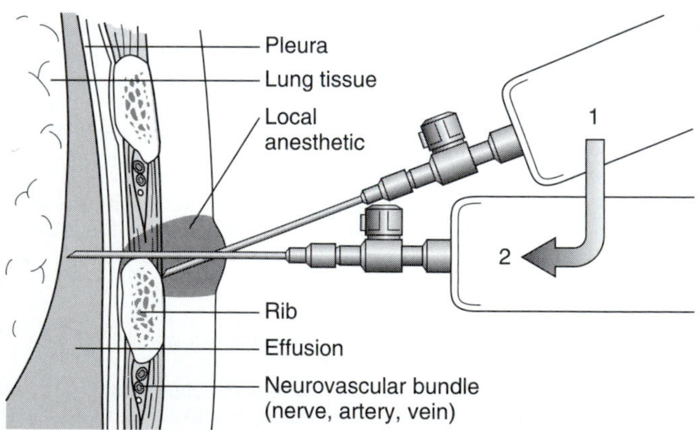

Figure 3–11. In a thoracentesis, the needle is passed over the top of the rib to avoid the neurovascular bundle. (Reproduced, with permission, from Gomella LG, ed. *Clinician's Pocket Reference.* 9th ed. McGraw-Hill; 2002.

is inserted into a vacuum drainage bottle. To avoid reexpansion pulmonary edema, *do not remove more than 1000–1500 cc per tap!*

7. Have the patient hum or do the Valsalva maneuver as you withdraw the needle. These actions increase intrathoracic pressure and decrease the chance of a pneumothorax. Bandage the site.
8. Obtain a chest x-ray to evaluate the fluid level and to rule out a pneumothorax. An expiratory film is best because a small pneumothorax is more likely to be visualized. Some authorities question whether routine chest radiography is necessary in asymptomatic patients after thoracentesis.
9. Send samples of pleural fluid for the following studies: pH, specific gravity, protein, LDH, glucose, cell count and differential, Gram's stain, and bacterial cultures. Optional lab studies are cytology, fungal, and AFB smears and cultures; amylase if you suspect an effusion secondary to pancreatitis (usually on the left); and a Sudan stain and triglycerides if a chylothorax is suspected. See Table 3–6, for the differential diagnosis.

TABLE 3–6. DIFFERENTIAL DIAGNOSIS OF PLEURAL FLUID.[1]

Transudate: Nephrosis, congestive heart failure, cirrhosis.

Exudate: Infection (parapneumonic, empyema, tuberculosis, viral, fungal, parasitic), malignancy, peritoneal dialysis, pancreatitis, chylothorax.

Lab Value	Transudate	Exudate
Specific gravity	<1.016	>1.016
Protein (pleural fluid)	<2.5 g/100 mL	>3 g/100 mL
Protein ratio (pleural fluid-to-serum ratio)	<0.5	>0.5
LDH ratio (pleural fluid-to-serum ratio)	<0.6	>0.6
Pleural fluid LDH	<200 IU	>200 IU
Fibrinogen (clot)	No	Yes
Cell count and differential	Low WBC count	WBC count > 2500/mL; suspect an inflammatory exudate (early polys, later monos)

Grossly bloody tap: Trauma, pulmonary infarction, tumor, and iatrogenic causes.

pH: The pH of pleural fluid is usually > 7.3. If between 7.2 and 7.3, suspect tuberculosis or malignancy or both. If < 7.2, suspect an empyema.

Glucose: Normal pleural fluid glucose is two-thirds serum glucose. If the pleural fluid glucose is *much, much* lower than the serum glucose, then consider empyema or rheumatoid arthritis (0–16 mg/100 mL) as the cause of the effusion.

Triglycerides and positive Sudan stain: Chylothorax.

[1] *Modified and reproduced with permission from Gomella LG, Lefor AT, eds.* Surgery On Call Reference. *3rd ed. McGraw-Hill; 2002.*

LDH = lactic dehydrogenase; WBC = white blood cells; polys = polymorphonuclear leukocytes; monos = monocytes.

Complications: Pneumothorax (5–10% incidence, of which 20% will require a chest tube), hemothorax, infection, pulmonary laceration, hypoxemia, vasovagal response, reexpansion pulmonary edema, laceration of spleen or liver.

REFERENCES

Aleman C, Alegre J, Armadans L et al: The value of chest roentgenography in the diagnosis of pneumothorax after thoracentesis. Am J Med 1999;107:340.

Ruhl TS: Thoracentesis. In: Pfenninger JL, Fowler GC, eds. *Procedures for Primary Care Physicians.* Mosby;1994:477.

IV. Fluids & Electrolytes

Daily maintenance requirements for the average 70-kg male are as follows:

Fluid	2000–2500 mL
Dextrose	100–200 g
Sodium	60–100 mEq
Potassium	40–60 mEq

These requirements can be met with an infusion of D5¼ NS with 20–30 mEq of potassium chloride per liter infused at 100 mL/hr. The preceding combination of fluid and electrolytes may differ depending on other clinical parameters such as congestive heart failure, cirrhosis, hyponatremia, hypernatremia, hyperkalemia, and renal insufficiency. Maintenance fluids should be used for only 48–72 hours, at which time more effective measures of nutritional support (enteral tube feedings) should be instituted. For patients with severe volume depletion, normal saline can be administered as rapidly as 500–1000 mL/hr until the patient is stabilized. For patients undergoing nasogastric suction, measured losses can be replaced every 4 hours with an equal volume of normal saline. Additional potassium may have to be added to the maintenance fluids to replace that lost with gastric suction. (See Tables 4–1 and 4–2.)

TABLE 4–1. COMPOSITION OF COMMONLY USED CRYSTALLOID SOLUTIONS.[1]

Fluid	Glucose (g/L)	Electrolytes (mEq/L)					kcal/L
		Na	Cl	K	Ca	HCO_3	
D5W (5% dextrose in water)	50	—	—	—	—	—	170
D10W (10% dextrose in water)	100	—	—	—	—	—	340
D20W (20% dextrose in water)	200	—	—	—	—	—	680
D50W (50% dextrose in water)	500	—	—	—	—	—	1700
½ NS (0.45% NaCl)	—	77	77	—	—	—	—
NS (0.9% NaCl)	—	154	154	—	—	—	—
3% NS	—	513	513	—	—	—	—
D5¼ NS	50	38	38	—	—	—	170
D5½ NS (0.45% NaCl)	50	77	77	—	—	—	170
D5% NS (0.9% NaCl)	50	154	154	—	—	—	170
D5LR (5% dextrose in lactated Ringer's)	50	130	110	4	3	27	180
Lactated Ringer's	—	130	110	4	3	27	<10

[1]*Modified and reproduced with permission from Gomella LG, ed.* Clinician's Pocket Reference. *9th ed.: McGraw-Hill; 2002.*
NS = normal saline.

TABLE 4–2. COMPOSITION AND DAILY PRODUCTION OF BODY FLUIDS.[1]

Fluid	Electrolytes (mEq/L)				Average Daily Production (mL)
	Na	Cl	K	HCO_3	
Sweat	50	40	5	0	Varies
Saliva	60	15	26	50	1500
Gastric juices	60–100	100	10	0	1500–2500
Duodenum	130	90	5	0–10	300–2000
Bile	145	100	5	15	100–300
Pancreatic juice	140	75	5	115	100–800
Ileum	140	100	2–8	30	100–9000
Diarrhea	120	90	25	45	—

[1]*Modified and reproduced with permission from Gomella LG, ed.* Clinician's Pocket Reference. *9th ed.: McGraw-Hill; 2002.*

V. Blood Component Therapy

■ RED BLOOD CELL TRANSFUSIONS

The blood supply in the United States has never been safer; however, transfusion with blood should be carefully considered and avoided whenever possible. Transfusions are indicated when:

1. Symptoms from acute blood loss have failed to respond to crystalloid infusions.
2. Symptoms from a chronic anemia have not improved with other therapeutic interventions.

Clinicians should not establish empiric, automatic transfusion thresholds.

■ ANEMIA

(See also Section I, Chapter 5, Anemia, p 27).

When confronted with a chronic anemia, the clinician must consider whether the Hgb and HcT accurately reflect the red blood cell (RBC) mass. The RBC mass is more important with respect to oxygen transport than the measured HcT or Hgb; however, a low Hgb or HcT usually reflects a low RBC mass. An increased plasma volume may result in a dilutional change in the Hgb and make an anemia appear more severe. Increased plasma volume may occur in congestive heart failure (CHF), pregnancy, and paraproteinemia.

Acute Blood Loss: In the setting of acute blood loss and hypotension, restoration of blood volume and tissue perfusion as well as improvement of oxygen-carrying capacity must be accomplished. You should use electrolyte solutions or colloids initially. Blood losses of 500–1000 mL in an adult do not usually require blood transfusion unless there is an underlying anemia or another medical condition requiring added oxygen-carrying capacity.

RBC Products—Availability and Indications

1. **Whole blood.** There are few indications for transfusion of whole blood today, except for transfusion of the massively bleeding patient when volume and oxygen-carrying capacity can be supplied in one product. Stored whole blood is not adequate replacement for platelets or labile coagulation factors.
2. **Packed RBCs.** Basically a unit of whole blood with two-thirds of the plasma removed. This has become the standard RBC product for most transfusions.
3. **Leukocyte-poor RBCs.** In this product, 70–90% of the leukocytes have been removed by a variety of techniques. Leukocyte-poor RBCs are used in patients with a history of repeated febrile reactions to

standard packed RBC transfusions. These reactions are usually due to leukocyte antigens. Leukocyte-poor RBCs are indicated for patients expected to require extensive blood product support. These products will decrease the risk of anti-allo platelet antibody formation.

4. **Washed RBCs.** Virtually all plasma and nonerythrocyte cellular elements are removed. Washed cells are indicated in patients with febrile reactions to leukocyte-poor RBCs, in patients with allergic reactions to plasma components (IgA deficiency), and in patients with paroxysmal nocturnal hemoglobinuria when exposure to complement may exacerbate the hemolytic process.
5. **Frozen stored RBCs.** Used primarily for autologous transfusion for elective surgery and to maintain availability of units for patients with alloantibodies to high-incidence blood group antigens.
6. **Cytomegalovirus (CMV)-negative products.** Patients undergoing organ and bone marrow transplantation require aggressive immunosuppressive therapy to ensure engraftment and avoid graft rejection. If these patients or candidates for organ or bone marrow transplantation are CMV-negative prior to their transplant, CMV-negative blood products will minimize the risk of CMV infection complicating their transplantation course.

Complications: See Section I, Chapter 62, Transfusion Reaction, p 338.

■ PLATELET TRANSFUSIONS

(See also Section I, Chapter 61, Thrombocytopenia, p 333).

Indications: Platelet transfusions are indicated for any patient with a major bleeding event involving a qualitative or quantitative platelet disorder. Prophylactic platelet transfusions are most commonly indicated in settings of decreased platelet production, such as aplastic anemia, acute leukemia, or chemotherapy- or radiation-induced bone marrow suppression. In these settings, many institutions empirically give transfusions to patients with platelet counts < 10,000. Individuals with fever, mucosal ulcerations, and planned invasive procedures are frequently supported with platelets to maintain counts > 20,000.

Individuals with thrombocytopenia on the basis of platelet destruction (either via antibodies or consumption) rarely benefit from prophylactic transfusion. In general, transfusion with ongoing platelet destruction is indicated only when there is bleeding of a microvascular nature greater than that expected.

The efficacy of platelet transfusion in the setting of platelet dysfunction is not well documented. Desmopressin (DDAVP) should be considered in this circumstance. Patients with lifelong quantitative or qualitative platelet disorders should not be transfused prophylactically solely on the basis of platelet count, bleeding time, or other platelet function studies. Overutilization of platelets increases the risk of alloimmunization and subsequent inadequate response to platelet transfusions. Likewise, patients with idiopathic thrombocytopenic purpura (ITP) should not be prophylactically transfused.

Complications

1. **Transmission of viral infections**
2. **Reactions to plasma components, RBCs, and WBCs.** Reactions to RBC antigens rarely cause a hemolytic transfusion reaction. They can cause alloimmunity and a potential for problems such as the use of Rh-positive platelets in an Rh-negative female. The patient should receive intravenous anti-D globulin (RhoGAM) if she is of childbearing age.
3. **Possible transmission of bacterial infections.** A potential problem because of the storage time and storage temperature of platelet concentrates.
4. **Development of alloimmunization.** This problem eventually develops in two-thirds of patients receiving multiple transfusions of platelets. May necessitate the use of HLA-matched platelets to achieve adequate post-transfusion counts.

■ PLASMA COMPONENT THERAPY

The following is a list of commonly available plasma products and selected remarks about indications and complications.

Fresh-Frozen Plasma

1. Contains all factors, but titers of factors VIII and V decline with long-term storage. Can be used for replacement of factor deficiencies, but problems include long turnaround time because of the need for thawing, and the potential volume of plasma needed to correct certain factor deficiencies.
2. Other side effects include urticaria, fever, nausea, headaches, and pruritus. These can usually be treated or prevented with antihistamines and antipyretics.
3. Transmission of viral infections is less likely than with the factor concentrates.

Single-Donor Plasma

1. Collected from one donor unit of whole blood. Levels of factors V and VIII decline appreciably with storage; single-donor plasma should not be used to replace these factors.
2. Risk of hepatitis and other infections is equivalent to the risk associated with transfusing a unit of whole blood.

Cryoprecipitate

1. Contains high levels of factor VIII, von Willebrand factor, and fibrinogen. Useful in factor VIII deficiency, von Willebrand's disease, fibrinogen disorders, and uremic bleeding.

2. Contains insignificant amounts of other coagulation factors. Most frequently used for hypofibrinogenemia related to conditions that cause consumptive coagulopathy. Therefore, most patients receiving cryoprecipitate will require other blood components.

Factor VIII Concentrate

1. Various preparations are available. Only genetically engineered preparations should be used so as to avoid transmitting HIV and viral hepatitis.
2. Use is limited to patients with factor VIII deficiency.

Vitamin K–Dependent Factor Concentrates

1. Contains factors II, VII, IX, and X; protein C; and protein S. Useful in these specific factor deficiencies and in patients with factor VIII inhibitors.
2. Risk of hepatitis and thromboembolic disease exists because of the presence of activated factors in some preparations.

Gamma Globulin. There are many different forms of intravenous and intramuscular gamma globulins available with a wide variety of indications and reactions.

1. **Indications**
   a. Nonspecific immunoglobulin for non-B hepatitis prophylaxis. Hepatitis B immunoglobulin is used for prophylaxis for hepatitis B. Specific immunoglobulins can also be used for postexposure prophylaxis for Varicella and rabies.
   b. Prophylactic or therapeutic intravenous use for inherited or acquired humoral immune deficiencies.
   c. Treatment of acute and chronic immune thrombocytopenic purpura (ITP).
2. **Reactions.** The following are adverse effects that might result from the administration of gamma globulin.
   a. **Anaphylactoid reaction.** An immediate reaction attributed to complement activation. Symptoms and signs may include flushing, chest tightness, dyspnea, fever, chills, nausea, vomiting, hypotension, and back pain. These are uncommon reactions with the currently available preparations but can occur with both intravenous and intramuscular administration. Therapy consists of discontinuation of the infusion and use of diphenhydramine (Benadryl), steroids, epinephrine, and vasopressors if necessary.
   b. **Inflammatory reaction.** This is characteristically a delayed reaction. Signs and symptoms may include headache, malaise, fever, chills, and nausea. The reaction disappears with discontinuation of gamma globulin therapy.

REFERENCES

Audet A-M, Goodnough LT: Practice strategies for elective red blood cell transfusion. Ann Intern Med 1992;116:403.

Fresh-Frozen Plasma, Cryoprecipitate, and Platelet Administration Practice Guidelines Development Task Force of the College of American Pathologists: Practice parameter for the use of fresh-frozen plasma, cryoprecipitate, and platelets. JAMA 1994;271:777.

Goodnough LT, Brecher ME, Kanter MH et al: Transfusion medicine—blood transfusion. N Engl J Med 1999;340:438.

McCullough J: Transfusion medicine. In: Handin RI, Lux SE, Stossel TP, eds. *Blood: Principles and Practice of Hematology.* Lippincott;1995:1947.

VI. Ventilator Management

1. INDICATIONS & SETUP

I. Indications

A. Ventilatory failure. A $PaCO_2 > 50$ Torr indicates ventilatory failure; however, many patients will have chronic ventilatory failure with renal compensation (retaining HCO_3^-). The absolute pH is often a better guide to determine the need for ventilatory assistance than $PaCO_2$. A significant acidemia suggests an acute respiratory acidosis or acute decompensation of a chronic respiratory acidosis. A respiratory acidosis with a rapidly falling pH or an absolute pH < 7.24 is an indication for ventilatory support.

The prototype of pure ventilatory failure is the drug overdose patient in whom there is a sudden loss of central respiratory drive with uncontrolled hypercarbia. Patients with sepsis, neuromuscular disease, and chronic obstructive pulmonary disease (COPD) may have hypercarbic ventilatory failure.

B. Hypoxemic respiratory failure. Inability to oxygenate is an important indication for ventilatory support. A $PaO_2 < 60$ Torr on > 50% inspired fraction of oxygen (FiO_2) constitutes hypoxemic respiratory failure. Newer nomenclature uses the PaO_2/FiO_2 (P/F) ratio to characterize hypoxemia. A P/F ratio < 200 is consistent with acute respiratory distress syndrome (ARDS), whereas a ratio between 200 and 300 is termed *acute lung injury.* Although these patients can sometimes be managed with higher FiO_2 delivery systems, such as partial or nonrebreather masks, or continuous positive airway pressure (CPAP) delivered by mask, they are at high risk for cardiopulmonary arrest. They should be closely monitored in an intensive care unit (ICU) if they are not intubated. Worsening of the respiratory status necessitates prompt intubation and ventilatory support.

The prototype disease for hypoxemic respiratory failure is ARDS, in which the high shunt fraction leads to refractory hypoxemia.

C. Mixed respiratory failure. Most patients have failure of both ventilation and oxygenation. The indications for ventilatory support remain the same as listed earlier.

An example of mixed respiratory failure is the COPD patient with an acute exacerbation. Bronchospasm alters the ventilation-perfusion ratio ($\dot{V}/\dot{Q}$) relationships, leading to worsening hypoxemia. Bronchospasm and accumulated secretions lead to a high work of breathing and consequent hypercarbia.

D. Neuromuscular disease with respiratory failure. This is actually a subcategory of ventilatory failure but deserves separate mention because of differing management. Hypercarbia occurs just before arrest; thus, criteria other than arterial blood gases (ABGs) are needed. Patients with myasthenia gravis, Guillain-Barré syndrome, and muscular dystrophy are at risk of respiratory failure.

1. Respiratory rates > 24/min are an early sign of respiratory failure. A progressive rise in the respiratory rate, or sustained respiratory rates > 35/min, are indications for ventilatory support.
2. Abdominal paradox indicates dyssynergy of chest wall muscles and diaphragms and impending respiratory failure. It is manifested by inward movement of the abdominal wall during inspiration rather than the normal outward motion.
3. A vital capacity < 15 mL/kg is associated with acute respiratory arrest as well as an inability to clear secretions. Similarly, a negative inspiratory force < –25 cm H_2O implies impending respiratory arrest.

   Guillain-Barré syndrome is the prototypic neuromuscular disease in which the preceding criteria require strict attention. A patient with Guillain-Barré syndrome should be closely observed and followed up with frequent vital capacity (VC) measurements. A rapidly falling VC, or VC < 1000 mL, requires respirator support.

II. Partial Ventilatory Assistance

A. **CPAP (continuous positive airway pressure)** may be administered by full face mask or nasal mask. Pressures of 5–15 cm H_2O may be used to recruit alveoli and improve oxygenation for refractory hypoxemia. CPAP has proven efficacy in respiratory failure due to pulmonary edema as well as in acute exacerbations of COPD. (It is thought to decrease work of breathing by splinting airways open and thus counteracting intrinsic positive end-expiratory pressure [PEEP].)

B. **BIPAP (bidirectional positive airway pressure)** may provide significant ventilatory assistance in patients with chronic neuromuscular diseases, COPD, or pneumonia; or for patients in whom intubation is not an option. Initial settings would be IPAP (inspiratory pressure) 12 cm; EPAP (expiratory pressure) 4 cm; Patient Assist Mode and backup rate, 12 breaths per minute. IPAP can then be titrated upward to increase the effective tidal volume. An experienced respiratory therapist is vital to the success of BIPAP. Starting at very low pressures and providing proper mask fit and a lot of reassurance are mandatory for success. Conventional ventilators can also be used to provide noninvasive ventilation via a face mask interface.

C. **CPAP or BIPAP** requires intensive respiratory therapy support for titration of O_2 and pressure as well as adjustments of the mask, since leaks are common. Necrosis of the bridge of the nose may occur.

D. **Contraindications.** Rapidly progressive respiratory failure, coma (inability to protect the airway), vomiting, pneumothorax, and gastric distension. Partial ventilatory support should be administered only in an ICU or stepdown unit.

III. Tracheal Intubation. See Section III, Chapter 7, Endotracheal Intubation, p 407. Endotracheal intubation is actually the most difficult and complication-ridden part of ventilator initiation. Skill and experience are required for correct placement. Aspiration, esophageal intubation, and right mainstem bronchus intubation are common complications. Bilateral breath sounds always need to be confirmed by chest auscultation in each axilla. An immediate postintubation portable chest x-ray (CXR) should be obtained. An inline CO_2 sensor can be used for rapid confirmation of tracheal intubation. Intubation can be accomplished by three routes:

A. Nasotracheal intubation. This can be accomplished blindly and in an awake patient. Intubation requires experience and adequate local anesthesia. Complications include intubation of the esophagus, nosebleeds, kinking of the endotracheal tube (ETT), and postobstructive sinusitis. A smaller ETT is usually required for nasotracheal versus orotracheal intubation; this leads to a higher work of breathing because of increased resistance, difficulties with adequate suctioning, and higher ventilation pressures. Nasotracheal ETTs are more comfortable than orotracheal ETTs; they are less damaging to the larynx because they are better stabilized in the airway. This type of intubation should be avoided in the presence of facial trauma.

B. Orotracheal intubation. Placement of orotracheal tubes requires normal neck mobility to allow hyperextension of the neck for direct visualization of the vocal cords. Larger ETTs can be placed via this route. Adequate local anesthesia or sedation is necessary for safe placement without aspiration.

C. Tracheostomy. Tracheostomy is a surgical procedure most often done acutely for upper airway obstruction; however, in patients who require more than 14–21 days of ventilatory support, a tracheostomy is recommended. Tracheostomy tubes facilitate the weaning process by decreasing tube resistance, as the tube is shorter and has a wider radius. Patients can eat with a tracheostomy, and find the tubes more comfortable than those used for tracheal intubation.

IV. Ventilator Setup

A. The ventilator. Contemporary ventilators are volume-cycled, pressure targeted, or time cycled. Elaborate alarm systems are present to alert personnel to inadequate minute ventilation or tidal volume, high peak pressure, disconnection of the ETT, and so forth.

Effective ventilation is measured by changes in $PaCO_2$. Minute ventilation ($\dot{V}_e$) can be calculated by tidal volume × breath rate. Thus, ventilation may be adjusted by changing the breath rate, the tidal volume, or both. Tidal volumes > 10 mL/kg may cause overdistension of alveoli and increase the risk of pneumothorax. Recent ARDS research suggests that a tidal volume of 5 cc/kg ideal body weight (IBW) is optimal. (It is thought that excessive stretch may lead to increased inflammatory response and alveolar leak.) Most initial tidal volumes are therefore set at 5–8 mL/kg IBW.

Oxygenation is adjusted by changing FiO_2. Prolonged $FiO_2 > 60\%$ may cause pulmonary fibrosis. Thus, down-adjustment to "safe levels" sufficient to maintain O_2 saturation > 90% should be attempted as indicated by ABGs. If an O_2 saturation > 90% cannot be maintained when decreasing the $FiO_2 < 60\%$, other means to increase oxygenation such as PEEP should be used.

The mode of ventilation should be specified:

1. **Assist control (AC) mode** allows the patient to trigger machine breaths once a threshold of inspiratory flow or effort is made. Each breath is a full machine breath. AC mode also supplies a backup rate in cases of apnea or paralysis. It is typically used in pulmonary edema states (both cardiogenic and noncardiogenic) as well as after cardiopulmonary resuscitation.
2. **Intermittent mandatory ventilation (IMV)** provides a set number of machine breaths per minute and allows the patient to make spontaneous breaths as well. Synchronized intermittent mandatory ventilation (SIMV) allows synchronization of the IMV breaths with patient efforts. As the rate is turned down, the patient assumes more and more of the work of breathing. Typically SIMV is used in patients with obstructive airways disease (COPD or asthma).
3. **Continuous positive airway pressure (CPAP)** allows completely spontaneous respirations while the patient is still connected to the ventilator. A set amount of continuous pressure may be applied as well (0–30 cm H_2O). It is almost always used in conjunction with pressure support.
4. **Pressure support.** Pressure support is an inspiratory boost given to augment spontaneous respiratory efforts. Thus, in CPAP mode or in SIMV, pressure support can be used to overcome the work of breathing imposed by the ventilatory system (endotracheal tube, tubing, demand valves) when a patient takes a spontaneous breath. Typically, an 8- to 10-cm pressure boost is used. Pressure support can also be used at higher levels during ventilator weaning (see Section VI, Chapter 4, Weaning, p 458).
5. **Pressure control.** Recent-model ventilators may be set to operate in a pressure-limited mode rather than volume-targeted. A set pressure boost is maintained for a measured time period in this mode. The primary goal is an improvement in oxygenation—often at the expense of ventilation (clearance of CO_2). Another goal is the limitation of peak airway pressures below 40 cm H_2O and thus minimization of barotrauma or overstretching of the lung. Pressure control is primarily used in ARDS. Often inverse ratio ventilation (increasing inspiratory time) is done simultaneously. Because this stimulates a breath-holding maneuver, it feels unnatural to patients, and they usually require deep sedation and/or paralysis in this mode. ***Caution:*** Pressure control should be used *only under supervision of ICU-trained faculty or fellows.*
6. **Airway pressure release ventilation (APRV)** is very similar to pressure control. However, the patient is able to breathe through-

out the machine cycles. Thus, deep sedation and paralysis can be avoided. Typical settings might be:

- P—high 30
- T (time)—high 3 seconds
- P—low 8
- T—low 0.5 seconds

APRV is used primarily in patients with ARDS.

7. **Initial ventilator settings** should be dictated by the underlying condition as well as by previous blood gas results. An example of the initial settings for a 70-kg patient after respiratory arrest would be:
   - FiO_2 1.0 (100%)
   - Assist control mode
   - Rate 18
   - Tidal volume 560 mL

   An attempt should be made to supply the patient with at least as much minute ventilation as was required prior to intubation. Thus, a patient with pulmonary edema, ARDS, or neuromuscular disease may require a minute ventilation rate of 14–22 L/min. The AC mode will generally be more comfortable and will alleviate the work of breathing to a large extent. Sample settings might be:
   - FiO_2 1.0
   - Assist control mode
   - Rate 22
   - Tidal volume 550 mL

   The patient with COPD, on the other hand, should not be overventilated initially. Such patients may have a chronically high bicarbonate because of renal compensation, and overventilation may cause a severe alkalosis. (A pH > 7.55 is felt to be severely arrhythmogenic as well as moving the oxyhemoglobin curve to the right, which impedes oxygen release to the tissues.) Sample settings might be:
   - FiO_2 0.5 (50%)
   - SIMV mode
   - Pressure support 10 cm
   - Rate 12
   - Tidal volume 600 mL

B. Additional setup requirements

1. **Restrain the patient's hands,** because one's natural reaction to the ETT upon awakening is to pull it out.
2. **Place a nasogastric tube** to decompress the stomach or to continue essential oral medications.
3. **Obtain a stat portable CXR** to confirm ETT placement and to reassess any underlying pulmonary disease. The tip of the ETT should be 3–4 cm above the carina.
4. **Treat any underlying pulmonary disease** (maximize bronchodilators in status asthmaticus or vasodilators and diuretics in pulmonary edema).

5. **Consider prophylactic measures.** Heparin 5000 U SC Q 12 hr may reduce the incidence of pulmonary embolism while the patient is on bed rest. Stress ulceration bleeding can be prevented by the use of any of the following: antacids; H_2 antagonists (cimetidine, ranitidine); sucralfate (Carafate); or tube feedings (enteral nutrition).
6. **Order other medications as needed,** such as morphine for pain and lorazepam (Ativan) for agitation.

2. ROUTINE MODIFICATION OF SETTINGS

Arterial blood gases (ABGs) should be monitored and adjusted to a normal pH (7.37–7.44) and a $PaO_2 > 60$ Torr on less than 60% O_2. Tachypnea should be investigated for adequacy of ventilation or for any other cause (eg, fever) prior to sedating the patient.

I. Adjusting PaO_2

A. To decrease: Inspired fraction of oxygen (FiO_2) should be decreased in increments of 10–20% every 30 minutes. The "rule of sevens" states that there will be a 7-Torr fall in PaO_2 for each 1% decrease in FiO_2.

B. To increase

1. **Ventilation** has some effect on PaO_2 (as shown by the alveolar air equation); therefore, correction of the respiratory acidosis will improve oxygenation.
2. **Positive end-expiratory pressure (PEEP)** can be added in increments of 2–4 cm H_2O. PEEP recruits previously collapsed alveoli, holds them open, and restores functional residual capacity (FRC) to a better physiologic level. It counteracts pulmonary shunts and will raise PaO_2. PEEP increases intrathoracic pressure and may thus impede venous return and decrease cardiac output. This is particularly true in the presence of volume depletion and shock. Consult your ICU staff or fellow if high PEEP is needed or if the blood pressure drops with PEEP adjustment.

II. Adjusting $PaCO_2$

A. To decrease

1. Increase the rate or tidal volume.
2. Check for leaks in the system.
3. Decrease CO_2 production by treating fever, minimizing shivering, and controlling agitation.

B. To increase

1. Decrease the rate.
2. You may have to switch from AC mode to SIMV mode to eliminate patient-driven central hyperventilation. Remember, every breath is a full machine breath in Assist Control mode!

3. An old and effective method is to place increased exhalation tubing to increase deadspace. The patient is then rebreathing his or her CO_2.

3. TROUBLESHOOTING

3A. AGITATION

I. **Problem.** The ventilator patient becomes agitated, struggles constantly, tries to pull out all tubes, and actively fights the respirator.

II. **Immediate Questions**

A. **Is the patient still properly connected?** Hypoxemia or hypercarbia resulting from disconnection of the respirator may result in agitation. A patient who can speak is probably no longer intubated.

B. **Review the ventilator flow and pressure waveforms.** Look for auto-PEEP. Failure of the expiratory flow to flatten at zero indicates airtrapping or auto-PEEP. This may cause increased work of breathing and agitation (an experienced respiratory therapist will be able to measure it for you and then apply external PEEP to counterbalance it). A double dip on the inspiratory flow curve usually indicates the patient has air hunger and wants a higher peak flow.

C. **What were the most recent ABGs?** Again, hypoxemia or hypercarbia can cause agitation. Adjusting the settings can correct either problem.

D. **What does the CXR show?** Atelectasis from mucous plugging or pneumothorax can occur spontaneously in asthma or as a result of barotrauma and can result in hypoxemia or hypercarbia. The endotracheal tube touching the carina almost always causes coughing and/or agitation.

E. **What is the underlying diagnosis? What are the current medications and IV fluids?** Agitation may be related to the underlying diagnosis or to a medication, and unrelated to the patient's respiratory status. Cimetidine (Tagamet) and narcotics can cause confusion, especially in the elderly. Multiple metabolic disturbances (eg, hyponatremia and hypernatremia) can lead to confusion and possibly agitation. See Section I, Chapter 13, Coma, Acute Mental Status Changes, p 72.

F. **What are the ventilator settings?** The ventilator setting may have been set incorrectly, resulting in hypoxemia or hypercarbia. A high sensitivity setting may make it impossible for the fatigued patient to trigger a breath. Barotrauma resulting in pneumothorax is associated with high PEEP settings, high tidal volumes, and peak inspiratory pressures > 45 cm.

III. **Differential Diagnosis**

A. **Causes of respiratory decompensation**

1. **Worsening of underlying pulmonary disease**
2. **Pneumothorax**

3. **Endotracheal tube displacement.** The tube may be outside the trachea, high in the glottis, or down the right mainstem bronchus.
4. **Mucous plugs.** May result in atelectasis and hypoxemia.
5. **Ventilator malfunction**
6. **Pulmonary embolism (PE).** Immobilization is a major risk for PE.
7. **Aspiration**
8. **Inadequate oxygenation or respiratory muscle fatigue**

B. **Sepsis**

C. **ICU psychosis**

D. **Medications.** Multiple medications such as digoxin (Lanoxin), lidocaine, theophylline, imipenem-cilastatin (Primaxin), diazepam (Valium) and other benzodiazepines, meperidine and other narcotics, and cimetidine may cause psychosis, especially in high doses or with decreased clearance states.

E. **Electrolyte imbalance.** Hyponatremia, hypernatremia, hypercalcemia, hypocalcemia, and hypophosphatemia can cause confusion, which can lead to agitation.

IV. Database

A. **Physical examination key points**

1. **Endotracheal tube.** Carefully check the patency, position, and function of the endotracheal tube (ETT).
2. **Vital signs.** Tachypnea may suggest hypoxemia. Tachycardia and hypertension can result from agitation or be associated with respiratory failure or an underlying problem such as myocardial infarction (MI). Hypotension may be due to auto-PEEP, volume depletion, sepsis, cardiogenic shock, tension pneumothorax, or massive PE. An elevated temperature suggests sepsis, ventilator-associated nosocomial pneumonia, or pulmonary emboli. Tachycardia, tachypnea, and fever may be associated with PE or MI. A pulsus paradoxus > 16 mm Hg implies severe respiratory distress or pericardial tamponade.
3. **HEENT.** Check for distended neck veins suggesting pericardial tamponade or congestive heart failure (CHF). Tracheal deviation may be caused by a tension pneumothorax.
4. **Chest.** Auscultate for bilateral breath sounds. Absent breath sounds on one side suggest pneumothorax or an improperly placed ETT. Bilaterally absent breath sounds can be secondary to either bilateral pneumothoraces or severe respiratory failure.
5. **Extremities.** Check for cyanosis.
6. **Skin.** Palpate for subcutaneous emphysema, which can result from a very high PEEP or may be seen in asthmatics.

B. **Laboratory data**

1. **Arterial blood gases.** To rule out hypoxemia and hypercarbia as well as severe acidosis or alkalosis.

2. **Electrolyte panel.** Including calcium and phosphorus.

C. **Radiologic and other studies.** A CXR to rule out atelectasis and pneumothorax and to evaluate underlying pulmonary pathology.

V. **Plan**

A. **Emergency management**

1. **Examine the patient** as outlined earlier. Carefully check the ETT function, ventilator connections, and chart.
2. **Suction the patient vigorously.** This confirms tube patency and clears out any mucous plugs.
3. **Bag the patient manually** to check for ease of ventilation. Marked difficulty can be seen with tension pneumothorax or mucus plugging. If auto-PEEP is suspected, use a slower rate and decrease the tidal volume. This allows trapped gas time to escape and thus will allow decreased intrathoracic pressure and increased venous return back to the heart.
4. **Obtain ABGs, electrolyte panel, and stat CXR.**
5. **If the patient appears cyanotic** or "air hungry," turn the inspired fraction of oxygen (FiO_2) to 1.0 and the ventilator mode to "Assist Control" (AC).
6. **If hypotension and unilaterally absent breath sounds** are found concomitantly, consider chest tube insertion for tension pneumothorax. Patients on ventilators can rapidly die of tension pneumothoraces.
7. **If you suspect ICU psychosis,** reassure the patient. Have a family member help reorient the patient. Often a familiar voice will work wonders! Ask the nurses to move the patient to a room with a window; this environmental feature has been shown to reduce ICU psychosis.
8. **Check the ventilator settings.** Perhaps too much effort is required to open the valves or to initiate a breath. Ask the respiratory therapist to lower the triggering sensitivity to 0.5 or 1.0 cm H_20. Experiment with adding a little more pressure support for patient comfort.
9. **If everything else is stable** and the patient is endangering himself or herself, sedate the patient. Haloperidol (Haldol) 0.5–2.0 mg IM or IV and lorazepam (Ativan) 0.5–2.0 mg IV are the currently recommended agents.

3B. HYPOXEMIA

I. **Problem.** The respirator patient requires > 60% FiO_2 to maintain a PaO_2 > 60 Torr.

II. **Immediate Questions**

A. **What is the sequence of ABGs?** In other words, is this an acute or a slowly developing change? A rapid deterioration implies an immediate life-threatening process such as a tension pneumothorax or a massive pulmonary embolism (PE).

B. What is the underlying diagnosis? A patient with long-bone fractures may develop fat embolus syndrome, a patient with sepsis may develop acute respiratory distress syndrome (ARDS), or a patient with head injury might develop neurogenic pulmonary edema.

C. What are the ventilator settings? Has a change been made recently? An error may have been made with the ventilator settings, or recent changes may have been made too aggressively in an attempt to wean the patient from the ventilator. Some patients are very sensitive to PEEP changes.

III. Differential Diagnosis

A. Shunts secondary to alveolar filling or by obstructed bronchi with consequent collapse

1. **Pneumonia**
2. **Pulmonary contusion**
3. **Atelectasis.** The endotracheal tube (ETT) may be placed too far in the right mainstem bronchus, or there may be mucous plugs.
4. **ARDS or cardiogenic pulmonary edema**

B. Cardiac level shunt. An acute ventricular septal defect, especially in the setting of an acute myocardial infarction (MI), may develop. Sudden pulmonary hypertension may occasionally lead to a patent foramen ovale and physiologic shunt at the atrial level. A tip-off to this is a worsening shunt and PaO_2 as positive end-expiratory pressure (PEEP) is increased.

C. Shunts secondary to pneumothorax

D. Ventilation/perfusion ($\dot{V}/\dot{Q}$) mismatch

1. **Bronchospasm**
2. **Pulmonary embolism**
3. **Aspiration.** Still possible, even when an ETT is in place.

E. Inadequate ventilation

1. **Ventilator disconnection or malfunction**
2. **Incorrect settings.** Has the patient recently been changed to intermittent mandatory ventilation (IMV), which has resulted in hypoventilation?
3. **Sedatives.** These can result in hypoxemia secondary to hypoventilation. Sedatives should be used cautiously, especially during weaning. Patients on ventilators may develop atelectasis due to failure to sigh or cough when sedated.
4. **Neuromuscular disease.** Hypophosphatemia or aminoglycosides can cause neuromuscular weakness, which can cause hypoxemia secondary to hypoventilation and lack of sighing.

IV. Database

A. Physical examination key points

1. **Endotracheal tube.** Confirm proper ETT position and listen for any leaks.

2. **Vital signs.** Tachypnea implies worsening of the respiratory status. Tachycardia can be associated with a variety of conditions including PE, sepsis, MI, and worsening of underlying pulmonary pathology. Fever can be seen with PE, MI, or an infection.
3. **Neck.** Stridor suggests upper airway obstruction.
4. **Chest.** Check for bilateral breath sounds, signs of consolidation, or new onset of wheezing. Unilateral breath sounds suggest a pneumothorax or possibly displacement of the ETT in one of the mainstem bronchi. Palpate the chest for new subcutaneous emphysema, which can occur in asthmatics or as a result of high PEEP.
5. **Heart.** New murmurs or a new S_3 or S_4 may be seen with an MI. A new systolic murmur may suggest a ventricular septal defect (VSD) or mitral regurgitation secondary to papillary muscle rupture.
6. **Extremities.** Check nailbeds for cyanosis from worsening pulmonary status. Also check legs for unilateral edema or other signs of phlebitis that point to PE.
7. **Skin.** Check for new rashes, which may suggest a drug or anaphylactic reaction.

B. Laboratory data

1. **Repeat ABGs or check oximetry** to assess accuracy of initial ABGs and progression of deterioration.
2. **Sputum appearance and Gram's stain** may direct antibiotic therapy if pneumonia is present.
3. **A Swan-Ganz catheter** will have to be in place to measure mixed venous oxygen saturation (SvO_2). SvO_2 is a direct reflection of oxygen delivery to the tissues and extraction of oxygen. The pulmonary artery catheter can also be used to determine the presence of an intracardiac shunt.

C. Radiologic and other studies

1. **Stat CXR.** To rule out atelectasis and pneumothorax, and to evaluate underlying pulmonary disease.
2. **Electrocardiogram.** An evolving MI may be evident. New right-axis deviation, right bundle branch block, P pulmonale, or an S wave in lead I, a Q wave in lead III, and a T wave in lead III ($S_1Q_3T_3$) suggest PE; however, these characteristic findings are often absent. Sinus tachycardia is the most common electrocardiographic finding with PE.
3. **$\dot{V}/\dot{Q}$ scan.** If clinical suspicion is high for PE.
4. **Swan-Ganz catheter.** To measure pulmonary capillary wedge pressure (PCWP) and to exclude a cardiac shunt as well as to measure cardiac output and maximum O_2 consumption.

V. Plan

A. Suction. Vigorously suction the patient to prove patency of the ETT and dislodge mucous plugs.

B. Treat underlying disorders

1. **Insert chest tube** for pneumothorax.
2. **Reassess choice of antibiotic agents.** A pneumonia secondary to *Legionella* requires erythromycin (1 g IV Q 6 hr) or another macrolide.
3. **Consider more vigorous chest physical therapy** or even bronchoscopy for recalcitrant mucous plugging or atelectasis.
4. **Maximize bronchodilators** if bronchospasm is the problem. Corticosteroids such as hydrocortisone 125 mg or methylprednisolone 60 mg should be added and given IV Q 6 hr. Aerosolized albuterol should be given at least Q 4 hr.
5. **Cardiogenic pulmonary edema** should be vigorously treated with afterload reduction and diuresis.

C. Optimize ventilator settings

1. **Correct any hypoventilation.** This may mean giving up on weaning, and using the "Assist Control" (AC) mode with the patient essentially controlled on a high minute ventilation.
2. **Increase FiO_2 to 100%.** Your first priority is to prevent anoxic brain or cardiac damage. You may then reduce the FiO_2 as other maneuvers further improve the PaO_2.
3. **PEEP will recruit unused, collapsed, or partially collapsed alveoli to overcome pulmonary shunts.** It should be added in 2–4 cm of H_2O increments while cardiac output and blood pressure are monitored.
4. **Oxygen consumption ($\dot{V}O_2$)** can be markedly reduced by administering a neuromuscular blocking agent as a last resort. Remember to provide adequate analgesia and sedation as well. Nerve stimulation studies should be done routinely to monitor the neuromuscular blockade; otherwise, these agents should be used for $<$ 24 hours.

D. Optimize hemodynamics

1. **Consider Swan-Ganz placement** when high levels of PEEP are in use, when shock of unclear cause is present, when a cardiac shunt is suspected, or when volume status is unclear.
2. **Correct volume excess** because it will obviously worsen CHF and ARDS.
3. **Volume depletion** will likewise alter both cardiac output and $\dot{V}/\dot{Q}$ ratios and may adversely affect oxygen delivery. A drop in blood pressure with the addition of PEEP almost always results from volume depletion.
4. **Correct anemia** so as to maximize O_2 delivery. Oxygen delivery to tissue depends on the hemoglobin as well as the cardiac output and SaO_2. If ARDS is present, red blood cell transfusions should either be washed or administered through leukocyte removal filters to prevent an exacerbation of the ARDS secondary to the transfusion.

5. **Correct low cardiac output** to maximize O_2 delivery. Inotropic agents (eg, dobutamine) and agents for afterload reduction (eg, IV nitroglycerin or nitroprusside) can be used.

E. **Prone positioning.** If the primary lung disorder is ARDS or acute lung injury, consider prone positioning of the patient. Up to 70% of patients will have a dramatic response. However, the nursing and respiratory therapy staff need experience in this technique since ETT dislodgement and unusual pressure sores may occur. Patients are left prone for 6–12 hours, flipped back supine for 1–2 hours, and then the cycle is repeated.

3C. HYPERCARBIA

I. **Problem.** The patient's $PaCO_2$ remains > 40 Torr. $PaCO_2$ is a direct reflection of both CO_2 production and alveolar ventilation. $PaCO_2$ increases when ventilation/perfusion ($\dot{V}/\dot{Q}$) mismatch worsens or deadspace increases.

II. **Immediate Questions**

A. **What is the sequence of arterial blood gases? In other words, is this an acute or a slowly developing change?** Rapid deterioration implies an immediate life-threatening process such as a tension pneumothorax or a massive pulmonary embolism.

B. **What is the underlying diagnosis?** Worsening of underlying pulmonary disease (pneumonia, atelectasis, or bronchospasm) can cause hypoventilation. Congestive heart failure (CHF) can cause $\dot{V}/\dot{Q}$ mismatch and CO_2 retention.

III. **Differential Diagnosis**

A. **Inadequate minute ventilation ($\dot{V}_e$)**

1. **Too low a rate, inadequate tidal volume, or both**
2. **Patient tiring during synchronized intermittent mandatory ventilation or weaning**
3. **Endotracheal tube (ETT) leak**
4. **Worsening bronchospasm**
5. **Pulmonary embolism (PE).** Keep in mind that immobilization is a major risk factor.

B. **Increased CO_2 production**

1. **High-carbohydrate feedings**
2. **Increased metabolism.** Causes include hyperthyroidism, fever, sepsis, and high work of breathing as well as rewarming after surgical procedures (a common but frequently overlooked cause of CO_2 production).

C. **Oversedation.** Decreases central ventilatory drive.

IV. **Database**

A. **Physical examination key points**

1. **Endotracheal tube.** Check ETT position and look for a leak.
2. **Vital signs.** Tachycardia can be associated with fever, sepsis, worsening bronchospasm, PE, and hyperthyroidism. Tachypnea can be seen with PE, worsening bronchospasm, or sepsis. Fever suggests infection but can also be seen with hyperthyroidism and PE.
3. **Chest.** Auscultate for new wheezes and look for inequality of breath sounds.
4. **Heart.** Listen for a new loud P_2, which suggests a PE.
5. **Extremities.** Check patient's legs for unilateral edema or other signs of thrombophlebitis.
6. **Musculoskeletal exam.** Check for signs of respiratory fatigue such as abdominal paradox or accessory muscle use.

B. **Laboratory data**

1. **Arterial blood gases.** Repeat ABGs or check oximetry to assess accuracy of initial ABGs and progression of deterioration.
2. **Complete blood count with differential.** An increased white blood count with an increase in banded neutrophils suggests an infection or sepsis.

C. **Radiologic and other studies.** With a CXR, proper ETT position can be ensured and new pulmonary infiltrates can be ruled out.

V. Plan

A. **Check position and functioning of ETT.** If there is a persistent leak, replace the tube.

B. **Verify proper ventilator function.** Check with particular care for leaky connections.

C. **Drugs.** Verify that the ordered sedatives are the drugs that were actually given and note time of last dose. If the patient is oversedated, you can either increase the minute ventilation ($\dot{V}_e$); or reverse sedation with naloxone (Narcan) 0.4 mg IV for narcotics or flumazenil (Romazicon) 1.0 mg IV over 5 minutes for benzodiazepines.

D. **Look for a source of sepsis.** Adjust antibiotics as indicated. Lower $\dot{V}O_2$ by treating fever with acetaminophen (Tylenol) or a cooling blanket.

E. **Review ventilator settings.** If the tidal volume is too low, deadspace ventilation will be present. Correct this condition by increasing the tidal volume. If the patient is tiring on a low synchronized intermittent mandatory ventilation (SIMV) rate, switch to either a higher rate or change to "Assist Control" (AC) mode.

F. **Review the patient's nutrition regimen.** If the patient is critically ill with bronchospasm or ARDS, you may be forced to reduce CO_2 production by decreasing the percentage of carbohydrates in tube feedings or IV hyperalimentation fluid.

3D. HIGH PEAK PRESSURES

I. **Problem.** The ventilator peak pressures remain consistently above 50 cm H_2O.

II. **Immediate Questions**

A. **Is this a new problem or has it developed progressively?** The answer to this question will be readily available on the respiratory therapy bedside flow sheet.

B. **What is the underlying diagnosis?** Severe status asthmaticus or acute respiratory distress syndrome (ARDS) can cause high ventilatory peak pressures.

C. **What are the most recent ABGs?** A decrease in the pO_2 or an increase in the pCO_2 may point to a worsening of the underlying pulmonary disease.

D. **Has endotracheal tube (ETT) function or position changed? Is it possible to suction the patient?** The tube could be kinked or plugged by secretions.

III. **Differential Diagnosis**

A. ETT
1. **Too small or obstructed** by secretions.
2. **Kinked,** especially if placed nasotracheally.
3. **Migration** down the right mainstem so that the entire tidal volume flows into one lung. This condition also increases coughing and anxiety.

B. **Incorrect ventilator settings**
1. **High tidal volume.** Tidal volumes > 10 mL/kg may increase distension pressure tremendously.
2. **High positive end-expiratory pressure.** PEEP should always be used at the lowest possible level.
3. **High minute ventilation.** A high minute ventilation may lead to the phenomenon of "auto-PEEP," in which the patient has inadequate time to exhale, leading to "stacked breaths." Auto-PEEP may cause hypotension because of high intrathoracic pressure decreasing venous return.

C. **Worsening lung disease.** Lung compliance decreases in all of the following:
1. **Severe status asthmaticus**
2. **Acute respiratory distress syndrome (ARDS)**
3. **Cardiogenic pulmonary edema**
4. **Interstitial lung disease**

D. **Uncooperative or agitated patient**
1. **Biting the ETT**
2. **Fighting the ventilator**

3. **Coughing**

E. **Abdominal distension.** The recently described abdominal compartment syndrome can lead to both inability to ventilate and hypotension. It is diagnosed by measuring intravesicular (bladder) pressure, and may result from severe ascites or intra-abdominal hemorrhage causing increased abdominal cavity pressure.

F. **Tension pneumothorax.** It is always imperative to exclude this as a cause of new onset of high peak pressures because death can occur quickly.

IV. Database

A. Physical examination key points

1. **ETT.** Check position to rule out migration down the right mainstem bronchus; check patency of the ETT.
2. **Vital signs.** Tachycardia and tachypnea can occur with worsening of the underlying pulmonary disease and with agitation. Hypotension and tachycardia are seen with tension pneumothorax, severe auto-PEEP, and the abdominal compartment syndrome.
3. **HEENT.** An increase in jugular venous distension (JVD) implies congestive heart failure (CHF). Tracheal deviation can be seen with tension pneumothorax.
4. **Chest.** Absent breath sounds, especially with hypotension, and unilateral hyperresonance to percussion point to tension pneumothorax. Rales suggest CHF.
5. **Heart.** An S_3 over the apex implies left ventricular dysfunction/CHF.
6. **Abdomen.** Examine for tenderness and distension.
7. **Extremities.** New cyanosis is consistent with worsening of underlying pulmonary disease. Edema will be seen with biventricular or right-sided heart failure.
8. **Skin.** Check for subcutaneous emphysema, which can be associated with barotrauma or with severe asthma.

B. Laboratory data

1. **Arterial blood gases.** Repeat ABGs or check oximetry to assess accuracy of initial ABGs and progression of deterioration.
2. **Complete blood count with differential.** An increased white blood count with an increase in banded neutrophils suggests an infection or sepsis.

C. Radiologic and other studies.
Use a stat portable CXR to check ETT position, rule out kinking, rule out pneumothorax, and assess any change in underlying pulmonary disease.

D. Ventilator.
Ask the respiratory therapist to measure "auto-PEEP" or check for it via the waveforms. **View the peak airway pressure pattern.** A rapid rise and fall suggests a kinked or obstructed ETT. Check the patient's mouth to be sure the patient is not biting the

tube. Suction the ETT to make sure it is not occluded and leading to artificially high pressures.

V. **Plan**

A. **Try to suction the patient.** If the patient is biting down, insert an oral airway or sedate the patient. If the patient is not biting down on the ETT but the suction tube will not go down the ETT, the ETT is kinked or blocked, possibly by a mucus plug, and must be replaced.

B. **Ambu bag the patient and confirm equal breath sounds.** Unequal breath sounds may result from a tension pneumothorax or from improper positioning of the ETT. Reposition the ETT if necessary. On an average-sized person, an oral ETT should not be in farther than 24 cm at the lip; however, there is considerable variability among patients, and the CXR should always be reviewed. If there is considerable resistance to bagging, a tension pneumothorax, auto-PEEP, or a mucus plug may be present.

C. **Place a chest tube** if a pneumothorax is present.

D. **Adjust the ventilator.** Try to reduce the PEEP to the minimum needed for adequate oxygenation. Try reducing high tidal volumes to 5 mL/kg body weight. Increase FiO_2 as needed to ensure adequate oxygenation.

E. **Sedation may have to be increased.**

F. **Consider switching to Airway Pressure Release Ventilation (APRV) or Pressure Control modes.** These modes exquisitely control high peak pressures while often improving oxygenation as well.

4. WEANING

I. **Requirements.** Once the underlying cause of respiratory failure has been corrected, it is time for the most arduous task of all: weaning the patient from the respirator.

A. **Stabilization.** The underlying disease is under optimum control.

B. **Initiation of weaning.** The process is begun in the early morning. Patients prefer to rest at night rather than work at breathing. Desirable conditions are:

1. **PaO_2 > 60 Torr on no PEEP; and $FiO_2 \leq 0.5$**
2. **Minute ventilation < 10 L/min**
3. **Negative inspiratory force more negative than –20 cm H_2O**
4. **Vital capacity > 800 mL**
5. **Tidal volume > 300 mL**
6. **Rapid shallow breathing index < 90 (60-second breath rate/tidal volume in liters).** This is the most predictive indicator of success.

II. **Weaning Techniques**

A. **T-piece (or T-tube bypass).** The patient is taken off the respirator for a limited period of time, and the endotracheal tube (ETT) is connected to a constant flow of O_2 (usually 40%). If the patient tolerates breathing independently for 2 hours, he or she is extubated immediately. In research studies, this technique has been the most rapid.

This technique, however, has important drawbacks. No alarms are available because the patient is totally disconnected from the ventilator. The technique is time-consuming for the respiratory therapists and nurses. Perhaps most important, it is much more work for the patient than breathing spontaneously without an ETT. This is due to the relatively small diameter of the tube. (Remember that resistance increases by the fourth power of the radius of a tube.) T-tube trials are thus usually limited to 2-hour trials or less.

B. Synchronized intermittent mandatory ventilation (SIMV). In this method, fewer and fewer machine breaths are given as the patient begins taking spontaneous breaths in the intervals. For example, a patient breathing at a rate of 14 in "Assist Control" (AC) mode is switched to SIMV mode, rate 14. The rate is then decreased to 10, to 6, to 4, and then to 0. Most physicians either place the patient on continuous positive airway pressure mode at this juncture or observe the patient briefly on a T-piece.

This method has several theoretical advantages over T-piece weaning. Backup alarms, including automatic rates in case of apnea, are in place. A graded assumption of work is done, allowing respiratory muscle "retraining"; however, this method has never been proven clearly superior to T-piece weaning. Moreover, there is still a high work of breathing because of the ETT resistance as well as the inherent resistance of the SIMV circuit valves.

One way to decrease the work of breathing with the SIMV weaning technique is to add pressure support (PS) to the system. *Pressure support* is a positive pressure boost that is initiated when a certain liter flow rate during inspiration is sensed by the respirator. It then supplies a set amount of positive pressure (and by Boyle's law, it also supplies some tidal volume). A PS level of 8–12 cm will overcome the increased work caused by the ETT resistance.

C. Continuous positive airway pressure and pressure support (PS). In this method, the patient is switched to the spontaneous breathing mode, which in some ventilators is the CPAP mode. In current usage, CPAP is equivalent to PEEP, except that it is used exclusively in spontaneously breathing mode. Anywhere from 0 to 30 cm pressure may be used, but generally the lowest level possible (usually 0–5 cm) is preferred. Pressure support may be used concomitantly to augment the patient's spontaneous breaths. It can then be progressively decreased as the patient increases tidal volumes. For example, PS levels of 25, then 20, then 15, and finally 10 can be used while monitoring the patient's breath rate, tidal volumes, and ABGs.

This method requires an alert, cooperative patient who is breathing spontaneously; if those conditions do not pertain, why wean anyway?

Machine backup functions remain in place in case of apnea or other inadequate parameters.

D. Extubation to BIPAP. Patients with advanced lung disease may never reach standard weaning criteria. Extubation to partial ventilatory support is often successful. It decreases risk of ventilator-associated pneumonia and saves the patient from having a tracheostomy tube.

III. Timing. Deciding when to extubate the patient is part of the art of medicine. Still, the fulfillment of certain criteria ensures success. The following weaning parameters (as discussed earlier) are acceptable:

A. Respiratory rate is < 30/min.

B. ABGs show a pH > 7.35 and adequate oxygenation on ≤ 50 FiO_2.

C. The patient is awake and alert.

D. A normal gag reflex is present.

E. The stomach is not distended.

IV. Postextubation care. After extubation, it is important to encourage the patient to cough frequently and forcefully. Respiratory therapy treatments should be continued. Incentive spirometry should be used several times an hour while the patient is awake to encourage deep breathing. The patient must be carefully observed for stridor, respiratory muscle fatigue, or other signs of failure. Oxygen should be given at the same level or at a level slightly higher than was given via the respirator prior to intubation. The ABGs should be checked 2–4 hours after extubation to confirm adequate ventilation and oxygenation.

REFERENCES

Albert RK: Prone ventilation (ARDS). Clin Chest Med 2000;21:511.

Glauser FL, Polatty C, Sessler CN: Worsening oxygenation in the mechanically ventilated patient: Causes, mechanisms and early detection. Am Rev Respir Dis 1988;138:458.

Luce JM et al: Intermittent mandatory ventilation. Chest 1981;79:678.

MacIntyre NR: Weaning from mechanical ventilatory support: Volume-assisting intermittent breaths versus pressure-assisting every breath. Respir Care 1988;33:121.

Marcy TW, Marini JJ: Respiratory distress in the ventilated patient. Clin Chest Med 1994;15:55.

Raoof S, Khan FA: *Mechanical Ventilation Manual.* American College of Physicians Press;1998.

Slutsky AS: ACCP consensus conference—Mechanical ventilation. Chest 1993;104:1833.

Tobin MJ: Mechanical ventilation. N Engl J Med 1994;330:1056.

VII. THERAPEUTICS

1. Classes of Generic Drugs, Minerals, Natural Products, & Vitamins
2. Generic Drugs: Indications, Actions, Dosage, Supplied, & Notes
3. Minerals: Indications/Effects, RDA/Dosage, Signs/Symptoms of Deficiency and Toxicity, and Other
4. Natural Products: Uses, Dose, Cautions, Adverse Effects, and Drug Interactions
5. Vitamins: Indications/Effects, RDA/Dosage, Signs/Symptoms of Deficiency and Toxicity, and Other
6. Tables
    1. Insulins
    2. Comparison of Glucocorticoids
    3. Angiotensin-Converting Enzyme Inhibitors
    4. Angiotensin Receptor Antagonists
    5. Antistaphylococcal Penicillins
    6. Extended-Spectrum Penicillins
    7. Beta-Adrenergic Blocking Agents
    8. First-Generation Cephalosporins
    9. Second-Generation Cephalosporins
    10. Third- and Fourth-Generation Cephalosporins
    11. Nonsteroidal Anti-Inflammatory Drugs
    12. Ophthalmic Agents
    13. Sulfonylurea Agents
    14. Proton Pump Inhibitors
    15. HMG-CoA Reductase Inhibitors
    16. Non-Antibiotic Drug Levels
    17. Therapeutic Drug Levels: Antibiotics
    18. Aminoglycoside Dosing in Adults: Every 8- or 12-Hour Dosing
    19. Aminoglycoside Dosing: Percentage of Loading Dose Required for Dosage Interval Selected
    20. Aminoglycoside Dosing: Once-Daily Dosing of Gentamicin and Tobramycin (*Not* Amikacin)

The Therapeutics Section is designed to serve as a quick reference to commonly used medications. You should be familiar with all of the indications, contraindications, side effects, and drug interactions of any medications that you prescribe. Such detailed information is beyond the scope of this manual and can be found in the package insert, *Physicians' Desk Reference* (*PDR*), or the American Hospital Formulary Service (AHFS).

Drugs in this section are listed in alphabetical order by generic names. Some of the more common trade names are listed for each medication.

Drugs under the control of the Drug Enforcement Agency (Schedule II-V controlled substances) are indicated by the symbol [C].

1. CLASSES OF GENERIC DRUGS, MINERALS, NATURAL PRODUCTS, & VITAMINS

Analgesic/Anti-Inflammatory/Antipyretic Agents

Acetaminophen
Acetaminophen with butalbital and caffeine
Acetaminophen with codeine
Aspirin
Aspirin with butalbital and caffeine
Aspirin with butalbital, caffeine, and codeine
Aspirin with codeine
Buprenorphine
Butorphanol
Capsaicin
Celecoxib
Cocaine
Codeine
Dezocine
Diclofenac sodium
Diflunisal
Etodolac
Fenoprofen
Fentanyl
Fentanyl transdermal system
Fentanyl, transmucosal
Flurbiprofen
Hydrocodone and acetaminophen
Hydrocodone and aspirin
Hydrocodone and ibuprofen
Hydromorphone
Ibuprofen
Indomethacin
Ketoprofen
Ketorolac
Meloxicam
Meperidine
Methadone
Morphine sulfate
Nabumetone
Nalbuphine
Naproxen
Oxaprozin
Oxycodone
Oxycodone and acetaminophen
Oxycodone and aspirin
Oxymorphone
Pentazocine
Piroxicam
Propoxyphene
Rofecoxib
Sulindac
Tolmetin
Tramadol

Antacids/Antigas

Aluminum carbonate
Aluminum hydroxide
Aluminum hydroxide with magnesium carbonate
Aluminum hydroxide with magnesium hydroxide
Aluminum hydroxide with magnesium hydroxide and simethicone
Aluminum hydroxide with magnesium trisilicate
Calcium carbonate
Dihydroxyaluminum sodium carbonate
Magaldrate
Simethicone

Antianxiety Agents

Alprazolam
Amoxapine
Buspirone
Chlordiazepoxide
Clorazepate
Diazepam
Doxepin
Hydroxyzine
Lorazepam
Meprobamate
Oxazepam
Zaleplon

Antiarrhythmics

Adenosine
Amiodarone
Digoxin
Diltiazem
Disopyramide
Dofetilide
Esmolol
Flecainide
Ibutilide
Lidocaine
Mexiletine
Procainamide
Propafenone
Quinidine
Sotalol
Tocainide
Verapamil

Antibiotics

Amikacin
Amoxicillin
Amoxicillin/potassium clavulanate
Ampicillin
Ampicillin/sulbactam
Atovaquone
Azithromycin
Aztreonam
Cefaclor
Cefadroxil
Cefamandole
Cefazolin
Cefdinir
Cefepime
Cefixime
Cefmetazole
Cefonicid
Cefoperazone
Cefotaxime
Cefotetan
Cefoxitin
Cefpodoxime
Cefprozil

Ceftazidime
Ceftibuten
Ceftizoxime
Ceftriaxone
Cefuroxime
Cephalexin
Cephapirin
Cephradine
Chloramphenicol
Ciprofloxacin
Clarithromycin
Clindamycin
Clofazimine
Cloxacillin
Cortisporin, otic
Dalfopristin/quinupristin
Dapsone
Demeclocycline
Dicloxacillin
Dirithromycin
Doxycycline
Erythromycin
Ethambutol
Fosfomycin
Gatifloxacin
Gentamicin
Imipenem/cilastatin
Isoniazid
Levofloxacin
Linezolid
Lomefloxacin
Loracarbef
Meropenem
Metronidazole
Mezlocillin
Moxifloxacin
Mupirocin
Nafcillin
Nalidixic acid
Neomycin sulfate
Nitrofurantoin
Norfloxacin
Ofloxacin
Oxacillin
Penicillin G aqueous
Penicillin G benzathine
Penicillin G procaine
Penicillin V
Pentamidine
Piperacillin
Piperacillin/tazobactam
Pyrazinamide
Quinupristin/dalfopristin
Rifabutin
Rifampin
Rifapentine
Silver sulfadiazine
Sparfloxacin
Streptomycin
Tetracycline
Ticarcillin
Ticarcillin/potassium clavulanate
Tobramycin
Trimethoprim
Trimethoprim/ sulfamethoxazole
Trimetrexate
Trovafloxacin
Vancomycin

Anticoagulant/Thrombolytic and Related Agents

Abciximab
Alteplase, recombinant (TPA)
Aminocaproic acid
Anistreplase
Antihemophilic Factor VIII
Aprotinin
Ardeparin
Argatroban
Bivalirudin
Cilostazol
Clopidogrel
Dalteparin
Danaparoid
Desmopressin (DDAVP)
Dipyridamole
Dipyridamole and aspirin
Enoxaparin
Heparin
Lepirudin
Pentoxifylline
Protamine sulfate
Reteplase
Streptokinase
Tenecteplase
Ticlopidine
Tinzaparin
Tirofiban
Urokinase
Warfarin

Anticonvulsants

Carbamazepine
Clonazepam
Diazepam
Ethosuximide
Fosphenytoin
Gabapentin
Lamotrigine
Levetiracetam
Lorazepam
Oxcarbazepine
Pentobarbital
Phenobarbital
Phenytoin
Tiagabine
Topiramate
Valproic acid
Zonisamide

Antidepressants

Amitriptyline
Amoxapine
Bupropion
Citalopram
Desipramine
Doxepin
Fluoxetine
Imipramine
Lithium carbonate
Maprotiline
Mirtazapine
Nefazodone
Nortriptyline
Paroxetine
Phenelzine
Sertraline
Trazodone
Venlafaxine

Antidiabetic Agents

Acarbose
Acetohexamide
Becaplermin
Chlorpropamide
Glimepiride
Glipizide

Glyburide
Glyburide micronized
Insulin
Metformin
Miglitol
Pioglitazone
Repaglinide
Rosiglitazone
Tolazamide
Tolbutamide

Antidiarrheal Agents

Bismuth subsalicylate
Diphenoxylate with atropine
Kaolin/Pectin
Lactobacillus
Loperamide
Octreotide

Antidotes

Acetylcysteine
Charcoal
Dexrazoxane
Digoxin immune Fab
Flumazenil
Fomepizole
Ipecac syrup
Mesna
Naloxone
Sodium polystyrene sulfonate
Succimer

Antiemetics

Buclizine
Chlorpromazine
Dimenhydrinate
Dolasetron
Dronabinol
Droperidol
Granisetron
Meclizine
Metoclopramide
Ondansetron
Prochlorperazine
Promethazine
Scopolamine
Thiethylperazine
Trimethobenzamide

Antifungal Agents

Amphotericin B
Amphotericin B cholesteryl
Amphotericin B lipid complex
Amphotericin B liposomal
Ciclopirox
Clotrimazole
Econazole
Fluconazole
Flucytosine
Itraconazole
Ketoconazole
Miconazole
Naftifine
Nystatin
Nystatin and triamcinolone
Oxiconazole
Terbinafine
Terconazole
Tioconazole
Triamcinolone and nystatin
Tolnaftate

Antigout Agents

Allopurinol
Colchicine
Probenecid
Sulfinpyrazone

Antihistamines

Azelastine
Cetirizine
Chlorpheniramine
Clemastine fumarate
Cyproheptadine
Diphenhydramine
Fexofenadine
Hydroxyzine
Loratadine
Terfenadine

Antihyperlipidemics

Atorvastatin
Cholestyramine
Colesevelam
Colestipol
Fenofibrate
Fluvastatin
Gemfibrozil
Lovastatin
Niacin
Pravastatin
Simvastatin

Antihypertensives

Acebutolol
Amlodipine
Atenolol
Benazepril
Betaxolol
Bisoprolol
Candesartan
Captopril
Carteolol
Carvedilol
Clonidine
Diltiazem
Doxazosin
Enalapril
Eprosartan
Felodipine
Fenoldopam
Fosinopril

Guanabenz
Guanadrel
Guanethidine
Guanfacine
Hydralazine
Irbesartan
Isradipine
Labetalol
Lisinopril
Losartan
Methyldopa
Metoprolol
Minoxidil
Moexipril
Nadolol
Nicardipine
Nifedipine
Nisoldipine
Nitroglycerin
Nitroprusside
Penbutolol
Perindopril
Pindolol
Prazosin
Propranolol
Quinapril
Ramipril
Telmisartan
Terazosin
Timolol
Trandolapril
Valsartan
Verapamil

Antineoplastic Agents and Related Medications

Aldesleukin (IL-2)
Altretamine
Amifostine
Aminoglutethimide
Anastrozole
Asparaginase
Bacillus Calmette-Guérin
Bexarotene
Bicalutamide
Bleomycin
Busulfan
Capecitabine
Carboplatin
Carmustine
Chlorambucil
Cisplatin
Cladribine
Cyclophosphamide
Cytarabine
Cytarabine liposome
Dacarbazine
Dactinomycin
Daunorubicin
Diethylstilbestrol
Docetaxel
Doxorubicin
Epirubicin
Estramustine
Etoposide
Exemestane
Floxuridine
Fludarabine phosphate
Fluorouracil
Fluorouracil, topical
Fluoxymesterone
Flutamide
Gemcitabine
Gemtuzumab ozagamicin
Goserelin
Hydroxyurea
Idarubicin
Ifosfamide
Irinotecan
Letrozole
Leuprolide
Levamisole
Lomustine
Mechlorethamine
Megestrol acetate
Melphalan
Mercaptopurine
Methotrexate
Mitomycin
Mitotane
Mitoxantrone
Nilutamide
Paclitaxel
Plicamycin
Procarbazine
Streptozocin
Tamoxifen citrate
Teniposide
6-Thioguanine
Thiotepa (See Triethylene-triphosphamide)
Topotecan
Trastuzumab
Triethylene-triphosphamide
Valrubicin
Vinblastine
Vincristine
Vinorelbine

Antiparkinsonism Agents

Amantadine
Benztropine
Bromocriptine
Carbidopa/levodopa
Entacapone
Pergolide
Pramipexole
Selegiline
Trihexyphenidyl

Antipsychotic Agents

Chlorpromazine
Clozapine
Fluphenazine
Haloperidol
Lithium carbonate
Mesoridazine
Molindone
Olanzapine
Perphenazine
Prochlorperazine
Quetiapine
Risperidone
Thioridazine
Thiothixine
Trifluoperazine

Antitussive, Decongestant, Expectorant, and Mucolytic Agents

Acetylcysteine
Benzonatate
Codeine
Dextromethorphan
Guaifenesin
Guaifenesin and codeine
Guaifenesin and dextromethorphan
Hydrocodone and guaifenesin
Hydrocodone and homatropine

Hydrocodone and pseudoephedrine
Hydrocodone, chlorpheniramine, phenylephrine, acetaminophen and caffeine
Phenylephrine
Pseudoephedrine

Antiviral Agents

Abacavir
Acyclovir
Amantadine
Amprenavir
Cidofovir
Delavirdine
Didanosine
Efavirenz
Famciclovir
Fomivirsen
Foscarnet
Ganciclovir
Imiquimod cream
Indinavir
Lamivudine
Lamivudine and zidovudine
Lopinavir and ritonavir
Nelfinavir
Nevirapine
Oseltamivir
Penciclovir
Ribavirin
Rimantadine
Ritonavir
Ritonavir and lopinavir
Saquinavir
Stavudine
Trifluridine
Valacyclovir
Zalcitabine
Zanamivir
Zidovudine
Zidovudine and lamivudine

Bronchodilators (Also see Respiratory and Nasal Inhalants)

Albuterol
Albuterol and ipratropium
Aminophylline
Bitolterol
Levalbuterol
Metaproterenol
Pirbuterol
Salmeterol
Terbutaline
Theophylline

Cardiovascular Agents

Acebutolol
Atenolol
Atropine
Bepridil
Candesartan
Cilostazol
Clopidogrel
Digoxin
Diltiazem
Dobutamine
Dopamine
Epoprostenol
Eprosartan
Eptifibatide
Ephedrine
Epinephrine
Esmolol
Hydralazine
Inamrinone
Irbesartan
Isoproterenol
Isosorbide dinitrate
Isosorbide mononitrate
Labetalol
Losartan
Metoprolol
Milrinone
Nadolol
Nicardipine
Nifedipine
Nimodipine
Nitroglycerin
Nitroprusside
Norepinephrine
Perindopril
Pindolol
Propranolol
Sodium polystyrene sulfonate
Telmisartan
Timolol
Tolazoline
Trandolapril
Valsartan
Verapamil

Cathartics/Laxatives

Bisacodyl
Docusate calcium
Docusate potassium
Docusate sodium
Glycerin suppositories
Lactulose
Magnesium citrate
Magnesium hydroxide
Mineral oil
Polyethylene glycol-electrolyte solution
Psyllium
Sorbitol

Dermatologic Agents

Acitretin
Anthralin
Bacitracin
Bacitracin and polymyxin B
Bacitracin, neomycin, and polymyxin B
Bacitracin, neomycin, polymyxin B, and hydrocortisone
Bacitracin, neomycin, polymyxin B, and lidocaine
Bexarotene
Calcipotriene
Clotrimazole
Clotrimazole and betamethasone
Dibucaine
Doxepin

Isotretinoin
Lactic acid and ammonium hydroxide
Neomycin and polymyxin B
Neomycin, bacitracin, and polymyxin B
Selenium sulfide
Silver nitrate
Triamcinolone and nystatin
Tazarotene
Tretinoin

Diuretics

Acetazolamide
Amiloride
Bumetanide
Chlorothiazide
Chlorthalidone
Ethacrynic acid
Furosemide
Hydrochlorothiazide
Hydrochlorothiazide and amiloride
Hydrochlorothiazide and spironolactone
Hydrochlorothiazide and triamterene
Indapamide
Mannitol
Metolazone
Spironolactone
Torsemide
Triamterene

Estrogens

Esterified estrogens
Esterified estrogens with methyltestosterone
Estradiol topical
Estradiol transdermal
Estrogen, conjugated
Estrogen, conjugated with methylprogesterone
Estrogen, conjugated methyltestosterone
Ethinyl estradiol
Norethindrone
Norgestrel
Oral contraceptives
Raloxifene

Gastrointestinal Agents

Balsalazide
Cimetidine
Dexpanthenol
Dicyclomine
Esomeprazole
Famotidine
Hyoscyamine
Hyoscyamine, atropine, scopolamine, and phenobarbital
Infliximab
Lactulose
Lansoprazole
Loperamide
Mesalamine enema
Metoclopramide
Misoprostol
Neomycin sulfate
Nizatidine
Octreotide
Olsalazine
Omeprazole
Pancreatin/pancrelipase
Pantoprazole
Paregoric
Propantheline
Rabeprazole
Sodium phosphate
Ranitidine
Sulfasalazine
Sucralfate
Vasopressin

Hormones/Synthetic Substitutes (Also see Estrogens and Thyroid/Antithyroid)

Aminoglutethimide
Betamethasone
Calcitonin
Cortisone
Desmopressin
Dexamethasone
Epoetin alfa (Erythropoietin)
Filgrastim (G-CSF)
Fludrocortisone acetate
Glucagon
Hydrocortisone
Insulin
Interferon alfa
Interferon alfa-2B
Interferon alfacon-1
Interferon beta-1b
Interferon gamma-1b
Levonorgestrel Implants
Medroxyprogesterone
Methylprednisolone
Metyrapone
Nicotine gum
Nicotine nasal spray
Nicotine, transdermal
Oxytocin
Pancreatin/pancrelipase
Prednisolone
Prednisone
Sargramostim (GM-CSF)
Steroids
Vasopressin

Immunosuppressive Agents

Antithymocyte globulin (ATG)
Azathioprine
Basiliximab
Cyclosporine
Daclizumab
Etanercept
Leflunomide
Methotrexate
Muromonab-CD3 (OKT-3)
Mycophenolate mofetil
Sirolimus
Tacrolimus (FK-506)
Thalidomide

Local Anesthetic Agents

Anusol
Bupivacaine
Dibucaine
Lidocaine
Lidocaine and prilocaine
Pramoxine and hydrocortisone

Muscle Relaxants

Atracurium
Baclofen
Diazepam
Metaxalone
Methocarbamol
Carisoprodol
Chlorzoxazone
Orphenadrine
Pancuronium
Rocuronium
Cyclobenzaprine
Dantrolene
Succinylcholine
Vecuronium

Ophthalmic Agents

Apraclonidine
Artificial tears
Betaxolol
Brimonidine
Brinzolamide
Carbachol
Chloramphenicol
Ciprofloxacin
Cortisporin
Demecarium
Dexamethasone
Dipivefrin
Dorzolamide
Dorzolamide and timolol
Echothiophate iodide
Erythromycin
Gentamicin
Gentamicin and prednisolone
Ketotifen
Latanoprost
Levobetaxolol
Levobunolol
Lodoxamide
Metipranolol
Naphazoline and antazoline
Naphazoline and pheniramine acetate
Neomycin
Neomycin and dexamethasone
Pemirolast
Pilocarpine
Prednisolone
Rimexolone
Sulfacetamide
Sulfacetamide and prednisolone
Timolol
Tobramycin
Tobramycin and dexamethasone

Otic Agents

Benzocaine and antipyrine
Ciprofloxacin
Cortisporin
Neomycin, colistin, and hydrocortisone
Neomycin, colistin, hydrocortisone, and thonzonium
Neomycin, polymyxin, and hydrocortisone
Polymyxin B and hydrocortisone
Ofloxacin
Triethanolamine

Plasma Volume Expanders

Albumin
Dextran 40
Hetastarch
Plasma protein fraction

Respiratory and Nasal Inhalants (Also see Bronchodilators)

Beclomethasone
Budesonide
Cromolyn sodium
Dexamethasone
Dornase alfa
Flunisolide
Fluticasone
Ipratropium
Montelukast
Nedocromil
Potassium iodide (see SSKI)
SSKI (see potassium iodide)
Triamcinolone
Zafirlukast
Zileuton

Sedatives/Hypnotics

Diphenhydramine
Estazolam
Flurazepam
Hydroxyzine
Midazolam
Quazepam
Secobarbital
Temazepam
Triazolam
Zolpidem

Supplements (Also see Minerals, Natural Products, and Vitamins)

Calcitrol
Calcium acetate
Calcium salts
Cholecalciferol
Cyanocobalamin (B_{12})
Ferric gluconate

Ferric gluconate complex
Ferrous sulfate
Folic acid
Iron dextran
Iron sucrose
Leucovorin
Magnesium oxide
Magnesium sulfate
Oprelvekin
Oral contraceptives
Phytonadione (vitamin K)
Potassium supplements
Pyridoxine (B_6)
Sodium bicarbonate
Thiamine (B_1)
Vitamin B_1 (thiamine)
Vitamin B_6 (pyridoxine)
Vitamin B_{12} (cyanocobalamin)
Vitamin K (phytonadione)

Thyroid/Antithyroid

Levothyroxine
Liothyronine
Methimazole
Potassium iodide (see SSKI)
Propylthiouracil
SSKI (see Potassium iodide)

Toxoids/Vaccines/Serums

Bacillus Calmette-Guérin
Cytomegalovirus immune globulin
Haemophilus B conjugate vaccine
Hepatitis A vaccine
Hepatitis B immune globulin
Hepatitis B vaccine
Immune globulin, intravenous
Influenza vaccine
Lyme disease vaccine
Pneumococcal vaccine, polyvalent
Tetanus immune globulin
Tetanus toxoid
Varicella vaccine

Urinary (and Genitourinary) Tract Agents

Alprostadil
Amino-cerv pH 5.5 cream
Ammonium aluminum sulfate
Belladonna and opium suppositories
Bethanechol
Dimethyl sulfoxide
Finasteride
Flavoxate
Hyoscyamine
Hyoscyamine, atropine, scopolamine, and phenobarbital
Mesna
Methenamine
Oxybutynin
Pentosan polysulfate sodium
Phenazopyridine
Sildenafil
Sodium citrate
Tamsulosin
Terazosin
Tolterodine

Miscellaneous

Alendronate
α-protease inhibitor
Cevimeline HCl
Demeclocycline
Diazoxide
Disulfiram
Edrophonium
Etidronate
Gallium nitrate
Lindane (γ benzene hexachloride)
Methylergonovine
Modafinil
Naltrexone
Naratriptan
Orlistat
Pamidronate
Permethrin
Physostigmine
Propofol
Risedronate
Rivastigmine
Rizatriptan
Sevelamer
Sibutramine
Silver nitrate
Sumatriptan
Tacrine
Zolmitriptan

Minerals (Also see under specific generic drugs)

Calcium
Chromium
Copper
Iron
Magnesium
Selenium
Zinc

Natural Products

Black cohosh
Chamomile
Dong quai
Echinacea
Ephedra/Ma huang
Feverfew

Garlic
Ginger
Ginkgo biloba
Ginseng
Glucosamine/Chondroitin sulfate
Kava kava
Melatonin
Saw palmetto
St. John's wort
Valerian
Yohimbine

Unsafe Herbs

Aconite
Calamus
Chaparral
"Chinese Herbal Mixtures"
Coltsfoot
Comfrey
Juniper
Licorice
Life Root
Ma-Huang/Ephedra
Pokeweed
Sassafras
Yohimbine

Vitamins (Also see under specific generic drugs)

Vitamin A
Folate
Thiamine
Vitamin B_6
Vitamin B_{12}
Vitamin C
Vitamin D
Vitamin E
Vitamin K

2. GENERIC DRUGS: INDICATIONS, ACTIONS, DOSAGE, SUPPLIED, & NOTES

Abacavir (Ziagen)

INDICATIONS: Treatment of HIV infection.
ACTIONS: Nucleoside reverse transcriptase inhibitor.
DOSAGE: 300 mg bid.
SUPPLIED: Tablets 300 mg; solution 20 mg/mL.
NOTES: May cause fatal hypersensitivity reactions, may manifest as respiratory symptoms. Discontinue immediately with symptoms of hypersensitivity (fever, skin rash, fatigue, nausea, vomiting, diarrhea, or abdominal pain); may cause lactic acidosis and hepatomegaly with steatosis.

Abciximab (Reopro)

INDICATIONS: Prevention of acute ischemic complications in patients undergoing percutaneous transluminal coronary angioplasty (PTCA).
ACTIONS: Inhibits platelet aggregation (GPII b/IIIa inhibitor).
DOSAGE: 0.25 mg/kg bolus administered 10–60 min prior to PTCA, then 0.125 μg/kg/min (to a maximum of 10 μg/min) continuous infusion for 12 hr.
SUPPLIED: Injection 2 mg/mL.
NOTES: Used concomitantly with heparin; may cause allergic reactions.

Acarbose (Precose)

INDICATIONS: Treatment of Type 2 diabetes mellitus.
ACTIONS: Alpha-glucosidase inhibitor; delays digestion of ingested carbohydrates, resulting in lower plasma glucose levels.
DOSAGE: 25–100 mg PO tid at the start of each meal.
SUPPLIED: Tablets 25 mg, 50 mg, 100 mg.
NOTES: May be taken concomitantly with sulfonylureas. Patients should swallow their dose with the first bite of each main meal. Adverse effects include abdominal pain, flatulence, and diarrhea. Avoid use in patients with inflammatory bowel disease, colonic ulceration, partial intestinal obstruction, or other chronic intestinal disease.

Acebutolol (Sectral) [See Table 7–7, pp 601-2]

Acitretin (Soriatane)

INDICATIONS: Severe psoriasis and other keratinization disorders (Lichen planus, etc).
ACTIONS: Retinoid-like activity.
DOSAGE: 25–50 mg PO q day, with main meal; can titrate upward if no response by 4 weeks to 75 mg/d.

SUPPLIED: Capsules 10 mg, 25 mg.
NOTES: Teratogenic, contraindicated in pregnancy; must be used with caution if at all in women of reproductive potential; check liver function tests since the drug can be hepatotoxic; response often takes 2–3 months.

Acetaminophen (Tylenol, Others)

INDICATIONS: Treatment of mild pain, headache, and fever.
ACTIONS: Non-narcotic analgesic; inhibits the synthesis of prostaglandins in the CNS and inhibits the hypothalamic heat-regulating center.
DOSAGE: 650 mg PO or PR Q 4–6 hr or 1000 mg PO Q 6 hr; do not exceed 4 g/24 hr.
SUPPLIED: Tablets 160 mg, 325 mg, 500 mg, 650 mg; liquid 100 mg/mL, 120 mg/2.5 mL, 120 mg/5 mL, 160 mg/5 mL, 167 mg/5 mL, 325 mg/5 mL, 500 mg/5 mL; suppositories 80, 120, 125, 300, 325, 650 mg.
NOTES: Decrease daily dose with alcohol use; overdose causes hepatotoxicity, which is treated with *N*-acetylcysteine; charcoal is not usually recommended; has no anti-inflammatory or platelet-inhibiting action.

Acetaminophen with Butalbital and Caffeine (Fioricet, Esgic, Others) [C]

INDICATIONS: Mild pain; headache, especially associated with stress.
ACTIONS: Non-narcotic analgesic with barbiturate.
DOSAGE: 1–2 tablets or capsules PO Q 4–6 hr prn.
SUPPLIED: Each tablet or capsule contains 325 mg acetaminophen, 40 mg caffeine, and 50 mg butalbital.
NOTES: Butalbital is habit-forming.

Acetaminophen with Codeine (Tylenol No. 1, No. 2, No. 3, No. 4) [C]

INDICATIONS: No. 1, No. 2, and No. 3 for relief of mild to moderate pain; No. 4 for relief of moderate to severe pain.
ACTIONS: Combined effects of acetaminophen and a narcotic analgesic.
DOSAGE: 1–2 tablets Q 3–4 hr prn (maximum dose of acetaminophen = 4 g/d).
SUPPLIED: Tablets 300 mg of APAP and codeine; capsules 325 mg of APAP and codeine; liquid acetaminophen 120 mg and codeine 12 mg per 5 mL.
NOTES: Codeine in No. 1 = 7.5 mg, No. 2 = 15 mg, No. 3 = 30 mg, No. 4 = 60 mg.

Acetazolamide (Diamox)

INDICATIONS: Diuresis, glaucoma, acute mountain sickness (treatment and prevention), refractory epilepsy.
ACTIONS: Carbonic anhydrase inhibitor; decreases renal excretion of hydrogen ions and increases renal excretion of sodium, potassium, bicarbonate, and water.
DOSAGE: *Diuretic*: 250–375 mg IV or PO Q 24 hr.

Glaucoma: 250–1000 mg PO Q 24 hr in divided doses.

Epilepsy: 8–30 mg/kg/d PO in divided doses.

Altitude sickness (treatment): 250 mg PO Q 8–12 hr or sustained-release 500 mg PO Q 12–24 hr.

Altitude sickness (prevention): 250 mg PO Q 8–12 hr or sustained-release 500 mg PO Q 12–24 hr starting 24–48 hr before ascent and 48 hr after highest ascent.

SUPPLIED: Tablets 125 mg, 250 mg; sustained-release capsules 500 mg; injection 500 mg per vial.
NOTES: Contraindicated in renal and hepatic failure, sulfa hypersensitivity; follow Na^+ and K^+; watch for metabolic acidosis; sustained-release dosage forms not recommended for use in epilepsy.

Acetohexamide (Dymelor) [See Table 7–13, p 610]

Acetylcysteine (Mucomyst, Mucosil)

INDICATIONS: Mucolytic agent as adjuvant therapy of chronic bronchopulmonary diseases and cystic fibrosis; as antidote to acetaminophen hepatotoxicity within 24 hr of ingestion.

ACTIONS: Splits disulfide linkages between mucoprotein molecular complexes; protects the liver by restoring glutathione levels in acetaminophen overdose.
DOSAGE: *Nebulizer:* 3–5 mL of 20% solution diluted with an equal volume of water or normal saline administered tid–qid.

Antidote: PO or NG: 140 mg/kg loading dose, then 70 mg/kg Q 4 hr for 17 doses. Dilute 1:3 in carbonated beverage or orange juice.
SUPPLIED: Solution 10%, 20%.
NOTES: Watch for bronchospasm when used by inhalation in asthmatics; activated charcoal will adsorb acetylcysteine when given PO for acute acetaminophen ingestion.

Acyclovir (Zovirax)

INDICATIONS: Treatment of herpes simplex and herpes zoster viral infections.
ACTIONS: Interferes with viral DNA synthesis.
DOSAGE: *Oral:*

- Initial genital herpes: 200 mg PO Q 4 hr while awake, for a total of 5 capsules per day for 10 days or 400 mg PO tid for 7–10 days.
- Chronic suppression: 400 mg PO bid.
- Intermittent therapy: Same as for initial treatment, except treat for 5 days, or 800 mg PO bid, initiated at the earliest prodrome.
- Herpes zoster: 800 mg PO 5 times per day for 7–10 days.

Intravenous: 5–10 mg/kg/dose IV Q 8 hr.

Topical initial herpes genitalis: Apply Q 3 hr (6 times per day) for 7 days.
SUPPLIED: Capsules 200 mg; tablets 400 mg, 800 mg; suspension 200 mg/5 mL; injection 500 mg per vial; ointment 5%.
NOTES: Adjust dose in renal insufficiency; oral better than topical for herpes genitalis.

Adenosine (Adenocard)

INDICATIONS: Treatment of paroxysmal supraventricular tachycardia, including that associated with Wolff-Parkinson-White syndrome.
ACTIONS: Class IV antiarrhythmic; slows conduction time through the AV node.
DOSAGE: 6 mg rapid IV bolus; may be repeated in 1–2 min; maximum 12 mg IV.
SUPPLIED: Injection 6 mg/2 mL.
NOTES: Doses > 12 mg are not recommended; caffeine and theophylline antagonize the effects of adenosine.

Albumin (Albuminar, Buminate, Albutein, Others)

INDICATIONS: Plasma volume expansion for shock resulting from burns, surgery, hemorrhage, or other trauma.
ACTIONS: Maintenance of plasma colloid oncotic pressure.
DOSAGE: Initial dose 25 g IV; subsequent infusions should depend on the clinical situation and response. No more than 250 g/48 hr.
SUPPLIED: Solution 5%, 25%.
NOTES: Contains 130–160 mEq Na^+/L. May precipitate pulmonary edema.

Albuterol (Proventil, Ventolin)

INDICATIONS: Treatment of bronchospasm in reversible obstructive airway disease; prevention of exercise-induced bronchospasm.
ACTIONS: Beta-adrenergic sympathomimetic bronchodilator; relaxes bronchial smooth muscle.
DOSAGE: *Metered-dose inhaler:* 2 inhalations Q 4–6 hr prn; *Rotacaps:* 1 inhaled Q 4–6 hr; oral: 2–4 mg PO tid–qid; *Nebulization:* 1.25–5 mg (0.25–1 cc of 0.5% solution in 2–3 cc of NS) tid–qid.
SUPPLIED: Tablets 2 mg, 4 mg; extended-release tablets 4 mg, 8 mg; syrup 2 mg/5 mL; metered-dose inhaler 90 μg/dose; Rotacaps 200 μg; solution for nebulization 0.083%, 0.5%.

Albuterol and Ipratropium (Combivent)

INDICATIONS: Management of COPD.

ACTIONS: Combination of beta-adrenergic bronchodilator and quaternary anticholinergic compound.
DOSAGE: 2 inhalations qid.
SUPPLIED: Metered-dose inhaler, 18 μg ipratropium/103 μg albuterol per puff.

Aldesleukin (IL-2) (Proleukin)

INDICATIONS: Renal cell carcinoma (RCC), melanoma.
ACTIONS: Acts via IL-2 receptor; numerous immunomodulatory effects.
DOSAGE: 600,000 IU/kg Q 8 hr for 14 doses (FDA-approved dose/schedule for RCC). Multiple continuous infusion and SC dosing schedules (including "high-dose" therapy with 24×10^6 IU/m^2 IV Q 8 hr on days 1–5 and 12–16).
SUPPLIED: Injection 1.1 mg/mL (22×10^6 IU).
NOTES: Toxicity includes flu-like syndrome (malaise, fever, chills), nausea and vomiting, diarrhea, and increased serum bilirubin. Capillary leak syndrome may develop with hypotension, pulmonary edema, fluid retention, and weight gain. Renal toxicity and mild hematologic toxicity (anemia, thrombocytopenia, leukopenia) and secondary eosinophilia may be seen. Cardiac toxicity (myocardial ischemia, atrial arrhythmias) may occur. Neurologic toxicity (CNS depression, somnolence, rarely coma, delirium). Pruritic skin rashes, urticaria, and erythroderma are common. Continuous-infusion schedules are less likely to result in severe hypotension and fluid retention.

Alendronate (Fosamax)

INDICATIONS: Treatment and prevention of osteoporosis, treatment of glucocorticoid-induced osteoporosis and Paget's disease.
ACTIONS: Inhibits normal and abnormal bone resorption.
DOSAGE: *Osteoporosis, treatment*: 10 mg PO once daily or 70 mg once weekly. *Glucocorticoid-induced osteoporosis, treatment:* 5 mg PO once daily; *Prevention:* 5 mg PO once daily or 35 mg once weekly. *Paget's disease:* 40 mg PO once daily.
SUPPLIED: Tablets 5 mg, 10 mg, 35 mg, 40 mg, 70 mg.
NOTES: Should be taken first thing in the morning with plain water (8 oz) at least 30 minutes prior to the first food or beverage of the day. Do not lie down for 30 minutes after taking. Adequate calcium and Vitamin D supplement is necessary.

Allopurinol (Zyloprim, Lopurin, Aloprim, Others)

INDICATIONS: Treatment of gout, hyperuricemia of malignancy, uric acid urolithiasis.
ACTIONS: Xanthine oxidase inhibitor, which decreases the production of uric acid.
DOSAGE: Initial dose 100 mg PO q day; usual 300 mg PO q day; maximum 800 mg/d. IV: 200–400 mg/m^2/d (maximum 600 mg/24 hr).
SUPPLIED: Tablets 100, 300 mg; injection 500 mg/30 mL.
NOTES: Aggravates acute gouty attack; do not begin until acute attack resolves; should be taken after meals. Intravenous administration of 6 mg/mL final concentration as single daily infusion or divided 6-, 8-, or 12-hour intervals. Dosage adjustment necessary in renal impairment.

Alpha$_1$ Protease Inhibitor (Prolastin)

INDICATIONS: Panacinar emphysema.
ACTIONS: Replacement of human alpha$_1$-protease inhibitor.
DOSAGE: 60 mg/kg IV once weekly.
SUPPLIED: Injection > 20 mg/mL.
NOTES: May cause delayed fever up to 12 hours after administration. Fever typically resolves over 24 hours.

Alprazolam (Xanax)[C]

INDICATIONS: Management of anxiety and panic disorders, and anxiety associated with depression.
ACTIONS: Benzodiazepine; antianxiety agent.
DOSAGE: 0.25–2 mg PO tid.

SUPPLIED: Tablets 0.25 mg, 0.5 mg, 1.0 mg, 2.0 mg.
NOTES: Reduce dose in elderly and debilitated patients; avoid abrupt discontinuation after prolonged use.

Alprostadil, Intracavernosal (Caverject, Edex)

INDICATIONS: Treatment of erectile dysfunction due to neurogenic, vasculogenic, or mixed etiology.
ACTIONS: Relaxes smooth muscles, dilates cavernosal arteries, increases lacunar spaces and entrapment of blood by compressing venules against tunica albuginea.
DOSAGE: 2.5–60 μg intracavernosal. Adjusted to individual needs.
SUPPLIED: *Caverject:* 6 vials of 5 μg, 10 μg, or 20 μg with or without diluent syringes; *Edex:* 5-μg, 10-μg, 20-μg, 40-μg vials with syringes.
NOTES: Penile pain is a common side effect; dosage must be titrated at physician's office. Patients should be informed of other side effects including priapism, penile fibrosis, and hematoma.

Alprostadil, Urethral Suppository (Muse)

INDICATIONS: Treatment of erectile dysfunction.
ACTIONS: Alprostadil (PGE_1) is absorbed through urethral mucosa. A portion of the administered dose is transported to the corpus cavernosa, where it acts as a vasodilator and smooth muscle relaxant.
DOSAGE: 125- to 1000-μg system 5–10 minutes prior to sexual activity.
SUPPLIED: 125 μg, 250 μg, 500 μg, 1000 μg with a transurethral delivery system.
NOTES: Hypotension, dizziness, syncope, penile pain, and priapism have been reported. Dose titration should be administered under the supervision of a physician.

Alteplase, Recombinant [t-PA] (Activase)

INDICATIONS: Treatment of acute myocardial infarction, pulmonary embolism, and acute ischemic stroke.
ACTIONS: A tissue plasminogen activator resulting in thrombolysis; inhibits local fibrinolysis by binding to fibrin in the thrombus.
DOSAGE: *AMI and PE:* 100 mg IV over 3 hr (10 mg over 2 min, then 50 mg over 1 hr, then 40 mg over 2 hr).
Stroke: 0.9 mg/kg (maximum 90 mg) infused over 60 minutes.
SUPPLIED: Powder for injection 50 mg, 100 mg.
NOTES: May cause bleeding; heparin should be given to prevent reocclusion; in AMI doses of > 150 mg are associated with intracranial bleeding.

Altretamine (Hexalen)

INDICATIONS: Epithelial ovarian cancer.
ACTIONS: Unknown; cytotoxic agent, possibly alkylating agent; inhibits nucleotide incorporation into DNA and RNA.
DOSAGE: Refer to specific protocols.
SUPPLIED: Capsules 50 mg, 100 mg.
NOTES: Toxicity, primarily vomiting, diarrhea, and cramps; neurologic toxicity (peripheral neuropathy, CNS depression); minimally myelosuppressive.

Aluminum Carbonate (Basaljel)

INDICATIONS: Hyperacidity (peptic ulcer, gastroesophageal reflux disease (GERD), etc); supplement to the management of hyperphosphatemia.
ACTIONS: Neutralizes gastric acid; binds phosphate.
DOSAGE: 2 capsules or tablets or 10 mL (in water) Q 2 hr prn.
SUPPLIED: Tablets, capsules, suspension.

Aluminum Hydroxide (Amphojel, Alternagel)

INDICATIONS: Hyperacidity (peptic ulcer, hiatal hernia, etc); supplement to the management of hyperphosphatemia.
ACTIONS: Neutralizes gastric acid; binds phosphate.

DOSAGE: 10–30 mL or 2 tablets PO Q 4–6 hr.
SUPPLIED: Tablets 300 mg, 600 mg; chewable tablets 500 mg; suspension 320 mg, 600 mg/5 mL.
NOTES: Can be used in renal failure; may cause constipation.

Aluminum Hydroxide with Magnesium Carbonate (Gaviscon)

INDICATIONS: Hyperacidity (peptic ulcer, hiatal hernia, etc).
ACTIONS: Neutralizes gastric acid.
DOSAGE: 15–30 PO PC and HS.
SUPPLIED: Liquid containing aluminum hydroxide 95 mg and magnesium carbonate 358 mg per 15 mL.
NOTES: Doses qid are best given after meals and at bedtime; may cause hypermagnesemia in renal insufficiency.

Aluminum Hydroxide with Magnesium Hydroxide (Maalox)

INDICATIONS: Hyperacidity (peptic ulcer, hiatal hernia, etc).
ACTIONS: Neutralizes gastric acid.
DOSAGE: 10–60 mL or 2–4 tablets PO qid or prn.
SUPPLIED: Tablets; suspension.
NOTES: Doses qid are best given after meals and at bedtime; may cause hypermagnesemia in renal insufficiency.

Aluminum Hydroxide with Magnesium Hydroxide and Simethicone (Mylanta, Mylanta II, Maalox Plus)

INDICATIONS: Hyperacidity with bloating.
ACTIONS: Neutralizes gastric acid.
DOSAGE: 10–60 mL or 2–4 tablets PO qid or prn.
SUPPLIED: Tablets; suspension.
NOTES: May cause hypermagnesemia in renal insufficiency; Mylanta II contains twice the amount of aluminum and magnesium hydroxide as Mylanta.

Aluminum Hydroxide with Magnesium Trisilicate (Gaviscon, Gaviscon-2)

INDICATIONS: Hyperacidity.
ACTIONS: Neutralizes gastric acid.
DOSAGE: Chew 2–4 tablets qid.
SUPPLIED: *Gaviscon:* aluminum hydroxide 80 mg and magnesium trisilicate 20 mg; *Gaviscon 2:* aluminum hydroxide 160 mg and magnesium trisilicate 40 mg.
NOTES: May cause hypermagnesemia in renal insufficiency.

Amantadine (Symmetrel)

INDICATIONS: Treatment or prophylaxis of influenza A viral infections, parkinsonism.
ACTIONS: Prevents release of infectious viral nucleic acid into the host cell; releases dopamine from intact dopaminergic terminals.
DOSAGE: *Influenza A:* 200 mg PO q day or 100 mg PO bid.
Parkinsonism: 100 mg PO q day–bid.
SUPPLIED: Capsules 100 mg; tablets 100 mg; solution 50 mg/5 mL.
NOTES: Reduce dose in renal insufficiency.

Amifostine (Ethyol)

INDICATIONS: Xerostomia prophylaxis for patients receiving radiation therapy for head and neck cancer or in patients with ovarian cancer or non-small cell lung cancer. Reduction of cumulative renal toxicity associated with repeated administration of cisplatin.
ACTIONS: Prodrug that is dephosphorylated by alkaline phosphatase to the pharmacologically active thiol metabolite.
DOSAGE: 910 mg/m^2 once daily as a 15-minute IV infusion 30 minutes prior to chemotherapy.
SUPPLIED: Vials containing 500 mg of lyophilized drug with 500 mg of mannitol, reconstituted in sterile NS.

NOTES: Toxicities include transient hypotension in > 60%, nausea and vomiting, flushing with hot or cold chills, dizziness, hypocalcemia, somnolence, and sneezing. This drug does not reduce the effectiveness of cyclophosphamide plus cisplatin chemotherapy.

Amikacin (Amikin)

INDICATIONS: Treatment of serious infections caused by gram-negative bacteria and mycobacterial infections.
ACTIONS: Aminoglycoside antibiotic; inhibits protein synthesis.
DOSAGE: 5–7.5 mg/kg/dose divided Q 8–24 hr based on renal function.
SUPPLIED: Injection 100 mg/2 mL, 500 mg/2 mL.
NOTES: May be effective against gram-negative bacteria resistant to gentamicin and tobramycin; monitor renal function carefully for dosage adjustments; monitor serum levels (see Table 7–17, p 613).

Amiloride (Midamor)

INDICATIONS: Hypertension and congestive heart failure (CHF).
ACTIONS: Potassium-sparing diuretic; interferes with potassium/sodium exchange in the distal tubules.
DOSAGE: 5–10 mg PO q day.
SUPPLIED: Tablets 5 mg.
NOTES: Hyperkalemia may occur; monitor serum potassium levels.

Aminocaproic Acid (Amicar)

INDICATIONS: Treatment of excessive bleeding resulting from systemic hyperfibrinolysis and urinary fibrinolysis.
ACTIONS: Inhibits fibrinolysis via inhibition of plasminogen activator substances.
DOSAGE: 5 g IV or PO (first hr) followed by 1–1.25 g/hr IV or PO;. maximum dose 18 g/m^2/d.
SUPPLIED: Tablets 500 mg; syrup 250 mg/mL; injection 250 mg/mL.
NOTES: Administer for 8 hr or until bleeding is controlled; contraindicated in disseminated intravascular coagulation; not for upper urinary tract bleeding.

Amino-Cerv pH 5.5 Cream

INDICATIONS: Mild cervicitis, postpartum cervicitis/cervical tears, post-cauterization, post-cryosurgery, and post-conization.
DOSAGE: 1 applicator full intravaginally Q HS for 2–4 weeks.
SUPPLIED: Vaginal cream.
NOTES: Contains 8.34% urea, 0.5% sodium propionate, 0.83% methionine, 0.35% cystine, 0.83% inositol, and benzalkonium chloride.

Aminoglutethimide (Cytadren)

INDICATIONS: Adrenal cortex carcinoma, Cushing's syndrome, breast cancer, and prostate cancer.
ACTIONS: Inhibits adrenal steroidogenesis and adrenal conversion of androgens to estrogens.
DOSAGE: 750–1500 mg/d in divided doses plus hydrocortisone 20–40 mg/d.
SUPPLIED: Tablets 250 mg.
NOTES: Toxicity includes adrenal insufficiency ("medical adrenalectomy"), hypothyroidism, masculinization, hypotension, vomiting, rare hepatotoxicity, rash, myalgia, and fever.

Aminophylline

INDICATIONS: Asthma and bronchospasm.
ACTIONS: Relaxes the smooth muscle of the bronchi and pulmonary blood vessels.
DOSAGE: *Acute bronchospasm:* Load 6 mg/kg IV, then 0.4–0.9 mg/kg/hr IV continuous infusion.
SUPPLIED: Tablets 100 mg, 200 mg; solution 105 mg/5 mL; suppositories 250, 500 mg; injection 25 mg/mL.

NOTES: Individualize dosage; signs of toxicity include nausea and vomiting, irritability, tachycardia, ventricular arrhythmias, and seizures; follow serum levels carefully (see Table 7–16, p 613); aminophylline is about 85% theophylline; erratic absorption with rectal doses.

Amiodarone (Cordarone, Pacerone)

INDICATIONS: Treatment of recurrent ventricular fibrillation or hemodynamically unstable ventricular tachycardia and supraventricular arrhythmias.
ACTIONS: Class III antiarrhythmic.
DOSAGE: *Ventricular arrhythmias:*

- *Intravenous:* 15 mg/min for 10 min, followed by 1 mg/min for 6 hr, then a maintenance dose of 0.5 mg/min continuous infusion OR
- Oral loading dose: 800–1600 mg/d PO for 1–3 weeks.
- Maintenance: 600–800 mg/d PO for 1 month, then 200–400 mg/d.

Supraventricular arrhythmias:

- *Intravenous:* 300 mg IV over 1 hr, then 20 mg/kg for 24 hr, then 600 mg PO q day for 1 week, then a maintenance dose of 100–400 mg q day OR
- *Oral:* Loading dose: 600–800 mg/d PO for 1–4 weeks.Maintenance dose: Gradually reduce dose to 100–400 mg q day.

SUPPLIED: Tablets 200 mg; injection 50 mg/mL.
NOTES: Average half-life is 53 days; potentially toxic effects include pulmonary fibrosis, liver failure, and ocular opacities, as well as exacerbation of arrhythmias; IV concentrations of 0.2 mg/mL should be administered via a central catheter.

Amitriptyline (Elavil, Others)

INDICATIONS: Depression, peripheral neuropathy, chronic pain, and tension and migraine headaches.
ACTIONS: Tricyclic antidepressant; inhibits reuptake of serotonin and norepinephrine by the presynaptic neuronal membrane.
DOSAGE: Initial dose 30–50 mg PO Q HS; may increase to 300 mg Q HS.
SUPPLIED: Tablets 10 mg, 25 mg, 50 mg, 75 mg, 100 mg, 150 mg; injection 10 mg/mL.
NOTES: Strong anticholinergic side effects; may cause urine retention and sedation; overdose can cause arrhythmias and seizures and may be fatal.

Amlodipine (Norvasc)

INDICATIONS: Treatment of hypertension, chronic stable angina, and vasospastic angina.
ACTIONS: Calcium channel blocking agent; produces relaxation of coronary vascular smooth muscle.
DOSAGE: 2.5–10 mg PO q day.
SUPPLIED: Tablets 2.5 mg, 5 mg, 10 mg.
NOTES: May be taken without regard to meals.

Ammonium Aluminum Sulfate (Alum)

INDICATIONS: Hemorrhagic cystitis when bladder irrigation fails.
ACTIONS: Astringent.
DOSAGE: 1–2% solution used with constant bladder irrigation with normal saline.
SUPPLIED: Powder for reconstitution.
NOTES: Can be used safely without anesthesia and in the presence of vesicoureteral reflux. Encephalopathy has been reported; obtain aluminum levels, especially in patients with renal insufficiency. Alum solution often precipitates and occludes catheters.

Amoxapine (Asendin)

INDICATIONS: Treatment of depression and anxiety.
ACTIONS: Tricyclic antidepressant; reduces reuptake of serotonin and norepinephrine.
DOSAGE: Initial dose, 150 mg PO Q HS or 50 mg PO tid; increase to 300 mg daily.
SUPPLIED: Tablets 25 mg, 50 mg, 100 mg, 150 mg.

NOTES: Reduce dose in elderly; taper slowly when discontinuing therapy.

Amoxicillin (Amoxil, Polymox, Others)

INDICATIONS: Treatment of infections resulting from susceptible gram-positive bacteria (streptococci) and gram-negative bacteria (*Haemophilus influenzae, Escherichia coli, Proteus mirabilis*).
ACTIONS: Beta-lactam antibiotic; inhibits cell wall synthesis.
DOSAGE: 250–500 mg PO tid or 500–875 mg bid.
SUPPLIED: Capsules 250 mg, 500 mg; chewable tablets 125 mg, 200 mg, 250 mg, 400 mg; suspension 125 mg/5 mL, 250 mg/5 mL; tablet 500 mg, 875 mg.
NOTES: Cross-hypersensitivity with penicillin; may cause diarrhea; skin rash is common; many hospital strains of *E coli* are resistant.

Amoxicillin and Clavulanic Acid (Augmentin)

INDICATIONS: Treatment of infections caused by beta-lactamase–producing strains of *Haemophilus influenzae, Staphylococcus aureus,* and *Escherichia coli.*
ACTIONS: Combination of a beta-lactam antibiotic and a beta-lactamase inhibitor.
DOSAGE: 250–500 mg PO Q 8 hr or 875 mg Q 12 hr.
SUPPLIED: (Expressed as amoxicillin/clavulanic acid) Tablets 250/125, 500/125 mg, 875/125 mg; chewable tablets 125/31.25, 200/28.5, 250/62.5 mg, 400/57 mg; suspension 125/31.25, 250/62.5 mg/5 mL, 200/28.5, 400/57 mg/5 mL.
NOTES: Do not substitute two 250-mg tablets for one 500-mg tablet or an overdose of clavulanic acid will occur; may cause diarrhea and GI intolerance.

Amphotericin B (Fungizone)

INDICATIONS: Treatment of severe, systemic fungal infections; oral and cutaneous candidiasis.
ACTIONS: Binds to ergosterol in the fungal membrane, altering membrane permeability.
DOSAGE: *Intravenous:* Test dose of 1 mg in adults, then 0.25–1.5 mg/kg/24 hr IV over 2–6 hr. Doses often range from 25 to 50 mg q day or every other day. Total dose varies with indication; *Oral:* 1 mL qid; *Topical:* Apply bid–qid for 1–4 weeks depending on infection.
SUPPLIED: Powder for injection 50 mg/vial; oral suspension 100 mg/mL; cream 3%, lotion 3%, ointment 3%.
NOTES: Monitor renal function; hypokalemia and hypomagnesemia may be seen from renal wasting; pretreatment with acetaminophen and antihistamines (Benadryl) helps minimize adverse effects associated with IV infusion.

Amphotericin B Cholesteryl (Amphotec)

INDICATIONS: Treatment of invasive fungal infection in persons refractory or intolerant to conventional amphotericin B.
ACTIONS: Binds to sterols in the cell membrane, resulting in changes in membrane permeability.
DOSAGE: Test dose of 1.6–8.3 mg, over 15–20 minutes, followed by a dose of 3–4 mg/kg/day. Infuse at a rate of 1 mg/kg/hr.
SUPPLIED: Powder for injection 50 mg, 100 mg per vial.
NOTES: Do *not* use in-line filter, final concentration 0.6 mg/mL.

Amphotericin B Lipid Complex (Abelcet)

INDICATIONS: Treatment of invasive fungal infection in persons refractory or intolerant to conventional amphotericin B.
ACTIONS: Binds to sterols in the cell membrane, resulting in changes in membrane permeability.
DOSAGE: 5 mg/kg/d IV administered as a single daily dose; infuse at a rate of 2.5 mg/kg/hr.
SUPPLIED: Injection 5 mg/mL.
NOTES: Filter solution with a 5-mm filter needle; do not mix in electrolyte-containing solutions. If infusion exceeds 2 hr, mix content of the bag.

Amphotericin B Liposomal (Ambisome)

INDICATIONS: Treatment of invasive fungal infection in persons refractory or intolerant to conventional amphotericin B.
ACTIONS: Binds to sterols in the cell membrane, resulting in changes in membrane permeability.
DOSE: 3–5 mg/kg/d, infused over 60–120 minutes.
SUPPLIED: Powder for injection 50 mg.

Ampicillin (Amcil, Omnipen, Others)

INDICATIONS: Treatment of susceptible gram-negative (*Shigella, Salmonella, E coli, H influenzae,* and *P mirabilis*) and gram-positive (streptococci) bacteria.
ACTIONS: Beta-lactam antibiotic; inhibits cell wall synthesis.
DOSAGE: 500 mg–2 g IM or IV Q 6 hr or 250–500 mg PO Q 6 hr.
SUPPLIED: Capsules 250 mg, 500 mg; suspension 100 mg/mL, 125 mg/5 mL, 250 mg/5 mL, 500 mg/5 mL; powder for injection 125 mg, 250 mg, 500 mg, 1 g, 2 g, 10 g per vial.
NOTES: Cross-hypersensitivity with penicillin; can cause diarrhea and skin rash; many hospital strains of *E coli* are now resistant.

Ampicillin-Sulbactam (Unasyn)

INDICATIONS: Treatment of infections caused by beta-lactamase–producing strains of *S aureus, Enterococcus, H influenzae, P mirabilis,* and *Bacteroides* spp.
ACTIONS: Combination of a beta-lactam antibiotic and a beta-lactamase inhibitor.
DOSAGE: 1.5–3.0 gm IM or IV Q 6 hr.
SUPPLIED: Powder for injection 1.5, 3.0 g per vial.
NOTES: 2:1 ratio of ampicillin:sulbactam; adjust dose in renal failure; observe for hypersensitivity reactions.

Amprenavir (Agenerase)

INDICATIONS: Management of HIV infection.
ACTIONS: Protease inhibitor, prevents the maturation of the virion to a mature viral particle.
DOSAGE: 1200 mg bid.
SUPPLIED: Capsules 50 mg, 150 mg; solution 15 mg/mL.
NOTES: Capsules and solution contain vitamin E exceeding the reference daily intake amounts; avoid high-fat meals with administration; has many drug interactions; can cause life-threatening rash; may cause hyperglycemia and fat redistribution; use with caution in persons with known sulfa allergy.

Anastrozole (Arimidex)

INDICATIONS: Treatment of breast cancer following tamoxifen.
ACTIONS: Selective nonsteroidal aromatase inhibitor, decreases levels of circulating estradiol concentrations.
DOSAGE: 1 mg once daily.
SUPPLIED: Tablets 1 mg.
NOTES: No detectable effect on adrenal corticosteroids or aldosterone; may increase cholesterol levels.

Anistreplase (Eminase)

INDICATIONS: Treatment of acute myocardial infarction.
ACTIONS: Thrombolytic agent; activates the conversion of plasminogen to plasmin, promoting thrombolysis.
DOSAGE: 30 U IV over 2–5 min.
SUPPLIED: Vials containing 30 U.
NOTES: May not be effective if re-administered > 5 days after the previous dose of anistreplase, streptokinase, or streptococcal infection because of the production of antistreptokinase antibody.

Anthralin (Anthraderm, Others)

INDICATIONS: Psoriasis.

ACTIONS: Keratolytic.
DOSAGE: Apply q day.
SUPPLIED: Cream, ointment 0.1; 0.2; 0.25; 0.4; 0.5; 1%.

Antihemophilic Factor (Factor VIII) (AHF) (Monoclate)

INDICATIONS: Treatment of classical hemophilia A.
ACTIONS: Provides Factor VIII needed to convert prothrombin to thrombin.
DOSAGE: 1 antihemophilic factor (AHF) unit/kg increases Factor VIII concentration in the body by ~ 2%. Units required = (kg) (desired Factor VIII increase as % normal) × (0.5).

- Prophylaxis of spontaneous hemorrhage: = 5% normal.
- Hemostasis following trauma or surgery: = 30% normal.
- Head injuries, major surgery, or bleeding: = 80–100% normal.

Note: Patient's percentage of normal level of factor VIII concentration must be ascertained prior to dosing for these calculations.
SUPPLIED: Check each vial for the number of units contained within the vial.
NOTES: AHF is not effective in controlling bleeding in patients with von Willebrand's disease.

Antithymocyte Globulin (ATG) (ATGAM)

INDICATIONS: Management of allograft rejection in transplant patients.
ACTIONS: Reduces the number of circulating, thymus-dependent lymphocytes.
DOSAGE: 10–15 mg/kg/d.
SUPPLIED: Injection 50 mg/mL.
NOTES: Do not administer to a patient with a prior history of severe systemic reaction to any other equine gamma globulin preparation; discontinue treatment if severe, unremitting thrombocytopenia or leukopenia occurs.

Anusol, Anusol-HC

INDICATIONS: Symptomatic relief of pain from external and internal hemorrhoids and anorectal surgery.
ACTIONS: Local anesthetic.
DOSAGE: One suppository Q AM, HS, and following each bowel movement; apply cream or ointment freely to anal area Q 6–12 hr.
SUPPLIED: Suppository, cream, ointment.
NOTES: Anusol-HC also contains hydrocortisone for anti-inflammatory effect.

Apraclonidine (Iopidine) [See Table 7–12, pp 608-9]

Aprotinin (Trasylol)

INDICATIONS: Reduction or prevention of blood loss in patients undergoing a coronary artery bypass graft.
ACTIONS: Protease inhibitor; antifibrinolytic.
DOSAGE: *High-dose:* 2 million KIU load, 2 million KIU for the pump prime dose, followed by 500,000 KIU/hr until surgery ends.

Low-dose: 1 million KIU load, 1 million KIU for the pump prime dose, followed by 250,000 KIU/hr until surgery ends.

Maximum total dose: 7 million KIU.
SUPPLIED: Injection 1.4 mg/mL (10,000 KIU/mL).
NOTES: 1000/KIU = 0.14 mg of aprotinin. All patients should receive a 1-mL IV test dose to assess for allergic reaction.

Ardeparin (Normiflo)

INDICATIONS: Prevention of DVT and PE following knee replacement.
ACTIONS: Low molecular weight heparin.
DOSAGE: 35–50 U/kg SC Q 12 hr. Begin the day of surgery and continue for up to 14 days.
SUPPLIED: Injection 5000 IU/0.5 mL, 10,000 IU/0.5 mL.
NOTES: Laboratory monitoring is not necessary.

Argatroban (Acova)

INDICATIONS: Prevention or treatment of thrombosis in patients with heparin-induced thrombocytopenia.
ACTIONS: A direct thrombin inhibitor, derived from L-arginine, which reversibly binds to the thrombin active site and inhibits thrombin-catalyzed or thrombin-induced reactions.
DOSAGE: 2 μg/kg/min administered as a continuous infusion. Adjust dose based on aPTT (Max dose 10 μg/kg/min). Initiate therapy at 0.5 μg/kg/min in patients with hepatic impairment.
SUPPLIED: 100 mg/mL solution in 2.5-mL vials.
NOTES: Monitor therapy using aPTT (adjust to achieve 1.5 to 3 times above baseline value—do not exceed 100 seconds). Steady state typically achieved 1–3 hours after initiation of therapy.

Artificial Tears (Tears Naturale, Others)

INDICATIONS: Dry eyes.
ACTIONS: Ocular lubricant.
DOSAGE: 1–2 drops tid–qid.
SUPPLIED: OTC solution.

L-Asparaginase (Elspar, Oncaspar)

INDICATIONS: Acute lymphocytic leukemia (in combination with other agents).
ACTIONS: Protein synthesis inhibitor.
DOSAGE: Refer to specific protocols.
SUPPLIED: Injection 10,000 IU.
NOTES: Toxicity includes hypersensitivity reactions in 20–35% (spectrum of urticaria to anaphylaxis), so a test dose is recommended; rare GI toxicity (mild nausea/anorexia, pancreatitis).

Aspirin (Bayer, St. Joseph, Others)

INDICATIONS: Mild pain, headache, fever, inflammation, prevention of emboli, and prevention of myocardial infarction.
ACTIONS: Prostaglandin inhibitor.
DOSAGE:

- Pain, fever: 325–650 mg Q 4–6 hr PO or PR.
- Rheumatoid arthritis: 3–6 g/d PO in divided doses.
- Platelet inhibitory action: 325 mg PO q day.
- Prevention of MI: 160–325 mg PO q day.

SUPPLIED: Tablets 325 mg, 500 mg; chewable tablets 81 mg; enteric-coated tablets 165 mg, 325 mg, 500 mg, 650 mg, 975 mg; sustained-release tablets 650 mg, 800 mg; effervescent tablets 325 mg, 500 mg; suppositories 120 mg, 200 mg, 300 mg, 600 mg.
NOTES: GI upset and erosion are common adverse reactions; discontinue use 1 week prior to surgery to avoid postoperative bleeding complications. See drug levels for salicylates (Table 7–16, p 613).

Aspirin and Butalbital Compound (Fiorinal, Lanorinal, Others) [C]

INDICATIONS: Tension headache, pain.
ACTIONS: Combination barbiturate and analgesic.
DOSAGE: 1–2 PO Q 4 hr prn, max 6 tablets/d.
SUPPLIED: *Capsules:* Fiorgen PF, Fiorinal, Lanorinal, Marnal: aspirin 325 mg/butalbital 50 mg/caffeine 40 mg; *Tablets:* Fiorinal, Lanorinal, Marnal: aspirin 325 mg/butalbital 50 mg/caffeine 40 mg.
NOTES: Butalbital can be habit forming.

Aspirin with Butalbital, Caffeine, and Codeine (Fiorinal With Codeine) [C]

INDICATIONS: Mild pain; headache, especially when associated with stress.
ACTIONS: Sedative analgesic, narcotic analgesic.
DOSAGE: 1–2 tablets (capsules) PO Q 4–6 hr prn.

SUPPLIED: Each capsule or tablet contains 325 mg aspirin, 40 mg caffeine, 50 mg of butalbital, codeine: No. 3 = 30 mg.
NOTES: Significant drowsiness associated with use.

Aspirin with Codeine (Empirin No. 2, No. 3, No. 4) [C]

INDICATIONS: Relief of mild to moderate pain.
ACTIONS: Combined effects of aspirin and codeine.
DOSAGE: 1–2 tablets PO Q 4–6 hr prn.
SUPPLIED: Tablets 325 mg of aspirin and codeine as below.
NOTES: Codeine in No. 2 = 15 mg, No. 3 = 30 mg, No. 4 = 60 mg.

Atenolol (Tenormin) [See Table 7–7, pp 601-2]

Atorvastatin (Lipitor) [See Table 7–15, p 612]

Atovaquone (Mepron)

INDICATIONS: Treatment of mild to moderate *Pneumocystis carinii* pneumonia, prevention of PCP.
ACTIONS: Inhibits nucleic acid and ATP synthesis.
DOSAGE: *Treatment:* 750 mg PO bid for 21 days; *Prevention:* 1500 mg PO once daily.
SUPPLIED: Suspension 750 mg/5 mL.
NOTES: Should be taken with meals.

Atracurium (Tracrium)

INDICATIONS: Adjunct to anesthesia to facilitate endotracheal intubation.
ACTIONS: Nondepolarizing neuromuscular blocker.
DOSAGE: 0.4–0.5 mg/kg IV bolus, then 0.08–0.1 mg/kg every 20–45 min prn.
SUPPLIED: Injection 10 mg/mL.
NOTES: Patient must be intubated and on controlled ventilation. Use adequate amounts of sedation and analgesia.

Atropine

INDICATIONS: Preanesthetic; symptomatic bradycardia and asystole.
ACTIONS: Antimuscarinic agent; blocks acetylcholine at parasympathetic sites.
DOSAGE: *Emergency cardiac care, bradycardia:* 0.5 mg IV Q 5 min up to 2.0 mg total; asystole 1.0 mg IV, repeat in 5 min.
Preanesthetic: 0.3–0.6 mg IM.
SUPPLIED: Tablets 0.3 mg, 0.4 mg, 0.6 mg; injection 0.05 mg/mL, 0.1 mg/mL, 0.3 mg/mL, 0.4 mg/mL, 0.5 mg/mL, 0.8 mg/mL, 1.0 mg/mL.
NOTES: Can cause blurred vision, urinary retention, and dried mucous membranes.

Azathioprine (Imuran)

INDICATIONS: Adjunct for the prevention of rejection following organ transplantation; rheumatoid arthritis; systemic lupus erythematosus.
ACTIONS: Immunosuppressive agent; antagonizes purine metabolism.
DOSAGE: 1–3 mg/kg IV or PO daily.
SUPPLIED: Tablets 50 mg; injection 100 mg/20 mL.
NOTES: May cause GI intolerance; do not administer vaccines to a patient taking azathioprine; injection should be handled with cytotoxic precautions. Interaction with allopurinol.

Azelastine (Astelin, Optivar)

INDICATIONS: Treatment of the symptoms of allergic rhinitis (rhinorrhea, sneezing, nasal pruritus); allergic conjunctivitis.
ACTIONS: A histamine H_1-receptor antagonist.
DOSAGE: *Nasal spray:* 2 sprays per nostril bid; *Ophthalmic solution:* 1 drop into each affected eye bid.

SUPPLIED: Nasal spray 137 μg/spray; ophthalmic solution 0.05%.

Azithromycin (Zithromax)

INDICATIONS: Treatment of acute bacterial exacerbations of chronic obstructive pulmonary disease (COPD), community-acquired pneumonia, pharyngitis, otitis media, skin and skin structure infections, nongonococcal urethritis, PID. Treatment and prevention of *Mycobacterium avium* complex (MAC) infections in HIV-infected persons.
ACTIONS: Macrolide antibiotic; inhibits protein synthesis.
DOSAGE: *Oral:*

- Respiratory tract: 500 mg PO on the first day, followed by 250 mg PO q day for 4 more days.
- Nongonococcal urethritis: 1 g as a single dose.
- Prevention of MAC: 1200 mg PO once a week.

Intravenous: 500 mg for at least 2 days, followed by 500 mg PO for total of 7–10 days.
SUPPLIED: Tablets 250 mg, 600 mg; suspension 1 g single-dose packet, 100 mg/5 mL, 200 mg/5 mL; injection 500 mg.
NOTES: Suspension should be taken on an empty stomach; tablets may be taken with or without food.

Aztreonam (Azactam)

INDICATIONS: Treatment of infections caused by aerobic gram-negative bacteria, including *Pseudomonas aeruginosa*.
ACTIONS: Monobactam antibiotic; inhibits cell wall synthesis.
DOSAGE: 1–2 g IV/IM Q 6–12 hr.
SUPPLIED: Injection 500 mg, 1 g, 2 g.
NOTES: Not effective against gram-positive or anaerobic bacteria; may be given to penicillin-allergic patients; dose adjust in renal impairment.

Bacillus Calmette-Guérin (Theracys, TICE BCG, Pacis)

INDICATIONS: Bladder carcinoma, tuberculosis prophylaxis.
ACTIONS: Immunomodulator.
DOSAGE: Bladder cancer, contents of 1 vial prepared and instilled in bladder for 2 hr. Repeat once weekly for 6 weeks; repeat 3, 6, 12, 18, and 24 months after the initial therapy.
SUPPLIED: Injection 27 mg (3.4 + 3 $\times 10^8$ CFU) per vial (TheraCys); 1–8 $\times 10^8$ CFU per vial (TICE BCG).
NOTES: Intravesical toxicity includes hematuria, urinary frequency, dysuria, and bacterial urinary tract infection.

Bacitracin, Topical (Baciguent); Bacitracin and Polymyxin B, Topical (Polysporin); Bacitracin, Neomycin, and Polymyxin B, Topical (Neosporin Ointment); Bacitracin, Neomycin, Polymyxin B, and Hydrocortisone, Topical (Cortisporin); Bacitracin, Neomycin, Polymyxin B, and Lidocaine, Topical (Clomycin)

INDICATIONS: Topical for prevention and treatment of minor cuts, scrapes, and burns.
ACTIONS: Topical antibiotic with added effects based on components (anti-inflammatory and analgesic).
DOSAGE: Apply sparingly bid–qid.
SUPPLIED: Bacitracin 500 U/g ointment.
Bacitracin 500 U/polymyxin B sulfate 10,000 U/g ointment and powder.
Bacitracin 400 U/neomycin/3.5 mg/polymyxin B 5000 U/g ointment.
Bacitracin 400 U/neomycin 3.5 mg/polymyxin B/10,000 U/hydrocortisone 10 mg/g ointment.
Bacitracin 500 U/neomycin 3.5 g/polymyxin B 5000 U/lidocaine 40 mg/g ointment.
NOTES: Systemic and irrigation forms of bacitracin available but not generally used due to potential toxicity.

Bacitracin, Ophthalmic (Ak-Tracin Ophthalmic) Bacitracin and Polymyxin B, Ophthalmic (Ak Poly Bac Ophthalmic Polysporin, Ophthalmic) Bacitracin, Neomycin, and Polymyxin B, Ophthalmic (Ak Spore Ophthalmic, Neosporin Ophthalmic) Bacitracin, Neomycin, Polymyxin B, and Hydrocortisone, Ophthalmic (Ak Spore Hc Ophthalmic, Cortisporin Ophthalmic)

INDICATIONS: Blepharitis, conjunctivitis, and prophylactic treatment of corneal abrasions.

ACTIONS: Topical antibiotic with added effects based on components (anti-inflammatory).

DOSAGE: Apply Q 3–4 hr into conjunctival sac.

SUPPLIED: See Topical equivalents this page.

Baclofen (Lioresal, Others)

INDICATIONS: Management of spasticity secondary to severe chronic disorders such as multiple sclerosis or spinal cord lesions, trigeminal neuralgia.

ACTIONS: Centrally acting skeletal muscle relaxant; inhibits transmission of both monosynaptic and polysynaptic reflexes at the spinal cord.

DOSAGE: Initial dose 5 mg PO tid; increase every 3 days to maximum effect; maximum 80 mg/d. *Intrathecal:* through implantable pump.

SUPPLIED: Tablets 10 mg, 20 mg; intrathecal injection 10 mg/20 mL, 10 mg/5 mL.

NOTES: Use caution in epileptics and neuropsychiatric disturbances; withdrawal may occur with abrupt discontinuation.

Balsalazide Disodium (Colazal)

INDICATIONS: Treatment of active ulcerative colitis.

ACTIONS: Cleaved in the colon to produce the anti-inflammatory drug, mesalamine (5-aminosalicylic acid).

DOSAGE: 2.25 g tid.

SUPPLIED: 750-mg capsules.

NOTES: Each daily dose of 6.75 g is equivalent to 2.4 g of mesalamine. Contraindicated in patients allergic to salicylates.

Basiliximab (Simulect)

INDICATIONS: Prevention of acute organ transplant rejections.

ACTIONS: Interleukin-2 receptor antagonists.

DOSAGE: 20 mg IV 2 hours prior to transplant, then 20 mg IV 4 days post transplant.

SUPPLIED: Injection 20 mg.

NOTES: Murine/human monoclonal antibody.

Becaplermin (Regranex Gel)

INDICATIONS: Diabetic foot ulcer.

ACTIONS: Recombinant human platelet derived growth factor (PDGF), enhanced formation of granulation tissue.

DOSAGE: Based on size of lesion; 1-⅓" ribbon from 2 g tube, ⅔" ribbon from 7.5 or 15 mg tube per square inch of ulcer; apply and cover with moist gauze; rinse after 12 hours; do not reapply; repeat process 12 hours later.

SUPPLIED: 0.01% gel in 2/7.5/15 g tubes.

NOTES: Should be used along with good wound care; wound must be vascularized.

Beclomethasone (Beconase, Vancenase Nasal Inhaler)

INDICATIONS: Allergic rhinitis refractory to conventional therapy with antihistamines and decongestants.

ACTIONS: Inhaled corticosteroid.

DOSAGE: 1 spray intranasally bid–qid; *Aqueous inhalation:* 1–2 sprays/nostril q day–bid.

SUPPLIED: Nasal metered-dose inhaler.

NOTES: Nasal spray delivers 42 μg/dose and 84 μg/dose.

Beclomethasone (Beclovent Inhaler, Vanceril Inhaler, QVAR)

INDICATIONS: Chronic asthma.

ACTIONS: Inhaled corticosteroid.
DOSAGE: 2–4 inhalations tid–qid (maximum 20/d); Vanceril double strength: 2 inhalations bid (maximum 10/d); QVAR (HFA preparation): 1–4 inhalations bid.
SUPPLIED: *Oral metered-dose inhaler:* 42 μg, 84 μg/inhalation; *QVAR:* 40, 80 μg/inhalation.
NOTES: Not effective for acute asthmatic attacks; may cause oral candidiasis, instruct patients to rinse their mouth after use.

Belladonna and Opium Suppositories (B & O Supprettes) [C]

INDICATIONS: Treatment of bladder spasms; moderate to severe pain.
ACTIONS: Antispasmodic.
DOSAGE: Insert 1 suppository rectally Q 6 hr prn.

- 15A = 30 mg of powdered opium; 16.2 mg of belladonna extract.
- 16A = 60 mg of powdered opium; 16.2 mg of belladonna extract.

SUPPLIED: Suppositories 15A, 16A.
NOTES: Anticholinergic side effects; caution patients about sedation, urinary retention, and constipation.

Benazepril (Lotensin) [See Table 7–3, p 598]

Benzocaine and Antipyrine (Auralgan)

INDICATIONS: Analgesia in severe otitis media.
ACTIONS: Anesthetic and local decongestant.
DOSAGE: Fill the ear and insert a moist cotton plug; repeat 1–2 hr prn.
SUPPLIED: Solution.
NOTES: Do not use with perforated eardrum.

Benzonatate (Tessalon Perles)

INDICATIONS: Symptomatic relief of cough.
ACTIONS: Anesthetizes the stretch receptors in the respiratory passages.
DOSAGE: 100 mg PO tid.
SUPPLIED: Capsules 100 mg.
NOTES: May cause sedation; do not chew or puncture the capsule.

Benztropine (Cogentin)

INDICATIONS: Treatment of parkinsonism and drug-induced extrapyramidal disorders.
ACTIONS: Partially blocks striatal cholinergic receptors.
DOSAGE: 0.5–6 mg PO, IM, or IV in divided doses per day.
SUPPLIED: Tablets 0.5 mg, 1.0 mg, 2.0 mg; injection 1 mg/mL.
NOTES: Anticholinergic side effects.

Bepridil (Vascor)

INDICATIONS: Treatment of chronic stable angina.
ACTIONS: Calcium channel blocking agent.
DOSAGE: 200–400 mg PO daily.
SUPPLIED: Tablets 200 mg, 300 mg, 400 mg.
NOTES: May cause agranulocytosis and serious ventricular arrhythmias, including torsades de pointes.

Betamethasone (Celestone) [See Table 7–2, p 597]

Betaxolol, Ophthalmic (Betoptic) [See Table 7–12, pp 607-9]

Betaxolol (Kerlone) [See Table 7–7, pp 601-2]

Bethanechol (Urecholine, Duvoid, Others)

INDICATIONS: Neurogenic atony of the bladder with urinary retention, acute postoperative and postpartum functional (nonobstructive) urinary retention.
ACTIONS: Stimulates cholinergic receptors in the smooth muscle of the bladder and GI tract.
DOSAGE: 10–50 mg PO tid–qid or 2.5–5 mg SC tid–qid and prn.

SUPPLIED: Tablets 5 mg, 10 mg, 25 mg, 50 mg; injection 5 mg/mL.
NOTES: Contraindicated in bladder outlet obstruction, asthma, and coronary artery disease; *do not* administer IM or IV.

Bexarotene (Targretin)

INDICATIONS: Treatment of cutaneous manifestations of cutaneous T-cell lymphoma in patients refractory to at least one prior systemic therapy.
ACTIONS: Selectively binds and activates retinoid X receptor subtypes.
DOSAGE: 300 mg/m^2/d. Taken as a single daily dose with a meal.
SUPPLIED: 75-mg capsules.
NOTES: Contraindicated in pregnancy; may cause hyperlipidemia, pancreatitis, increased LFTs, hypothyroidism, and leukopenia.

Bicalutamide (Casodex)

INDICATIONS: Advanced prostate cancer (in combination with gonadotropin-releasing hormone agonists such as leuprolide or goserelin).
ACTIONS: Nonsteroidal antiandrogen.
DOSAGE: 50 mg/d.
SUPPLIED: Capsules 50 mg.
NOTES: Toxicity includes hot flashes, loss of libido, impotence, diarrhea, nausea and vomiting, gynecomastia, and LFT elevation.

Bisacodyl (Dulcolax)

INDICATIONS: Constipation; preoperative bowel preparation.
ACTIONS: Stimulates peristalsis.
DOSAGE: 5–15 mg PO or 10 mg PR prn.
SUPPLIED: Enteric-coated tablets 5 mg; suppositories 10 mg.
NOTES AND CAUTIONS: *Do not* use with an acute abdomen or bowel obstruction; instruct patient *not* to chew tablets; *do not* administer within 1 hour of giving antacids or milk.

Bismuth Subsalicylate (Pepto-Bismol)

INDICATIONS: Indigestion, nausea, and diarrhea. In combination for the treatment of *Helicobacter pylori* infection.
ACTIONS: Antisecretory and anti-inflammatory effects.
DOSAGE: 2 tablets or 30 mL PO prn (up to 8 doses/24 hr).
SUPPLIED: Chewable tablets 262 mg; liquid 262 mg/15 mL, 524 mg/15 mL.
NOTES: May turn tongue and stools black.

Bisoprolol (Zebeta) [See Table 7–7, pp 601-2]

Bitolterol (Tornalate)

INDICATIONS: Prophylaxis and treatment of asthma and reversible bronchospasm.
ACTIONS: Sympathomimetic bronchodilator; stimulates beta$_2$-adrenergic receptors in the lungs.
DOSAGE: 2 inhalations Q 8 hr.
SUPPLIED: Aerosol 0.8%.

Bivalirudin (Angiomax)

INDICATIONS: An anticoagulant in patients with unstable angina undergoing percutaneous transluminal coronary angioplasty (PTCA).
ACTIONS: A specific and reversible direct thrombin inhibitor.
DOSAGE: A 1 mg/kg IV bolus, followed by a 2.5 mg/kg/hr IV infusion for 4 hours, then if needed a 0.2 mg/kg/hr continuous infusion for up to 20 hours. Should be administered with 300–325 mg of aspirin.
SUPPLIED: 250 mg per vial after reconstitution.
NOTES: Adjust dose in patients with renal impairment.

Bleomycin Sulfate (Blenoxane)

INDICATIONS: Testicular carcinomas, Hodgkin's and non-Hodgkin's lymphomas, cutaneous lymphomas, and squamous cell carcinomas of the head and neck, larynx, cervix, skin, and penis.
ACTIONS: Induces breakage (*scission*) of single- and double-stranded DNA.
DOSAGE: Refer to specific protocols.
NOTES: Toxicity includes hyperpigmentation (skin staining) and hypersensitivity (rash to anaphylaxis); test dose of 1 mg (U) recommended, especially in lymphoma patients; fever in 50%; lung toxicity (idiosyncratic and dose-related); pneumonitis may progress to fibrosis. Serious lung toxicity is most likely when the total dose exceeds 400 mg (U).

Brimonidine (Alphagan) [See Table 7–12, pp 607-9]

Brinzolamide (Azopt) [See Table 7–12, pp 607-9]

Bromocriptine (Parlodel)

INDICATIONS: Treatment of Parkinson's syndrome; treatment of hyperprolactinemia.
ACTIONS: Acts directly on the striatal dopamine receptors; inhibits prolactin secretion.
DOSAGE: Initial dose 1.25 mg PO bid; titrate to effect.
SUPPLIED: Tablets 2.5 mg; capsules 5 mg.
NOTES: Nausea and vertigo are common side effects.

Buclizine (Bucladin-S Softabs)

INDICATIONS: Control of nausea, vomiting, and dizziness of motion sickness.
ACTIONS: Centrally acting antiemetic.
DOSAGE: 50 mg dissolved in the mouth bid; 50 mg PO prophylactically 30 min prior to travel.
SUPPLIED: Tablets 50 mg.
NOTES: Not safe in pregnancy; contains tartrazine; observe the patient for allergic reactions.

Budesonide (Rhinocort, Pulmicort)

INDICATIONS: Management of allergic and nonallergic rhinitis, management of asthma.
ACTIONS: Steroid.
DOSAGE:

- Intranasal: 2 sprays in each nostril bid or 4 sprays per nostril q day.
- Aqueous: 1 spray/nostril q day.
- Oral inhaled: 1–4 inhalations twice daily.

SUPPLIED: Metered-dose inhaler, Turbuhaler, nasal inhaler, and aqueous spray.
NOTES: May cause oral candidiasis; instruct patients to rinse their mouth after use.

Bumetanide (Bumex)

INDICATIONS: Management of edema from CHF, hepatic cirrhosis, and renal disease.
ACTIONS: Loop diuretic; inhibits reabsorption of sodium and chloride in the ascending loop of Henle and the distal renal tubule.
DOSAGE: 0.5–2.0 mg PO daily; 0.5–1.0 mg IV Q 8–24 hr (max 10 mg/d).
SUPPLIED: Tablets 0.5 mg, 1 mg, 2 mg; injection 0.25 mg/mL.
NOTES: Monitor fluid and electrolyte status during treatment.

Bupivacaine (Marcaine)

INDICATIONS: Peripheral nerve block.
ACTIONS: Local anesthetic.
DOSAGE: Dose is dependent on the procedure, vascularity of the tissues, depth of anesthesia, and degree of muscle relaxation required.
SUPPLIED: Injection 0.25%, 0.5%, 0.75%.

Buprenorphine (Buprenex) [C]

INDICATIONS: Relief of moderate to severe pain.
ACTIONS: Opiate agonist-antagonist.

DOSAGE: 0.3–0.6 mg IM or slow IV push Q 6 hr prn.
SUPPLIED: Injection 0.324 mg/mL (= 0.3 mg of buprenorphine).
NOTES: May induce withdrawal syndrome in opioid-dependent patients.

Bupropion (Wellbutrin, Zyban)

INDICATIONS: Treatment of depression, adjunct to smoking cessation.
ACTIONS: Weak inhibitor of neuronal uptake of serotonin and norepinephrine; inhibits the neuronal reuptake of dopamine.
DOSAGE:

- Depression: 100–450 mg/d divided bid–tid.
- Smoking cessation: 150 mg daily for 3 days, then 150 mg twice daily for 8–12 weeks.

SUPPLIED: Tablets 75 mg, 100 mg; SR tablets 100, 150 mg.
NOTES: Has been associated with seizures; avoid use of alcohol and other CNS depressants.

Buspirone (Buspar)

INDICATIONS: Short-term relief of anxiety.
ACTIONS: Antianxiety agent; selectively antagonizes CNS serotonin receptors.
DOSAGE: 5–10 mg PO tid. Increase dose to desired response; usual daily dose is 20–30 mg. Do not exceed 60 mg/d.
SUPPLIED: Tablets 5 mg, 10 mg, 15 mg.
NOTES: No abuse potential. No physical or psychological dependence.

Busulfan (Myleran)

INDICATIONS: Chronic myelogenous leukemia, preparative regimens for allogeneic and autologous bone marrow transplantation in high doses.
ACTIONS: Alkylating agent.
DOSAGE: Refer to specific protocols.
NOTES: Toxicity includes myelosuppression, pulmonary fibrosis, nausea (high-dose therapy), gynecomastia, adrenal insufficiency, hyperpigmentation of the skin.

Butorphanol (Stadol) [C]

INDICATIONS: Treatment of moderate to severe pain and headaches.
ACTIONS: Opiate agonist-antagonist with central analgesic actions.
DOSAGE:

- Pain: 1–4 mg IM or IV every 3–4 hr prn.
- Headaches: 1 spray in 1 nostril, may be repeated once if pain not relieved in 60–90 min.

SUPPLIED: Injection 1, 2 mg/mL; nasal spray 10 mg/mL.
NOTES: May induce withdrawal syndrome in opioid-dependent patients.

Calcipotriene (Dovonex)

INDICATIONS: Plaque psoriasis.
ACTIONS: Keratolytic.
DOSAGE: Apply bid.
SUPPLIED: Cream 0.005%, ointment 0.005%, solution 0.005%.

Calcitonin (Cibacalcin, Miacalcin)

INDICATIONS: Paget's disease of bone; hypercalcemia; osteogenesis imperfecta; postmenopausal osteoporosis.
ACTIONS: Polypeptide hormone.
DOSAGE:

- Paget's (salmon form): Initial dose 100 U/d IM/SC, maintenance 50 U/d or 50–100 U Q 1–3 days.
- Paget's (human form): Initial dose 0.5 mg/d; maintenance 0.5 mg 2–3 times/wk or 0.25 mg/d, max 0.5 mg bid.

- Hypercalcemia (salmon calcitonin): 4 U/kg IM/SC Q 12 hr; increase to 8 U/kg Q 12 hr, max Q 6 hr.
- Osteoporosis (salmon calcitonin): 100 U/d IM/SC; *Intranasal:* 200 U = 1 nasal spray/d.

SUPPLIED: Spray, nasal 200 units/activation; injection Human (Cibacalcin), 0.5 mg/vial; Salmon, 200 units/mL (2 mL).
NOTES: Human (Cibacalcin) and salmon forms; human only approved for Paget's bone disease.

Calcitriol (Rocaltrol)

INDICATIONS: Reduction of elevated parathyroid hormone levels, hypocalcemia associated with dialysis.
ACTIONS: 1,25 dihydroxycholecalciferol, a vitamin D analogue.
DOSAGE:

- Renal failure: 0.25 μg PO q day increase 0.25 μg/d every 4–6 wk prn; 0.5 μg 3 times a week IV, increase as needed.
- Hypoparathyroidism: 0.5–2.0 μg/d.

SUPPLIED: Injection 1, 2 μg/mL (in 1-mL volume); capsules 0.25, 0.5 μg.
NOTES: Monitor dosing to keep calcium levels within normal range.

Calcium Acetate (Calphron, Phos-Ex, Phoslo)

INDICATIONS: ESRD-associated hyperphosphatemia.
ACTIONS: Calcium supplement to treat ESRD hhyperphosphatemia without aluminum.
DOSAGE: 2–4 tablets PO with meals.
SUPPLIED: Capsule (*Phos-Ex*): 500 mg (125 mg elemental calcium); Tablets (*Calphron and Phos-Lo*): 667 mg (169 mg elemental calcium).
NOTES: Can cause hypercalcemia; monitor levels.

Calcium Carbonate (Tums, Alka-Mints)

INDICATIONS: Hyperacidity associated with peptic ulcer disease, hiatal hernia, etc.
ACTIONS: Neutralizes gastric acid.
DOSAGE: 500 mg to 2 g PO prn.
SUPPLIED: Chewable tablets 350 mg, 420 mg, 500 mg, 550 mg, 750 mg, 850 mg; suspension.
NOTES: Calcium carbonate contains 40% elemental calcium (20 mEq calcium per gram).

Calcium Salts

INDICATIONS: Electromechanical dissociation secondary to hypocalcemia or calcium channel blocker toxicity, life-threatening hypocalcemia, symptomatic hypocalcemia.
ACTIONS: Dietary supplement; increased myocardial contractility, binding phosphate.
DOSAGE: *Replacement:* 1–2 g PO Q day.
Cardiac emergencies: Calcium chloride 0.5–1.0 g IV Q 10 min or calcium gluconate 1–2 g IV Q 10 min.
Hyperphosphatemia in end-stage renal disease: 2 tablets with each meal.
SUPPLIED: *Oral:* Tablets 500 mg, 650 mg, 975 mg, 1 g; *IV:* calcium chloride injection 10% (100 mg/mL); calcium gluconate injection 10% (100 mg/mL).
NOTES: Calcium chloride contains 270 mg (13.6 mEq) elemental calcium per gram, and calcium gluconate contains 90 mg (4.5 mEq) elemental calcium per gram.

Candesartan (Atacand) [See Table 7–4, p 599]

Capecitabine (Xeloda)

INDICATIONS: Treatment of patients with metastatic breast cancer resistant to both paclitaxel and an anthracycline-containing chemotherapy regimen.
ACTIONS: Enzymatically converted to 5-fluorouracil. Inhibitor of thymidylate synthetase.
DOSAGE: Refer to specific protocols.
NOTES: Adjust in renal impairment; may cause nausea, vomiting, diarrhea, stomatitis, hand-and-foot syndrome, neutropenia, and fever.

Capsaicin (Capsin, Zostrix, Others)

INDICATIONS: Topical therapy of pain due to postherpetic neuralgia, chronic neuralgia, arthritis, diabetic neuropathy, postoperative pain, psoriasis, intractable pruritus.
ACTIONS: Topical analgesic.
DOSAGE: Apply tid–qid.
SUPPLIED: OTC creams, gel, lotions, roll-ons.

Captopril (Capoten) [See Table 7–3, p 598]

Carbachol (Isopto Carbachol) [See Table 7–12, pp 607-9]

Carbamazepine (Tegretol)

INDICATIONS: Treatment of epilepsy and trigeminal neuralgia.
ACTIONS: Anticonvulsant.
DOSAGE: Initial dose 200 mg PO bid; increase by 200 mg/d; usual 800–1200 mg/d in divided doses.
SUPPLIED: Tablets 200 mg; chewable tablets 100 mg; XR tablets 100 mg, 200 mg, 400 mg; suspension 100 mg/5 mL.
NOTES: Can cause severe hematologic side effects; monitor CBC; monitor serum levels (see Table 7–16, p 613); generic products are not interchangeable.

Carbidopa/Levodopa (Sinemet)

INDICATIONS: Treatment of Parkinson's disease.
ACTIONS: Increases CNS levels of dopamine.
DOSAGE: 25/100 bid–qid; titrate as needed (maximum 200/2000 mg/d).
SUPPLIED: Tablets (mg of carbidopa/mg of levodopa): 10/100, 25/100, 25/250; tablets SR (mg of carbidopa/mg of levodopa): 25/100, 50/200.
NOTES: May cause psychiatric disturbances, orthostatic hypotension, dyskinesias, and cardiac arrhythmias.

Carboplatin (Paraplatin)

INDICATIONS: Ovarian cancer, lung cancer (small cell and non-small cell), head and neck cancer, testicular cancer, brain cancers, and allogeneic and autologous transplantation in high doses.
ACTIONS: DNA cross-linker; forms DNA-platinum adducts.
DOSAGE: Refer to specific protocols.
NOTES: Toxicity includes myelosuppression, nausea and vomiting, diarrhea, nephrotoxicity, hematuria, neurotoxicity, and hepatic enzyme elevations; physiologic dosing based on either Calvert's or Egorin's formula allows larger doses to be given with reduced toxicity.

Carisoprodol (Soma)

INDICATIONS: Adjunct to sleep and physical therapy for the relief of painful musculoskeletal conditions.
ACTIONS: Centrally acting muscle relaxant.
DOSAGE: 350 mg PO tid–qid.
SUPPLIED: Tablets 350 mg.
NOTES: Avoid alcohol and other CNS depressants; available in combination with aspirin or codeine.

Carmustine (BCNU, BICNU)

INDICATIONS: Primary brain tumors, melanoma, Hodgkin's and non-Hodgkin's lymphomas, multiple myeloma, and preparative regimens for allogeneic and autologous bone marrow transplantation in high doses.
ACTIONS: Alkylating agent; forms DNA cross-links; inhibitor of DNA synthesis.
DOSAGE: Refer to specific protocols.
NOTES: Toxicity includes myelosuppression (especially leukocytes and platelets), phlebitis, facial flushing, hepatic and renal dysfunction, pulmonary fibrosis, and optic neuroretinitis. Hematologic toxicity may persist up to 4–6 weeks after administration.

Carteolol (Cartrol) [See Table 7–7, pp 601-2]

Carteolol (Ocupress) [See Table 7–12, pp 607-9]

Carvedilol (Coreg) [See Table 7–7, pp 601-2]

Cefaclor (Ceclor) [See Table 7–9, p 603]

Cefadroxil (Duricef, Ultracef) [See Table 7–8, p 603]

Cefamandole (Mandol) [See Table 7–9, p 603]

Cefazolin (Ancef, Kefzol) [See Table 7–8, p 603]

Cefdinir (Omnicef) [See Table 7–10, p 604]

Cefepime (Maxipime) [See Table 7–10, p 604]

Cefixime (Suprax) [See Table 7–10, p 604]

Cefmetazole (Zefazone) [See Table 7–9, p 603]

Cefonicid (Monocid) [See Table 7–9, p 603]

Cefoperazone (Cefobid) [See Table 7–10, p 604]

Cefotaxime (Claforan) [See Table 7–10, p 604]

Cefotetan (Cefotan) [See Table 7–9, p 603]

Cefoxitin (Mefoxin) [See Table 7–9, p 603]

Cefpodoxime (Vantin) [See Table 7–10, p 604]

Cefprozil (Cefzil) [See Table 7–9, p 603]

Ceftazidime (Fortaz, Ceptaz, Tazidime, Tazicef) [See Table 7–10, p 604]

Ceftibuten (Cedax) [See Table 7–10, p 604]

Ceftizoxime (Cefizox) [See Table 7–10, p 604]

Ceftriaxone (Rocephin) [See Table 7–10, p 604]

Cefuroxime (Ceftin, Zinacef) [See Table 7–9, p 603]

Celecoxib (Celebrex) [See Table 7–11, pp 605-6]

Cephalexin (Keflex, Keftab) [See Table 7–8, p 603]

Cephapirin (Cefadyl) [See Table 7–8, p 603]

Cephradine (Velosef) [See Table 7–8, p 603]

Cetirizine (Zyrtec)

INDICATIONS: Treatment of allergic rhinitis and chronic urticaria.
ACTIONS: Non-sedating antihistamine.
DOSAGE: 10 mg/d.
SUPPLIED: Tablets 5, 10 mg; syrup 5 mg/5 mL.

Cevimeline HCl (Evoxac)

INDICATIONS: Treatment of symptoms of dry mouth in patients with Sjögren's syndrome.
ACTIONS: A cholinergic agonist.
DOSAGE: 30 mg PO tid.
SUPPLIED: Capsules 30 mg.

NOTES: May cause excessive sweating, salivation, rhinitis, nausea, visual disturbances, and alteration in cardiac conduction and/or heart rate. Use with caution in patients with a history of nephrolithiasis or cholelithiasis. Contraindicated in patients with uncontrolled asthma.

Charcoal, Activated (Superchar, Actidose, Liqui-Char)

INDICATIONS: Emergency treatment in poisoning by most drugs and chemicals.
ACTIONS: Adsorbent detoxicant.
DOSAGE: *Acute intoxication:* 30–100 g/dose.
Gastrointestinal dialysis: 25–50 g Q 4–6 hr.
SUPPLIED: Powder, liquid.
NOTES: Administer with a cathartic; some liquid dosage forms are in sorbitol base. Protect airway in lethargic or comatose patient.

Chlorambucil (Leukeran)

INDICATIONS: Chronic lymphocytic leukemia, Hodgkin's disease, Waldenström's macroglobulinemia.
ACTIONS: Alkylating agent.
DOSAGE: Refer to specific protocol.
NOTES: Toxicity includes myelosuppression, CNS stimulation, nausea and vomiting, drug fever, skin rash, chromosomal damage that can result in secondary leukemias, alveolar dysplasia, and pulmonary fibrosis.

Chloramphenicol (Chloromycetin)

INDICATIONS: Serious infections caused by gram-positive and gram-negative aerobic and anaerobic bacteria. Can be used to treat *Enterococcus* resistant to ampicillin and vancomycin.
ACTION: Interferes with protein synthesis.
DOSAGE: 50–100 mg/kg/d IV in four divided doses.
SUPPLIED: Powder for injection.
NOTES AND CAUTION: Aplastic anemia has been associated with the use of this drug; monitor hematology lab results closely. Reduce dosage with hepatic impairment. *Pseudomonas aeruginosa* is almost universally resistant.

Chloramphenicol, Ophthalmic (Chloromycetin Ophthalmic) [See Table 7–12, pp 607-9]

Chlordiazepoxide (Librium) [C]

INDICATIONS: Anxiety, tension, alcohol withdrawal, and preoperative apprehension.
ACTIONS: Benzodiazepine; antianxiety agent.
DOSAGE: *Mild anxiety:* 5–10 mg PO tid–qid or prn.
Severe anxiety: 25–50 mg IM, IV, or PO 3–4 times a day or prn.
Alcohol withdrawal: 50–100 mg IM or IV; repeat in 2–4 hr if needed, up to 300 mg in 24 hr; gradually taper the daily dosage.
SUPPLIED: Capsules 5 mg, 10 mg, 25 mg; tablets 10 mg, 25 mg; injection 100 mg.
NOTES: Reduce dose in the elderly; absorption of IM doses can be erratic.

Chlorothiazide (Diuril)

INDICATIONS: Hypertension, edema, congestive heart failure.
ACTIONS: Thiazide diuretic.
DOSAGE: 500 mg–1.0 g PO or IV q day–bid.
SUPPLIED: Tablets 250 mg, 500 mg; suspension 250 mg/5 mL; injection 500 mg/vial.
NOTES: Contraindicated in anuria.

Chlorpheniramine (Chlor-Trimeton, Others)

INDICATIONS: Allergic reactions.
ACTIONS: Antihistamine.
DOSAGE: 4 mg PO or IV Q 4–6 hr or 8–12 mg PO bid of sustained release.
SUPPLIED: Tablets 4 mg; chewable tablets 2 mg; tablets SR 8 mg, 12 mg; syrup 2 mg/5 mL; injection 10 mg/mL, 100 mg/mL.
NOTES: Anticholinergic side effects and sedation are common.

Chlorpromazine (Thorazine)

INDICATIONS: Psychotic disorders, apprehension, intractable hiccups, control of nausea and vomiting.
ACTIONS: Phenothiazine antipsychotic, antiemetic.
DOSAGE: *Acute anxiety, agitation:* 10–25 mg PO or PR bid–tid.
Severe symptoms: 25 mg IM, can repeat in 1 hour; then 25–50 mg PO or PR tid.
Hiccups: 25–50 mg PO bid–tid.
SUPPLIED: Tablets 10 mg, 25 mg, 50 mg, 100 mg, 200 mg; Capsules sustained-release 30 mg, 75 mg, 150 mg, 200 mg, 300 mg; syrup 10 mg/5 mL; concentrate 30 mg/mL, 100 mg/mL; suppositories 25 mg, 100 mg; injection 25 mg/mL.
NOTES: Beware of extrapyramidal side effects, and sedation; drug has alpha-adrenergic blocking properties.

Chlorpropamide (Diabinese) [See Table 7–13, p 610]

Chlorthalidone (Hygroton, Others)

INDICATIONS: Hypertension, edema associated with congestive heart failure.
ACTIONS: Thiazide diuretic.
DOSAGE: 50–100 mg PO q day.
SUPPLIED: Tablets 15 mg, 25 mg, 50 mg, 100 mg.
NOTES: Contraindicated in anuric patients.

Chlorzoxazone (Paraflex, Parafon Forte DSC, Others)

INDICATIONS: Adjunct to rest and physical therapy for the relief of discomfort associated with acute, painful musculoskeletal conditions.
ACTIONS: Centrally acting skeletal muscle relaxant.
DOSAGE: 250–500 mg PO tid–qid.
SUPPLIED: Tablets 250 mg, 500 mg; caplets 250 mg, 500 mg.

Cholecalciferol [Vitamin D_3] (Delta D)

INDICATIONS: Dietary supplement for treatment of vitamin D deficiency.
ACTIONS: Enhances intestinal calcium absorption.
DOSAGE: 400–1000 IU PO daily.
SUPPLIED: Tablets 400, 1000 IU.
NOTES: 1 mg of cholecalciferol = 40,000 IU of vitamin D activity.

Cholestyramine (Questran)

INDICATIONS: Adjunctive therapy for the reduction of serum cholesterol in patients with primary hypercholesterolemia; relief of pruritus associated with partial biliary obstruction.
ACTIONS: Binds bile acids in the intestine to form insoluble complexes.
DOSAGE: Individualize the dose; 4 g q day–bid (increase to max 24 g/d and 6 doses per day).
SUPPLIED: 4 g of cholestyramine resin/9 g of powder; *With aspartame:* 4 g resin/5 g of powder.
NOTES: Mix 4 g of cholestyramine in 2–6 oz of noncarbonated beverage; take other medications 1–2 hr before or 6 hr after cholestyramine.

Ciclopirox (Loprox)

INDICATIONS: Tinea pedis, tinea cruris, tinea corporis, cutaneous candidiasis, tinea versicolor.
ACTIONS: Antifungal antibiotic.
DOSAGE: *Adults and children younger than 10 years:* massage into affected area bid.
SUPPLIED: Cream 1%, gel 1%, lotion 1%.

Cidofovir (Vistide)

INDICATIONS: Treatment of cytomegalovirus retinitis.
ACTIONS: Selective inhibition of viral DNA synthesis.
DOSAGE:

- Treatment: 5 mg/kg IV once a week for 2 weeks, administered with probenecid.
- Maintenance: 5 mg/kg IV once every two weeks, administered with probenecid.

- Probenecid: 2 g PO 3 hours prior to cidofovir, and then 1 g PO at 2 hours and 8 hours after cidofovir.

SUPPLIED: Injection 75 mg/mL.
NOTES: Dose adjust in renal impairment, hydrate patient with normal saline prior to each infusion; causes renal toxicity.

Cilostazol (Pletal)

INDICATIONS: Reduction of symptoms of intermittent claudication.
ACTIONS: Phosphodiesterase III inhibitor. Increases cAMP in platelets and blood vessels, leading to inhibition of platelet aggregation and vasodilation.
DOSAGE: 100 mg PO bid, taken ½ hour before or 2 hours after breakfast and dinner.
SUPPLIED: Tablets 50 mg, 100 mg.
NOTES: Contraindicated in patients with congestive heart failure of any severity. Dosage adjustment may be necessary when used in conjunction with other drugs known to inhibit CYP3A4 and CYP2C19.

Cimetidine (Tagamet, Others)

INDICATIONS: Duodenal ulcer; ulcer prophylaxis in hypersecretory states such as trauma, burns, surgery; and gastroesophageal reflux disease (GERD).
ACTIONS: Histamine-2 receptor antagonist.
DOSAGE: *Active ulcer:* 2400 mg/d IV continuous infusion or 300 mg IV Q 6 hr; 400 mg PO bid or 800 mg Q HS; *Maintenance therapy:* 400 mg PO Q HS.
GERD: 800 mg PO bid; maintenance 800 mg PO HS.
SUPPLIED: Tablets 200 mg, 300 mg, 400 mg, 800 mg; liquid 300 mg/5 mL; injection 300 mg/2 mL.
NOTES: Extend dosing interval with renal insufficiency; decrease dose in the elderly. Many drug interactions.

Ciprofloxacin, Ophthalmic (Ciloxan) [See Table 7–12, pp 607-9]

Ciprofloxacin (Cipro)

INDICATIONS: Broad-spectrum activity against a variety of gram-positive and gram-negative aerobic bacteria.
ACTIONS: Quinolone antibiotic; inhibits DNA gyrase.
DOSAGE: 250–750 mg PO Q 12 hr or 200–400 mg IV Q 12 hr.
SUPPLIED: Tablets 100 mg, 250 mg, 500 mg, 750 mg; suspension 5 g/100 mL, 10 g/100 mL; injection 200 mg, 400 mg.
NOTES: Little activity against streptococci; drug interactions with theophylline, caffeine, sucralfate, warfarin, and antacids; nausea, vomiting, and abdominal discomfort are common side effects; take on empty stomach; *contraindicated in pregnancy.*

Ciprofloxacin, Otic (Cipro HC Otic)

INDICATIONS: Otitis externa.
ACTIONS: Quinolone antibiotic; inhibits DNA gyrase.
DOSAGE: 1–2 ggt in ear/s bid for 7 days.
SUPPLIED: Suspension ciprofloxacin 0.2% and hydrocortisone 1%.

Cisplatin (Platinol AQ)

INDICATIONS: Testicular cancers, small cell and non-small cell lung cancers, bladder cancer, ovarian cancer, breast cancer, penile cancer, osteosarcoma, head and neck cancer, pediatric brain tumors.
ACTIONS: DNA binding; intra-strand cross-linking; formation of DNA adducts.
DOSAGE: Refer to specific protocols.
NOTES: Toxicity includes allergic reactions, nausea and vomiting, nephrotoxicity (exacerbated by concurrent administration of other nephrotoxic drugs and minimized by saline infusion and mannitol diuresis), high-frequency hearing loss in approximately 30%, peripheral "stocking-glove"-type neuropathy, cardiotoxicity (ST-T–wave changes), hypomagnesemia, mild myelosuppression, and hepatotoxicity. Renal impairment is dose-related and cumulative.

Citalopram (Celexa)

INDICATIONS: Treatment of depression.
ACTIONS: Selective serotonin reuptake inhibitor.
DOSAGE: Initial 20 mg per day, may be increased to 40 mg per day.
SUPPLIED: Tablets 20 mg, 40 mg.
NOTES: May cause insomnia or hypersomnia and sexual dysfunction.

Cladribine (Leustatin)

INDICATIONS: Hairy cell leukemia (HCL).
ACTIONS: Induces DNA strand breakage and interference with DNA repair enzymes and DNA synthesis.
DOSAGE: Refer to specific protocols.
NOTES: Toxicity includes myelosuppression; T-lymphocyte suppression may be prolonged (26–34 weeks). Fever occurs in 46% (probably related to tumor lysis); infections are common (especially at lung and IV catheter sites); rash is common (50%) in patients treated for HCL.

Clarithromycin (Biaxin)

INDICATIONS: Treatment of upper and lower respiratory tract infections, skin and skin structure infections, *Helicobacter pylori* infections, and infections caused by non-tuberculosis (atypical) *Mycobacterium*. Prevention of *Mycobacterium avium* complex (MAC) infections in HIV-infected individuals.
ACTIONS: Macrolide antibiotic; inhibits protein synthesis.
DOSAGE: 250–500 mg PO bid or 1000 mg (2 × 500 mg ER tab) q day.
Mycobacterium: 500–1000 mg PO bid.
SUPPLIED: Tablets 250 mg, 500 mg; suspension 125 mg/5 mL, 250 mg/5 mL; extended-release tablet 500 mg.
NOTES: Increases theophylline and carbamazepine levels; avoid concurrent use with cisapride; causes metallic taste.

Clemastine Fumarate (Tavist)

INDICATIONS: Allergic rhinitis.
ACTIONS: Antihistamine.
DOSAGE: 1.34 mg bid to 2.68 mg tid, maximum 8.04 mg/d.
SUPPLIED: Tablets 1.34 mg, 2.68 mg; syrup 0.67 mg/5 mL.

Clindamycin (Cleocin, Cleocin-T)

INDICATIONS: Susceptible strains of streptococci, pneumococci, staphylococci, and gram-positive and gram-negative anaerobes; no activity against gram-negative aerobes; bacterial vaginosis; topical for severe acne and vaginal infections.
ACTIONS: Bacteriostatic; interferes with protein synthesis.
DOSAGE: *Oral:* 150–450 mg PO qid.
Intravenous: 300–600 mg IV Q 6 hr or 900 mg IV Q 8 hr.
Vaginal: 1 applicatorful Q HS for 7 days.
Topical: Apply 1% gel, lotion, or solution bid.
SUPPLIED: Capsules 75 mg, 150 mg, 300 mg; suspension 75 mg/5 mL; injection 300 mg/2 mL; vaginal cream 2%.
NOTES: Beware of diarrhea that may represent pseudomembranous colitis caused by *Clostridium difficile.*

Clofazimine (Lamprene)

INDICATIONS: Treatment of leprosy, and as part of combination therapy for *Mycobacterium avium* complex in HIV patients.
ACTIONS: Bactericidal, inhibits DNA synthesis.
DOSAGE: 100–300 mg PO Q day.
SUPPLIED: Capsules 50 mg, 100 mg.
NOTES: To be taken with meals. May change skin pigmentation to pink or brownish-black; may cause skin dryness and GI intolerance.

Clonazepam (Klonopin) [C]

INDICATIONS: Lennox-Gastaut syndrome, akinetic and myoclonic seizures, absence seizures.
ACTIONS: Benzodiazepine anticonvulsant.
DOSAGE: 1.5 mg/d PO in 3 divided doses; increase by 0.5–1.0 mg/d every 3 days prn up to 20 mg/d.
SUPPLIED: Tablets 0.5 mg, 1.0 mg, 2.0 mg.
NOTES: CNS side effects including sedation.

Clonidine, Oral (Catapres)

INDICATIONS: Hypertension; opioid, alcohol, and tobacco withdrawal.
ACTIONS: Centrally acting alpha-adrenergic stimulant.
DOSAGE: 0.1 mg PO bid adjusted daily by 0.1- to 0.2-mg increments (maximum 2.4 mg/d).
SUPPLIED: Tablets 0.1 mg, 0.2 mg, 0.3 mg.
NOTES: Dry mouth, drowsiness, sedation occur frequently. More effective for hypertension when combined with diuretics; rebound hypertension can occur with abrupt cessation of doses above 0.2 mg bid.

Clonidine, Transdermal (Catapres TTS)

INDICATIONS: Hypertension.
ACTIONS: Centrally acting alpha-adrenergic stimulant.
DOSAGE: Apply one patch every 7 days to a hairless area on the upper arm or torso; titrate according to individual therapeutic requirements.
SUPPLIED: TTS-1, TTS-2, TTS-3 (programmed to deliver 0.1 mg, 0.2 mg, 0.3 mg respectively of clonidine per day, for 1 week).
NOTES: Doses > two TTS-3 are usually not associated with increased efficacy. May take 2–3 days before steady-state levels are achieved.

Clopidogrel (Plavix)

INDICATIONS: Reduction of atherosclerotic events.
ACTIONS: Inhibits platelet aggregation.
DOSAGE: 75 mg once daily.
SUPPLIED: Tablet 75 mg.
NOTES: Prolongs bleeding time, use with caution in persons at risk of bleeding from trauma, etc.

Clorazepate (Tranxene) [C]

INDICATIONS: Acute anxiety disorders, acute alcohol withdrawal symptoms, adjunctive therapy in partial seizures.
ACTIONS: Benzodiazepine; antianxiety agent.
DOSAGE: 15–60 mg/d PO in single or divided doses.

Elderly and debilitated patients: Initiate therapy at 7.5–15 mg/d in divided doses.

Alcohol withdrawal: Day 1: Initial dose 30 mg; followed by 30–60 mg in divided doses; Day 2: 45–90 mg in divided doses; Day 3: 22.5–45 mg in divided doses; Day 4: 15–30 mg in divided doses.

SUPPLIED: Tablets 3.75 mg, 7.5 mg, 11.25 mg, 15 mg, 22.5 mg.
NOTES: Monitor patients with renal and hepatic impairment, since drug may accumulate; CNS depressant effects.

Clotrimazole (Lotrimin, Mycelex)

INDICATIONS: Treatment of candidiasis and tinea infections.
ACTIONS: Antifungal agent; alters cell wall permeability.
DOSAGE: *Oral:* One troche dissolved slowly in the mouth 5 times a day for 14 days.

Vaginal:

- Cream: 1 applicator full Q HS for 7–14 days OR
- Tablets: 100 mg vaginally Q HS for 7 days; or 200 mg (2 tablets) vaginally Q HS for 3 days; or 500-mg tablet vaginally HS × 1.

Topical: Apply twice daily for 10–14 days.

SUPPLIED: Cream 1%; solution 1%; lotion 1%; troche 10 mg; vaginal tablets 100 mg, 500 mg; vaginal cream 1%.
NOTES: Oral prophylaxis commonly used in immunosuppressed patients.

Clotrimazole and Betamethasone (Lotrisone)

INDICATIONS: Fungal skin infections.
ACTIONS: Imidazole antifungal and anti-inflammatory.
DOSAGE: Apply and gently massage into the area twice a day from 2 to 4 weeks.
SUPPLIED: Cream 15 g, 45 g.

Cloxacillin (Cloxapen, Tegopen) [See Table 7–5, p. 600]

Clozapine (Clozaril)

INDICATIONS: Severe schizophrenia that does not respond to standard therapy.
ACTIONS: Tricyclic "atypical" antipsychotic agent.
DOSAGE: Initial dose 25 mg q day–bid; increase dose to 300–450 mg/d over 2 weeks. Maintain the patient at the lowest dose possible.
SUPPLIED: Tablets 25 mg, 100 mg.
NOTES: Monitor blood counts frequently (weekly for the first 6 months, then every other week) because of the risk of agranulocytosis. May also cause drowsiness and seizures.

Cocaine [C]

INDICATIONS: Topical anesthetic for mucous membranes.
ACTIONS: Narcotic analgesic, local vasoconstrictor.
DOSAGE: Apply topically the lowest amount of topical solution that provides relief; 1 mg/kg max.
SUPPLIED: Topical solution and viscous preparations 4,10% powder, soluble tablet (135 mg) for solution.

Codeine [C]

INDICATIONS: Mild to moderate pain; symptomatic relief of cough.
ACTIONS: Narcotic analgesic; depresses the cough reflex.
DOSAGE: *Analgesic:* 15–60 mg PO or IM qid prn.
Antitussive: 10–20 mg PO Q 4 hr prn; maximum 120 mg/d.
SUPPLIED: Tablets 15 mg, 30 mg, 60 mg; solution 15 mg/5 mL; injection 30 mg/mL, 60 mg/mL.
NOTES: Most often used in combination with acetaminophen for pain or with agents such as terpin hydrate as an antitussive; 120 mg IM equivalent to 10 mg of morphine IM.

Colchicine

INDICATIONS: Treatment of acute gout.
ACTIONS: Inhibits migration of leukocytes; reduces production of lactic acid by leukocytes.
DOSAGE: *Acute gout:* Initial dose 0.5–1.2 mg PO, then 0.5–0.6 mg every 1–2 hr until relief or GI side effects develop (maximum 8 mg/d). Do not repeat for 3 days.
IV: 1–3 mg, then 0.5 mg Q 6 hr until relief (max 4 mg/d). Do not repeat for 7 days.
Prophylaxis: PO: 0.5–0.6 mg q day or 3–4 times weekly.
SUPPLIED: Tablets 0.5 mg, 0.6 mg; injection 1 mg/2 mL.
NOTES: Use caution in elderly and patients with renal impairment. Colchicine 1–2 mg IV within 24–48 hr of an acute attack can be diagnostic and therapeutic in monoarticular arthritis.

Colesevelam (Welchol)

INDICATIONS: Reduction of LDL and total cholesterol.
ACTIONS: Bile acid sequestrant.
DOSAGE: 3 tablets PO twice daily with meals.
SUPPLIED: Tablet 625 mg.

Colestipol (Colestid)

INDICATIONS: Adjunctive therapy for the reduction of serum cholesterol in patients with primary hypercholesterolemia.
ACTIONS: Binds bile acids in the intestine to form an insoluble complex.
DOSAGE: *Granules:* 5–30 g/d divided into 2–4 doses; *Tablets:* 2–16 g/d q day–bid.

SUPPLIED: Tablets 1 g; granules.
NOTES: Do not use dry powder; mix with beverages, soups, cereals, etc.

Cortisone (Cortone) [See Table 7–2, p 597]

Cortisporin Ophthalmic [See Table 7–12, pp 607-9]

Cortisporin Otic

INDICATIONS: Treatment of superficial bacterial infections of the external auditory canal by organisms sensitive to neomycin or polymyxin; suspension may also be used in the treatment of infections in the mastoid and fenestrated cavities.
ACTIONS: Topical antibiotic combination.
DOSAGE: 4 drops instilled into external auditory canal 3–4 times daily.
SUPPLIED: Otic solution, otic suspension.
NOTES: Use suspension in cases of ruptured eardrum.

Cromolyn Sodium (Intal, Nasalcrom, Opticrom)

INDICATIONS: Adjunct to the prophylaxis of asthma; prevention of exercise-induced asthma; allergic rhinitis; ophthalmic allergic manifestations.
ACTIONS: Antiasthmatic; mast cell stabilizer.
DOSAGE: *Inhalation:* 20 mg (as powder in capsule) inhaled qid or metered-dose inhaler 2 puffs qid.
Oral: 200 mg 4 times a day 15–20 min before meals, up to 400 mg 4 times a day.
Nasal instillation: Spray once in each nostril 2–6 times daily.
Ophthalmic: 1–2 drops in each eye 4–6 times daily.
SUPPLIED: Oral concentrate 100 mg/5 mL; solution for nebulization 20 mg/2 mL; metered-dose inhaler; nasal solution 40 mg/mL; ophthalmic solution 4%.
NOTES: Has no benefit in acute situations; may require 2–4 weeks for maximal effect in perennial allergic disorders.

Cyanocobalamin (Vitamin B_{12})

INDICATIONS: Pernicious anemia and other vitamin B_{12} deficiency states.
ACTIONS: Dietary supplement of vitamin B_{12}.
DOSAGE: 100 μg IM or SC q day for 7 days, then 100 μg IM twice a week for 1 month, then 100 μg weekly for 1 month, then 1000 μg IM monthly.
SUPPLIED: Tablets 25 μg, 50 μg, 100 μg, 250 μg, 500 μg, 1000 μg; injection 30 μg/mL, 100 μg/mL, 1000 μg/mL.
NOTES: Oral absorption highly erratic, altered by many drugs and not recommended; for use with hyperalimentation.

Cyclobenzaprine (Flexeril)

INDICATIONS: Adjunct to rest and physical therapy for the relief of muscle spasm associated with acute painful musculoskeletal conditions.
ACTIONS: Centrally acting skeletal muscle relaxant; reduces tonic somatic motor activity.
DOSAGE: 10 mg PO 2–4 times per day.
SUPPLIED: Tablets 10 mg.
NOTES: Do not use for longer than 2–3 weeks; has sedative and anticholinergic properties.

Cyclophosphamide (Cytoxan, Neosar)

INDICATIONS: Hodgkin's and non-Hodgkin's lymphomas, multiple myeloma, breast cancer, ovarian cancer, mycosis fungoides, neuroblastoma, retinoblastoma, acute leukemias, small cell lung cancer, and allogeneic and autologous transplantation in high doses; severe rheumatologic disorders.
ACTIONS: Converted to acrolein and phosphoramide mustard, the active alkylating moieties.
DOSAGE: Refer to specific protocols.
NOTES: Toxicity includes myelosuppression (leukopenia and thrombocytopenia); sterile hemorrhagic cystitis, syndrome of inappropriate antidiuretic hormone (SIADH), alopecia, and anorexia; nausea and vomiting are common. Hepatotoxicity and rarely interstitial pneumonitis

may occur. Irreversible testicular atrophy may occur. Cardiotoxicity is rare. Second malignancies (bladder cancer and acute leukemias) have been reported; cumulative risk of 3.5% at 8 years, 10.7% at 12 years. Preventive measures to avoid hemorrhagic cystitis are often applied in high-dose regimens and may include continuous bladder irrigation and Mesna uroprotection.

Cyclosporine (Sandimmune, Neoral)

INDICATIONS: Prophylaxis of organ rejection in kidney, liver, heart, and bone marrow transplants in conjunction with adrenal corticosteroids.
ACTIONS: Immunosuppressant; reversible inhibition of immunocompetent lymphocytes.
DOSAGE: *Oral:* 15 mg/kg/d beginning 12 hr prior to transplant; after 2 weeks, taper the dose by 5 mg/week to 5–10 mg/kg/d.
IV: If the patient is unable to take the drug orally, give ⅓ of the oral dose IV.
SUPPLIED: Capsules 25 mg, 50 mg, 100 mg; oral solution 100 mg/mL; injection 50 mg/mL.
NOTES: May elevate blood urea nitrogen and creatinine, which may be confused with renal transplant rejection; should be administered in glass containers; has many drug interactions; Neoral and Sandimmune are not interchangeable.

Cyproheptadine (Periactin)

INDICATIONS: Allergic reactions; especially good for itching.
ACTIONS: Phenothiazine antihistamine.
DOSAGE: 4–20 mg PO divided Q 8 hr; maximum 0.5 mg/kg/d.
SUPPLIED: Tablets 4 mg; syrup 2 mg/5 mL.
NOTES: Anticholinergic side effects and drowsiness are common; may stimulate appetite in some patients.

Cytarabine [ARA-C] (Cytosar-U)

INDICATIONS: Acute leukemias, chronic myelogenous leukemia, non-Hodgkin's lymphoma, and intrathecal administration for leukemic meningitis or prophylaxis.
ACTIONS: Antimetabolite; interferes with DNA synthesis.
DOSAGE: Refer to specific protocols.
NOTES: Toxicity includes myelosuppression, nausea and vomiting, diarrhea, stomatitis, flu-like syndrome, rash of the palms and soles of the feet, and hepatic dysfunction. Toxicity of high-dose regimens (conjunctivitis) ameliorated by corticosteroid ophthalmic solution, cerebellar dysfunction, and noncardiogenic pulmonary edema.

Cytarabine Liposome (Depocyt)

INDICATIONS: Treatment of lymphomatous meningitis.
ACTIONS: Antimetabolite; interferes with DNA synthesis.
DOSAGE: 50 mg intrathecal every 14 days for 5 doses; followed by 50 mg intrathecal every 28 days for 4 doses.
SUPPLIED: Intrathecal injection 50 mg/5 mL.

Cytomegalovirus Immune Globulin [CMV-IVIG] (Cytogam)

INDICATIONS: Attenuation of primary CMV disease associated with transplantation.
ACTIONS: Provides exogenous IgG antibodies to CMV.
DOSAGE: Administered for 16 weeks post transplant; see product information for dosing schedule.
SUPPLIED: Injection 50 ± 10 mg/mL.

Dacarbazine (DTIC)

INDICATIONS: Melanoma, Hodgkin's disease, sarcoma.
ACTIONS: Alkylating agent; antimetabolite activity as a purine precursor; inhibits synthesis of protein, RNA, and especially DNA.
DOSAGE: Refer to specific protocols.
NOTES: Toxicity includes moderate myelosuppression, severe nausea and vomiting, hepatotoxicity, flu-like syndrome, hypotension with high-dose therapy, photosensitivity, alopecia, facial flushing, facial paresthesias, urticaria, and phlebitis at the injection site.

Daclizumab (Zenapax)

INDICATIONS: Prevention of acute organ rejection.
ACTIONS: IL-2 receptor antagonists.
DOSAGE: 1 mg/kg IV per dose; first dose prior to transplant followed by 4 doses 14 days apart post transplant.
SUPPLIED: Injection 5 mg/mL.

Dactinomycin (Cosmegen)

INDICATIONS: Choriocarcinoma, Wilms' tumor, Kaposi's sarcoma, Ewing's sarcoma, rhabdomyosarcoma, and testicular cancer.
ACTIONS: DNA intercalating agent.
DOSAGE: Refer to specific protocols.
NOTES: Toxicity includes myelosuppression, immunosuppression, nausea and vomiting, alopecia, acneiform skin changes and hyperpigmentation, radiation recall phenomenon, phlebitis and tissue damage with extravascular extravasation, and hepatotoxicity.

Dalfopristin/Quinupristin (Synercid)

INDICATIONS: Treatment of infections caused by vancomycin-resistant *Enterococcus faecium* (VREF); complicated skin and skin structure infections caused by *Staphylococcus aureus* and *Streptococcus pyogenes.*
ACTIONS: A streptogramin antimicrobial agent. Acts on the bacterial ribosome to inhibit protein synthesis.
DOSAGE: 7.5 mg/kg IV Q 8–12 hours (administer over 60 minutes).
SUPPLIED: 500 mg (150 mg quinupristin and 350 mg dalfopristin) per 10-mL vial.
NOTES: Significantly inhibits CYP3A4 isoenzymes. Use with caution when coadministered with drugs metabolized by this isoenzyme (eg, cyclosporine). May cause venous irritation, elevation in bilirubin, and arthralgias/myalgias.

Dalteparin (Fragmin)

INDICATIONS: Treatment of unstable angina, non-Q-wave MI, prevention of ischemic complications due to clot formation in patients on concurrent aspirin, prevention of deep venous thrombosis (DVT) following surgery.
ACTIONS: Low molecular weight heparin.
DOSAGE: *Angina/MI:* 120 IU/kg (maximum 10,000 IU) SC Q 12 hr with aspirin.
DVT prophylaxis: 2500–5000 IU SC 1–2 hours prior to surgery, then once daily for 5–10 days.
Systemic anticoagulation: 200 IU/kg SC once daily or 100 IU/kg SC twice daily.
SUPPLIED: Injection 2500 IU (16 mg/0.2 mL), 5000 IU (32 mg/0.2 mL), 10,000 (64 mg/mL).
NOTES: Predictable antithrombotic effects eliminate need for laboratory monitoring.

Danaparoid (Orgaron)

INDICATIONS: Prophylaxis of deep venous thrombosis (DVT) which may lead to PE, in patients undergoing hip replacement surgery.
ACTIONS: Antithrombotic agent that acts by inhibition of factor Xa and IIa.
DOSAGE: 750 anti-Xa units bid administered by SC injection beginning 1–4 hours preoperatively and starting no sooner than 2 hours post surgery.
SUPPLIED: Ampoules and prefilled syringes 0.6 mL (750 anti-Xa units).
NOTES: aPTT monitoring is not necessary. Increased risk of epidural or spinal hematoma in patients receiving epidural/spinal anesthesia.

Dantrolene (Dantrium)

INDICATIONS: Treatment of clinical spasticity resulting from upper motor neuron disorders such as spinal cord injuries, strokes, cerebral palsy, or multiple sclerosis; treatment of malignant hyperthermic crisis.
ACTIONS: Skeletal muscle relaxant.
DOSAGE: *Spasticity:* Initial dose 25 mg PO q day; titrate to effect by 25 mg up to a maximum dose of 100 mg PO qid prn.

Malignant hyperthermia:

- Treatment: Continuous rapid IV push beginning at 1 mg/kg until symptoms subside or 10 mg/kg is reached.
- Post-crisis follow-up: 4–8 mg/kg/d in 3–4 divided doses for 1–3 days to prevent recurrence.

SUPPLIED: Capsules 25 mg, 50 mg, 100 mg; powder for injection 20 mg per vial.
NOTES: Monitor ALT and AST closely.

Dapsone (Avlosulfon)

INDICATIONS: Treatment and prevention of *P carinii* pneumonia; toxoplasmosis prophylaxis; leprosy.
ACTIONS: Unknown; bactericidal.
DOSAGE: 50–100 mg PO q day.
SUPPLIED: Tablets 25 mg, 100 mg.
NOTES: Absorption is enhanced by an acidic environment.

Daunorubicin (Daunomycin, Cerubidine)

INDICATIONS: Acute leukemias.
ACTIONS: DNA intercalating agent; inhibits topoisomerase II; generates oxygen free radicals.
DOSAGE: Refer to specific protocols.
NOTES: Toxicity includes myelosuppression, mucositis, nausea and vomiting, alopecia, radiation recall phenomenon, hepatotoxicity (hyperbilirubinemia), tissue necrosis on extravascular extravasation, and cardiotoxicity (1–2% risk of congestive heart failure with a cumulative dose of 550 mg/m^2).

Delavirdine (Rescriptor)

INDICATIONS: Treatment of HIV infection.
ACTIONS: Non-nucleoside reverse transcriptase inhibitor.
DOSAGE: 400 mg PO tid.
SUPPLIED: Tablets 100 mg.
NOTES: Inhibits cytochrome P-450 enzymes. Numerous drug interactions.

Demecarium (Humorsol) [See Table 7–12, pp 607-9]

Demeclocycline (Declomycin)

INDICATIONS: Treatment of syndrome of inappropriate antidiuretic hormone (SIADH).
ACTIONS: Antagonizes the action of ADH on renal tubules.
DOSAGE: 300–600 mg PO Q 12 hr.
SUPPLIED: Capsules 150 mg; tablets 150 mg, 300 mg.
NOTES: Reduce dose in renal failure. May cause diabetes insipidus.

Desipramine (Norpramin)

INDICATIONS: Treatment of endogenous depression, chronic pain, peripheral neuropathy.
ACTIONS: Tricyclic antidepressant; increases synaptic concentration of serotonin or norepinephrine in the CNS.
DOSAGE: 25–200 mg/d in single or divided doses; usually as a single HS dose (maximum 300 mg/d).
SUPPLIED: Tablets 10 mg, 25 mg, 50 mg, 75 mg, 100 mg, 150 mg; capsules 25 mg, 50 mg.
NOTES: Many anticholinergic side effects, including blurred vision, urinary retention, and dry mouth.

Desmopressin (DDAVP, Stimate)

INDICATIONS: Diabetes insipidus (intranasal and parenteral administration); bleeding due to hemophilia A, Type I von Willebrand's disease, and uremia (parenteral administration).
ACTIONS: Synthetic analogue of vasopressin, a naturally occurring human antidiuretic hormone; increases factor VIII.
DOSAGE: *Diabetes insipidus:*

- Intranasal 0.1–0.4 mL (10–40 μg) daily in 2–3 divided doses.
- Parenteral 0.5–1 mL (2–4 μg) daily in 2 divided doses. When converting from intranasal to parenteral dosing, use 1/10th of intranasal dose.

Hemophilia A, von Willebrand's disease (Type I), and uremia: 0.3 μg/kg diluted to 50 mL with NSS infused slowly over 15–30 min.

SUPPLIED: Tablets 0.1 mg, 0.2 mg; injection 4 μg/mL; nasal solution 0.1 mg/mL, 1.5 mg/mL.

NOTES: In very young and old patients, adjust fluid intake to avoid water intoxication and hyponatremia.

Dexamethasone (Decadron) [See Table 7–2, p 597]

Dexamethasone, Nasal (Dexacort Phosphate Turbinaire)

INDICATIONS: Chronic nasal inflammation and/or allergic rhinitis.

ACTIONS: Anti-inflammatory corticosteroid.

DOSAGE: 2 sprays per nostril bid–tid, max 12 sprays per day.

SUPPLIED: Aerosol, 84 μg/activation.

Dexamethasone Ophthalmic (AK-DEX Ophthalmic, Decadron Ophthalmic, Others) [See Table 7–12, pp 607-9]

Dexpanthenol (Ilopan-Choline Oral, Ilopan)

INDICATIONS: Minimize paralytic ileus, treat postoperative distension.

ACTIONS: Cholinergic agent.

DOSAGE: *Relief of gas:* 2–3 tablets PO tid.

Prevention of postoperative ileus: 250–500 mg IM stat, repeat in 2 hours, then Q 6 hr as needed.

Ileus: IM: 500 mg stat, repeat in 2 hours, followed by doses Q 6 hr, if needed.

SUPPLIED: Injection; tablets 50 mg; cream.

NOTES: Do not use if obstruction is suspected.

Dexrazoxane (Zinecard)

INDICATIONS: Prevention of anthracycline-induced cardiomyopathy in metastatic breast cancer therapy.

ACTIONS: Chelates heavy metals; binds intracellular iron and prevents anthracycline-induced free radical generation.

DOSAGE: 10:1 ratio of dexrazoxane to doxorubicin, 30 min prior to each dose of anthracycline.

SUPPLIED: Injection 10 mg/mL.

NOTES: Toxicity includes myelosuppression (especially leukopenia), fever, infection, stomatitis, alopecia, diarrhea, and nausea and vomiting. Mild elevations of hepatic transaminases and local pain at the site of injection occur less frequently.

Dextran 40 (Rheomacrodex)

INDICATIONS: Plasma expander for adjunctive therapy in shock, prophylaxis of deep venous thrombosis (DVT) and thromboembolism, and adjunct in peripheral vascular surgery.

ACTIONS: Expands plasma volume; decreases blood viscosity.

DOSAGE: *Shock:* 10 mL/kg infused rapidly with a maximum dose of 20 mL/kg in the first 24 hr; total daily dosage beyond 24 hr should not exceed 10 mL/kg and should be discontinued after 5 days.

Prophylaxis of DVT and thromboembolism: 10 mL/kg IV on the day of surgery followed by 500 mL daily for 2–3 days, then 500 mL IV every 2–3 days based on the patient's risk factors for up to 2 weeks.

SUPPLIED: 10% dextran 40 in 0.9% sodium chloride or in 5% dextrose.

NOTES: Observe for hypersensitivity reactions; monitor renal function and electrolytes.

Dextromethorphan (Mediquell, Benylin DM)

INDICATIONS: To control nonproductive cough.

ACTIONS: Depresses the cough center in the medulla.

DOSAGE: 10–30 mg PO Q 4–8 hr prn (max 120 mg/24 hr).
SUPPLIED: Capsules 30 mg; lozenges 2.5 mg/mL, 5 mg/mL, 7.5 mg/mL, 15 mg/mL; syrup 15 mg/15 mL, 10 mg/5 mL; liquid 10 mg/15 mL, 3.5 mg/5 mL, 7.5 mg/5 mL, 15 mg per 5 mL; sustained-action liquid 30 mg/5 mL.
NOTES: May be found in combination products with guaifenesin.

Dezocine (Dalgan)

INDICATIONS: Relief of moderate to severe pain.
ACTIONS: Narcotic agonist-antagonist.
DOSAGE: 5–20 mg IM or 2.5–10 mg IV Q 2–4 hr prn.
SUPPLIED: Injection 5 mg/mL, 10 mg/mL, 15 mg/mL.
NOTES: May cause withdrawal in patients dependent on narcotics. Not recommended for patients younger than 18 years.

Diazepam (Valium, Others) [C]

INDICATIONS: Anxiety, alcohol withdrawal, muscle spasm, status epilepticus, panic disorders, amnesia, and preoperative sedation.
ACTIONS: Benzodiazepine.
DOSAGE:

- Status epilepticus: 5–10 mg every 10–20 min to a maximum dose of 30 mg in an 8-hr period.
- Anxiety, muscle spasm: 2–10 mg PO bid–qid or IM/IV Q 3–4 hr prn.
- Preoperative: 5–10 mg PO or IM 20–30 min before procedure; can be given IV just prior to procedure.
- Alcohol withdrawal: Initial dose 2–5 mg IV, then 5–10 mg every 5–10 min, not to exceed 100 mg in 1 hr. May require up to 1000 mg in a 24-hr period for severe withdrawal symptoms. Titrate to agitation; avoid excessive sedation; may lead to aspiration and/or respiratory arrest.

SUPPLIED: Tablets 2 mg, 5 mg, 10 mg; solution 1 mg/mL, 5 mg/mL; injection 5 mg/mL; gel for rectal delivery 5 mg/mL.
NOTES: Do not exceed 5 mg/min IV, as respiratory arrest can occur; absorption of IM dose may be erratic.

Diazoxide (Hyperstat, Proglycem)

INDICATIONS: Management of hypoglycemia caused by hyperinsulinism.
ACTIONS: Inhibits pancreatic insulin release.
DOSAGE: 3–8 mg/kg/24 hr PO divided Q 8–12 hr.
SUPPLIED: Injection 15 mg/mL; capsules 50 mg; oral suspension 50 mg/mL.
NOTES: Sodium retention and hyperglycemia frequently occur; possible thiazide diuretic cross-hypersensitivity; cannot be titrated.

Dibucaine (Nupercainal)

INDICATIONS: Hemorrhoids and minor skin conditions.
ACTIONS: Topical anesthetic.
DOSAGE: Insert into rectum with applicator bid and after each bowel movement; apply sparingly to skin.
SUPPLIED: Ointment with rectal applicator 1%; cream 0.5%.

Diclofenac (Cataflam, Voltaren) [See Table 7–11, pp 605-6, and Table 7–12, pp 607-9]

Dicloxacillin (Dynapen, Dycill) [See Table 7–5, p 600]

Dicyclomine (Bentyl)

INDICATIONS: Treatment of functional irritable bowel syndromes.
ACTIONS: Smooth muscle relaxant.
DOSAGE: 20 mg PO qid; titrate to a maximum dose of 160 mg/d or 20 mg IM Q 6 hr.

SUPPLIED: Capsules 10 mg, 20 mg; tablets 20 mg; syrup 10 mg/5 mL; injection 10 mg/mL.
NOTES: Anticholinergic side effects may limit dose.

Didanosine [ddI] (Videx)

INDICATIONS: Treatment of HIV infection in patients who are zidovudine-intolerant.
ACTIONS: Nucleoside antiretroviral agent.
DOSAGE:

- ≥ 60 kg: 400 mg PO q day or 200 mg PO bid.
- < 60 kg: 250 mg PO q day or 125 mg PO bid.

SUPPLIED: Delayed-release capsules 125 mg, 200 mg, 250 mg, 400 mg; chewable tablets 25 mg, 50 mg, 100 mg, 150 mg, 200 mg; powder packets 100 mg, 167 mg, 250 mg; powder for solution 2 g, 4 g.
NOTES: Reconstitute powder with water; side effects include pancreatitis, peripheral neuropathy, diarrhea, and headache; take 2 tablets for each administration. Dose-adjust in renal impairment; do not mix powder with fruit juice or other acidic beverages.

Diethylstilbestrol (DES)

INDICATIONS: Treatment of breast and prostate cancer.
ACTIONS: Hormone; antineoplastic.
DOSAGE: 50 mg PO tid; may be increased to 200 mg PO tid depending on patient tolerance.
SUPPLIED: Tablets 1 mg, 5 mg, 50 mg.

Diflunisal (Dolobid) [See Table 7–11, pp 605-6]

Digoxin (Lanoxin, Lanoxicaps)

INDICATIONS: Congestive heart failure, atrial fibrillation and flutter, paroxysmal atrial tachycardia.
ACTIONS: Positive inotrope, increases refractory period of AV node.
DOSAGE: *PO digitalization:* 0.50–0.75 mg PO; then 0.25 mg PO Q 6–8 hr until total dose is between 1.0 and 1.5 mg or until therapeutic effect at lower dose.
IV digitalization: 0.25–0.50 mg or IV; then 0.25 mg Q 4–6 hr until total dose of ~ 1 mg.
Daily maintenance: 0.125–0.500 mg PO, or IV q day (average daily dose 0.125–0.250 mg).
SUPPLIED: Capsules 0.05 mg, 0.1 mg, 0.2 mg; tablets 0.125 mg, 0.25 mg, 0.5 mg; elixir 0.05 mg/mL; injection 0.1 mg/mL, 0.25 mg/mL.
NOTES: Can cause heart block; low potassium can potentiate toxicity; reduce dose in renal failure. Symptoms of toxicity include nausea, vomiting, headache, fatigue, visual disturbances (yellow–green halos around lights), cardiac arrhythmias (See Table 7–16, Non-Antibiotic Drug Levels, p 613); IM injection can be painful, has erratic absorption, and should not be used. Therapeutic levels: 0.5–2.0 ng/mL.

Digoxin Immune FaB (Digibind)

INDICATIONS: Treatment of life-threatening digoxin intoxication.
ACTIONS: Antigen-binding fragments bind digoxin, inactivating it prior to elimination through the urine.
DOSAGE: Based on serum level and patient's weight; see dosing charts provided with the drug.
SUPPLIED: Injection 38 mg/vial.
NOTES: Each vial will bind approximately 0.6 mg of digoxin; in renal failure redosing may be required after several days due to breakdown of the immune complex.

Dihydroxyaluminum Sodium Carbonate (Rolaids)

INDICATIONS: Heartburn, gastroesophageal reflux, and acid indigestion.
ACTIONS: Neutralizes gastric acid.
DOSAGE: 1–2 tablets prn.
SUPPLIED: Chewable tablets, 334 mg.

Diltiazem (Cardizem, Dilacor, Tiazac)

INDICATIONS: Treatment of angina pectoris, prevention of reinfarction, hypertension, atrial fibrillation or flutter, and paroxysmal supraventricular tachycardia.
ACTIONS: Calcium channel blocking agent.
DOSAGE: *Oral:* Initial dose 30 mg PO qid; titrate to 180–360 mg/d in 3–4 divided doses prn.

- Sustained-release: 60–120 mg PO bid; titrate to effect; maximum dose 360 mg/d.
- Continuous dose: (CD or XR) 120–360 mg q day (maximum 480 mg/d).

IV: 0.25 mg/kg IV bolus over 2 min; may repeat the dose in 15 min at 0.35 mg/kg. May begin continuous infusion of 5–15 mg/hr.
SUPPLIED: Tablets 30 mg, 60 mg, 90 mg, 120 mg; SR capsules 60 mg, 90 mg, 120 mg; CD or XR capsules 120 mg, 180 mg, 240 mg, 300 mg, 360 mg, 420 mg; injection 5 mg/mL.
NOTES: Contraindicated in sick sinus syndrome, AV block, and hypotension; Cardizem CD, Dilacor XR, and Tiazac are not interchangeable.

Dimenhydrinate (Dramamine, Other)

INDICATIONS: Prevention and treatment of nausea, vomiting, dizziness, or vertigo of motion sickness.
ACTIONS: Antiemetic.
DOSAGE: 50–100 mg PO Q 4–6 hr to a maximum of 400 mg/d; 50 mg IM/IV prn.
SUPPLIED: Tablets 50 mg; chewable tablets 50 mg; liquid 12.5 mg/4 mL, 12.5 mg/5 mL, 15.62 mg/5 mL; injection 50 mg/mL.
NOTES: Anticholinergic side effects.

Dimethyl Sulfoxide [DMSO] (RIMSO 50)

INDICATIONS: Interstitial cystitis.
ACTIONS: Unknown.
DOSAGE: Intravesical, 50 mL, retain for 15 min; repeat Q 2 wk until relief.
SUPPLIED: 50% solution in 50 mL.

Diphenhydramine (Benadryl, Others)

INDICATIONS: Allergic reactions, motion sickness, potentiate narcotics, sedation, cough suppression, treatment of extrapyramidal reactions.
ACTIONS: Antihistamine, antiemetic.
DOSAGE: 25–50 mg PO, IV, or IM bid–tid.
SUPPLIED: Tablets and capsules 25 mg, 50 mg; chewable tablets 12.5 mg; elixir 12.5 mg/5 mL; syrup 12.5 mg/5 mL; liquid 6.25 mg/5 mL, 12.5 mg/5 mL; injection 50 mg/mL.
NOTES: Anticholinergic side effects, including dry mouth and urinary retention; causes sedation; increase dosing interval in moderate to severe renal failure.

Diphenoxylate With Atropine (Lomotil) [C]

INDICATIONS: Diarrhea.
ACTIONS: A constipating meperidine congener, reduces GI motility.
DOSAGE: Initial dose 5 mg PO tid–qid until under control; then 2.5–5.0 mg PO bid.
SUPPLIED: Tablets 2.5 mg diphenoxylate/0.025 mg atropine; liquid 2.5 mg diphenoxylate/0.025 mg atropine per 5 mL.
NOTES: Atropine-type side effects (headache, drowsiness).

Dipivefrin (Propine) [See Table 7–12, pp 607-9]

Dipyridamole (Persantine)

INDICATIONS: Prevention of postoperative thromboembolic disorders.
ACTIONS: Antiplatelet activity.
DOSAGE: 75–100 mg PO tid–qid.
SUPPLIED: Tablets 25 mg, 50 mg, 75 mg.
NOTES: Aspirin potentiates the antiplatelet effects. Drug may cause nausea and vomiting.

Dipyridamole and Aspirin (Aggrenox)

INDICATIONS: Prevention of stroke in patients who have had a transient ischemic attack (TIA) or ischemic stroke due to thrombosis.
ACTIONS: Antiplatelet activity.
DOSAGE: One capsule (25 mg/200 mg) PO bid.
SUPPLIED: Capsule 25 mg aspirin/200 mg extended-release dipyridamole.
NOTES: Instruct patient to swallow capsule whole and do not chew it. Not interchangeable with the individual components of aspirin and dipyridamole.

Dirithromycin (Dynabac)

INDICATIONS: Treatment of bronchitis, community-acquired pneumonia, and skin and skin structure infections.
ACTIONS: Macrolide antibiotic.
DOSAGE: 500 mg PO q day.
SUPPLIED: Tablets 250 mg.
NOTES: Absorption is enhanced when taken with food.

Disopyramide (Norpace)

INDICATIONS: Suppression and prevention of premature ventricular contractions.
ACTIONS: Class 1A antiarrhythmic.
DOSAGE: 400–800 mg/d divided Q 6 hr for regular-release products and Q 12 hr for sustained-release products.
SUPPLIED: Capsules 100 mg, 150 mg; sustained-release capsules 100 mg, 150 mg.
NOTES: Has anticholinergic side effects (urinary retention); negative inotropic properties may induce congestive heart failure; decrease dose in impaired hepatic function and renal dysfunction.

Disulfiram (Antabuse)

INDICATIONS: Alcohol consumption deterrent.
ACTIONS: Blocks oxidation of alcohol to produce unpleasant reaction when alcohol is consumed.
DOSAGE: 500 mg PO q day for 1–2 weeks, then 250 mg PO q day.
SUPPLIED: Tablets 250 mg, 500 mg.
NOTES: Instruct patients to avoid all hidden forms of alcohol (cough syrup, mouthwashes, sauces, etc); CBC and LFTs should be checked periodically.

Dobutamine (Dobutrex)

INDICATIONS: Short-term use in patients with cardiac decompensation secondary to depressed contractility.
ACTIONS: Positive inotropic agent.
DOSAGE: Continuous IV infusion of 2.5–15 μg/kg/min; rarely 40 μg/kg/min may be required; titrate according to response.
SUPPLIED: Injection 250 mg/20 mL.
NOTES: Monitor ECG for increase in heart rate, blood pressure, and increased ectopic activity; monitor pulmonary wedge pressure and cardiac output if possible.

Docetaxel (Taxotere)

INDICATIONS: Breast cancer (anthracycline-resistant), ovarian cancer, lung cancer.
ACTIONS: Antimitotic agent; promotes microtubular aggregation; semisynthetic toxoid.
DOSAGE: Refer to specific protocols.
NOTES: Toxicities include myelosuppression, neuropathy, and nausea and vomiting; fluid retention syndrome with cumulative doses of 300–400 mg/m^2 without corticosteroid preparation and post-treatment and 600–800 mg/m^2 with corticosteroid preparation. Hypersensitivity reactions may occur, but only rarely with corticosteroid preparation. Decrease dose with increased bilirubin levels.

Docusate Calcium (Surfak, Others) (See Docusate Sodium)

Docusate Potassium (Dialose) (See Docusate Sodium)

Docusate Sodium (Doss, Colace, Others)

INDICATIONS: Constipation-prone patient; adjunct to painful anorectal conditions (hemorrhoids).

ACTIONS: Softens stools.
DOSAGE: 50–500 mg PO q day.
SUPPLIED: *Calcium:* Capsules 50 mg, 240 mg.
Potassium: Capsules 100 mg, 240 mg.
Sodium: Capsules 50 mg, 100 mg, 240 mg, 250 mg; syrup 50 mg/15 mL, 60 mg/15 mL; liquid 150 mg/15 mL; solution 50 mg/mL.
NOTES: No significant side effects; no laxative action.

Dofetilide (Tikosyn)

INDICATIONS: Conversion to and maintenance of normal sinus rhythm in patients with atrial fibrillation or flutter.
ACTIONS: Class III antiarrhythmic agent.
DOSAGE: The dosage is individualized based on calculated creatinine clearance and QTc.

- Cl_{cr} > 60 mL/min: 500 μg PO bid.
- Cl_{cr} = 40–60 mL/min: 250 μg PO bid.
- Cl_{cr} = 20 – < 40 mL/min: 125 μg PO bid.

Determine QTc 2–3 hours after first dose. If increase in QTc is ≤ 15%, continue current dose. If QTc increase is > 15% or > 500 msec (550 msec in patients with ventricular conduction abnormalities), adjust dose as follows:

Starting Dose	Adjusted Dose
500 μg PO bid	250 μg PO bid
250 μg PO bid	125 μg PO bid
125 μg PO bid	125 μg PO q day

Continue to check QTc 2–3 hours after each subsequent dose (for a minimum of 3 days). If at any time QTc increases to > 500 msec (550 msec in patients with ventricular conduction abnormalities), discontinue dofetilide.
SUPPLIED: Capsules 125 μg, 250 μg, 500 μg.
NOTES: Contraindicated if baseline QTc is greater than 440 msec (500 msec in patients with ventricular conduction abnormalities) or Cl_{cr} is < 20 mL/min. Concomitant use of verapamil, cimetidine, trimethoprim, or ketoconazole is contraindicated. Avoid use with other drugs that prolong the QT interval. Class I or III antiarrhythmic agents should be withheld for at least 3 half-lives prior to dosing with dofetilide. Amiodarone level should be < 0.3 mg/L prior to dosing with dofetilide. May cause serious ventricular arrhythmias including torsades de pointes.

Dolasetron (Anzemet)

INDICATIONS: Prevention of nausea and vomiting associated with chemotherapy.
ACTIONS: 5-HT_3 receptor antagonist.
DOSAGE: *IV:* 1.8 mg/kg IV as a single dose 30 min prior to chemotherapy.
Oral: 100 mg PO as a single dose 1 hr prior to chemotherapy.
SUPPLIED: Tablets 50 mg, 100 mg; injection 20 mg/mL.
NOTES: May cause prolongation of the QT interval.

Dopamine (Intropin, Dopastat)

INDICATIONS: Short-term use in patients with cardiac decompensation secondary to decreased contractility; increases organ perfusion.
ACTIONS: Positive inotropic agent with dose-related response.

- 2–10 μg/kg/min beta-effects (increases cardiac output and renal perfusion).
- 10–20 μg/kg/min alpha-effects (peripheral vasoconstriction, pressor).
- > 20 μg/kg/min peripheral and renal vasoconstriction.

DOSAGE: 5 μg/kg/min by continuous infusion, titrated by increments of 5 μg/kg/min to a maximum of 50 μg/kg/min based on effect.
SUPPLIED: Injection 40 mg/mL, 80 mg/mL, 160 mg/mL.

NOTES: Dosage > 10 μg/kg/min may decrease renal perfusion; monitor urinary output; monitor ECG for increases in heart rate, BP, and ectopic activity; monitor pulmonary capillary wedge pressure and cardiac output if possible.

Dornase Alfa (Pulmozyme)

INDICATIONS: To reduce the frequency of respiratory infections in patients with cystic fibrosis.
ACTIONS: An enzyme that selectively cleaves DNA.
DOSAGE: 2.5 mg inhaled once daily.
SUPPLIED: Solution for inhalation, 1 mg/mL.
NOTES: To be used with recommended nebulizer.

Dorzolamide (Trusopt) [See Table 7–12, pp 607-9]

Dorzolamide and Timolol (Cosopt) [See Table 7–12, pp 607-9]

Doxazosin (Cardura)

INDICATIONS: Treatment of hypertension and benign prostatic hyperplasia.
ACTIONS: Alpha$_1$-adrenergic blocker; relaxation of bladder neck smooth muscle fibers.
DOSAGE: *Hypertension:* Initial dose 1 mg PO q day; may be increased to 16 mg PO q day.
BPH: Initial dose 1 mg PO q day, may be increased to 8 mg PO q day.
SUPPLIED: Tablets 1 mg, 2 mg, 4 mg, 8 mg.
NOTES: Doses > 4 mg increase the likelihood of excessive postural hypotension.

Doxepin (Sinequan, Adapin)

INDICATIONS: Treatment of depression, anxiety, chronic pain.
ACTIONS: Tricyclic antidepressant; increases the synaptic concentrations of serotonin or norepinephrine in the CNS.
DOSAGE: 25–150 mg PO q day, usually Q HS, but can be in divided doses.
SUPPLIED: Capsules 10 mg, 25 mg, 50 mg, 75 mg, 100 mg, 150 mg; oral concentrate 10 mg/mL.
NOTES: Anticholinergic, CNS, and cardiovascular side effects.

Doxepin Topical (Zonalon)

INDICATIONS: Short-term treatment of pruritus (atopic dermatitis or lichen simplex chronicus).
ACTIONS: Tricyclic antidepressant; increases the synaptic concentrations of serotonin or norepinephrine.
DOSAGE: Apply thin coating qid 8 days max.
SUPPLIED: Cream 5%.
NOTES: Apply to limited areas to avoid systemic toxicity (anticholinergic, CNS, and cardiovascular side effects).

Doxorubicin (Adriamycin, Rubex)

INDICATIONS: Acute leukemias, Hodgkin's and non-Hodgkin's lymphomas, breast cancer, soft tissue and osteosarcomas, Ewing's sarcoma, Wilms' tumor, neuroblastoma, bladder cancer, ovarian cancer, gastric cancer, thyroid cancer, lung cancer.
ACTIONS: DNA intercalating agent; inhibitor of DNA topoisomerases I and II.
DOSAGE: Refer to specific protocols.
NOTES: Toxicity includes myelosuppression; extravasation leads to tissue damage; venous streaking and phlebitis may occur, as well as nausea and vomiting, diarrhea, mucositis, and radiation recall phenomenon. Cardiomyopathy rare but dose-related; limit of 550 mg/m^2 cumulative dose (400 mg/m^2 if prior history of mediastinal irradiation).

Doxycycline (Vibramycin)

INDICATIONS: Broad-spectrum antibiotic, including activity against *Rickettsiae, Chlamydia,* and *Mycoplasma pneumoniae.*
ACTIONS: Tetracycline; interferes with protein synthesis.
DOSAGE: 100 mg PO Q 12 hr on the first day, then 100 mg PO q day–bid or 100 mg IV Q 12 hr.

SUPPLIED: Tablets 50 mg, 100 mg; capsules 20 mg, 50 mg, 100 mg; syrup 50 mg/5 mL; suspension 25 mg/5 mL; injection 100 mg per vial, 200 mg per vial.
NOTES: Useful for chronic bronchitis; tetracycline of choice for patients with renal impairment.

Dronabinol (Marinol) [C]

INDICATIONS: Nausea and vomiting associated with cancer chemotherapy; appetite stimulation.
ACTIONS: Antiemetic.
DOSAGE: *Antiemetic:* 5–15 mg/m^2/dose Q 4–6 hr prn.
Appetite stimulant: 2.5 mg PO before lunch and supper.
SUPPLIED: Capsules 2.5 mg, 5 mg, 10 mg.
NOTES: Principal psychoactive substance present in marijuana; many CNS side effects.

Droperidol (Inapsine)

INDICATIONS: Nausea and vomiting; premedication for anesthesia.
ACTIONS: Tranquilization, sedation, and antiemetic.
DOSAGE: *Nausea:* 2.5–5 mg IV or IM Q 3–4 hr prn.
Premedication: 2.5–10 mg IV, 30–60 min pre-op.
SUPPLIED: Injection 2.5 mg/mL.
NOTES: May cause drowsiness, moderate hypotension, occasionally tachycardia, and possible QT prolongation.

Econazole (Spectazole)

INDICATIONS: Treatment of most tinea, cutaneous *Candida,* and tinea versicolor infections.
ACTIONS: Topical antifungal.
DOSAGE: Apply to affected areas bid (q day for tinea versicolor) for 2–4 weeks.
SUPPLIED: Topical cream 1%.
NOTES: Relief of symptoms and clinical improvement may be seen early in treatment, but the course of therapy should be carried out to avoid recurrence.

Echothiophate Iodide (Phospholine Iodide) [See Table 7–12, pp 607-9]

Edrophonium (Tensilon)

INDICATIONS: Diagnosis of myasthenia gravis; acute myasthenic crisis; curare antagonist.
ACTIONS: Anticholinesterase.
DOSAGE: *Test for myasthenia gravis:* 2 mg IV in 1 min; if tolerated, give 8 mg IV; a positive test is a brief increase in strength.
SUPPLIED: Injection 10 mg/mL.
NOTES: Can cause severe cholinergic effects; keep atropine available.

Efavirenz (Sustiva)

INDICATIONS: Management of HIV infections.
ACTIONS: Antiretroviral agent, non-nucleoside reverse transcriptase inhibitor.
DOSAGE: 600 mg PO once daily.
SUPPLIED: Capsules 50 mg, 100 mg, 200 mg.
NOTES: Take at bedtime, may cause CNS detachment, somnolence, vivid dreams, dizziness; may cause rash. Dose may be divided to minimize vivid dreams.

Enalapril (Vasotec) [See Table 7–3, p 598]

Enoxaparin (Lovenox)

INDICATIONS: Prevention of deep venous thrombosis (DVT); treatment of DVT and pulmonary embolus; unstable angina and non-Q-wave MI.
ACTIONS: Low molecular weight heparin.
DOSAGE: *DVT prevention:* 30 mg SC twice daily or 40 mg SC Q 24 hr.
DVT/PE treatment: 1 mg/kg SC Q 12 hr or 1.5 mg/kg SC Q 24 hr.
Angina: 1 mg/kg SC Q 12 hr.
SUPPLIED: Injection 10 mg/0.1 mL (30-mg, 40-mg, 60-mg, 80-mg, 100-mg syringes).
NOTES: Does not significantly affect bleeding time, platelet function, prothrombin time, or aPTT.

Entacapone (Comtan)

INDICATIONS: Treatment of Parkinson's disease.
ACTIONS: Selective and reversible inhibitor of catechol-*o*-methyltransferase (COMT).
DOSAGE: 200 mg administered concurrently with each levodopa/carbidopa dose to a maximum of 8 times per day.
SUPPLIED: Tablets 200 mg.

Ephedrine

INDICATIONS: Treatment of hypotension.
ACTIONS: Sympathomimetic that stimulates both alpha and beta receptors.
DOSAGE: 25–50 mg IM or IV Q 10 min to maximum 150 mg/d or 25–50 mg PO Q 3–4 hr prn.
SUPPLIED: Injection 25 mg/mL, 50 mg/mL; capsules 25 mg, 50 mg; syrup 11 mg per 5 mL, 20 mg per 5 mL.

Epinephrine (Adrenalin, Sus-Phrine, Others)

INDICATIONS: Cardiac arrest, anaphylactic reactions, acute asthma.
ACTIONS: Beta-adrenergic agonist with some alpha effects.
DOSAGE: *Emergency cardiac care:* 0.5–1.0 mg (5–10 mL of 1:10,000) IV Q 5 min to response.

Anaphylaxis: 0.3–0.5 mL of 1:1000 dilution SC; may repeat Q 10–15 min to maximum of 1 mg/dose and 5 mg/d.

Asthma: 0.3–0.5 mL of 1:1000 dilution SC repeated at 20 min to 4-hr intervals; OR 1 inhalation (metered dose) repeated in 1–2 min; OR suspension 0.1–0.3 mL SC for extended effect.
SUPPLIED: Injection 1:1000, 1:2000, 1:10,000, 1:100,000; suspension for injection: 1:200; aerosol; solution for inhalation.
NOTES: Sus-Phrine offers sustained action; in acute cardiac settings can be given via endotracheal tube if a central line is not available.

Epirubicin (Ellence)

INDICATIONS: Adjuvant therapy in patients with evidence of axillary node tumor involvement following resection of primary breast cancer.
ACTIONS: An anthracycline cytotoxic agent.
DOSAGE: Refer to individual protocols.
NOTES: *Toxicity:* mucositis, alopecia, myelosuppression, cardiotoxicity, secondary acute myelogenous leukemia, severe tissue necrosis if extravasation occurs.

Epoetin Alfa [Erythropoietin] (Epogen, Procrit)

INDICATIONS: Treatment of anemia associated with chronic renal failure, zidovudine treatment in HIV-infected patients, and patients receiving cancer chemotherapy; reduction in transfusions associated with surgery.
ACTIONS: Erythropoietin supplementation.
DOSAGE: 50–150 U/kg 3 times weekly; adjust the dose every 4–6 weeks as needed.

Surgery: 300 U/kg/d for 10 days prior to surgery.
SUPPLIED: Injection 2000 U/mL, 3000 U/mL, 4000 U/mL, 10,000 U/mL, 20,000 U/mL.
NOTES: May cause hypertension, headache, tachycardia, nausea, and vomiting; store in refrigerator.

Epoprostenol (Flolan)

INDICATIONS: Treatment of pulmonary hypertension.
ACTIONS: Dilates the pulmonary and systemic arterial vascular beds; inhibits platelet aggregation.
DOSAGE: 4 ng/kg/min IV continuous infusion; make dosage adjustments based on clinical status and package insert guidelines.
SUPPLIED: Injection 0.5 mg, 1.5 mg.
NOTES: Availability through a pharmacy benefit manager (PBM).

Eprosartan (Teveten) [See Table 7–4, p 599]

Eptifibatide (Integrilin)

INDICATIONS: Treatment of acute coronary syndrome.
ACTIONS: Glycoprotein IIb/IIIa inhibitor.
DOSAGE: 180 μg/kg IV bolus, followed by 2 μg/kg/min continuous infusion.
SUPPLIED: Injection 0.75 mg/mL, 2 mg/mL.

Erythromycin (E-Mycin, Ilosone, Erythrocin, Others)

INDICATIONS: Infections caused by group A streptococci (*Streptococcus pyogenes*), alpha-hemolytic streptococci, and *N gonorrhoeae* infections in penicillin-allergic patients, *S pneumoniae, M pneumoniae,* and Legionnaire's disease.
ACTIONS: Bacteriostatic; interferes with protein synthesis.
DOSAGE: 250–500 mg PO qid or 500 mg–1 g IV qid.
SUPPLIED:

- *Powder for injection as lactobionate and gluceptate salts:* 500 mg, 1 g.
- *Base:* Tablets 250 mg, 333 mg, 500 mg; capsules 250 mg.
- *Estolate:* Tablets 500 mg; capsules 250 mg; suspension 125 mg/5 mL, 250 mg/5 mL.
- *Stearate:* Tablets: 250 mg, 500 mg.
- *Ethylsuccinate:* Chewable tablets 200 mg; tablets 400 mg; suspension 200 mg per 5 mL, 400 mg per 5 mL.

NOTES: Frequent mild GI disturbances; estolate salt is associated with cholestatic jaundice; erythromycin base not well absorbed from the GI tract; some forms, such as PCE, are better tolerated with respect to GI irritation.

Erythromycin, Ophthalmic (Ilotycin) [See Table 7–12, pp 607-9]

Esomeprazole Magnesium (Nexium) [See Table 7–14, p 611)

Esmolol (Brevibloc)

INDICATIONS: Supraventricular tachycardia, noncompensatory sinus tachycardia.
ACTIONS: Beta-adrenergic blocking agent, class II antiarrhythmic.
DOSAGE:

- Initiate treatment with 500 μg/kg load over 1 min, then 50 μg/kg/min for 4 min.
- If inadequate response, repeat loading dose and follow with maintenance infusion of 100 μg/kg/min for 4 min; continue titration process by repeating loading dose followed by incremental increases in the maintenance dose of 50 μg/kg/min for 4 min until desired heart rate is reached or a decrease in blood pressure occurs.
- Average dose is 100 μg/kg/min.

SUPPLIED: Injection 10 mg/mL, 250 mg/mL.
NOTES: Monitor closely for hypotension; decreasing or discontinuing infusion will reverse hypotension in about a minute.

Estazolam (Prosom) [C]

INDICATIONS: Insomnia.
ACTIONS: Benzodiazepine, sedative-hypnotic.
DOSAGE: 1–2 mg PO Q HS prn.
SUPPLIED: Tablets 1 mg, 2 mg.

Esterified Estrogens (Estratab, Menest)

INDICATIONS: Vasomotor symptoms, atrophic vaginitis, or kraurosis vulvae associated with menopause; female hypogonadism.
ACTIONS: Estrogen supplementation.
DOSAGE: *Menopause:* 0.3–1.25 mg daily, administered cyclically 3 weeks on and 1 week off. *Hypogonadism:* 2.5 mg PO q day–tid.
SUPPLIED: Tablets 0.3 mg, 0.625 mg, 1.25 mg, 2.5 mg.

Esterified Estrogens with Methyltestosterone (Estratest)

INDICATIONS: Moderate to severe vasomotor symptoms associated with menopause; postpartum breast engorgement.
ACTIONS: Estrogen and androgen supplementation.
DOSAGE: 1 tablet q day for 3 weeks, then 1 week off.
SUPPLIED: Tablets (estrogen/methyltestosterone) 0.625 mg/1.25 mg, 1.25 mg/2.5 mg.

Estradiol (Estrace)

INDICATIONS: Atrophic vaginitis and kraurosis vulvae associated with menopause, vasomotor symptoms.
ACTIONS: Estrogen supplementation.
DOSAGE: *Oral:* 1–2 mg per day, adjust the dose as necessary to control symptoms.
Vaginal cream: 2–4 g daily for 2 weeks, then 1 g 1–3 times a week.
SUPPLIED: Tablets 0.5 mg, 1 mg, 2 mg; vaginal cream.

Estradiol, Transdermal (Estraderm, Others)

INDICATIONS: Severe vasomotor symptoms associated with menopause; female hypogonadism.
ACTIONS: Estrogen supplementation.
DOSAGE: 0.1 mg/d patch once or twice weekly depending on product utilized; adjust the dose as necessary to control symptoms.
SUPPLIED: Transdermal patches (delivers mg per 24 hr) 0.025, 0.0375, 0.05, 0.075, 0.1.

Estramustine Phosphate (Estracyte, EMCYT)

INDICATIONS: Advanced prostate cancer.
ACTIONS: Antimicrotubule agent; weak estrogenic and antiandrogenic activity.
DOSAGE: 14 mg/kg/d in 3–4 divided doses.
SUPPLIED: Capsules 140 mg.
NOTES: Toxicity includes nausea and vomiting; exacerbation of preexisting congestive heart failure; gynecomastia in 20–100%.

Estrogen, Conjugated (Premarin)

INDICATIONS: Moderate to severe vasomotor symptoms associated with menopause; atrophic vaginitis; palliative therapy of advanced prostatic carcinoma; prevention of estrogen deficiency-induced osteoporosis.
ACTIONS: Hormonal replacement.
DOSAGE: 0.3–1.25 mg/d PO cyclically; prostatic carcinoma requires 1.25–2.5 mg PO tid.
SUPPLIED: Tablets 0.3 mg, 0.625 mg, 0.9 mg, 1.25 mg, 2.5 mg; injection 25 mg/mL.
NOTES: Do not use in pregnancy; associated with an increased risk of endometrial carcinoma, gallbladder disease, thromboembolism, and possibly breast cancer; generic products are not equivalent.

Estrogen, Conjugated—Synthetic (Cenestin)

INDICATIONS: Treatment of moderate to severe vasomotor symptoms associated with menopause.
ACTIONS: Hormonal replacement.
DOSAGE: 0.625–1.25 mg PO q day.
SUPPLIED: Tablets 0.625 mg, 0.9 mg, 1.25 mg.
NOTES: Do not use in pregnancy; associated with an increased risk of endometrial carcinoma, gallbladder disease, thromboembolism, and possibly breast cancer.

Estrogen, Conjugated with Methylprogesterone (Premarin with Methylprogesterone)

INDICATIONS: Vasomotor symptoms associated with menopause.
ACTIONS: Estrogen and androgen combination.
DOSAGE: 1 tablet q day.

SUPPLIED: Tablets containing 0.625 mg of estrogen, conjugated, and 5 mg of methylprogesterone.

Estrogen, Conjugated with Methyltestosterone (Premarin with Methyltestosterone)

INDICATIONS: Moderate to severe vasomotor symptoms associated with menopause; postpartum breast engorgement.
ACTIONS: Estrogen and androgen combination.
DOSAGE: 1 tablet q day for 3 weeks, then 1 week off.
SUPPLIED: Tablets (estrogen/methyltestosterone) 0.625 mg/5 mg, 1.25 mg/10 mg.

Etanercept (Enbrel)

INDICATIONS: Treatment of signs and symptoms and delaying structural damage in patients with moderately to severely active rheumatoid arthritis.
ACTIONS: Binds tumor necrosis factor (TNF), thus blocking its interaction at TNF receptors.
DOSAGE: 25 mg given SC twice weekly (separated by at least 72–96 hours).
SUPPLIED: *Dose tray:* Contains 25 mg single-use vial of etanercept and 1 syringe of sterile bacteriostatic water for injection.
NOTES: Serious infections and sepsis have been reported. Avoid use in patients with active infections or with underlying conditions that predispose them to infection.

Ethacrynic Acid (Edecrin)

INDICATIONS: Edema, congestive heart failure, and ascites; any time rapid diuresis is desired.
ACTIONS: Loop diuretic; inhibits reabsorption of sodium and chlorine in the ascending loop of Henle and the distal renal tubule.
DOSAGE: 50–200 mg PO q day or 50 mg IV prn.
SUPPLIED: Tablets 25 mg, 50 mg; powder for injection: 50 mg.
NOTES: Contraindicated in anuria; severe side effects have been reported.

Ethambutol (Myambutol)

INDICATIONS: Pulmonary tuberculosis and other mycobacterial infections.
ACTIONS: Inhibits cellular metabolism.
DOSAGE: 15–25 mg/kg PO daily as a single dose.
SUPPLIED: Tablets 100 mg, 400 mg.
NOTES: May cause vision changes and GI upset.

Ethinyl Estradiol (Estinyl, Feminone)

INDICATIONS: Vasomotor symptoms associated with menopause; female hypogonadism.
ACTIONS: Estrogen supplementation.
DOSAGE: 0.02–1.5 mg/d divided q day–tid.
SUPPLIED: Tablets 0.02 mg, 0.05 mg, 0.5 mg.

Ethosuximide (Zarontin)

INDICATIONS: Management of seizures.
ACTIONS: Anticonvulsant; increases the seizure threshold.
DOSAGE: Initial dose 500 mg PO divided bid; increase by 250 mg/d every 4–7 days as needed. (max 1500 mg/d).
SUPPLIED: Capsules 250 mg; syrup 250 mg/5 mL.
NOTES: Blood dyscrasias as well as CNS and GI side effects may occur; use caution in patients with renal or hepatic impairment. See Table 7–16, Non-Antibiotic Drug Levels, p 613.

Etidronate Disodium (Didronel)

INDICATIONS: Treatment of hypercalcemia of malignancy and hypertropic ossification.
ACTIONS: Inhibition of normal and abnormal bone resorption.
DOSAGE: 5–20 mg/kg/d, may be given in divided doses; (Duration of therapy 3–6 months); 7.5 mg/kg/day IV infusion over 2 hours.
SUPPLIED: Tablets 200 mg, 400 mg; injection.
NOTES: GI intolerance may be decreased by dividing oral daily doses.

Etodolac (Lodine) [See Table 7–11, pp 605-6]

Etoposide [VP-16] (VePesid)

INDICATIONS: Testicular cancer, non-small cell lung cancers, Hodgkin's and non-Hodgkin's lymphomas, pediatric acute lymphocytic leukemia, allogeneic and autologous bone marrow transplantation in high doses.
ACTIONS: Topoisomerase II inhibitor.
DOSAGE: Refer to specific protocols.
NOTES: Toxicity includes myelosuppression, nausea and vomiting, and alopecia; hypotension may occur if infused too rapidly; anaphylaxis or lesser hypersensitivity reactions (wheezing) rarely occurs; potential for secondary leukemias.

Exemestane (Aromasin)

INDICATIONS: Treatment of advanced breast cancer in postmenopausal women whose disease has progressed following tamoxifen therapy.
ACTIONS: An irreversible, steroidal aromatase inhibitor, which lowers circulating estrogen concentrations.
DOSAGE: 25 mg PO q day after a meal.
SUPPLIED: Tablet 25 mg.
NOTES: May cause hot flashes, nausea, fatigue.

Famciclovir (Famvir)

INDICATIONS: Management of acute herpes zoster (shingles), genital herpes infections.
ACTIONS: Inhibits viral DNA synthesis.
DOSAGE: *Zoster:* 500 mg PO Q 8 hr.
Simplex: 125–250 mg PO bid.
SUPPLIED: Tablets 125 mg, 250 mg, 500 mg.

Famotidine (Pepcid)

INDICATIONS: Short-term treatment of active duodenal ulcer and benign gastric ulcer; maintenance therapy for duodenal ulcer, hypersecretory conditions, gastroesophageal reflux disease (GERD), and heartburn.
ACTIONS: H_2-antagonist; inhibits gastric acid secretion.
DOSAGE: *Ulcer:* 20–40 mg PO HS or 20 mg IV Q 12 hr.
Hypersecretory: 20–160 mg PO Q 6 hr.
GERD: Treatment: 20 mg PO bid for 4–6 weeks; maintenance: 20 mg PO HS.
Heartburn: 10 mg PO prn.
SUPPLIED: Tablets 10 mg, 20 mg, 40 mg; chewable tablets 10 mg; suspension 40 mg/5 mL; injection 10 mg/mL.
NOTES: Decrease dose in renal insufficiency.

Felodipine (Plendil)

INDICATIONS: Treatment of hypertension and congestive heart failure.
ACTIONS: Calcium channel blocking agent.
DOSAGE: 5–20 mg PO q day.
SUPPLIED: Extended-release tablets 2.5 mg, 5 mg, 10 mg.
NOTES: Closely monitor BP in elderly patients and patients with impaired hepatic function; doses of > 10 mg should not be used in these patients. Bioavailability is increased when administered with grapefruit juice.

Fenofibrate (Tricor)

INDICATIONS: Treatment of hypertriglyceridemia.
ACTIONS: Inhibits triglyceride synthesis.
DOSAGE: Initial dose 54–160 mg q day.
SUPPLIED: Capsules 54 mg, 160 mg.
NOTES: Take with meals to increase bioavailability; may cause cholecystitis; monitor LFTs.

Fenoldopam (Corlopam)

INDICATIONS: Treatment of hypertensive emergency.
ACTIONS: Rapid-acting vasodilator.
DOSAGE: Initial dose 0.03–0.1 μg/kg/min IV continuous infusion, titrate to effect every 15 minutes with 0.05–0.1 μg/kg/min increments.
SUPPLIED: Injection 10 mg/mL.
NOTES: Avoid concurrent use with beta-blockers.

Fenoprofen (Nalfon) [Table 7–11, pp 605-6]

Fentanyl (Sublimaze) [C]

INDICATIONS: Short-acting analgesic used in conjunction with anesthesia.
ACTIONS: Narcotic.
DOSAGE: 0.025–0.15 mg/kg IV/IM titrated to effect.
SUPPLIED: Injection 0.05 mg/mL.
NOTES: Causes significant sedation; 0.1 mg of fentanyl is equivalent to 10 mg of morphine IM.

Fentanyl, Transdermal (Duragesic) [C]

INDICATIONS: Management of chronic pain.
ACTIONS: Narcotic.
DOSAGE: Apply a patch to the upper torso every 72 hr. Dose is calculated from the narcotic requirements for the previous 24 hr.
SUPPLIED: Transdermal patches that deliver 25 μg/hr, 50 μg/hr, 75 μg/hr, 100 μg/hr.
NOTES: 0.1 mg of fentanyl is equivalent to 10 mg of morphine IM.

Fentanyl, Transmucosal System (Actiq, Fentanyl Oralet) [C]

INDICATIONS: Induction of anesthesia and breakthrough cancer pain.
ACTIONS: Narcotic.
DOSAGE: *Anesthesia:* 5–15 μg/kg.
Pain: 200 μg consumed over 15 min, titrate to desired effect.
SUPPLIED: Lozenges 100 μg, 200 μg, 300 μg, 400 μg; lozenges on stick: 200 μg, 400 μg, 600 μg, 800 μg, 1200 μg, 1600 μg.

Ferrous Gluconate (Fergon, Others)

INDICATIONS: Iron deficiency anemia and iron supplementation.
ACTIONS: Dietary supplementation.
DOSAGE: 100–200 mg of elemental iron per day.
SUPPLIED: Tablets 240 (27 mg iron), 325 mg (36 mg iron).
NOTES: 12% elemental iron; may turn stool and urine dark.

Ferric Gluconate Complex (Ferrlecit)

INDICATIONS: Treatment of iron deficiency in patients receiving supplemental erythropoietin therapy.
ACTIONS: Supplemental iron.
DOSAGE: Give test dose of 2 mL (25 mg iron) infused over 1 hour. If no reaction, 125 mg (10 mL) IV over 1 hour until favorable hematocrit is achieved. Usual cumulative dose is 1 g iron administered over 8 sessions.
SUPPLIED: Injection 12.5 mg/mL elemental iron.
NOTES: Dosage is expressed as mg elemental iron; may be infused during dialysis.

Ferrous Sulfate

INDICATIONS: Iron deficiency anemia and iron supplementation.
ACTIONS: Dietary supplementation.
DOSAGE: 100–200 mg of elemental iron per day.
SUPPLIED: Tablets 187 mg, 200 mg, 324 mg; slow-release caplets and tablets 160 mg; drops 75 mg/0.6 mL; elixir 220 mg/5 mL; syrup 90 mg/5 mL.
NOTES: May turn stools and urine dark; can cause GI upset and constipation; vitamin C taken with ferrous sulfate will increase the absorption of iron, especially in patients with atrophic gastritis.

Fexofenadine (Allegra)

INDICATIONS: Relief of allergic rhinitis.
ACTIONS: Antihistamine.
DOSAGE: 60 mg twice daily or 180 mg q day.
SUPPLIED: Capsules 60 mg, 180 mg tablet; also available in combination with pseudoephedrine (60 mg fexofenadine/120 mg pseudoephedrine).

Filgrastim [G-CSF] (Neupogen)

INDICATIONS: To decrease the incidence of infection in febrile neutropenic patients, and treatment of chronic neutropenia.
ACTIONS: Recombinant granulocyte colony-stimulating factor.
DOSAGE: 5 μg/kg/d SC or IV as a single daily dose.
SUPPLIED: Injection 300 μg/mL.
NOTES: May cause bone pain. Discontinue therapy when ANC > 10,000.

Finasteride (Proscar, Propecia)

INDICATIONS: Treatment of benign prostatic hyperplasia and androgenetic alopecia.
ACTIONS: Inhibits 5-α reductase.
DOSAGE: *BPH:* 5 mg PO q day.
Alopecia: 1 mg PO q day.
SUPPLIED: Tablets 1 mg, 5 mg.
NOTES: Will decrease prostate-specific antigen levels; may take 3–6 months to see effect on urinary symptoms.

Flavoxate (Urispas)

INDICATIONS: Symptomatic relief of dysuria, urgency, nocturia, suprapubic pain, urinary frequency, and incontinence.
ACTIONS: Counteracts smooth muscle spasm of the urinary tract.
DOSAGE: 100–200 mg PO tid–qid.
SUPPLIED: Tablets 100 mg.
NOTES: May cause drowsiness, blurred vision, and dry mouth.

Flecainide (Tambocor)

INDICATIONS: Prevention of paroxysmal atrial fibrillation/flutter and paroxysmal supraventricular tachycardia (PSVT), treatment of life-threatening ventricular arrhythmias.
ACTIONS: Class 1C antiarrhythmic.
DOSAGE: 100 mg PO Q 12 hr; increase in increments of 50 mg Q 12 hr every 4 days to a maximum of 400 mg/d.
SUPPLIED: Tablets 50 mg, 100 mg, 150 mg.
NOTES: May cause new or worsened arrhythmias; therapy should be initiated in the hospital; may dose Q 8 hr if the patient is intolerant or uncontrolled at 12-hr intervals; drug interactions with propranolol, digoxin, verapamil, and disopyramide; may cause congestive heart failure.

Floxuridine (FUDR)

INDICATIONS: Colon carcinoma, pancreatic carcinoma, liver cancer, biliary tract cancers, and adenocarcinoma of the GI tract metastatic to the liver.
ACTIONS: Inhibitor of thymidylate synthase; interferes with DNA synthesis (S phase-specific).
DOSAGE: Refer to specific protocols.
NOTES: Toxicity includes myelosuppression, nausea and vomiting, anorexia, abdominal cramps, diarrhea, mucositis, alopecia, skin rash, and hyperpigmentation; rare neurotoxicity (blurred vision, depression, nystagmus, vertigo, and lethargy). Intra-arterial catheter-related problems (ischemia, thrombosis, bleeding, and infection) may occur.

Fluconazole (Diflucan)

INDICATIONS: Oropharyngeal and esophageal candidiasis, cryptococcal meningitis, *Candida* infections of the lungs, peritoneum, and urinary tract; prevention of candidiasis in bone marrow transplant patients on chemotherapy or radiation; *Candida* vaginitis.
ACTIONS: Antifungal; inhibits fungal cytochrome P-450 sterol demethylation.
DOSAGE: *Usual:* 100–400 mg PO or IV q day.
Vaginitis: 150 mg PO as single dose.
SUPPLIED: Tablets 50 mg, 100 mg, 150 mg, 200 mg; suspension 10 mg/mL, 40 mg/mL; injection 2 mg/mL.
NOTES: Adjust dose in renal insufficiency. Oral dosing produces the same blood levels as intravenously; therefore, the oral route should be used whenever possible.

Flucytosine (Ancobon)

INDICATIONS: Serious infections caused by susceptible strains of *Candida* or *Cryptococcus.*
ACTIONS: Antifungal.
DOSAGE: 50–150 mg/kg/d divided Q 6 hr.
SUPPLIED: Capsules 250 mg, 500 mg.
NOTES: May cause nausea, vomiting, and diarrhea. Instruct patient to take capsules a few at a time over 15 min.

Fludarabine Phosphate (Flamp, Fludara)

INDICATIONS: Chronic lymphocytic leukemia, low-grade lymphoma, mycosis fungoides.
ACTIONS: Inhibits ribonucleotide reductase; blocks DNA polymerase-induced DNA repair.
DOSAGE: Refer to specific protocols.
NOTES: Toxicity includes myelosuppression, nausea and vomiting, diarrhea, and hepatic transaminase elevations; severe CNS toxicity occurs only rarely in leukemic patients and pulmonary toxicity.

Fludrocortisone Acetate (Florinef)

INDICATIONS: Partial treatment for adrenocortical insufficiency.
ACTIONS: Mineralocorticoid replacement.
DOSAGE: 0.05–0.2 mg PO q day.
SUPPLIED: Tablets 0.1 mg.
NOTES: For adrenal insufficiency, must be used in conjunction with a glucocorticoid supplement; dosage changes based on plasma renin activity.z

Flumazenil (Romazicon)

INDICATIONS: For complete or partial reversal of the sedative effects of benzodiazepines (diazepam, etc).
ACTIONS: Benzodiazepine receptor antagonist.
DOSAGE: 0.2 mg IV over 15 sec; dose may be repeated if the desired level of consciousness is not obtained, to a maximum dose of 1 mg.
SUPPLIED: Injection 0.1 mg/mL.
NOTES: Does not reverse narcotics.

Flunisolide (AeroBid, Nasalide)

INDICATIONS: Chronic treatment for asthma; relief of seasonal or perennial allergic rhinitis.
ACTIONS: Topical steroid.
DOSAGE: *Metered-dose inhaler:* 2–4 inhalations bid.
Nasal: 2 sprays in each nostril 2 × daily.
SUPPLIED: Metered-dose aerosol 250 mg; nasal spray 0.025%.
NOTES: May cause oral candidiasis; instruct patients to rinse their mouth after use; not for acute asthma attack.

Fluorometholone (FML, Flarex) [See Table 7–12, pp 607-9]

Fluorouracil (5-FU) (Adrucil)

INDICATIONS: Colorectal cancer, bladder cancer, gastric cancer, pancreatic cancer, anal cancer, head and neck cancer, breast cancer, and topical application for basal cell carcinoma of the skin.

ACTIONS: Inhibitor of thymidylate synthetase (interferes with DNA synthesis, S phase–specific).

DOSAGE: Refer to specific protocol.

NOTES: Toxicity includes stomatitis, esophagitis, diarrhea, anorexia, and nausea and vomiting. Myelosuppression includes leukocytopenia, thrombocytopenia, and anemia; rash, dry skin, and photosensitivity occur frequently. Tingling in the hands and feet followed by pain (palmar-plantar erythrodysesthesia) may occur; phlebitis and discoloration may occur at injection sites.

Fluorouracil, Topical (5-FU) (Efudex)

INDICATIONS: Basal cell carcinoma of the skin, actinic and solar keratosis.

ACTIONS: Inhibitor of thymidylate synthetase (interferes with DNA synthesis, S phase–specific).

DOSAGE: Apply 5% cream bid for 4–6 weeks.

SUPPLIED: Cream 1%, 5%; solution 1%, 2%, 5%.

NOTES: Toxicity: rash, dry skin, and photosensitivity.

Fluoxetine (Prozac, Sarafem)

INDICATIONS: Treatment of depression, obsessive-compulsive disorders, bulimia, premenstrual dysphoric disorder (PMDD).

ACTIONS: Selective serotonin reuptake inhibitor.

DOSAGE: *Depression:* Initial dose, 20 mg PO q day; titrate to a maximum of 80 mg/24 hr; doses of > 20 mg/d should be divided.

Bulimia: 60 mg once daily in the morning.

PMDD: 20 mg q day.

SUPPLIED: Capsules 10 mg, 20 mg; tablets 10 mg; solution 20 mg/5 mL.

NOTES: May cause nausea, nervousness, and weight loss; hepatic failure dosage adjustment. Can cause insomnia or hypersomnia and sexual dysfunction.

Fluoxymesterone (Halotestin) [C]

INDICATIONS: Androgen-responsive metastatic breast cancer.

ACTIONS: Inhibition of secretion of luteinizing hormone and follicle-stimulating hormone by feedback inhibition.

DOSAGE: Refer to specific protocol.

NOTES: Toxicity includes virilization, amenorrhea and menstrual irregularities, hirsutism, alopecia and acne, nausea, and cholestasis. *Hematologic notes:* Toxicity includes suppression of clotting factors II, V, VII, and X and polycythemia. Increased libido, headache, and anxiety occur.

Fluphenazine (Prolixin, Permitil)

INDICATIONS: Psychotic disorders.

ACTIONS: Phenothiazine antipsychotic; blocks postsynaptic mesolimbic dopaminergic receptors in the brain.

DOSAGE: 0.5–10 mg/d in divided doses PO Q 6–8 hr; average maintenance 5.0 mg/d or 1.25 mg IM initially; then 2.5–10 mg/d in divided doses Q 6–8 hr prn.

SUPPLIED: Tablets 1 mg, 2.5 mg, 5 mg, 10 mg; concentrate 5 mg/mL; elixir 2.5 mg/5 mL; injection 2.5 mg/mL; Depo injection 25 mg/mL.

NOTES: Reduce dose in the elderly; monitor liver functions; may cause drowsiness. Do not administer concentrate with caffeine, tannic acid, or pectin-containing products.

Flurazepam (Dalmane) [C]

INDICATIONS: Treatment of insomnia.

ACTIONS: Benzodiazepine.

DOSAGE: 15–30 mg PO Q HS prn.
SUPPLIED: Capsules 15 mg, 30 mg.
NOTES: Reduce dose in the elderly.

Flurbiprofen (Ansaid, Ocufen) [See Table 7–11, pp 605-6, or see Table 7–12, p 607–608]

Flutamide (Eulexin)

INDICATIONS: Advanced prostate cancer (in combination with gonadotropin-releasing hormone [GnRH] agonists such as leuprolide or goserelin); with radiation for localized prostate cancer.
ACTIONS: Nonsteroidal antiandrogen.
DOSAGE: Refer to specific protocol.
NOTES: Toxicity includes hot flashes, loss of libido, impotence, diarrhea, nausea and vomiting, and gynecomastia; follow LFTs.

Fluticasone Nasal (Flonase)

INDICATIONS: Seasonal allergic rhinitis.
ACTIONS: Topical steroid.
DOSAGE: 1–2 sprays in each nostril once daily.
SUPPLIED: Nasal spray 50 μg per actuation.

Fluticasone Oral (Flovent, Flovent Rotadisk)

INDICATIONS: Chronic treatment of asthma.
ACTIONS: Topical steroid.
DOSAGE: 2–4 puffs bid.
SUPPLIED: *Multidose inhaler:* 44 μg, 110 μg, or 220 μg per activation; *Rotadisk dry powder:* 50 μg, 100 μg, and 250 μg per activation.
NOTES: May cause oral candidiasis; instruct patients to rinse their mouth after use. Counsel patients carefully on use of delivery system.

Fluvastatin (Lescol) [See Table 7–15, p 612]

Fluvoxamine (Luvox)

INDICATIONS: Treatment of obsessive-compulsive disorder.
ACTIONS: Elective serotonin inhibitor.
DOSAGE: Initial 50 mg as single HS dose; may be increased to 300 mg per day in divided doses.
SUPPLIED: Tablets 25 mg, 50 mg, 100 mg.
NOTES: Divide doses of > 100 mg; numerous drug interactions.

Folic Acid

INDICATIONS: Treatment of megaloblastic anemia, all women of childbearing years, adjunct to be taken with folate antagonists.
ACTIONS: Dietary supplementation.
DOSAGE: *Supplement:* 0.4 mg PO q day.
Pregnancy: 0.8 mg PO q day.
Folate deficiency: 1.0 mg PO q day–tid.
SUPPLIED: Tablets 0.1 mg, 0.4 mg, 0.8 mg, 1.0 mg; injection 5 mg/mL.
NOTES: Recommended for all women of childbearing years; will decrease fetal neural tube defects by 50%.

Fomepizole (Antizol)

INDICATIONS: Antidote for ethylene glycol and methanol toxicity.
ACTIONS: Complexes and inactivates alcohol dehydrogenase.

DOSAGE: 15 mg/kg IV load, followed by 10 mg/kg Q 12 hr for 4 doses, then 15 mg/kg Q 12 hr until ethylene glycol levels < 20 mg/dL.
SUPPLIED: 1 g/mL (1.5-mL vials).
NOTES: Dosage adjustment for hemodialysis.

Fomivirsen (Vitravene)

INDICATIONS: Cytomegalovirus retinitis in AIDS patients refractory to or intolerant of other treatments.
ACTIONS: Ophthalmic antiviral.
DOSAGE: 330 μg intravitreal injection every other week for 2 doses, followed by maintenance doses of 330 μg every 4 weeks.
SUPPLIED: 6.6 mg/mL (0.25 mL solution for injection).
NOTES: Intraocular pressure commonly increases; do not use within 2 weeks of cidofovir.

Foscarnet (Foscavir)

INDICATIONS: Treatment of cytomegalovirus; acyclovir-resistant herpes infections.
ACTIONS: Inhibits viral DNA polymerase and reverse transcriptase.
DOSAGE: *Induction:* 60 mg/kg IV Q 8 hr for 14–21 days.
Maintenance: 90–120 mg/kg IV q day (Mon–Fri).
SUPPLIED: Injection 24 mg/mL.
NOTES: Dosage must be adjusted for renal function; nephrotoxic; monitor ionized calcium closely; administer through a central line.

Fosfomycin (Monurol)

INDICATIONS: Treatment of uncomplicated urinary tract infection.
ACTIONS: Inhibits bacterial cell wall synthesis.
DOSAGE: 3 gm PO dissolved in 90–120 mL of water as single dose.
SUPPLIED: Granule packets 3 g.
NOTES: May take 2–3 days for symptoms to improve.

Fosinopril (Monopril) [See Table 7–3, p 598]

Fosphenytoin (Cerebyx)

INDICATIONS: Treatment of status epilepticus.
ACTION: Inhibits seizure spread in the motor cortex.
DOSAGE: *Loading:* 15–20 mg PE/kg.
Maintenance: 4–6 mg PE/kg/d.
SUPPLIED: Injection.
NOTES: Dosed as phenytoin equivalents; requires 15 min to convert the prodrug fosphenytoin to phenytoin; administer at < 150 mg PE/min to prevent hypotension. Dosage adjustment/plasma monitoring may be necessary in hepatic impairment.

Furosemide (Lasix)

INDICATIONS: Treatment of congestive heart failure, edema, hypertension.
ACTIONS: Loop diuretic; inhibits sodium and chloride reabsorption in the ascending loop of Henle and the distal renal tubule.
DOSAGE: 20–80 mg PO or IV q day–bid.
SUPPLIED: Tablets 20 mg, 40 mg, 80 mg; solution 10 mg/mL, 40 mg/5 mL; injection 10 mg/mL.
NOTES: Monitor for hypokalemia; use with caution in hepatic disease; high doses of the IV form may cause ototoxicity.

Gabapentin (Neurontin)

INDICATIONS: Adjunctive therapy in the treatment of partial seizures.
ACTIONS: Anticonvulsant.
DOSAGE: 900–1800 mg/d PO in 3 divided doses.
SUPPLIED: Capsules 100 mg, 300 mg, 400 mg.

NOTES: It is not necessary to monitor serum gabapentin levels; dosage adjustment in renal impairment.

Gallium Nitrate (Ganite)

INDICATIONS: Treatment of bladder cancer and lymphoma and hypercalcemia related to malignancy.
ACTIONS: Inhibits resorption of calcium from bone; antitumor activity.
DOSAGE: Refer to specific protocol.
NOTES: Can cause renal insufficiency; may cause hypocalcemia, hypophosphatemia, and decreased bicarbonate; < 1% of patients developed acute optic neuritis. For bladder cancer, used in combination with vinblastine and ifosfamide.

Ganciclovir (Cytovene, Vitrasert)

INDICATIONS: Treatment and prevention of cytomegalovirus (CMV) retinitis and prevention of CMV disease in transplant recipients.
ACTIONS: Inhibits viral DNA synthesis.
DOSAGE: *IV:* 5 mg/kg IV Q 12 hr for 14–21 days, then maintenance of 5 mg/kg IV q day for 7 days/week or 6 mg/kg IV q day for 5 days/week.
PO: Following induction, 1000 mg PO tid.
Prevention: 1000 mg PO tid.
Ocular implant: One implant every 5–8 months.
SUPPLIED: Capsules 250 mg, 500 mg; injection 500 mg; ocular implant 4.5 mg.
NOTES: Not a cure for CMV; granulocytopenia and thrombocytopenia are the major toxicities; injection should be handled with cytotoxic precautions; take capsules with food. Implant confers no systemic benefit; dosage adjustment in renal impairment.

Gatifloxacin (Tequin)

INDICATIONS: Treatment of acute exacerbation of chronic bronchitis, sinusitis, community-acquired pneumonia, urinary tract infections.
ACTIONS: Quinolone antibiotic, inhibits DNA-gyrase.
DOSAGE: 400 mg PO or IV once daily.
SUPPLIED: Tablets 200 mg, 400 mg; injection.
NOTES: Avoid use with antacids; do NOT use in children < 18 years or in pregnant or lactating women; reliable activity against *S pneumoniae;* dosage adjustment in renal impairment.

Gemcitabine (Gemzar)

INDICATIONS: Pancreatic cancer, gastric cancer, and lung cancer.
ACTIONS: Antimetabolite; inhibits ribonucleotide reductase; produces false nucleotide base inhibiting DNA synthesis.
DOSAGE: Refer to specific protocol.
NOTES: Toxicities include myelosuppression, nausea and vomiting, diarrhea, drug fever, and skin rash.

Gemfibrozil (Lopid)

INDICATIONS: Treatment of hypertriglyceridemia, and to reduce the risk of coronary heart disease.
ACTIONS: Lipid-regulating agent.
DOSAGE: 1200 mg/d PO in 2 divided doses 30 min before the morning and evening meals.
SUPPLIED: Tablets 600 mg; capsules 300 mg.
NOTES: Monitor serum lipids during therapy; cholelithiasis may occur secondary to treatment; may enhance the effect of warfarin; concurrent use with the HMG-CoA reductase inhibitors may cause hepatic injury or rhabdomyolysis.

Gemtuzumab Ozagamicin (Mylotarg)

INDICATIONS: Relapsed CD33+ acute myelogenous leukemia in patients >60 years who are poor candidates for chemotherapy.
ACTIONS: Monoclonal antibody linked to calicheamicin; selective for myeloid cells.

DOSAGE: Refer to specific protocol.
NOTES: Premedicate with diphenhydramine and acetaminophen.

Gentamicin (Garamycin, G-Mycitin, Others)

INDICATIONS: Serious infections caused by susceptible *Pseudomonas, Proteus, E coli, Klebsiella, Enterobacter,* and *Serratia,* and for initial treatment of gram-negative sepsis.
ACTIONS: Bactericidal; inhibits protein synthesis.
DOSAGE: See Aminoglycoside Dosing (See Table 7–18, p 614, Table 7–19, p 615, and Table 7–20, pp 616-17).
SUPPLIED: Injection 10 mg/mL, 40 mg/mL; intrathecal preservative free 2 mg/mL.
NOTES: Nephrotoxic and ototoxic; decrease dose with renal insufficiency; monitor creatinine clearance and serum concentration for dosage adjustments (See Table 7–17, p 613).

Gentamicin, Ophthalmic (Garamycin, Genoptic, Gentacidin, Gentak, Others) [See Table 7–12, pp 607-9]

Gentamicin, Topical (Garamycin, G-Mycitin)

INDICATIONS: Skin infections caused by susceptible organisms.
ACTIONS: Bactericidal; inhibits protein synthesis.
DOSAGE: Adults apply tid–qid.
SUPPLIED: Cream 0.1%, ointment 0.1%.

Gentamicin and Prednisolone, Ophthalmic (Pred-G Opthalmic) [See Table 7–12, p 607-9]

Glimepiride (Amaryl) [See Table 7–13, p 610]

Glipizide (Glucotrol) [See Table 7–13, p 610]

Glucagon

INDICATIONS: Treatment of severe hypoglycemic reactions in diabetic patients with sufficient liver glycogen stores or beta-blocker overdose.
ACTIONS: Accelerates liver gluconeogenesis.
DOSAGE: *Usual:* 0.5–1.0 mg SC, IM, or IV; repeat after 20 min prn.
Beta-blocker overdose: 3–10 mg IV; repeat in 10 min prn; may be given as a continuous infusion.
SUPPLIED: Injection 1 mg.
NOTES: Administration of glucose IV is necessary; ineffective in states of starvation, adrenal insufficiency, or chronic hypoglycemia.

Glyburide (Diabeta, Micronase) [See Table 7–13, p 610]

Glyburide Micronized (Glynase) [See Table 7–13, p 610]

Glycerin Suppository

INDICATIONS: Constipation.
ACTIONS: 1 adult suppository PR prn.
SUPPLIED: Suppositories (adult, infant); liquid 4 mL/applicatorful.

Goserelin (Zoladex)

INDICATIONS: Advanced prostate cancer and with radiation for localized prostate cancer; endometriosis.
ACTIONS: Slow-release form of LHRH agonist, thereby inhibiting the release of gonadotropin, decreasing testosterone levels.
DOSAGE: Refer to specific protocol.
NOTES: Toxicity includes hot flashes, decreased libido, gynecomastia, and transient exacerbation of cancer-related bone pain ("flare reaction" 7–10 days after first dose).

Granisetron (Kytril)

INDICATIONS: Prevention of nausea and vomiting.

ACTIONS: Serotonin receptor antagonist.
DOSAGE: 10 µg/kg IV 30 min prior to initiation of chemotherapy; OR 1 mg PO 1 hr prior to chemotherapy, then 12 hr after.
SUPPLIED: Tablets 1 mg; injection 1 mg/mL.

Guaifenesin (Robitussin, Others)

INDICATIONS: Symptomatic relief of dry, nonproductive cough.
ACTIONS: Expectorant.
DOSAGE: 200–400 mg (10–20 mL) PO Q 4 hr (max 2.4 g/d).
SUPPLIED: Tablets 100 mg, 200 mg, 1200 mg; sustained-release tablets 600 mg; capsules 200 mg; sustained-release capsules 300 mg; liquid 100 mg/5 mL, 200 mg/5 mL.

Guaifenesin and Codeine (Robitussin AC, Brontex, Others) [C]

INDICATIONS: Symptomatic relief of dry, nonproductive cough.
ACTIONS: Antitussive with expectorant.
DOSAGE: 10 mL or 1 tablet PO Q 6–8 hr.
SUPPLIED: Brontex tablet 10 mg codeine; Brontex liquid 2.5 mg codeine/5 mL; others 10 mg codeine/5 mL.

Guaifenesin and Dextromethorphan (Many OTC Brands)

INDICATIONS: Cough due to upper respiratory irritation.
ACTIONS: Antitussive with expectorant.
DOSAGE: 10 mL PO Q 6 hr.
SUPPLIED: Guaifenesin/dextromethorphan dose: 100 mg/5 mg per 5 mL; 100 mg/10 mg per 5 mL; 100 mg/15 mg per 5 mL.

Guanfacine (Tenex)

INDICATIONS: Hypertension.
ACTIONS: Centrally acting alpha-adrenergic agonist.
DOSAGE: Initial dose, 1 mg Q HS; increase by 1 mg/24-hr increments to a maximum of 3 mg/24 hr; split the dose bid if BP increases at the end of the dosing interval.
SUPPLIED: Tablets 1 mg, 2 mg.
NOTES: Concomitant use with a thiazide diuretic is recommended; sedation and drowsiness are common; rebound hypertension may occur with abrupt cessation of therapy.

Haemophilus B Conjugate Vaccine (ProHIBIT, Comvax, Others)

INDICATIONS: Routine immunization of children against diseases caused by *Haemophilus influenzae* type B and others at high risk (splenectomy).
ACTIONS: Active immunization against *Haemophilus B.*
DOSAGE: 0.5 mL (25 mg) IM in deltoid or vastus lateralis.
SUPPLIED: Injection 7.5 µg/0.5 mL, 10 µg/0.5 mL, 15 µg/0.5 mL, 25 µg/0.5 mL.
NOTES: Booster not required; observe for anaphylaxis.

Haloperidol (Haldol)

INDICATIONS: Management of psychotic disorders, agitation, Tourette's syndrome.
ACTIONS: Antipsychotic, neuroleptic.
DOSAGE: *Moderate symptoms:* 0.5–2.0 mg PO bid–tid.
Severe symptoms or agitation: 3–5 mg PO bid–tid; OR 1–5 mg IM Q 4 hr prn (maximum 100 mg/d).
SUPPLIED: Tablets 0.5 mg, 1 mg, 2 mg, 5 mg, 10 mg, 20 mg; concentrate liquid 2 mg/mL; injection 5 mg/mL; decanoate injection 50 mg/mL, 100 mg/mL.
NOTES: Can cause extrapyramidal symptoms and hypotension; reduce dose in the elderly.

Heparin

INDICATIONS: Treatment and prevention of venous thrombosis and pulmonary emboli, atrial fibrillation with emboli formation, acute arterial occlusion, unstable angina, acute myocardial infarction.
ACTIONS: Acts with antithrombin III to inactivate thrombin and inhibit thromboplastin formation.

DOSAGE: *Prophylaxis:* 3000–5000 U SC Q 8–12 hr.

Treatment of thrombosis: Load dose of 50–80 U/kg IV, then 10–20 U/kg IV QH (adjust based on partial thromboplastin time [PTT]).

SUPPLIED: Injection 10 U/mL, 100 U/mL, 1000 U/mL, 2000 U/mL, 2500 U/mL, 5000 U/mL, 7500 U/mL, 10,000 U/mL, 20,000 U/mL, 40,000 U/mL.

NOTES: Follow PTT, thrombin time, or activated clotting time to assess effectiveness; heparin has little effect on the prothrombin time (PT); with proper dose, PTT is about 1.5–2 × the control; can cause thrombocytopenia; follow platelet counts.

Hepatitis A Vaccine (Havrix, Vaqta)

INDICATIONS: Prevention of hepatitis A in individuals at high risk, such as travelers, those in certain professions, or those practicing high-risk behavior.

ACTIONS: Provides active immunity.

DOSAGE: *Havrix:* 1440 EL.U. as a single IM dose.

Vaqta: 50 U as a single IM dose.

SUPPLIED: Injection 720 EL.U./0.5 mL, 1440 EL.U./1 mL.; 50 U/mL.

NOTES: Booster is recommended 6–12 months after primary vaccination.

Hepatitis B Immune Globulin (Hyperhep, H-BIG)

INDICATIONS: Exposure to HBsAg-positive materials such as blood, plasma, or serum (accidental needle-stick, mucous membrane contact, or oral ingestion).

ACTIONS: Passive immunization.

DOSAGE: 0.06 mL/kg IM to a maximum of 5 mL; within 24 hr of needle-stick or percutaneous exposure; within 14 days of sexual contact; repeat 1 and 6 months after exposure.

SUPPLIED: Injection.

NOTES: Administered in gluteal or deltoid muscle; if exposure continues, the patient should also receive the hepatitis B vaccine.

Hepatitis B Vaccine (Engerix-B, Recombivax HB)

INDICATIONS: Prevention of hepatitis B.

ACTIONS: Active immunization.

DOSAGE: 3 IM doses of 1 mL each, the first 2 given 1 month apart, the third 6 months after the first.

SUPPLIED: *Engerix-B:* Injection 20 μg/mL.

Recombivax HB: Injection 10 and 40 μg/mL.

NOTES: IM should be administered in the deltoid; may cause fever, injection site soreness; derived from recombinant DNA technology.

Hetastarch (Hespan)

INDICATIONS: Plasma volume expansion as an adjunct in the treatment of shock and leukapheresis.

ACTIONS: Synthetic colloid with actions similar to those of albumin.

DOSAGE: *Volume expansion:* 500–1000 mL (do not exceed 1500 mL/d) IV at a rate not to exceed 20 mL/kg/hr.

Leukapheresis: 250–700 mL.

SUPPLIED: Injection 6 g/100 mL.

NOTES: Hetastarch is *not* a substitute for blood or plasma; contraindicated in patients with severe bleeding disorders, severe congestive heart failure, or renal failure with oliguria or anuria.

Hydralazine (Apresoline, Others)

INDICATIONS: Treatment of moderate to severe hypertension.

ACTIONS: Peripheral vasodilator.

DOSAGE: Begin at 10 mg PO qid, then increase to 25 mg qid to a maximum of 300 mg/d.

SUPPLIED: Tablets 10 mg, 25 mg, 50 mg, 100 mg; injection 20 mg/mL.

NOTES: Use cautiously with impaired hepatic function and coronary artery disease. Compensatory sinus tachycardia can be eliminated with the addition of a beta-blocker. Chronically high doses can cause SLE-like syndrome. Supraventricular tachycardia can occur following IM administration; dosage adjustment in renal impairment.

Hydrochlorothiazide (HydroDIURIL, Esidrix, Others)

INDICATIONS: Edema, hypertension, congestive heart failure.
ACTIONS: Thiazide diuretic; inhibits sodium reabsorption in the distal tubule.
DOSAGE: 25–100 mg PO q day in single or divided doses.
SUPPLIED: Tablets 25 mg, 50 mg, 100 mg; capsules 12.5 mg; oral solution: 50 mg/5 mL.
NOTES: Hypokalemia is frequent; hyperglycemia, hyperuricemia, hyperlipidemia, and hyponatremia are common side effects.

Hydrochlorothiazide and Amiloride (Moduretic)

INDICATIONS: Hypertension; adjunctive therapy for CHF.
ACTIONS: Combined effects of a thiazide diuretic and a potassium-sparing diuretic.
DOSAGE: 1–2 tablets PO q day.
SUPPLIED: Tablets (amiloride/hydrochlorothiazide) 5 mg/50 mg.
NOTES: Hypokalemia, hyperkalemia, hyperglycemia, hyperuricemia, hyperlipidemia, and hyponatremia are common side effects.

Hydrochlorothiazide and Spironolactone (Aldactazide)

INDICATIONS: Edema (congestive heart failure, cirrhosis); hypertension.
ACTIONS: Combined effects of a thiazide diuretic and a potassium-sparing diuretic.
DOSAGE: 25–200 mg each component per day in divided doses.
SUPPLIED: Tablets (hydrochlorothiazide/spironolactone) 25 mg/25 mg, 50 mg/50 mg.
NOTES: Hypokalemia, hyperkalemia, hyperglycemia, hyperuricemia, hyperlipidemia, and hyponatremia are common side effects.

Hydrochlorothiazide and Triamterene (Dyazide, Maxzide)

INDICATIONS: Edema; hypertension.
ACTIONS: Combined effects of a thiazide diuretic and a potassium-sparing diuretic.
DOSAGE: *Dyazide:* 1–2 capsules PO q day–bid.
Maxzide: 1 tablet PO q day.
SUPPLIED: (triamterene/HCTZ) 37.5 mg/25 mg, 50 mg/25 mg, 75 mg/50 mg.
NOTES: HCTZ component in Maxzide is more bioavailable than Dyazide; can cause hyperkalemia as well as hypokalemia; follow serum potassium levels. Hyperglycemia, hyperuricemia, hyperlipidemia, and hyponatremia are common side effects.

Hydrocodone and Acetaminophen (Lorcet, Vicodin, Others) [C]

INDICATIONS: Moderate to severe pain; hydrocodone has antitussive properties.
ACTIONS: Narcotic analgesic with non-narcotic analgesic.
DOSAGE: 1–2 capsules or tablets PO Q 4–6 hr prn.
SUPPLIED: Many different combinations; specify hydrocodone/acetaminophen dose: capsules 5/500; tablets 2.5/500, 5/400, 5/500, 7.5/400, 10/400, 7.5/500, 7.5/650, 7.5/750, 10/325, 10/400, 10/500, 10/650; elixir and solution (fruit punch flavored) 2.5 mg hydrocodone/167 mg acetaminophen per 5 mL.

Hydrocodone and Aspirin (Lortab ASA, Others) [C]

INDICATIONS: Moderate to severe pain.
ACTIONS: Narcotic analgesic with nonsteroidal anti-inflammatory.
DOSAGE: 1–2 PO Q 4–6 hr prn.
SUPPLIED: 5 mg hydrocodone/500 mg aspirin per tablet.

Hydrocodone and Guaifenesin (Hycotuss Expectorant, Others) [C]

INDICATIONS: Nonproductive cough associated with respiratory infection.
ACTIONS: Expectorant plus cough suppressant.
DOSAGE: 5 mL Q 4 hr, PC and HS.
SUPPLIED: Hydrocodone 5 mg/guaifenesin 100 mg/5 mL.

Hydrocodone and Homatropine (Hycodan, Others) [C]

INDICATIONS: Relief of cough.
ACTIONS: Combination antitussive.
DOSAGE: Dose based on hydrocodone 5–10 mg Q 4–6 hr.
SUPPLIED: Syrup 5-mg hydrocodone/5 mL; tablet 5-mg hydrocodone.

Hydrocodone and Ibuprofen (Vicoprofen) [C]

INDICATIONS: Moderate to severe pain (less than 10 d).
ACTIONS: Narcotic with nonsteroidal anti-inflammatory.
DOSAGE: 1–2 tablets Q 4–6 hr prn.
SUPPLIED: Tablets 7.5 mg hydrocodone/200 mg ibuprofen.

Hydrocodone and Pseudoephedrine (Entuss-D, Histussin-D, Others) [C]

INDICATIONS: Cough and nasal congestion.
ACTIONS: Narcotic cough suppressant with decongestant.
DOSAGE: 5 mL qid, prn.
SUPPLIED: *Entuss-D*: 5-mg hydrocodone/30 mg pseudoephedrine/5 mL; *Histussin-D:* 5-mg hydrocodone/60 mg pseudoephedrine/5 mL.

Hydrocodone, Chlorpheniramine, Phenylephrine, Acetaminophen, and Caffeine (Hycomine) [C]

INDICATIONS: Cough and symptoms of upper respiratory infections.
ACTIONS: Narcotic cough suppressant with decongestants and analgesic.
DOSAGE: 1 PO, Q 4 hr, prn.
SUPPLIED: Hydrocodone 5 mg/chlorpheniramine 2 mg/phenylephrine 10 mg/acetaminophen 250 mg/caffeine 30 mg/tablet.

Hydrocortisone [See Table 7–2, p 597]

Hydrocortisone, Rectal (Anusol-HC Suppository, Cortifoam Rectal, Proctocort, Others)

INDICATIONS: Adjunct to painful anorectal conditions; radiation proctitis, management of ulcerative colitis.
ACTIONS: Anti-inflammatory steroid.
DOSAGE: *Adults:* Ulcerative colitis 10–100 mg rectally q day/bid for 2–3 weeks.
SUPPLIED: Hydrocortisone acetate rectal aerosol 90 mg/applicator; suppository 25 mg; hydrocortisone base rectal cream 1% and 2.5%; rectal suspension: 100 mg/60 mL.

Hydromorphone (Dilaudid) [C]

INDICATIONS: Management of moderate to severe pain.
ACTIONS: Narcotic analgesic.
DOSAGE: 1–4 mg PO, IM, IV, or PR Q 4–6 hr prn; 3 mg PR Q 6–8 hr prn.
SUPPLIED: Tablets 1 mg, 2 mg, 3 mg, 4 mg, 8 mg; liquid 5 mg/mL; injection 1 mg/mL, 2 mg/mL, 4 mg/mL, 10 mg/mL; suppositories: 3 mg.
NOTES: 1.5 mg IM is equivalent to 10 mg of morphine IM; side effects include sedation, dizziness, GI upset.

Hydroxyurea (Hydrea, Droxia)

INDICATIONS: Chronic myelogenous leukemia (CML), polycythemia vera, head and neck cancer, ovarian cancer, melanoma, colon cancer, acute leukemia, sickle cell anemia, HIV.
ACTIONS: Probable inhibitor of the ribonucleotide reductase system.
DOSAGE: 50–75 mg/kg for WBC counts of > 100,000 cells/mL; 20–30 mg/kg in refractory CML. *HIV:* 1000–1500 mg daily in single or divided doses.
SUPPLIED: Capsules 200 mg, 300 mg, 400 mg, 500 mg.
NOTES: Toxicity includes myelosuppression (primarily leukopenia), nausea and vomiting, rashes, facial erythema, radiation recall reactions, and renal dysfunction; dosage adjustment in renal dysfunction.

Hydroxyzine (Atarax, Vistaril)

INDICATIONS: Anxiety, tension, sedation, itching.
ACTIONS: Antihistamine, anxiety.
DOSAGE: *Anxiety or sedation:* 50–100 mg PO or IM qid or prn (maximum 600 mg/d). *Itching:* 25–50 mg PO or IM tid–qid.
SUPPLIED: Tablets 10 mg, 25 mg, 50 mg, 100 mg; capsules 25 mg, 50 mg, 100 mg; syrup 10 mg/5 mL; suspension 25 mg/5 mL; injection 25, 50 mg/mL.
NOTES: Useful in potentiating the effects of narcotics; not for IV use; drowsiness and anticholinergic effects are common.

Hyoscyamine (Anaspaz, Cystospaz, Levsin, Others)

INDICATIONS: Spasm associated with GI and bladder disorders.
ACTIONS: Anticholinergic, antispasmodic.
DOSAGE: Tablets 0.125–0.25 mg (1–2 tablets) 3–4 × a day, AC and HS; sustained-release capsule 1 Q 12 hr.
SUPPLIED: Capsules sustained-release (Cystospaz-M, Levsinex).

Hyoscyamine, Atropine, Scopolamine, and Phenobarbital (Donnatal, Others)

INDICATIONS: Irritable bowel, spastic colitis, peptic ulcer, spastic bladder.
DOSAGE: Tablets 0.125–0.25 mg (1–2 tablets) 3–4 × a day, sustained-release capsule 1 capsule Q 12 hr, 5–10 mL; elixir 3–4 × a day or Q 8 hr.

Ibuprofen (Motrin, Rufen, Advil, Others) [See Table 7–11, pp 605-6]

Ibutilide (Corvert)

INDICATIONS: Rapid conversion of atrial fibrillation or flutter.
ACTIONS: Class III antiarrhythmic agent.
DOSAGE: 0.01 mg/kg (maximum 1 mg) IV infusion over 10 minutes. May be repeated once.
SUPPLIED: Injection 0.1 mg/mL.
NOTES: Do not administer Class I or III antiarrhythmics concurrently or within 4 hours of ibutilide infusion.

Idarubicin (Idamycin)

INDICATIONS: Acute myelocytic leukemia (in combination with cytarabine), chronic myelogenous leukemia in blast crisis, and acute lymphocytic leukemia.
ACTIONS: DNA intercalating agent; inhibits DNA topoisomerases I and II.
DOSAGE: Refer to specific protocol.
NOTES: Toxicity includes myelosuppression, cardiotoxicity, nausea and vomiting, mucositis, alopecia, and irritation at sites of intravenous administration; rare changes in renal and hepatic function; dosage adjustment in renal or hepatic dysfunction.

Ifosfamide (Ifex, Holoxan)

INDICATIONS: Lung cancer (small cell and non-small cell), soft tissue sarcoma, testicular cancer, non-Hodgkin's lymphoma.
ACTIONS: Alkylating agent.
DOSAGE: Refer to specific protocol.
NOTES: Toxicity includes hemorrhagic cystitis, nephrotoxicity, nausea and vomiting, mild to moderate leukopenia, lethargy and confusion, alopecia, and hepatic enzyme elevations; dosage adjustment in renal impairment.

Imipenem-Cilastatin (Primaxin)

INDICATIONS: Treatment of serious infections caused by a wide variety of susceptible bacteria; inactive against *S aureus,* group A and B streptococci, and others.
ACTIONS: Bactericidal; interferes with cell wall synthesis.
DOSAGE: 250–500 mg (imipenem) IV Q 6 hr.
SUPPLIED: Injection (imipenem/cilastatin) 250 mg/250 mg, 500 mg/500 mg.

NOTES: Seizures may occur if drug accumulates; adjust dosage for renal insufficiency to avoid drug accumulation if calculated creatinine clearance is < 70 mL/min.

Imipramine (Tofranil)

INDICATIONS: Treatment of depression, panic attacks, enuresis, chronic pain.
ACTIONS: Tricyclic antidepressant; increases synaptic concentration of serotonin and/or norepinephrine in the CNS.
DOSAGE: *Hospitalized patient:* Start at 100 mg/24 hr PO in divided doses; can increase over several weeks to 250–300 mg/24 hr.
Outpatient: Maintenance dose of 50–150 mg PO Q HS, not to exceed 200 mg/24 hr.
SUPPLIED: Tablets 10 mg, 25 mg, 50 mg; capsules 75 mg, 100 mg, 125 mg, 150 mg.
NOTES: Do not use with monoamine oxidase inhibitors; less sedation than with amitriptyline.

Imiquimod Cream, 5% (Aldara)

INDICATIONS: Treatment of external genital warts.
ACTIONS: Exact mechanism unknown; may induce cytokines.
DOSAGE: Applied 3 × a week; leave on skin for 6–10 hours and wash off with soap and water; use for a maximum of 16 weeks.
SUPPLIED: Single-dose packets (250 mg of the cream).
NOTES: Local skin reactions are common.

Immune Globulin, Intravenous (Gamimmune N, Sandoglobulin, Gammar IV)

INDICATIONS: IgG antibody deficiency disease states such as congenital agammaglobulinemia, common variable hypogammaglobulinemia, and bone marrow transplantation (BMT); idiopathic thrombocytopenic purpura (ITP).
ACTIONS: IgG supplementation.
DOSAGE: *Immunodeficiency:* 100–200 mg/kg IV monthly at a rate of 0.01–0.04 mL/kg/min to a maximum of 400 mg/kg/dose.
ITP: 400 mg/kg/dose IV q day for 5 days.
BMT: 500 mg/kg/week.
SUPPLIED: Injection.
NOTES: Adverse effects are associated mostly with the rate of infusion.

Inamrinone (Inocor)

INDICATIONS: Short-term management of low cardiac output states and pulmonary hypertension.
ACTIONS: Positive inotrope with vasodilator activity.
DOSAGE: Initial dose give IV bolus of 0.75 mg/kg over 2–3 min followed by a maintenance dose of 5–10 μg/kg/min.
SUPPLIED: Injection 5 mg/mL.
NOTES: Not to exceed 10 mg/kg/d; incompatible with dextrose-containing solutions; monitor for fluid and electrolyte changes and renal function during therapy.

Indapamide (Lozol)

INDICATIONS: Treatment of hypertension and congestive heart failure.
ACTIONS: Thiazide diuretic; enhances sodium, chloride, and water excretion in the proximal segment of the distal tubule.
DOSAGE: 1.25–5.0 mg PO q day.
SUPPLIED: Tablets 1.25 mg, 2.5 mg.
NOTES: Doses > 5 mg do not have additional effects on lowering BP.

Indinavir (Crixivan)

INDICATIONS: Treatment of HIV infection when antiretroviral therapy is indicated.
ACTIONS: Protease inhibitor; inhibits maturation of immature noninfectious virions to mature infectious virus.
DOSAGE: 800 mg PO Q 8 hr.
SUPPLIED: Capsules 200 mg, 400 mg.

NOTES: Use in combination with other antiretroviral agents; take on an empty stomach; may cause nephrolithiasis; drink six 8-oz glasses of water per day. Numerous drug interactions; dosage adjustment in hepatic impairment.

Indomethacin (Indocin) [See Table 7–11, pp 605-6]

Infliximab (Remicade)

INDICATIONS: Treatment of moderate to severe Crohn's disease; rheumatoid arthritis (in combination with methotrexate).
ACTIONS: IgG1κ neutralizes the biological activity of TNF-α.
DOSAGE: *Crohn's disease:* 5 mg/kg IV infusion, may follow with subsequent doses given at 2 and 6 weeks after initial infusion.
Rheumatoid arthritis: 3 mg/kg IV infusion at 0, 2, and 6 weeks, followed by every 8 weeks.
SUPPLIED: Injection.
NOTES: May cause hypersensitivity reaction, made up of human constant and murine variable regions; patients are predisposed to infection. Active tuberculosis may develop soon after initiating therapy with infliximab. Screening for latent tuberculosis before initiating therapy is recommended.

Influenza Vaccine (Fluzone, Fluogen, Flushield, Fluvirin)

INDICATIONS: Prevention of influenza in high-risk populations (chronic medical conditions such as heart disease, lung disease, or diabetes; residents of chronic care facilities; and any person over 50 years of age). Health care workers or members of households who may come into contact with the above patients are also encouraged to be immunized.
ACTIONS: Active immunization to inactivated virus grown in eggs.
DOSAGE: 0.5 mL/dose IM. Optimal time for vaccination in the United States is October–November, since protection begins 1–2 weeks after vaccination and lasts up to 6 months.
SUPPLIED: Each year, specific polyvalent influenza vaccines are manufactured based on predictions of the strains likely to be active in the influenza season. The flu season is generally from December through the spring in the United States.
NOTES: Soreness at the injection site and fever or malaise are common after injection; severe reactions are rare. Whole or split virus is usually given to adults.

Insulin [See Table 7–1, p 597]

INDICATIONS: Type 1 and type 2 diabetes mellitus that cannot be controlled by diet and/or oral hypoglycemic agents; adjunct to the management of acute life-threatening hyperkalemia.
ACTIONS: Insulin supplementation.
DOSAGE: Usually given SC but can also be given IV or IM (only regular insulin can be given IV).
SUPPLIED: See Table 7–1, p 597.
NOTES: The highly purified insulins provide an increase in free insulin; monitor patients closely for several weeks when changing doses.

Interferon Alfa (Roferon-A, Intron A)

INDICATIONS: Treatment of hairy cell leukemia, Kaposi's sarcoma, multiple myeloma, chronic myelogenous leukemia, renal cell carcinoma, bladder cancer, melanoma, chronic hepatitis C.
ACTIONS: Direct antiproliferative action against tumor cells; modulation of the host immune response.
DOSAGE: Dictated by treatment protocol.
Alfa-2a (Roferon): 3 million IU daily for 16–24 weeks SC or IM.
Alfa-2b (Intron A): 2 million IU/m^2 IM or SC 3 × a week for 2–6 months; intravesical 50–100 million IU in 50 mL normal saline weekly × 6.
SUPPLIED: Injectable forms.
NOTES: May cause flu-like symptoms; fatigue is common; anorexia occurs in 20–30% of patients; neurotoxicity may occur at high doses; neutralizing antibodies can occur in up to 40% of patients receiving prolonged therapy.

Interferon Alpha-2B and Ribavirin Combination (Rebetron)

INDICATIONS: Treatment of chronic hepatitis C in patients with compensated liver disease who have relapsed following alpha interferon therapy.
ACTIONS: Combination antiviral agents.
DOSAGE: 3 million units Intron A SC 3 × a week with 1000–1200 mg of Rebetol PO divided bid dose for 24 weeks; if patient weighs < 75 kg, give 1000 mg of Rebetol per day.
SUPPLIED: Combination pack if < 75 kg:

- 6 vials Intron A (3 million units/0.5 mL) with 6 syringes and alcohol swabs; 70 Rebetol capsules.
- One 18 million units multidose vial of Intron A injection (22.5 million U/3.8 mL; 3 million units/0.5 mL) and 6 syringes and alcohol swabs; 70 Rebetol capsules.
- One 18 million IU Intron A injection multidose pen (22.5 million IU per 1.5 mL; 3 million IU/0.2 mL) and 6 disposable needles and alcohol swabs; 70 Rebetol capsules.
- For patients weighing > 75 kg: identical except for 84 Rebetol capsules per pack.

NOTES: Patients must be instructed in self-administration of SC Intron A.

Interferon Alfacon-1 (Infergen)

INDICATIONS: Management of chronic hepatitis C.
ACTIONS: Biologic response modifier.
DOSAGE: 9 μg SC 3 times per week.
SUPPLIED: Injection 9, 15 μg.
NOTES: At least 48 hours should elapse between injections.

Interferon Beta-1b (Betaseron)

INDICATIONS: Management of multiple sclerosis.
ACTIONS: Biologic response modifier.
DOSAGE: 0.25 mg SC every other day.
SUPPLIED: Powder for injection 0.3 mg.
NOTES: May cause flu-like syndrome.

Interferon Gamma-1b (Actimmune)

INDICATIONS: Management of chronic granulomatous disease.
ACTIONS: Biologic response modifier.
DOSAGE: 50 mg/m^2 SC 3 × weekly.
SUPPLIED: Injection 100 mg.
NOTES: 100 mg = 3 million U; may cause flu-like syndrome.

Ipecac Syrup

INDICATIONS: To induce vomiting in the treatment of drug overdose and certain cases of poisoning.
ACTIONS: Irritation of the GI mucosa; stimulation of the chemoreceptor trigger zone.
DOSAGE: 15–30 mL PO, followed by 200–300 mL of water; if no emesis occurs in 20 min, may repeat × 1.
SUPPLIED: Syrup 15 mL, 30 mL.
NOTES: Do not use for ingestion of petroleum distillates or strong acid, base, or other corrosive or caustic agents; not for use in comatose or unconscious patients; caution in CNS depressant overdose.

Ipratropium (Atrovent)

INDICATIONS: Management of bronchospasm associated with chronic obstructive pulmonary disease, bronchitis, and emphysema; rhinorrhea.
ACTIONS: Synthetic anticholinergic agent similar to atropine.
DOSAGE: *Metered-dose inhaler:* 2–4 puffs qid.
Nasal: 2 sprays in each nostril 2–3 × daily.

SUPPLIED: Metered-dose inhaler 18 μg/dose; solution for inhalation 0.02%; nasal spray 0.03%, 0.06%.
NOTES: Not for initial treatment of acute episodes of bronchospasm.

Irbesartan (Avapro) [See Table 7–4, p 599]

Irinotecan (Camptosar)

INDICATIONS: Advanced colorectal cancer; lung cancer.
ACTIONS: Topoisomerase I inhibitor; interferes with DNA synthesis.
DOSE: Refer to specific protocol.
NOTES: Toxicities include myelosuppression, diarrhea (acute or subacute), nausea, vomiting, abdominal cramping, and alopecia. Diarrhea is dose-limiting in many studies; acute diarrhea associated with crampy abdominal pain can be successfully treated with atropine; subacute diarrhea is treated with loperamide (Imodium). Diarrhea appears to be correlated to levels of metabolite SN-38.

Iron Dextran (Dexferrum, Infed)

INDICATIONS: Iron deficiency when oral supplementation is not possible.
ACTIONS: Parenteral iron supplementation.
DOSAGE: Based on estimate of iron deficiency , given IM/IV. Give a 0.5-mL test dose prior to starting iron dextran.

$$\begin{aligned}&\text{Total replacement dose (mL)}\\&= 0.0476 \times \text{weight (kg)}\\&\quad \times (\text{desired hemoglobin (g / dL)}\\&\quad - \text{measured hemoglobin (g / dL)}\\&\quad + 1\text{ mL / per 5 kg weight (max 14 mL)}\end{aligned}$$

Maximum daily dose: 100 mg iron.
SUPPLIED: Injection 50 mg (Fe) per mL.
NOTES: Test dose must be administered since anaphylaxis is common. Iron dextran may be given deep IM using the "Z-track" technique, although IV administration is preferred.

Iron Sucrose (Venofer)

INDICATIONS: Iron deficiency anemia in patients undergoing chronic hemodialysis who are receiving supplemental erythropoietin therapy.
ACTIONS: Iron replacement.
DOSAGE: 5 mL (100 mg) IV during dialysis, given no faster than 1 mL (20 mg) per minute.
SUPPLIED: 20 mg elemental iron per mL, 5-mL vials.
NOTES: Most patients require cumulative doses of 1000 mg; anaphylaxis and significant hypotension may follow administration.

Isoniazid (INH)

INDICATIONS: Treatment and prophylaxis of *Mycobacterium* infections.
ACTIONS: Bactericidal; interferes with mycolic acid synthesis, thus disrupting the bacterial cell wall.
DOSAGE: *Active tuberculosis (TB):* 5 mg/kg/24 hr PO or IM q day (usually 300 mg/d).
Prophylaxis: 300 mg PO q day for 6–12 months.
SUPPLIED: Tablets 50 mg, 100 mg, 300 mg; syrup 50 mg/5 mL; injection 100 mg/mL.
NOTES: Can cause severe hepatitis. Isoniazid is given with other antituberculous drugs for active TB; consult *MMWR* for the latest recommendations on the treatment and prophylaxis of TB. Prophylaxis is usually with INH alone and treatment for active TB includes INH plus two or three other antituberculous drugs pending drug sensitivity results. IM route is rarely used. To prevent peripheral neuropathy, can give pyridoxine 50–100 mg/d. Dosage adjustment in hepatic impairment.

Isoproterenol (Isuprel, Medihaler-ISO)

INDICATIONS: Shock, cardiac arrest, and AV nodal block; antiasthmatic.
ACTIONS: $Beta_1$- and $beta_2$-receptor stimulant.
DOSAGE: *Shock:* 1–4 mg/min IV infusion; titrate to effect.
AV nodal block: 20–60 mg IV push; may repeat every 3–5 min; 1–5 mg/min IV infusion maintenance.
Inhalation: 1–2 inhalations 4–6 × daily.
SUPPLIED: Metered-dose inhaler; solution for nebulization: 0.5%, 1%; injection 0.02 mg/mL, 0.2 mg/mL.
NOTES: Contraindications include tachycardia; pulse > 130 BPM may induce ventricular arrhythmias.

Isosorbide Dinitrate (Isordil, Sorbitrate)

INDICATIONS: Treatment and prevention of angina pectoris.
ACTIONS: Relaxation of vascular smooth muscle.
DOSAGE: *Acute angina:* 5–10 mg PO (chewable tablet) Q 2–3 hr or 2.5–10 mg SL prn Q 5–10 min. > 3 doses should not be given in less than a 15- to 30-min period.
Angina prophylaxis: 5–60 mg PO tid.
SUPPLIED: Tablets 5 mg, 10 mg, 20 mg, 30 mg, 40 mg; sustained-release tablets 40 mg; sublingual tablets 2.5 mg, 5 mg, 10 mg; chewable tablets 5 mg, 10 mg; sustained-release capsules 40 mg.
NOTES: Nitrates should not be given on a chronic Q 6 hr or qid basis because of development of tolerance; can cause headaches; usually need to give a higher oral dose to achieve the same results as with sublingual forms.

Isosorbide Mononitrate (ISMO, Imdur)

INDICATIONS: Prevention of angina pectoris.
ACTIONS: Causes relaxation of the vascular smooth muscle.
DOSAGE: 20 mg PO bid, with the 2 doses given 7 hr apart or extended-release (Imdur) 30–120 mg PO q day.
SUPPLIED: Tablets 10 mg, 20 mg; extended-release 30 mg, 60 mg, 120 mg.

Isotretinoin (13-*cis* Retinoic Acid) (Accutane)

INDICATIONS: Severe acne unresponsive to conventional therapy.
ACTIONS: Retinoic acid derivative.
DOSAGE: 0.5–2 mg/kg/d PO divided bid.
SUPPLIED: Capsules 10 mg, 20 mg, 40 mg.
NOTES: Contraindicated in pregnancy and lactation; isolated reports of depression, psychosis, suicidal thoughts; dosage adjustment in hepatic impairment.

Isradipine (DynaCirc)

INDICATIONS: Treatment of hypertension and congestive heart failure.
ACTIONS: Calcium channel blocking agent.
DOSAGE: 2.5–10 mg PO bid.
SUPPLIED: Capsules 2.5 mg, 5.0 mg; tablets CR 5, 10 mg.

Itraconazole (Sporanox)

INDICATIONS: Treatment of systemic fungal infections caused by *Aspergillus, Blastomyces,* and *Histoplasma.*
ACTIONS: Inhibits synthesis of ergosterol.
DOSAGE: 200 mg PO or IV q day–bid.
SUPPLIED: Capsules 100 mg; solution 10 mg/mL; injection 10 mg/mL .
NOTES: Administer with meals or cola; should not be used concurrently with H_2-antagonist, omeprazole, antacids; numerous other drug interactions (a potent CYP3A4 inhibitor). Watch for signs/symptoms of CHF with IV use.

Kaolin-Pectin (Kaodene, KAO-SPEN, Kapectolin)

INDICATIONS: Treatment of diarrhea.

ACTIONS: Adsorbent demulcent.
DOSAGE: 60–120 mL PO after each loose stool or Q 3–4 hr prn.
SUPPLIED: Multiple OTC forms.
NOTES: Also available with opium (Parepectolin).

Ketoconazole (Nizoral)

INDICATIONS: Systemic fungal infections: candidiasis, chronic mucocutaneous candidiasis, blastomycosis, coccidioidomycosis, histoplasmosis, and paracoccidioidomycosis; topical cream for localized fungal infections due to dermatophytes and yeast; short-term treatment of prostate cancer where rapid reduction of testosterone is needed (ie, spinal cord compression).
ACTIONS: Inhibits fungal cell wall synthesis.
DOSAGE: *Oral:* 200 mg PO q day; increase to 400 mg PO q day for serious infections.
Prostate cancer: 400 mg PO tid (short term).
Topical: Apply to the affected area once daily (cream or shampoo).
SUPPLIED: Tablets 200 mg; topical cream 2%; shampoo 2%.
NOTES: Systemic use associated with hepatotoxicity; monitor LFTs. Avoid concurrent use with any agent increasing gastric pH (preventing absorption of ketoconazole); avoid concurrent use with cisapride. Ketoconazole may enhance activity of oral anticoagulants; may react with alcohol to produce a disulfiram-like reaction; numerous other drug interactions.

Ketoprofen (Orudis, Oruvail) [See Table 7–11, pp 605-6]

Ketorolac (Toradol) [See Table 7–11, pp 605-6]

Ketorolac Ophthalmic (Acular) [See Table 7–12, pp 607-9]

Ketotifen (Zaditor) [See Table 7–12, pp 607-9]

Labetalol (Trandate, Normodyne) (Also See Table 7–7, pp 601-2]

INDICATIONS: Hypertension and hypertensive emergencies.
ACTIONS: Alpha- and beta-adrenergic blocking agent.
DOSAGE: *Hypertension:* Initial dose, 100 mg PO bid; then 200–400 mg PO bid.
Hypertensive emergency: 20–80 mg IV bolus, then 2 mg/min IV infusion, titrated to effect.
SUPPLIED: Tablets 100 mg, 200 mg, 300 mg; injection 5 mg/mL.

Lactic Acid and Ammonium Hydroxide [Ammonium Lactate] (LAC-Hydrin)

INDICATIONS: Severe xerosis and ichthyosis.
ACTIONS: Emollient moisturizer.
DOSAGE: Apply bid.
SUPPLIED: Lactic acid 12% with ammonium hydroxide.

Lactobacillus (Lactinex Granules)

INDICATIONS: Control of diarrhea, especially after antibiotic therapy.
ACTIONS: Replaces normal intestinal flora.
DOSAGE: 1 packet, 2 capsules, or 4 tablets with meals or liquids tid–qid.
SUPPLIED: Tablets; capsules; enteric-coated capsules; powder in packets.

Lactulose (Chronulac, Cephulac)

INDICATIONS: Hepatic encephalopathy; laxative.
ACTIONS: Acidifies the colon, allowing ammonia to diffuse into the colon.
DOSAGE: *Acute hepatic encephalopathy:* 30–45 mL PO Q 1 hr until soft stools are observed, then tid–qid; adjust the dosage every 1–2 days to produce 2–3 soft stools q day.
Chronic laxative therapy: 30–45 mL PO tid–qid; adjust the dosage every 1–2 days to produce 2–3 soft stools q day.
Rectally: 200 g diluted with 700 mL of water instilled into the rectum.
SUPPLIED: Syrup 10 g/15 mL.
NOTES: Can cause severe diarrhea and life-threatening hypernatremia with an excessive number of stools per day.

Lamivudine (Epivir, Epivir-HBV)

INDICATIONS: Treatment of HIV infection when therapy is warranted based on clinical and/or immunologic evidence of disease progression; chronic hepatitis B.
ACTIONS: Inhibits HIV reverse transcriptase, resulting in viral DNA chain termination.
DOSAGE: *HIV:* 150 mg PO bid.
HBV: 100 mg once daily.
SUPPLIED: Tablets 100 mg, 150 mg; solution 5 mg/mL, 10 mg/mL.
NOTES: Used in combination with zidovudine; adjust dose for renal dysfunction.

Lamotrigine (Lamictal)

INDICATIONS: Treatment of partial seizures.
ACTIONS: Phenyltriazine antiepileptic.
DOSAGE: Initial dose 50 mg PO once daily, followed by 50 mg PO bid for 2 weeks, then maintenance dose of 300–500 mg/d in two divided doses.
SUPPLIED: Tablets 25 mg, 100 mg, 150 mg, 200 mg; chewable tablets 5 mg, 25 mg.
NOTES: May cause rash and photosensitivity; the value of therapeutic monitoring has not been established; interacts with other antiepileptics.

Lansoprazole (Prevacid) [See Table 7–14, p 611]

Latanoprost (Xalatan) [See Table 7–12, pp 607-9]

Leflunomide (Arava)

INDICATIONS: Treatment of active rheumatoid arthritis.
ACTIONS: Inhibits pyrimidine synthesis.
DOSAGE: Initial 100 mg q day for 3 days, followed by 10–20 mg q day.
SUPPLIED: Tablets 10 mg, 20 mg, 100 mg.
NOTES: **DO NOT USE** during pregnancy, category X; monitor serum transaminase levels during initial therapy.

Lepirudin (Refludan)

INDICATIONS: Management of heparin-induced thrombocytopenia.
ACTIONS: Direct inhibitor of thrombin.
DOSAGE: Bolus 0.4 mg/kg IV, followed by 0.15 mg/kg continuous infusion.
SUPPLIED: Injection 50 mg.
NOTES: Adjust dose based on aPTT ratio; maintain aPTT ratio of 1.5–2.0.

Letrozole (Femara)

INDICATIONS: Treatment of advanced breast cancer.
ACTIONS: Nonsteroidal inhibitor of the aromatase enzyme system.
DOSAGE: Refer to specific protocol.
NOTES: Requires periodic CBC, thyroid function, electrolyte, liver function, and renal monitoring.

Leucovorin (Wellcovorin)

INDICATIONS: Overdose of folic acid antagonist; augmentation of 5-fluorouracil (5-FU).
ACTIONS: Reduced folate source; circumvents the action of folate reductase inhibitors (ie, methotrexate).
DOSAGE: *Methotrexate (MTX) rescue:* 10 mg/m^2/dose IV or PO Q 6 hr for 72 hours until MTX level < 10^{-8} molar.
5-FU: 200 mg/m^2/d IV 1–5 days during daily 5-FU treatment or 500 mg/m^2/week with weekly 5-FU therapy. *Adjunct to antimicrobials:* 5–15 mg PO q day.
SUPPLIED: Tablets 5 mg, 15 mg, 25 mg; injection.
NOTES: Many different dosing schedules exist for leucovorin rescue following MTX therapy.

Leuprolide (Lupron)

INDICATIONS: Treatment of prostate cancer, endometriosis, central precocious puberty (CPP).

ACTIONS: Luteinizing hormone (LH)-releasing hormone agonist; paradoxically inhibits release of gonadotropin, resulting in decreased LH and testosterone levels.
DOSAGE: *Prostate:* 7.5 mg IM Q 28 days or 22.5 mg IM Q 3 months of depot preparation. *Endometriosis* (depot only): 3.75 mg IM as a single monthly dose.
SUPPLIED: Injection 5 mg/mL; depot preparation 3.75 mg, 7.5 mg, 11.25 mg, 15 mg, 22.5 mg, 30 mg.
NOTES: Toxicity includes hot flashes, gynecomastia, nausea and vomiting, constipation, anorexia, dizziness, headache, insomnia, paresthesias, peripheral edema, and bone pain (transient "flare reaction" at 7–14 days after the first dose due to testosterone surge).

Levalbuterol (Xopenex)

INDICATIONS: Treatment and prevention of bronchospasm.
ACTIONS: Sympathomimetic bronchodilator.
DOSAGE: 0.63–1.25 mg nebulized Q 6–8 hr.
SUPPLIED: Solution for inhalation 0.63 mg/3 mL, 1.25 mg/3 mL.
NOTES: Therapeutically active R-isomer of albuterol.

Levamisole (Ergamisol)

INDICATIONS: Adjuvant therapy of Dukes C colon cancer (in combination with 5-FU).
ACTIONS: Multiple poorly understood immunostimulatory effects.
DOSAGE: Refer to specific protocol.
NOTES: Toxicity includes nausea and vomiting, diarrhea, abdominal pain, taste disturbance, anorexia, hyperbilirubinemia, disulfiram-like reaction with alcohol ingestion, minimal bone marrow depression, fatigue, fever, and conjunctivitis.

Levetiracetam (Keppra)

INDICATIONS: Treatment of partial onset seizures.
ACTIONS: Unknown.
DOSAGE: 500 mg PO bid, may be increased to a maximum of 3000 mg/d.
SUPPLIED: Tablets 250 mg, 500 mg, 750 mg.
NOTES: May cause dizziness and somnolence; may impair coordination; requires renal dosage adjustment.

Levobetaxolol (Betaxon) [See Table 7–12, pp 607-9]

Levobunolol (A-K Beta, Betagan) [See Table 7–12, pp 607-9]

Levocabastine (Livostin) [See Table 7–12, pp 607-9]

Levofloxacin (Levaquin)

INDICATIONS: Treatment of lower respiratory tract infections, sinusitis, and urinary tract infections.
ACTIONS: Quinolone antibiotic, inhibits DNA gyrase.
DOSAGE: 250–500 mg PO or IV once daily.
SUPPLIED: Tablets 250 mg, 500 mg; injection 5 mg/mL, 25 mg/mL.
NOTES: Reliable activity against *S pneumoniae,* drug interactions with cation-containing products; renal dosage adjustment.

Levonorgestrel Implant (Norplant)

INDICATIONS: Prevention of pregnancy.
DOSAGE: Implant 6 capsules in the mid forearm.
SUPPLIED: Kits containing 6 implantable capsules, each containing 36 mg.
NOTES: Prevents pregnancy for up to 5 years; capsules may be removed if pregnancy is desired.

Levothyroxine (Synthroid)

INDICATIONS: Hypothyroidism.
ACTIONS: Supplementation of L-thyroxine.
DOSAGE: Initial dose 25–50 μg/d PO or IV; increase by 25–50 μg/d every month; usual dose 100–200 μg/d.

SUPPLIED: Tablets 25 μg, 50 μg, 75 μg, 88 μg, 100 μg, 112 μg, 125 μg, 150 μg, 175 μg, 200 μg, 300 μg; injection 200 μg, 500 μg.
NOTES: Titrate dosage based on clinical response and thyroid function tests; dosage can be increased more rapidly in young to middle-aged patients.

Lidocaine (Anestacon Topical, Xylocaine, Others)

INDICATIONS: Local anesthetic; treatment of cardiac arrhythmias.
ACTIONS: Anesthetic; class IB antiarrhythmic.
DOSAGE: *Antiarrhythmic: Endotracheal:* 5 mg/kg; follow with 0.5 mg/kg in 10 min if effective.
IV Load: 1 mg/kg/dose bolus over 2–3 min; repeat in 5–10 min up to 200–300 mg/hr; continuous infusion of 20–50 μg/kg/min or 1–4 mg/min.
Topical: Apply max 3 mg/kg/dose.
Local injection anesthetic: Max 4.5 mg/kg.
SUPPLIED: Injection (local): 0.5%, 1%, 1.5%, 2%, 4 %, 10%, 20%; injection IV 1% (10 mg/mL), 2% (20 mg/mL); admixture 4%, 10%, 20%; IV infusion 0.2%, 0.4%; cream 2%; gel 2%, 2.5%, ointment 2.5%, 5%; liquid 2.5%; solution 2%, 4%; viscous 2%.
NOTES: Endotracheal doses should be diluted to 1–2 mL with normal saline. Epinephrine may be added for local anesthesia to prolong effect and help decrease bleeding. *Do not* use lidocaine with epinephrine on the digits, ears, or nose because vasoconstriction may cause necrosis. For IV forms, dosage reduction is required with liver disease or congestive heart failure. Dizziness, paresthesias, and convulsions are associated with toxicity; see Table 7–16, p 613, for drug levels.

Lidocaine/Prilocaine (EMLA)

INDICATIONS: Topical anesthetic; adjunct to phlebotomy or invasive dermal procedures.
ACTIONS: Topical anesthetic.
DOSAGE: *Cream and anesthetic disc (1 g/10 cm^2):* Thick layer of cream 2–2.5 g applied to intact skin and covered with an occlusive dressing (Tegaderm) for at least 1 hr.
Anesthetic disc: 1 g per 10 cm^2 for at least 1 hr.
SUPPLIED: Cream 2.5% lidocaine/2.5% prilocaine; anesthetic disc (1 g).
NOTES: Not for ophthalmic use; use with caution in patients at risk of methemoglobinemia; longer contact time gives greater effect.

Lindane (Kwell)

INDICATIONS: Treatment of head lice, crab lice, scabies.
ACTIONS: An ectoparasiticide and ovicide.
DOSAGE: *Cream or lotion:* Apply a thin layer after bathing and leave in place for 8–12 hr, pour on laundry.
Shampoo: Apply 30 mL and develop a lather with warm water for 4 min; comb out nits.
SUPPLIED: Lotion 1%; shampoo 1%.
NOTES: Caution patient about overuse; drug may be absorbed into blood; repeat in 7 days if necessary.

Linezolid (Zyvox)

INDICATIONS: Infections caused by gram-positive bacteria, including vancomycin-resistant and methicillin-resistant strains.
ACTIONS: Inhibits bacterial protein synthesis.
DOSAGE: 400–600 mg IV or PO Q 12 hr.
SUPPLIED: Injection 2 mg/mL; tablets 400 mg, 600 mg; suspension 100 mg/5 mL.
NOTES: A reversible inhibitor of MAO; avoid foods that contain tyramine; avoid cough and cold products containing pseudoephedrine. Myelosuppression may occur; monitor CBC weekly.

Liothyronine (Cytomel)

INDICATIONS: Hypothyroidism.
ACTIONS: T_3 replacement.
DOSAGE: Initial dose of 25 μg/24 hr, then titrate every 1–2 weeks according to clinical response and thyroid function tests to maintenance dose of 25–100 μg PO q day.
Myxedema coma: 25–50 μg IV.

SUPPLIED: Tablets 5 µg, 25 µg, 50 µg; injection 10µg/mL.
NOTES: Reduce dose in the elderly; monitor thyroid function tests.

Lisinopril (Prinivil, Zestril) [See Table 7–3, p 598]

Lithium Carbonate (Eskalith, Others)

INDICATIONS: Manic episodes of manic-depressive illness; maintenance therapy in recurrent disease.
ACTIONS: Effects a shift toward intraneuronal metabolism of catecholamines.
DOSAGE: *Acute mania:* 600 mg PO tid or 900 mg sustained-release bid.
Maintenance: 300 mg PO tid–qid.
SUPPLIED: Capsules 150 mg, 300 mg, 600 mg; tablets 300 mg; sustained-release tablets 300 mg, 450 mg; syrup 300 mg/5 mL.
NOTES: Dosage must be titrated; follow serum levels (see Table 7–16, page 613). Common side effects are polyuria, tremor; contraindicated in patients with severe renal impairment. Sodium retention or diuretic use may potentiate toxicity.

Lodoxamide (Alomide Ophthalmic) [See Table 7–12, pp 607-9]

Lomefloxacin (Maxaquin)

INDICATIONS: Treatment of urinary tract infections and lower respiratory tract infections caused by gram-negative bacteria; prophylaxis in transurethral procedures.
ACTIONS: Quinolone antibiotic; inhibits DNA gyrase.
DOSAGE: 400 mg PO q day.
SUPPLIED: Tablets 400 mg.
NOTES: May cause photosensitivity; renal dosage adjustment.

Lomustine (CCNU, CeeNU)

INDICATIONS: Hodgkin's lymphoma; primary brain tumors.
ACTIONS: Nitrosourea alkylating agent.
DOSAGE: Refer to specific protocol.
NOTES: Toxicity includes myelosuppression, renal injury, anorexia, nausea and vomiting, stomatitis, pulmonary fibrosis, and hepatotoxicity. High lipid solubility translates into excellent penetration into the CNS.

Loperamide (Imodium)

INDICATIONS: Treatment of diarrhea.
ACTIONS: Slows intestinal motility.
DOSAGE: Initial dose, 4 mg PO; then 2 mg after each loose stool, up to 16 mg/d.
SUPPLIED: Capsules 2 mg; tablets 2 mg; liquid 1 mg/5 mL, 1 mg/mL.
NOTES: Do not use in acute diarrhea caused by *Salmonella, Shigella,* or *C difficile.*

Lopinavir/Ritonavir (Kaletra)

INDICATIONS: HIV-1 infection.
ACTIONS: Combination protease inhibitor.
DOSAGE: 3 capsules or 5 mL PO bid with food.
SUPPLIED: 133.3 mg lopinavir/33.3 mg ritonavir capsules; 80 mg lopinavir/20 mg ritonavir per mL solution.
NOTES: Ritonavir inhibits metabolism of lopinavir; may inhibit metabolism of other drugs, including HMG CoA reductase inhibitors, midazolam, St. John's Wort. Adverse effects are similar to those of other protease inhibitors.

Loracarbef (Lorabid) [See Table 7–9, p 603]

Loratadine (Claritin)

INDICATIONS: Treatment of allergic rhinitis.
ACTIONS: Non-sedating antihistamine.
DOSAGE: 10 mg PO once daily.
SUPPLIED: Tablets 10 mg; syrup 1 mg/mL.

NOTES: Should be taken on an empty stomach.

Lorazepam (Ativan, Others) [C]

INDICATIONS: Anxiety and anxiety mixed with depression; preoperative sedation; control of status epilepticus; antiemetic; alcohol withdrawal.
ACTIONS: Benzodiazepine; antianxiety agent.
DOSAGE: *Anxiety:* 1–10 mg/d PO in 2–3 divided doses.

Preoperative sedation: 0.05 mg/kg to a maximum of 4 mg IM 2 hr prior to surgery.

Insomnia: 2–4 mg PO Q HS.

Status epilepticus: 4 mg/dose IV may be repeated at 10- to 15-min intervals; usual total dose 8 mg.

Antiemetic: 0.5–2 mg IV or PO Q 4–6 hr prn.

Alcohol withdrawal: 2–5 mg IV or 1–2 mg PO initially depending on the severity. Subsequent dosing will depend on type of management and symptoms (See Section I, Chapter 16, Delirium Tremens (DTs): Major Alcohol Withdrawal, V, p 95).

SUPPLIED: Tablets 0.5 mg, 1 mg, 2 mg; solution, oral concentrate 2 mg/mL; injection 2 mg/mL, 4 mg/mL.
NOTES: Decrease dose in elderly. Do not administer IV faster than 2 mg/min or 0.05 mg/kg/min. Effects of drug may not be apparent for as long as 10 min when given IV.

Losartan (Cozaar) [See Table 7–4, p 599]

Lovastatin (Mevacor) [See Table 7–15, p 612]

Lyme Disease Vaccine (Lymerix)

INDICATION: Prevention of Lyme disease.
ACTION: Provides active immunity against *B burgdorferi.*
DOSAGE: 30 μg/0.5 mL IM administered at 0, 1, and 12 months.
SUPPLIED: Vaccine 30 μg/0.5 mL.

Magaldrate (Riopan, Lowsium)

INDICATIONS: Hyperacidity associated with peptic ulcer, gastritis, and hiatal hernia.
ACTIONS: Low-sodium antacid.
DOSAGE: 5–10 mL PO between meals and HS.
SUPPLIED: Suspension.
NOTES: < 0.3 mg of sodium per tablet or teaspoon. *Do not* use in renal insufficiency due to magnesium content.

Magnesium Citrate

INDICATIONS: Vigorous bowel preparation; constipation.
ACTIONS: Cathartic laxative.
DOSAGE: 120–240 mL PO prn.
SUPPLIED: Effervescent solution.
NOTES: Do not use in renal insufficiency or intestinal obstruction.

Magnesium Hydroxide (Milk of Magnesia)

INDICATIONS: Constipation.
ACTIONS: Saline laxative.
DOSAGE: 15–30 mL PO prn.
SUPPLIED: Tablets 311 mg; liquid 400 mg/5 mL, 800 mg/5 mL.
NOTES: Do not use in renal insufficiency or intestinal obstruction.

Magnesium Oxide (MAG-Ox 400, Others)

INDICATIONS: Replacement for low plasma levels.
ACTIONS: Magnesium supplementation.
DOSAGE: 400–800 mg/d divided q day–qid.
SUPPLIED: Capsules 140 mg; tablets 400 mg.
NOTES: May cause diarrhea. Do not use in renal insufficiency or intestinal obstruction.

Magnesium Sulfate

INDICATIONS: Replacement for low plasma levels; refractory hypokalemia and hypocalcemia; pre-eclampsia and premature labor.
ACTIONS: Magnesium supplement.
DOSAGE: *Supplement:* 1–2 g IM or IV; repeat dosing based on response and continued hypomagnesemia.
Pre-eclampsia, premature labor: 4 g load, then 1–4 g/hr IV infusion.
SUPPLIED: Injection 100 mg/mL, 125 mg/mL, 250 mg/mL, 500 mg/mL; oral solution 500 mg/mL; granules 40 mEq/5 g.
NOTES: Reduce dose with low urine output or renal insufficiency.

Mannitol

INDICATIONS: Treatment of cerebral edema, oliguria, anuria, myoglobinuria.
ACTIONS: Osmotic diuretic.
DOSAGE: *Diuresis:* 0.2 g/kg/dose IV over 3–5 min; if no diuresis within 2 hr, discontinue.
Cerebral edema: 0.25 g/kg/dose IV push, repeated at 5-min intervals prn; increase incrementally to 1 g/kg/dose prn for increased intracranial pressure.
SUPPLIED: Injection 5%, 10%, 15%, 20%, 25%.
NOTES: Use cautiously with congestive heart failure or volume overload.

Mechlorethamine (Mustargen)

INDICATIONS: Hodgkin's and non-Hodgkin's lymphoma, cutaneous T-cell lymphoma (mycosis fungoides), lung cancer, chronic lymphocytic leukemia, chronic myelogenous leukemia, malignant pleural effusions.
ACTIONS: Alkylating agent (bifunctional).
DOSAGE: Refer to specific protocol.
NOTES: Toxicity includes myelosuppression, thrombosis, or thrombophlebitis at the site of injection; tissue damage with extravasation (sodium thiosulfate may be used topically to treat); nausea and vomiting; skin rash; amenorrhea; and sterility. High rates of sterility (especially in men) and secondary leukemia in patients treated for Hodgkin's disease. Highly volatile; must be administered within 30–60 min of preparation.

Meclizine (Antivert)

INDICATIONS: Motion sickness; vertigo associated with diseases of the vestibular system.
ACTIONS: Antiemetic, anticholinergic, and antihistaminic properties.
DOSAGE: 25 mg PO tid–qid prn.
SUPPLIED: Tablets 12.5 mg, 25 mg, 50 mg; chewable tablets 25 mg; capsules 25 mg, 30 mg.
NOTES: Drowsiness, dry mouth, and blurred vision commonly occur.

Medroxyprogesterone (Provera, Depo Provera, Cycrin)

INDICATIONS: Secondary amenorrhea and abnormal uterine bleeding caused by hormonal imbalance; contraception; endometrial cancer.
ACTIONS: Progestin supplement.
DOSAGE:

- *Secondary amenorrhea:* 5–10 mg PO q day for 5–10 days.
- *Abnormal uterine bleeding:* 5–10 mg PO q day for 5–10 days beginning on the 16th or 21st day of the menstrual cycle.
- *Contraception:* 150 mg IM every 3 months.
- *Endometrial cancer:* 400–1000 mg IM Q week.

SUPPLIED: Tablets 2.5 mg, 5 mg, 10 mg; Depo-injection 100 mg/mL, 150 mg/mL, 400 mg/mL.
NOTES: Contraindicated in patients with histories of past thromboembolic disorders or hepatic disease. If used for contraception, obtain pregnancy test if the last injection was over 3 months ago.

Megestrol Acetate (Megace)

INDICATIONS: Treatment of breast and endometrial cancers; appetite stimulant in cancer and HIV-related cachexia.

ACTIONS: Hormone; progesterone analogue.
DOSAGE: *Cancer:* 40–320 mg/d PO in divided doses.
Appetite regulation: 800 mg PO q day.
SUPPLIED: Tablets 20 mg, 40 mg; solution 40 mg/mL.
NOTES: May induce deep venous thrombosis; do not abruptly discontinue therapy.

Meloxicam (Mobic) [See Table 7–11, pp 605-6]

Melphalan (Alkeran, L-PAM)

INDICATIONS: Multiple myeloma, breast cancer, testicular cancer, ovarian cancer, melanoma, and allogenic and autologous bone marrow transplantation (BMT) in high doses.
ACTIONS: Alkylating agent (bifunctional).
DOSAGE: Refer to specific protocol.
NOTES: Toxicity includes myelosuppression (leukopenia and thrombocytopenia), secondary leukemia, alopecia, dermatitis, stomatitis, and pulmonary fibrosis; very rare hypersensitivity reactions.

Meperidine (Demerol) [C]

INDICATIONS: Relief of moderate to severe pain.
ACTIONS: Narcotic analgesic.
DOSAGE: 50–150 mg PO or IM Q 3–4 hr prn.
SUPPLIED: Tablets 50 mg, 100 mg; syrup 50 mg/mL; injection 10 mg/mL, 25 mg/mL, 50 mg/mL, 75 mg/mL, 100 mg/mL.
NOTES: 75 mg IM = 10 mg of morphine IM; beware of respiratory depression; reduces seizure threshold; should not be used in renal failure; reduce dose in elderly and with renal impairment.

Meprobamate (Equinil, Miltown)

INDICATIONS: Short-term relief of anxiety.
ACTIONS: Mild tranquilizer; antianxiety.
DOSAGE: 400 mg PO tid–qid up to 2400 mg/d; sustained release 400–800 mg PO bid.
SUPPLIED: Tablets 200 mg, 400 mg, 600 mg; sustained-release capsules 200 mg, 400 mg.
NOTES: May cause drowsiness; adjust dose for renal impairment.

Mercaptopurine (6-MP) (Purinethol)

INDICATIONS: Acute leukemias, second-line treatment of chronic myelogenous leukemia and non-Hodgkin's lymphoma and immunosuppressant therapy for autoimmune diseases (Crohn's disease).
ACTIONS: Antimetabolite; mimics hypoxanthine.
DOSAGE: Refer to specific protocol.
NOTES: Toxicity includes mild hematologic toxicity; uncommon GI toxicity, except mucositis, stomatitis, and diarrhea. Rash, fever, eosinophilia, jaundice, and hepatitis have been reported. Concurrent allopurinol therapy requires a 67–75% dose reduction of 6-MP because of interference with metabolism by xanthine oxidase.

Meropenem (Merrem)

INDICATIONS: Treatment of serious infections caused by a wide variety of bacteria including intra-abdominal and polymicrobic; bacterial meningitis.
ACTIONS: Carbapenem; inhibition of cell wall synthesis.
DOSAGE: 1 g IV Q 8 hr.
SUPPLIED: Injection.
NOTES: Adjust dose for renal function; less seizure potential than imipenem.

Mesalamine (Rowasa, Asacol, Pentasa)

INDICATIONS: Treatment of mild to moderate distal ulcerative colitis, proctosigmoiditis, or proctitis.
ACTIONS: Unknown; may topically inhibit prostaglandins.
DOSAGE: *Retention enema:* At bedtime daily or insert 1 suppository bid.

Oral: 800–1000 mg PO 3–4 × a day.

SUPPLIED: Tablets 400 mg; capsules 250 mg; suppository 500 mg; rectal suspension 4 g/60 mL.

Mesna (Mesnex)

INDICATIONS: Reduction of the incidence of ifosfamide- and cyclophosphamide-induced hemorrhagic cystitis.

ACTIONS: Antidote.

DOSAGE: 20% of the ifosfamide dose (w/w) or cyclophosphamide dose IV at 15 min prior to and 4 and 8 hr after chemotherapy.

SUPPLIED: Injection 100 mg/mL.

Mesoridazine (Serentil)

INDICATIONS: Schizophrenia, acute and chronic alcoholism, chronic brain syndrome.

ACTIONS: Phenothiazine antipsychotic.

DOSAGE: Initial dose 25–50 mg PO or IV tid; titrate to a maximum of 300–400 mg/d.

SUPPLIED: Tablets 10 mg, 25 mg, 50 mg, 100 mg; oral concentrate 25 mg/mL; injection 25 mg/mL.

NOTES: Low incidence of extrapyramidal side effects.

Metaproterenol (Alupent, Metaprel)

INDICATIONS: Bronchodilator for asthma and reversible bronchospasm.

ACTIONS: Sympathomimetic bronchodilator.

DOSAGE: *Inhalation:* 1–3 inhalations Q 3–4 hr to a maximum of 12 inhalations Q 24 hr; allow at least 2 min between inhalations.

Oral: 20 mg Q 6–8 hr.

SUPPLIED: Aerosol 75 mg, 150 mg; solution for inhalation 0.4%, 0.6%, 5%; tablets 10 mg, 20 mg; syrup 10 mg/5 mL.

NOTES: Fewer $beta_1$-effects than isoproterenol and is longer acting.

Metaxalone (Skelaxin)

INDICATIONS: Relief of painful musculoskeletal conditions.

ACTIONS: Centrally acting skeletal muscle relaxant.

DOSAGE: 800 mg PO 3–4 × a day.

SUPPLIED: Tablets 400 mg.

Metformin (Glucophage)

INDICATIONS: Treatment of non-insulin-dependent diabetes mellitus.

ACTIONS: Decreases hepatic glucose production; decreases intestinal absorption of glucose; improves insulin sensitivity.

DOSAGE: Initial dose of 500 mg PO bid; dose may be increased to a maximum daily dose of 2500 mg. XR: 500–2000 mg PO Q pm.

SUPPLIED: Tablets 500 mg, 850 mg, 1000 mg; XR tablets 500 mg.

NOTES: Administer with the morning and evening meals. May cause lactic acidosis. *Do not use metformin* if serum creatinine is > 1.3 in females or > 1.4 in males; withhold prior to and following IV contrast studies; contraindicated in hypoxemic conditions, including acute congestive heart failure and sepsis.

Methadone (Dolophine) [C]

INDICATIONS: Severe pain; detoxification and maintenance of narcotic addiction.

ACTIONS: Narcotic analgesic.

DOSAGE: 5–10 mg IM Q 3–8 hr or 5–15 mg PO Q 8 hr; titrate as needed.

SUPPLIED: Tablets 5 mg, 10 mg, 40 mg; oral solution 5 mg/5 mL, 10 mg/5 mL; oral concentrate 10 mg/mL; injection 10 mg/mL.

NOTES: Equianalgesic with parenteral morphine; long half-life; increase dose slowly to avoid respiratory depression.

Methenamine (Hiprex, Urex, Others)

INDICATIONS: Suppression or elimination of bacteriuria associated with chronic and recurrent infections of the urinary tract.

DOSAGE: *Hippurate:* 1 g bid.
Mandelate: 1 g qid PC and HS.

SUPPLIED: Methenamine hippurate (Hiprex, Urex): 1 g tablet; Methenamine mandelate 500 mg and 1 g enteric-coated tablet.

NOTES: Contraindicated in patients with renal insufficiency, severe hepatic disease, and severe dehydration.

Methimazole (Tapazole)

INDICATIONS: Hyperthyroidism; preparation for thyroid surgery or radiation.

ACTIONS: Blocks the formation of T_3 and T_4.

DOSAGE: Initial dosage 15–60 mg/d PO divided tid; maintenance dosage 5–15 mg PO q day.

SUPPLIED: Tablets 5 mg, 10 mg.

NOTES: Follow up on the patient clinically and with thyroid function tests.

Methocarbamol (Robaxin)

INDICATIONS: Relief of discomfort associated with painful musculoskeletal conditions.

ACTIONS: Centrally acting skeletal muscle relaxant.

DOSAGE: 1.5 g PO qid for 2–3 days; then 1 g PO qid maintenance therapy; IV form rarely indicated.

SUPPLIED: Tablets 500 mg, 750 mg; injection 100 mg/mL.

NOTES: Can discolor urine; may cause drowsiness or GI upset; contraindicated in patients with myasthenia gravis.

Methotrexate (Folex, Rheumatrex)

INDICATIONS: Treatment of acute lymphoblastic and myelogenous leukemias, leukemic meningitis, trophoblastic tumors (chorioepithelioma, choriocarcinoma, chorioadenoma destruens, hydatidiform mole), breast cancer, Burkitt's lymphoma, mycosis fungoides, osteosarcoma, head and neck cancer, Hodgkin's and non-Hodgkin's lymphoma, lung cancer, psoriasis, and rheumatoid arthritis.

ACTIONS: Inhibits dihydrofolate reductase-mediated generation of tetrahydrofolate.

DOSAGE: *Cancer:* Refer to specific protocol.
Rheumatoid arthritis: 7.5 mg/week PO as a single dose each week; OR 2.5 mg Q 12 hr PO for 3 doses each week.

SUPPLIED: Tablets 2.5 mg; injection 2.5 mg/mL, 25 mg/mL; preservative-free injection 25 mg/mL.

NOTES: Toxicity includes myelosuppression, nausea and vomiting, anorexia, mucositis, diarrhea, hepatotoxicity (transient and reversible; may progress to atrophy, necrosis, fibrosis, cirrhosis), rashes, dizziness, malaise, blurred vision, renal failure, pneumonitis, and, rarely, pulmonary fibrosis. Chemical arachnoiditis and headache may occur with intrathecal delivery. "High-dose" therapy requires leucovorin rescue to prevent severe hematologic and mucosal toxicity. Monitor blood counts and methotrexate levels carefully.

Methyldopa (Aldomet)

INDICATIONS: Treatment of essential hypertension.

ACTIONS: Centrally acting antihypertensive.

DOSAGE: 50–500 mg PO bid–tid (maximum 2–3 g/d); OR 250 mg–1 g IV Q 6–8 hr.

SUPPLIED: Tablets 125 mg, 250 mg, 500 mg; oral suspension 50 mg/mL; injection 50 mg/mL.

NOTES: Do not use methyldopa in the presence of liver disease. May discolor urine. Initial transient sedation or drowsiness are frequent side effects.

Methylergonovine (Methergine)

INDICATIONS: Prevention and treatment of postpartum hemorrhage caused by uterine atony.

ACTIONS: Ergotamine derivative.

DOSAGE: 0.2 mg IM after delivery of placenta; may repeat dose at 2- to 4-hr intervals or 0.2–0.4 mg PO Q 6–12 hr for 2–7 days.

SUPPLIED: Injectable forms; tablets 0.2 mg.

NOTES: IV doses should be given over a period of not less than 1 min with frequent BP monitoring.

Methylprednisolone (Solu-Medrol) [See Table 7–2, p 597]

Metipranolol (Optipranolol) [See Table 7-12, pp 607-9]

Metoclopramide (Reglan, Octamide)

INDICATIONS: Relief of diabetic gastroparesis; symptomatic gastroesophageal reflux disease; relief of cancer chemotherapy-induced nausea and vomiting.

ACTIONS: Stimulates motility of the upper GI tract and blocks dopamine in the chemoreceptor trigger zone.

DOSAGE: *Diabetic gastroparesis:* 10 mg PO 30 min AC and HS for 2–8 weeks prn; OR same dose given IV for 10 days, then switch to PO.

Reflux: 10–15 mg PO 30 min AC and HS.

Antiemetic: 1–3 mg/kg/dose IV 30 min prior to antineoplastic agent, then Q 2 hr for 2 doses, then Q 3 hr for 3 doses.

SUPPLIED: Tablets 5 mg, 10 mg; syrup 5 mg/5 mL; solution 10 mg/mL; injection 5 mg/mL.

NOTES: Dystonic reactions common with high doses; can be treated with IV diphenhydramine. Metoclopramide can also be used to facilitate small bowel intubation and radiologic evaluation of the upper GI tract.

Metolazone (Diulo, Zaroxolyn)

INDICATIONS: Mild to moderate essential hypertension; edema of renal disease or cardiac failure.

ACTIONS: Thiazide-like diuretic; inhibits reabsorption of sodium in the distal tubules.

DOSAGE: *Hypertension:* 2.5–5 mg PO daily.

Edema: 5–20 mg PO daily.

SUPPLIED: Tablets 0.5 mg, 2.5 mg, 5 mg, 10 mg.

NOTES: Monitor fluid and electrolyte status of the patient during treatment.

Metoprolol (Lopressor, Toprol XL) [See Table 7–7, pp 601-2]

Metronidazole (Flagyl, Metrogel)

INDICATIONS: Amebiasis, trichomoniasis, *C difficile, H pylori,* anaerobic infections, and bacterial vaginosis.

ACTIONS: Interferes with DNA synthesis.

DOSAGE:

- *Anaerobic infections:* 500 mg IV Q 6–8 hr.
- *Amebic dysentery:* 750 mg PO q day for 5–10 days.
- *Trichomoniasis:* 250 mg PO tid for 7 days or 2 g PO in a single dose.
- *C difficile:* 500 mg PO or IV Q 8 hr for 7–10 days.
- *Bacterial vaginosis:* 1 applicatorful intravaginally bid or 500 mg PO bid for 7 days.
- *Acne rosacea and skin:* apply bid.

SUPPLIED: Tablets 250 mg, 500 mg; tablets ER 750 mg; capsules 375 mg; topical lotion and gel 0.75%; vaginal gel 0.75% (5 g per applicator; 37.5 mg in 70-g tube).

NOTES: For *Trichomonas* infections, also treat the patient's partner. Reduce dose in patients with renal and hepatic failure. Metronidazole has no activity against aerobic bacteria; use in combination in serious mixed infections. Drug may cause a disulfiram-like reaction; avoid concurrent use of alcohol.

Metyrapone (Metopirone)

INDICATIONS: Diagnostic test for hypothalamic-pituitary adrenocorticotropic hormone (ACTH) function.

ACTIONS: Inhibits adrenocortical synthesis by blocking 11-beta hydroxylase.

DOSAGE: *Metapyrone test:*

- *Day 1:* Control period: Collect 24-hr urine to measure 17-hydroxycorticosteroids (17-OHCS) or 17-ketogenic steroids (17-KSG).
- *Day 2:* ACTH test: 50 U of ACTH infused over 8 hr; measure 24-hr urinary steroids.

- *Days 3–4:* Rest period.
- *Day 5:* Administer metyrapone 750 mg PO Q 4 hr for 6 doses; give with milk or a snack.

SUPPLIED: Tablets 250 mg.
NOTES: Normal 24-hr urine 17-OHCS is 3–12 mg; following ACTH, it increases to 15–45 mg/24 hr; normal response to metyrapone is a twofold to fourfold increase in 17-OHCS excretion. Drug interactions with phenytoin, cyproheptadine, and estrogens may lead to subnormal response.

Mexiletine (Mexitil)

INDICATIONS: Suppression of symptomatic ventricular arrhythmias; diabetic neuropathy.
ACTIONS: Class IB antiarrhythmic.
DOSAGE: Administer with food or antacids; 200–300 mg PO Q 8 hr; do not exceed 1200 mg/d.
SUPPLIED: Capsules 150 mg, 200 mg, 250 mg.
NOTES: Not to be used in cardiogenic shock or second- or third-degree AV block if no pacemaker is present. Drug may worsen severe arrhythmias. Monitor liver function during therapy; drug interactions with hepatic enzyme inducers and suppressors, may require dosage changes.

Mezlocillin (Mezlin) [See Table 7–6, p 600]

Miconazole (Monistat, Others)

INDICATIONS: Severe systemic fungal infections, including coccidioidomycosis, candidiasis, *Cryptococcus,* and others; various tinea forms; cutaneous candidiasis; vulvovaginal candidiasis; tinea versicolor.
ACTIONS: Fungicidal; alters permeability of the fungal cell membrane.
DOSAGE: *Dermatologic use:* Apply to affected area twice daily for 2–4 weeks.
Intravaginal: Insert 1 applicatorful or suppository at bedtime for 7 days.
Systemic use: Intravenous 200–3600 mg/d divided into Q 8-hr dosing.
SUPPLIED: Topical cream 2%; lotion 2%; powder 2%; spray 2%; vaginal suppository 100 mg, 200 mg; vaginal cream 2%.
NOTES: Antagonistic to amphotericin B in vivo.

Midazolam (Versed) [C]

INDICATIONS: Preoperative sedation; conscious sedation for short procedures; induction of general anesthesia.
ACTIONS: Short-acting benzodiazepine.
DOSAGE: 1–5 mg IV or IM; titrate dose to effect.
SUPPLIED: Injection 1 mg/mL, 5 mg/mL; syrup 2 mg/mL.
NOTES: Monitor the patient for respiratory depression. Midazolam may produce hypotension in conscious sedation.

Miglitol (Glyset)

INDICATIONS: Treatment of Type 2 diabetes mellitus.
ACTIONS: Alpha-glucosidase inhibitor; delays the digestion of ingested carbohydrates.
DOSAGE: Initial dose 25 mg PO three × daily taken at the first bite of each meal; maintenance dose 50–100 mg three × daily with meals.
SUPPLIED: Tablets 25 mg, 50 mg, 100 mg.
NOTES: May be used alone or in combination with sulfonylureas.

Milrinone (Primacor)

INDICATIONS: Treatment of congestive heart failure.
ACTIONS: Positive inotrope and vasodilator, with little chronotropic activity.
DOSAGE: Loading dose of 50 μg/kg, followed by a continuous infusion of 0.375–0.75 μg/kg/min.
SUPPLIED: Injection 1 μg/mL.
NOTES: Carefully monitor fluid and electrolyte status; adjust dose in renal impairment.

Mineral Oil

INDICATIONS: Constipation.
ACTIONS: Emollient laxative.
DOSAGE: 5–45 mL PO prn.
SUPPLIED: Liquid.

Minoxidil (Loniten, Rogaine)

INDICATIONS: Severe hypertension; treatment of male and female pattern baldness.
ACTIONS: Peripheral vasodilator; stimulates vertex hair growth.
DOSAGE: *Oral:* 2.5–10 mg PO bid–qid.
Topical: Apply twice daily to the affected area.
SUPPLIED: Tablets 2.5 mg, 10 mg; topical solution (Rogaine) 2%.
NOTES: Pericardial and pleural effusions and volume overload may occur with oral use; hypertrichosis after chronic use.

Mirtazapine (Remeron)

INDICATIONS: Treatment of depression.
ACTIONS: Tetracyclic antidepressant.
DOSAGE: 15 mg PO Q HS, up to 45 mg Q HS.
SUPPLIED: Tablets 15 mg, 30 mg, 45 mg.
NOTES: Do not increase dose at intervals of less than 1–2 weeks. Drug may cause agranulocytosis.

Misoprostol (Cytotec)

INDICATIONS: Prevention of NSAID-induced gastric ulcers.
ACTIONS: Synthetic prostaglandin with both antisecretory and mucosal protective properties.
DOSAGE: 200 μg PO qid with meals. If GI side effects occur, may reduce dose to 100 μg qid or 200 μg bid.
SUPPLIED: Tablets 100 μg, 200 μg.
NOTES AND CAUTION: Contraindicated during pregnancy; misoprostol can cause miscarriage with potentially dangerous bleeding. GI side effects are common.

Mitomycin C (Mutamycin)

INDICATIONS: Adenocarcinomas of the stomach, pancreas, colon, and breast; non-small cell lung cancer; head and neck cancer; cervical cancer; squamous cell carcinoma of the anus; and bladder cancer (intravesically).
ACTIONS: Alkylating agent; may also generate oxygen free radicals, which induce DNA strand breaks.
DOSAGE: Refer to specific protocol.
NOTES: Toxicity includes myelosuppression, which may persist up to 3–8 weeks after a dose and may be cumulative (minimized by a lifetime dose < 50–60 mg/m^2). Other toxicities are nausea and vomiting, anorexia, stomatitis, and renal toxicity. Microangiopathic hemolytic anemia (similar to hemolytic-uremic syndrome) with progressive renal failure may occur. Veno-occlusive disease of the liver, interstitial pneumonia, and alopecia (rarely) may occur; extravasation reactions can be severe. Adjust dose in renal impairment.

Mitotane (Lysodren)

INDICATIONS: Palliative treatment of inoperable adrenal cortex carcinoma.
ACTIONS: Exact action unclear; induces mitochondrial injury in adrenocortical cells.
DOSAGE: Refer to specific protocol.
NOTES: Toxicity includes anorexia, nausea and vomiting, and diarrhea. Acute adrenal insufficiency may be precipitated by physical stresses (shock, trauma, infection), in which case corticosteroid replacement is necessary. Allergic reactions (rare), visual disturbances, hemorrhagic cystitis, albuminuria, hematuria, hypertension or hypotension, minor aches, and fever also may occur.

Mitoxantrone (Novantrone)

INDICATIONS: Treatment of acute myelogenous leukemia (with cytarabine), acute lymphocytic leukemia, chronic myelogenous leukemia, breast and prostate cancer, non-Hodgkin's lymphoma.
ACTIONS: DNA intercalating agent; inhibitor of DNA topoisomerase II.
DOSAGE: Refer to specific protocol.
NOTES: Toxicity includes myelosuppression, nausea and vomiting, stomatitis, alopecia (infrequent), cardiotoxicity. The cumulative dose should not exceed 160 mg/m^2 in patients who have received mediastinal radiation therapy or 120 mg/m^2 in patients who have received prior anthracycline therapy; dosage adjustment for hepatic failure may be warranted.

Modafinil (Provigil)

INDICATIONS: Narcolepsy.
ACTIONS: Possible mechanisms include altered dopamine and norepinephrine release, decreased GABA-mediated neurotransmission.
DOSAGE: 200 mg PO Q morning.
SUPPLIED: Tablets 100 mg, 200 mg.
NOTES: Consider lower doses in elderly patients, reduce dose by 50% in patients with hepatic impairment; use with caution in patients with cardiovascular disease.

Moexipril (Univasc) [See Table 7—3, p 598]

Molindone (Moban)

INDICATIONS: Management of psychotic disorders.
ACTIONS: Piperazine phenothiazine.
DOSAGE: 50–75 mg/d, titrating up to 225 mg daily if necessary.
SUPPLIED: Tablets 5 mg, 10 mg, 25 mg, 50 mg, 100 mg; concentrate 20 mg/mL.

Montelukast (Singulair)

INDICATIONS: Prophylaxis and treatment of chronic asthma.
ACTIONS: Leukotriene receptor antagonist.
DOSAGE: 10 mg PO daily taken in the evening.
SUPPLIED: Tablets 10 mg; chewable tablets 4 mg, 5 mg.
NOTES: NOT for acute asthma attacks.

Morphine (Roxanol, Duramorph, MS Contin) [C]

INDICATIONS: Relief of severe pain.
ACTIONS: Narcotic analgesic.
DOSAGE: *Oral:* 10–30 mg Q 4 hr prn; sustained-release tablets 30–60 mg Q 8–12 hr.
IV/IM: 2–15 mg Q 2–6 hr.
SUPPLIED: Tablets 10 mg, 15 mg, 30 mg; sustained-release tablets 15 mg, 30 mg, 60 mg; solution 10 mg, 20 mg, 100 mg; suppositories 5, 10, 20 mg; injection 2 mg/mL, 4 mg/mL, 5 mg/mL, 8 mg/mL, 10 mg/mL, 15 mg/mL; preservative-free injection 0.5 mg/mL, 1 mg/mL.
NOTES: Morphine has many narcotic side effects; may require scheduled dosing to relieve severe chronic pain. Duramorph and MS Contin are commonly used sustained-release forms.

Moxifloxacin (Avelox)

INDICATIONS: Treatment of acute sinusitis, acute bronchitis, community-acquired pneumonia.
ACTIONS: Quinolone; inhibits DNA gyrase.
DOSAGE: 400 mg once daily.
SUPPLIED: Tablets 400 mg.
NOTES: Active against gram-negative bacteria and *Streptococcus pneumoniae;* interactions with products containing Mg, Ca, Al, and Fe and Class IA and III antiarrhythmic agents.

Mupirocin (Bactroban)

INDICATIONS: Treatment of impetigo; eradication of methicillin-resistant *Staphylococcus aureus* (MRSA) nasal carrier state.

ACTIONS: Inhibits bacterial protein synthesis.
DOSAGE: *Topical:* Apply small amount to affected area.
Nasal: Apply twice daily in the nostrils.
SUPPLIED: Ointment 2%; cream 2%.
NOTES: *Do not* use concurrently with other nasal products.

Muromonab-CD3 (Orthoclone OKT3)

INDICATIONS: Treatment of acute rejection following organ transplantation.
ACTIONS: Blocks T-cell function.
DOSAGE: 5 mg IV q day for 10–14 days.
SUPPLIED: Injection 5 mg/5 mL.
NOTES: Muromonab is a murine antibody; may cause significant fever and chills after the first dose; requires close patient monitoring for anaphylaxis or pulmonary edema.

Mycophenolate Mofetil (Cellcept)

INDICATIONS: Prevention of organ rejection following transplantation.
ACTIONS: Inhibits immunologically mediated inflammatory responses.
DOSAGE: 1 g PO bid.
SUPPLIED: Capsules 250 mg, 500 mg; injection 500 mg.
NOTES: Used in conjunction with corticosteroids and cyclosporin.

Nabumetone (Relafen) [See Table 7–11, pp 605-6]

Nadolol (Corgard) [See Table 7–7, pp 601-2]

Nafcillin (Nafcil, Unipen, Nallpen) [See Table 7–5, p 600]

Naftifine (Naftin)

INDICATIONS: Tinea cruris and tinea corporis.
ACTIONS: Antifungal antibiotic.
DOSAGE: Apply bid.
SUPPLIED: 1% cream, gel.

Nalbuphine (Nubain)

INDICATIONS: Treatment of moderate to severe pain; preoperative and obstetrical analgesia.
ACTIONS: Narcotic agonist-antagonist; inhibits ascending pain pathways.
DOSAGE: 10–20 mg IM or IV Q 4–6 hr prn; maximum of 160 mg per day; single maximum dose, 20 mg.
SUPPLIED: Injection 10 mg/mL, 20 mg/mL.
NOTES: Nalbuphine causes CNS depression and drowsiness. Use with caution in patients receiving opiate drugs.

Nalidixic Acid (NegGram)

INDICATIONS: Urinary tract infections caused by susceptible strains of *Proteus, Klebsiella, Enterobacter,* and *E coli* but not *Pseudomonas.*
ACTIONS: Inhibits bacterial RNA and DNA synthesis.
DOSAGE: *Treatment dose:* 1 g PO qid.
Suppressive dose: 500 mg PO qid.
SUPPLIED: Tablets 250 mg, 500 mg, 1 g; oral suspension 250 mg/5 mL.
NOTES: Resistance emerges within 48 hr in a significant percentage of trials. Nalidixic acid may enhance the effect of oral anticoagulants; may cause CNS adverse effects that reverse on discontinuation of the drug; has decreased effect with concurrent use of antacids.

Naloxone (Narcan)

INDICATIONS: Reversal of narcotic effect.
ACTIONS: Competitive narcotic antagonist.
DOSAGE: 0.4–2.0 mg IV, IM, or SC every 5 min; maximum total dose of 10 mg.
SUPPLIED: Injection 0.4 mg/mL, 1.0 mg/mL.

NOTES: May precipitate acute withdrawal in addicts; if no response after 10 mg, suspect a non-narcotic cause.

Naltrexone (Revia)

INDICATIONS: Treatment of alcoholism and narcotic addiction.
ACTIONS: Competitively binds to opioid receptors.
DOSAGE: 50 mg PO q day.
SUPPLIED: Tablets 50 mg.
NOTES: May cause hepatotoxicity; do not give until patient is opioid free for 7–10 days.

Naphazoline and Antazoline (Albalon-A Ophthalmic, Others) [See Table 7–12, pp 607-9]

Naphazoline and Pheniramine Acetate (Naphcon A) [See Table 7–12, pp 607-9]

Naproxen (Aleve, Naprosyn, Anaprox) [See Table 7–11, pp 605-6]

Naratriptan (Amerge)

INDICATIONS: Treatment of acute migraine attacks.
ACTIONS: Serotonin 5-HT_1 receptor antagonist.
DOSAGE: 1–2.5 mg PO once; may be repeated once in 4 hours.
SUPPLIED: Tablets 1 mg, 2.5 mg.
NOTES: Contraindicated in patients with severe renal impairment; adjust dose in patients with renal dysfunction; avoid use in patients with angina, ischemic heart disease, uncontrolled hypertension, and ergot administration.

Nedocromil (Tilade)

INDICATIONS: Management of patients with mild to moderate asthma.
ACTIONS: Anti-inflammatory agent.
DOSAGE: 2 inhalations 4 × a day.
SUPPLIED: Metered-dose inhaler.

Nedocromil Sodium (Alocril) [See Table 7–12, pp 607-9]

Nefazodone (Serzone)

INDICATIONS: Treatment of depression.
ACTIONS: Inhibits neuronal uptake of serotonin and norepinephrine.
DOSAGE: Initial dose 100 mg PO bid; usual effective range is 300–600 mg/d in 2 divided doses.
SUPPLIED: Tablets 100 mg, 150 mg, 200 mg, 250 mg.
NOTES: May cause postural hypotension and allergic reactions. Many drug interactions, potent CYP3A4 inhibitor.

Nelfinavir (Viracept)

INDICATIONS: Treatment of HIV infection.
ACTIONS: Protease inhibitor; results in formation of immature, non-infectious virion.
DOSAGE: 750 mg PO tid or 1250 mg PO bid.
SUPPLIED: Tablets 250 mg; oral powder.
NOTES: Food necessary to increase absorption; interacts with St. John's wort.

Neomycin, Bacitracin, and Polymyxin B (Neosporin Ointment) (See Bacitracin, Neomycin, and Polymixin, p 483]

Neomycin, Colistin, and Hydrocortisone (Cortisporin-TC Otic Drops) Neomycin, Colistin, Hydrocortisone, and Thonzonium (Cortisporin-TC Otic Suspension)

INDICATIONS: External otitis, infections of mastoidectomy, and fenestration cavities.
ACTIONS: Antibiotic and anti-inflammatory.

DOSAGE: 4–5 ggt in the ear/s tid–qid.
SUPPLIED: Otic drops and suspension.

Neomycin and Dexamethasone (AK-NEO-DEX Ophthalmic, Neodecadron Ophthalmic) [See Table 7–12, pp 607-9]

Neomycin, Polymyxin B (Neosporin Cream)

INDICATIONS: Infection in minor cuts, scrapes, and burns.
ACTIONS: Bactericidal antibiotic.
DOSAGE: Apply bid–qid.
SUPPLIED: Cream neomycin 3.5 mg/polymyxin B 10,000 U/g.
NOTES: Different than Neosporin ointment.

Neomycin, Polymyxin-B, and Dexamethasone (Maxitrol) [See Table 7–12, pp 607-9]

Neomycin, Polymyxin Bladder Irrigant

INDICATIONS: Continuous irrigant for prophylaxis against bacteriuria and gram-negative bacteremia associated with indwelling catheter use.
ACTIONS: Bactericidal antibiotic.
DOSAGE: 1-mL irrigant added to 1 L of 0.9% NaCl; continuous irrigation of the bladder with 1–2 L of solution per 24 hr.
SUPPLIED: Ampoules 1 mL, 20 mL.
NOTES: Potential for bacterial or fungal superinfection; slight possibility for neomycin-induced ototoxicity or nephrotoxicity.

Neomycin, Polymyxin, and Hydrocortisone (Cortisporin Ophthalmic and Otic) [Also see Table 7–12, pp 607-9]

INDICATIONS: Ocular and otic bacterial infections.
ACTIONS: Antibiotic and anti-inflammatory.
DOSAGE: *Otic:* 3–4 drops in the ear 3–4 × a day.
Ophthalmic: Apply a thin layer to the eye or 1 drop 1-4 × per day.
SUPPLIED: Otic suspension; ophthalmic solution; ophthalmic ointment.

Neomycin, Polymyxin-B and Prednisolone (Poly-Pred Ophthalmic) [See Table 7–12, pp 607-9]

Neomycin Sulfate

INDICATIONS: Hepatic coma and preoperative bowel preparation.
ACTIONS: Aminoglycoside; suppresses GI bacterial flora.
DOSAGE: 3–12 g/24 hr PO in 3–4 divided doses.
SUPPLIED: Tablets 500 mg; oral solution 125 mg/5 mL.
NOTES: Part of the Condon bowel prep.

Nevirapine (Viramune)

INDICATIONS: Treatment of HIV infection.
ACTIONS: Non-nucleoside reverse transcriptase inhibitor.
DOSAGE: Initial dose 200 mg once daily for 14 days; then 200 mg bid.
SUPPLIED: Tablets 200 mg; suspension 50 mg/5 mL.
NOTES: May cause life-threatening rash; give without regard to food.

Niacin (Nicolar, Niaspan)

INDICATIONS: Adjunctive therapy in patients with significant hyperlipidemia who do not respond adequately to diet and weight loss.
ACTIONS: Inhibits lipolysis; decreases esterification of triglycerides; increases lipoprotein lipase activity.
DOSAGE: 1–6 g in divided doses tid; maximum of 9 g/d; *ER:* 500–2000 mg/d Q HS.

SUPPLIED: Sustained-release capsules 125 mg, 250 mg, 300 mg, 400 mg, 500 mg; tablets 25 mg, 50 mg, 100 mg, 250 mg, 500 mg; sustained-release tablets 150 mg, 250 mg, 500 mg, 750 mg; elixir 50 mg/5 mL. Extended-release tablets 500 mg, 750 mg, 1000 mg.
NOTES: Patients may have upper body and facial flushing and warmth following dose. Drug may cause hepatitis, exacerbate peptic ulcer disease and gout, and worsen glucose control in patients with diabetes mellitus.

Nicardipine (Cardene)

INDICATIONS: Treatment of chronic stable angina and hypertension; prophylaxis of migraine.
ACTIONS: Calcium channel blocking agent.
DOSAGE: *Oral:* 20–40 mg PO tid.
Sustained-release: 30–60 mg PO bid.
IV: 5 mg/hr IV continuous infusion; increase by 2.5 mg/hr Q 15 min to maximum 15 mg/hr.
SUPPLIED: Capsules 20 mg, 30 mg; sustained-release capsules 30 mg, 45 mg, 60 mg; injection 2.5 mg/mL.
NOTES: Oral-to-IV conversion: 20 mg tid = 0.5 mg/hr, 30 mg tid = 1.2 mg/hr, 40 mg tid = 2.2 mg/hr; adjust dose in renal or hepatic impairment.

Nicotine Gum (Nicorette, Nicorette DS)

INDICATIONS AND ACTIONS: See Nicotine, Transdermal (below).
DOSAGE: 9–12 pieces/d prn. Maximum 30 pieces per day.
SUPPLIED: *Nicorette:* 2 mg (96 pieces/box).
Nicorette DS: 4 mg/piece.
NOTES: For maximum effect, patients must stop smoking and perform behavior modification.

Nicotine Nasal Spray (Nicotrol NS)

INDICATIONS: Aid to smoking cessation for the relief of nicotine withdrawal.
ACTIONS: Provides systemic delivery of nicotine.
DOSAGE: 0.5 mg/actuation; 1–2 sprays per hr, not to exceed 10 sprays per hr.
SUPPLIED: Nasal inhaler 10 mg/mL.
NOTES: For maximum effect, patients must stop smoking and perform behavior modification.

Nicotine, Transdermal (Habitrol, Nicoderm, Nicotrol, ProStep)

INDICATIONS: Aid to smoking cessation for the relief of nicotine withdrawal.
ACTIONS: Provides systemic delivery of nicotine.
DOSAGE: Individualized to the patient's needs; apply 1 patch (14–22 mg q day), and taper over 6 weeks.
SUPPLIED: *Habitrol and Nicoderm:* 7 mg, 14 mg, 21 mg of nicotine/24 hr.
Nicotrol: 5 mg/24 hr, 10 mg/24 hr, 15 mg/24 hr.
ProStep: 11 mg/24 hr, 22 mg/24 hr.
NOTES: Nicotrol patch is to be worn for 16 hr to mimic smoking patterns; others are worn for 24 hr. For maximum effect, patients must stop smoking and perform behavior modification.

Nifedipine (Procardia, Procardia XL, Adalat, Adalat CC)

INDICATIONS: Vasospastic or chronic stable angina and hypertension; tocolytic.
ACTIONS: Calcium channel blocking agent.
DOSAGE: *Sustained-release tablets:* 30–90 mg once daily.
Tocolysis: 10–20 mg PO Q 4–6 hr.
SUPPLIED: Capsules 10 mg, 20 mg; sustained-release tablets 30 mg, 60 mg, 90 mg.
NOTES: Headaches are common on initial treatment, also lower-extremity edema is common. Reflex tachycardia may occur with regular-release dosage forms. Adalat CC and Procardia XL are *not* interchangeable dosage forms. Sublingual administration not advisable.

Nilutamide (Nilandron)

INDICATIONS: Combination with surgical castration for the treatment of metastatic prostate cancer.
ACTIONS: Nonsteroidal anti-androgen.
DOSAGE: 300 mg/d in divided doses for the first 30 days, then 150 mg/d.

SUPPLIED: Tablets 50 mg.

NOTES: Toxicity can include hot flashes, loss of libido, impotence, diarrhea, nausea, vomiting, gynecomastia, hepatic dysfunction (follow LFTs), and interstitial pneumonitis.

Nimodipine (Nimotop)

INDICATIONS: Prevention of vasospasm following subarachnoid hemorrhage.

ACTIONS: Calcium channel blocking agent.

DOSAGE: 60 mg PO Q 4 hr for 21 days.

SUPPLIED: Capsules 30 mg.

NOTES: Contents of capsule may be extracted and administered down a nasogastric tube if the capsule cannot be swallowed whole; dosage adjustment in hepatic failure.

Nisoldipine (Sular)

INDICATIONS: Treatment of hypertension.

ACTIONS: Calcium channel blocker.

DOSAGE: 10–60 mg PO once daily.

SUPPLIED: Extended-release tablets 10 mg, 20 mg, 30 mg, 40 mg.

NOTES: Do not take with grapefruit juice or high-fat meal; lower starting doses in elderly or in patients with hepatic impairment.

Nitrofurantoin (Macrodantin, Furadantin, Macrobid)

INDICATIONS: Prevention and treatment of urinary tract infections.

ACTIONS: Bacteriostatic; interferes with carbohydrate metabolism.

DOSAGE: *Suppression:* 50–100 mg PO q day.
Treatment: 50–100 mg PO qid.

SUPPLIED: Capsules and tablets 50 mg, 100 mg; sustained-release capsules 100 mg; suspension 25 mg/5 mL.

NOTES: GI side effects common; drug should be taken with food, milk, or antacid. Macrocrystals (Macrodantin) cause less nausea than other forms of the drug; avoid using nitrofurantoin if CrCl < 50 mL/min.

Nitroglycerin (Nitrostat, Nitrolingual, Nitro-Bid Ointment, Nitro-Bid IV, Nitrodisc, Transderm-Nitro, Others)

INDICATIONS: Angina pectoris, acute and prophylactic therapy, congestive heart failure, BP control.

ACTIONS: Relaxation of vascular smooth muscle.

DOSAGE:

- *Sublingual:* 1 tablet every 5 min SL prn for 3 doses.
- *Translingual:* 1–2 metered doses sprayed onto the oral mucosa Q 3–5 min, maximum 3 doses.
- *Oral:* 2.5–9 mg tid.
- *Intravenous:* 5–20 μg/min, titrated to effect.
- *Topical:* Apply 1–2 inches of ointment to the chest wall Q 6 hr, then wipe off at night.
- *Transdermal:* 5- to 20-cm patch q day.

SUPPLIED: Sublingual tablets 0.3 mg, 0.4 mg, 0.6 mg; translingual spray 0.4 mg/dose; sustained-release capsules 2.5 mg, 6.5 mg, 9 mg, 13 mg; sustained-release tablets 2.6 mg, 6.5 mg, 9.0 mg; injection 0.5 mg/mL, 5 mg/mL, 10 mg/mL; ointment 2%; transdermal patches 2.5 mg/24 hr, 5 mg/24 hr, 7.5 mg/24 hr, 10 mg/24 hr, 15 mg/24 hr; buccal controlled release 1 mg, 2 mg, 3 mg.

NOTES: Tolerance to nitrates will develop with chronic use after 1–2 weeks; this can be avoided by providing a nitrate-free period each day. Shorter-acting nitrates should be used on a tid basis, and long-acting patches and ointment should be removed before bedtime to prevent the development of tolerance.

Nitroprusside (Nipride, Nitropress)

INDICATIONS: Pulmonary edema.

ACTIONS: Reduces systemic vascular resistance.

DOSAGE: 0.5–10 μg/kg/min IV infusion, titrated to desired effect; usual dose 3 μg/kg/min.
SUPPLIED: Injection 10 mg/mL, 25 mg/mL.
NOTES: Thiocyanate, the metabolite, is excreted by the kidney; thiocyanate toxicity occurs at plasma levels of 5–10 mg/dL; more likely to occur when used for > 2–3 days.

Nizatidine (Axid)

INDICATIONS: Treatment of duodenal ulcers, gastroesophageal reflux (GERD), and heartburn.
ACTIONS: H_2-receptor antagonist.
DOSAGE: *Active ulcer:* 150 mg PO bid OR 300 mg PO Q HS; maintenance dose 150 mg PO Q HS.
GERD: 300 mg PO bid × 4–8 weeks; maintenance dose 300 mg PO Q HS.
SUPPLIED: Capsules 75 mg, 150 mg, 300 mg.
NOTES: Dosage adjustment in renal impairment.

Norepinephrine (Levophed)

INDICATIONS: Acute hypotensive states.
ACTIONS: Peripheral vasoconstrictor acting on both the arterial and venous beds.
DOSAGE: 8–12 μg/min IV, titrated to desired effect.
SUPPLIED: Injection 1 mg/mL.
NOTES: Correct blood volume depletion as much as possible prior to initiation of vasopressor therapy. Drug may interact with tricyclic antidepressants to produce severe profound hypertension. Infuse into large vein to avoid extravasation; phentolamine 5–10 mg/10 mL NS may be injected locally as an antidote to extravasation.

Norethindrone Acetate/Ethinyl Estradiol (FemHRT)

INDICATIONS: Treatment of moderate to severe vasomotor symptoms associated with menopause; prevention of osteoporosis.
ACTIONS: Hormone replacement.
DOSAGE: 1 tablet q day.
SUPPLIED: 1 mg norethindrone/5 μg ethinyl estradiol tablets.
NOTES: Use in women with intact uterus.

Norfloxacin (Noroxin)

INDICATIONS: Treatment of complicated and uncomplicated urinary tract infections caused by a wide variety of gram-negative bacteria, prostatitis, and infectious diarrhea.
ACTIONS: Quinolone, inhibits DNA gyrase.
DOSAGE: *Usual:* 400 mg PO bid.
Gonorrhea: 800 mg as single dose.
Conjunctivitis: 1–2 gtts qid.
SUPPLIED: Tablets 400 mg; ophthalmic solution 0.3%.
NOTES AND CAUTION: *Not* for use in pregnancy; drug interactions with antacids, theophylline, and caffeine. Good concentrations in the kidney and urine, poor blood levels. *Do not* use in urosepsis; adjust dosage in renal impairment.

Norgestrel (Ovrette)

INDICATIONS: Prevention of pregnancy.
ACTIONS: Prevent follicular maturation and ovulation.
DOSAGE: Tablet q day; begin day 1 of menses.
SUPPLIED: Tablet 0.075 mg.
NOTES: Progestin-only products have higher risk of failure in prevention of pregnancy.

Nortriptyline (Aventyl, Pamelor)

INDICATIONS: Treatment of endogenous depression.
ACTIONS: Tricyclic antidepressant; increases the synaptic concentrations of serotonin and/or norepinephrine in the CNS.
DOSAGE: 25 mg PO tid–qid. Doses > 150 mg/d not recommended.
Elderly: 10–25 mg Q HS.
SUPPLIED: Capsules 10 mg, 25 mg, 50 mg, 75 mg; solution 10 mg/5 mL.

NOTES: Drug has many anticholinergic side effects, including blurred vision, urinary retention, and dry mouth; maximum effect seen after 2 weeks of therapy.

Nystatin (Mycostatin, Nilstat, Others)

INDICATIONS: Treatment of mucocutaneous *Candida* infections (thrush, vaginitis).
ACTIONS: Alters membrane permeability.
DOSAGE: *Oral:* 400,000–600,000 U PO "swish and swallow" qid.
Intravaginal: 1 tablet per vagina Q HS for 2 weeks.
Topical: Apply 2–3 × daily to the affected area.
SUPPLIED: Oral suspension 100,000 U/mL; oral tablets 500,000 U; troches 200,000 U; vaginal tablets 100,000 U; topical cream and ointment 100,000 U/g.
NOTES: Nystatin is not absorbed orally; therefore, is not effective for systemic infections.

Octreotide (Sandostatin)

INDICATIONS: Suppresses or inhibits severe diarrhea associated with carcinoid and neuroendocrine tumors of the intestinal tract; treatment of bleeding esophageal varices.
ACTIONS: Long-acting peptide that mimics the natural hormone somatostatin.
DOSAGE: 100–600 μg/d SC in 2–4 divided doses; initiate at 50 μg q day–bid.
SUPPLIED: Injection 0.05 mg/mL, 0.1 mg/mL, 0.2 mg/mL, 0.5 mg/mL, 1 mg/mL.
NOTES: May cause nausea, vomiting, and abdominal discomfort.

Ofloxacin (Floxin, Ocuflox Ophthalmic)

INDICATIONS: Treatment of infections of the lower respiratory tract, skin and skin structure, and urinary tract; prostatitis; uncomplicated gonorrhea; and *Chlamydia* infections; topical for bacterial conjunctivitis; otltis externa in adults.
ACTIONS: Bactericidal; inhibits DNA gyrase.
DOSAGE: *Usual:* 200–400 mg PO bid or IV Q 12 hr.
Ophthalmic: 1–2 drops in eye(s) Q 2–4 hr for 2 days, then qid for 5 additional days.
Otic: 10 drops in ear bid for 10 days.
SUPPLIED: Tablets 200 mg, 300 mg, 400 mg; injection 20 mg/mL, 40 mg/mL; ophthalmic 0.3%.
NOTES: Drug may cause nausea and vomiting, diarrhea, insomnia, and headache. Ofloxacin interacts with antacids, sucralfate, and aluminum-, calcium-, magnesium-, iron-, or zinc-containing products, which decrease its absorption; should be taken on an empty stomach. Drug may increase theophylline levels; adjust dosage in patients with renal impairment. Ophthalmic form may be used to treat otitis externa.

Olanzapine (Zyprexa)

INDICATIONS: Treatment of psychotic disorders.
ACTIONS: Dopamine and serotonin antagonist.
DOSAGE: 5–10 mg/d; titrate up to maximum of 20 mg per day.
SUPPLIED: Tablet 5 mg, 7.5 mg, 10 mg.
NOTES: May take many weeks to titrate to therapeutic dose; cigarette smoking will decrease levels.

Olsalazine (Dipentum)

INDICATIONS: Maintenance of remission of ulcerative colitis.
ACTIONS: Topical anti-inflammatory activity.
DOSAGE: 500 mg PO bid.
SUPPLIED: Capsules 250 mg.
NOTES: Take olsalazine with food; may cause diarrhea.

Omeprazole (Prilosec) [See Table 7–14, p 611]

Ondansetron (Zofran)

INDICATIONS: Prevention of nausea and vomiting associated with cancer chemotherapy; prevention of postoperative nausea and vomiting.
ACTIONS: Serotonin receptor antagonist.

DOSAGE: *Chemotherapy:* 0.15 mg/kg/dose IV prior to chemotherapy; then repeated 4 and 8 hr after the first dose; OR 4–8 mg PO tid; administer first dose 30 min prior to chemotherapy.

Post-op: 4 mg IV immediately before induction of anesthesia or post-op.

SUPPLIED: Tablets 4 mg, 8 mg; injection 2 mg/mL.

NOTES: Drug may cause diarrhea and headache; should be administered on a schedule, *not* prn.

Oprelvekin (Neumega)

INDICATIONS: Prevention of severe thrombocytopenia due to chemotherapy.

ACTIONS: Promotes proliferation and maturation of megakaryocytes.

DOSAGE: 50 µg/kg SC q day for 10–21 days.

SUPPLIED: Injection.

NOTES: Interleukin-11.

Oral Contraceptives, Biphasic, Monophasic, Triphasic, Progestin Only

INDICATIONS: Birth control and regulation of anovulatory bleeding.

ACTIONS: *Birth control:* Suppress LH surge, prevent ovulation. Progestins thicken cervical mucus, inhibit fallopian tubule cilia, decrease endometrial thickness, and hence decrease chances of fertilization.

Anovulatory bleeding: Cyclic hormones mimic the body's natural cycle and help to regulate the endometrial lining, resulting in regular bleeding every 28 days; may also reduce uterine bleeding and dysmenorrhea.

DOSAGE: 28-day-cycle pills are taken every day. 21-day-cycle pills are taken every day, no pills taken during the last 7 days of the cycle (during the menstrual period).

SUPPLIED: 28-day-cycle pills (21 hormonally active pills + 7 placebo/iron supplementation); 21-day-cycle pills (21 hormonally active pills).

NOTES AND CAUTIONS:

- OCPs if taken correctly are 99.9% effective for preventing pregnancy, but do not protect against STDs; encourage use of additional barrier birth control. OCPs over long periods of time can decrease risk of ectopic pregnancy, benign breast disease, and future development of ovarian and uterine cancer.
- *Absolute contraindications:* Undiagnosed abnormal vaginal bleeding, pregnancy, estrogen-dependent malignancy, hypercoagulation disorders, liver disease, complicated migraine headaches, and smokers > 35 years old.
- *Relative contraindications:* Migraine headaches, hypertension, diabetes, sickle cell disease, and gallbladder disease.
- *Prescribing OCPs for menstrual cycle control:* Start with a monophasic pill. The pill should be taken for 3 months before switching to another brand. If abnormal bleeding continues, change to pill with higher estrogen dose.
- *Prescribing OCPs for birth control:* Choose pill that has the most beneficial side effect profile for that particular patient. Side effects of OCPs are numerous and due to symptoms of estrogen excess or progesterone deficiency. However, each pill has a unique side effect profile that may be found in the package insert and therefore may be tailored to a specific patient.
- *Common OCPs side effects:* Intramenstrual bleeding/oligomenorrhea/amenorrhea, increased appetite/weight gain, loss of libido, fatigue/depression/mood swings, mastalgia, headaches, melasma, increased vaginal discharge, acne/greasy skin, corneal edema, nausea.

Orlistat (Xenical)

INDICATIONS: Management of obesity in patients with BMI ≥ 30 kg/m^2 or ≥ 27 kg/m^2 in presence of other risk factors.

ACTIONS: Reversible inhibitor of gastric and pancreatic lipases.

DOSAGE: 120 mg PO tid with a fat-containing meal.

SUPPLIED: Capsules 120 mg.

NOTES: *Do not* administer if meal contains no fat. GI effects increase with higher-fat meals. Supplement with fat-soluble vitamins; use caution in patients with nephrolithiasis.

Orphenadrine (Norflex)

INDICATIONS: Treatment of muscle spasms.
ACTIONS: Central atropine-like effects cause indirect skeletal muscle relaxation, euphoria, and analgesia.
DOSAGE: 100 mg PO bid, 60 mg IM/IV Q 12 hr.
SUPPLIED: Tablets 100 mg; sustained-release tablets 100 mg; injection 30 mg/mL.

Oseltamivir (Tamiflu)

INDICATIONS: Treatment of influenza A and B.
ACTIONS: Inhibition of viral neuraminidase.
DOSAGE: 75 mg twice daily for 5 days.
SUPPLIED: Capsule 75 mg.
NOTES: Initiate within 36 hr of symptom onset; reduce dose in renal impairment.

Oxacillin (Bactocill) [See Table 7–5, p 600]

Oxaprozin (Daypro) [See Table 7–11, pp 605-6]

Oxazepam (Serax) [C]

INDICATIONS: Anxiety; acute alcohol withdrawal; anxiety with depressive symptoms.
ACTIONS: Benzodiazepine.
DOSAGE: 10–15 mg PO tid–qid. Severe anxiety and alcohol withdrawal may require up to 30 mg qid.
SUPPLIED: Capsules 10 mg, 15 mg, 30 mg; tablets 15 mg.
NOTES: Oxazepam is one of the metabolites of diazepam (Valium); avoid abrupt discontinuation.

Oxcarbazepine (Trileptal)

INDICATIONS: Treatment of partial seizures.
ACTIONS: Produce blockage of voltage-sensitive sodium channels, resulting in stabilization of hyperexcited neural membranes.
DOSAGE: 300 mg twice daily; increase dose weekly to a usual dose of 1200–2400 mg/d.
SUPPLIED: Tablets 150 mg, 300 mg, 600 mg.
NOTES: Drug may cause clinically significant hyponatremia; has possible cross-sensitivity to carbamazepine.

Oxiconazole (Oxistat)

INDICATIONS: Tinea pedis; tinea cruris; tinea corporis.
ACTIONS: Antifungal antibiotic.
DOSAGE: Apply bid.
SUPPLIED: 1% cream, lotion.

Oxybutynin (Ditropan, Ditropan XL)

INDICATIONS: Symptomatic relief of urgency, nocturia, and incontinence associated with neurogenic or reflex neurogenic bladder.
ACTIONS: Direct antispasmodic effect on smooth muscle; increases bladder capacity.
DOSAGE: 5 mg PO tid–qid.
Extended-release: 5 mg PO q day; can titrate up to 30 mg PO q day.
SUPPLIED: Tablets 5 mg; extended-release tablets 5 mg, 10 mg, 15 mg; syrup 5 mg/5 mL.
NOTES: Anticholinergic side effects.

Oxycodone (Dihydrohydroxycodeinone) (OxyContin, OxyiR, Roxicodone)

INDICATIONS: Moderate to severe pain, normally used in combination with non-narcotic analgesics.
ACTIONS: Narcotic analgesic.

DOSAGE: 5 mg PO Q 6 hr prn.
SUPPLIED: Capsule immediate release: (OxyIR) 5 mg.
Tablet immediate release (Percolone): 5 mg.
Tablet controlled release (OxyContin): 10 mg, 20 mg, 40 mg, 80 mg.
Liquid controlled release: 5 mg/5 mL.
Solution concentrate controlled release: 20 mg/mL.
NOTES: Usually prescribed in combination with acetaminophen or aspirin; OxyContin is useful for chronic cancer pain. In some parts of the United States, OxyContin is highly sought after as a drug of abuse. The tablets can be crushed and snorted or injected.

Oxycodone and Acetaminophen (Percocet, Tylox) [C]

INDICATIONS: Management of moderate to severe pain.
ACTIONS: Narcotic analgesic.
DOSAGE: 1–2 tablets/capsules PO Q 4–6 hr prn.
SUPPLIED: *Percocet tablet:* oxycodone/acetaminophen 2.5 mg/325 mg; 5 mg/325 mg; 7.5 mg/325 mg; 10 mg/650 mg.
Tylox capsule: 5 mg of oxycodone, 500 mg of acetaminophen.
Solution: 5 mg of oxycodone and 325 mg of acetaminophen per 5 mL.
NOTES: Acetaminophen maximum dose of 4 g per day.

Oxycodone and Aspirin (Percodan, Percodan-Demi) [C]

INDICATIONS: Moderate to moderately severe pain.
ACTIONS: Narcotic analgesic with nonsteroidal anti-inflammatory.
DOSAGE: 1–2 tablets/capsules PO Q 4–6 hr prn.
SUPPLIED: *Percodan:* 4.5-mg oxycodone hydrochloride 0.38-mg oxycodone terephthalate, 325-mg aspirin.
Percodan-Demi: 2.25-mg oxycodone hydrochloride, 0.19-mg oxycodone terephthalate, 325-mg aspirin.

Oxymorphone (Numorphan) [C]

INDICATIONS: Treatment of moderate to severe pain, sedative.
ACTIONS: Narcotic analgesic.
DOSAGE: 0.5 mg IM, SC, IV initially, 1–1.5 mg Q 4–6 hr prn.
Rectal: 5 mg Q 4–6 hr prn.
SUPPLIED: Injection 1 mg/mL, 1.5 mg/mL; suppository 5 mg.
NOTES: Chemically related to hydromorphone.

Oxytocin (Pitocin, Syntocinon)

INDICATIONS: Induction of labor and control of postpartum hemorrhage; promotion of milk letdown in lactating woman.
ACTIONS: Stimulates muscular contractions of the uterus, stimulates milk flow during nursing.
DOSAGE: 0.001–0.002 U/min IV infusion; titrate to desired effect, to a maximum of 0.02 U/min.
Breastfeeding: 1 spray in both nostrils 2–3 min before feeding.
SUPPLIED: Injection 10 U/mL; nasal solution 40 U/mL.
NOTES: Can cause uterine rupture and fetal death; monitor vital signs closely; nasal form for breastfeeding only.

Paclitaxel (Taxol)

INDICATIONS: Treatment of ovarian and breast cancer.
ACTIONS: Mitotic spindle poison promotes microtubule assembly and stabilization against depolymerization.
DOSAGE: Refer to specific protocol.
NOTES: Toxicity includes hypersensitivity reactions (dyspnea, hypotension, urticaria, rash) usually within 10 min of starting infusion; these can be minimized by corticosteroid, antihistamine (H_1 and H_2 antagonist) pretreatment. Myelosuppression, peripheral neuropathy, transient ileus, myalgia, bradycardia, hypotension, mucositis, diarrhea, nausea and vomiting, fever, rash, headache, and phlebitis also can occur. Hematologic toxicity is schedule-dependent;

leukopenia is dose-limiting by 24-hr infusion; neurotoxicity is dose-limiting by short (1- to 3-hr) infusion. This agent must be infused in glass or polyolefin containers using polyethylene-lined tubing sets. Use of polyvinyl chloride infusion sets will result in leaching of plasticizer.

Pamidronate (Aredia)

INDICATIONS: Treatment of hypercalcemia of malignancy and Paget's disease; palliation of symptomatic bone metastases.
ACTIONS: Inhibition of normal and abnormal bone resorption.
DOSAGE: *Hypercalcemia:* 60 mg IV over 4 hr OR 90 mg IV over 24 hr.
Paget's disease: 30 mg IV daily for 3 days.
SUPPLIED: Powder for injection 30 mg, 60 mg, 90 mg.
NOTES: Toxicity includes fever, tissue irritation at the site of injection, uveitis, fluid overload, hypertension, abdominal pain, nausea and vomiting, constipation, urinary tract infection, bone pain, hypokalemia, hypocalcemia, hypomagnesemia, and hypophosphatemia; slow infusion rate necessary.

Pancreatin/Pancrelipase (Pancrease, Cotazyme, Creon, Ultrase)

INDICATIONS: For patients deficient in exocrine pancreatic secretions (cystic fibrosis, chronic pancreatitis, other pancreatic insufficiency), and for steatorrhea of malabsorption syndrome.
ACTIONS: Pancreatic enzyme supplementation.
DOSAGE: 1–3 capsules (tablets) with meals and snacks; dosage may be increased up to 8 capsules (tablets).
SUPPLIED: Capsules; tablets.
NOTES: Instruct patient to avoid antacids, and not to crush or chew enteric-coated products. Drug may cause nausea, abdominal cramps, or diarrhea; dosage is dependent on digestive requirements of patient.

Pancuronium (Pavulon)

INDICATIONS: Aids in the management of patients on mechanical ventilation.
ACTIONS: Nondepolarizing neuromuscular blocker.
DOSAGE: 2–4 mg IV Q 2–4 hr prn.
SUPPLIED: Injection 1 mg/mL, 2 mg/mL.
NOTES: Patient must be intubated and on controlled ventilation; use an adequate amount of sedation or analgesia; adjust dose for renal or hepatic impairment.

Pantoprazole (Protonix) [See Table 7–14, p 611]

Paregoric [C]

INDICATIONS: Diarrhea, pain, neonatal opiate withdrawal syndrome.
ACTIONS: Narcotic.
DOSAGE: 5–10 mL PO q day–qid prn.
NOTES: Contains opium; drug is for short-term use only.

Paroxetine (Paxil)

INDICATIONS: Treatment of depression, obsessive-compulsive disorder, panic disorder, social anxiety disorder.
ACTIONS: Serotonin reuptake inhibitor.
DOSAGE: 10–60 mg PO as a single daily dose.
SUPPLIED: Tablets 10 mg, 20 mg, 30 mg, 40 mg; suspension 10 mg/5 mL.
NOTES: Should be administered in the morning; may cause insomnia or hypersomnia and sexual dysfunction.

Pemirolast (Alamast) [See Table 7–12, pp 607-9]

Penbutolol (Levatol) [See Table 7–7, pp 601-2]

Penciclovir (Denavir)

INDICATIONS: Treatment of herpes simplex.
ACTIONS: Competitive inhibitor of DNA polymerase.

DOSAGE: Apply topically at first sign of lesions, then Q 2 hr for 4 days.
SUPPLIED: Cream 1%.

Penicillin G, Aqueous (Potassium or Sodium) (Pfizerpen, Pentids)

INDICATIONS: Most gram-positive infections (except penicillin-resistant staphylococci), including streptococci, *N meningitidis,* syphilis, clostridia, and some coliforms.
ACTIONS: Bactericidal; inhibits cell wall synthesis.
DOSAGE: 400,000–800,000 U PO qid; IV doses vary greatly depending on indications; range from 1.2 to 24 million U/d in divided doses Q 4 hr.
SUPPLIED: Tablets 200,000 U, 250,000 U, 400,000 U, 800,000 U; suspension 200,000 U/5 mL, 400,000 U/5 mL; powder for injection.
NOTES: Beware of hypersensitivity reactions. Dosage adjustment in renal impairment.

Penicillin G Benzathine (Bicillin)

INDICATIONS: Useful as a single-dose treatment regimen for streptococcal pharyngitis, rheumatic fever and glomerulonephritis prophylaxis, and syphilis.
ACTIONS: Bactericidal; inhibits cell wall synthesis.
DOSAGE: 1.2–2.4 million U deep IM injection every 2–4 weeks.
SUPPLIED: Injection 300,000 U/mL, 600,000 U/mL.
NOTES: Has sustained action with detectable levels up to 4 weeks; considered the drug of choice for treatment of noncongenital syphilis. Bicillin L-A contains the benzathine salt only; Bicillin C-R contains a combination of the benzathine and procaine (300,000 U procaine with 300,000 U benzathine per milliliter or 900,000 U of benzathine with 300,000 U of procaine per 2 milliliters).

Penicillin G Procaine (Wycillin, Others)

INDICATIONS: Moderately severe infections caused by penicillin G-sensitive organisms that respond to low, persistent serum levels.
ACTIONS: Bactericidal; inhibits cell wall synthesis.
DOSAGE: 0.6–4.8 million U/d in divided doses Q 12–24 hr.
SUPPLIED: Injection 300,000 U/mL, 500,000 U/mL, 600,000 U/mL.
NOTES: A long-acting parenteral penicillin; provides measurable blood levels up to 15 hr. Give probenecid at least 30 min prior to administration of penicillin to prolong action.

Penicillin V (Pen-Vee K, Veetids, Others)

INDICATIONS: Most gram-positive infections, including streptococci, *N meningitidis,* syphilis, clostridia, and some coliforms.
ACTIONS: Bactericidal; inhibits cell wall synthesis.
DOSAGE: 250–500 mg PO Q 6 hr.
SUPPLIED: Tablets 125 mg, 250 mg, 500 mg; suspension 125 mg/5 mL, 250 mg/5 mL.
NOTES: A well-tolerated oral penicillin; 250 mg = 400,000 U of penicillin G.

Pentamidine (Pentam 300, NebuPent)

INDICATIONS: Treatment and prevention of *P carinii* pneumonia.
ACTIONS: Inhibits DNA, RNA, phospholipid, and protein synthesis.
DOSAGE: *Treatment:* 4 mg/kg/24 hr IV daily for 14–21 days.
Prevention: 300 mg once every 4 weeks, administered via Respirgard II nebulizer.
SUPPLIED: Injection 300 mg/vial; aerosol 300 mg.
NOTES: Monitor patient for severe hypotension following IV administration. Drug is associated with pancreatic islet cell necrosis leading to hypoglycemia and hyperglycemia. Monitor hematology lab results for leukopenia and thrombocytopenia. IV route requires dosage adjustment in renal impairment.

Pentazocine (Talwin) [C]

INDICATIONS: Management of moderate to severe pain.
ACTIONS: Partial narcotic agonist-antagonist.
DOSAGE: 30 mg IM or IV; 50–100 mg PO Q 3–4 hr prn.

SUPPLIED: Tablets 50 mg (with naloxone 0.5 mg); injection 30 mg/mL.
NOTES: 30–60 mg IM equianalgesic to 10 mg of morphine IM. Drug is associated with considerable dysphoria; adjust dosage in patients with renal impairment.

Pentobarbital (Nembutal, Others) [C]

INDICATIONS: Insomnia, convulsions, induced coma following severe head injury.
ACTIONS: Barbiturate.
DOSAGE: *Sedative:* 20–40 mg PO or PR Q 6–12 hr.
Hypnotic: 100–200 mg PO or PR Q HS prn.
Induced coma: Loading dose 5–10 mg/kg IV, then maintenance 1–3 mg/kg/hr IV continuous infusion to keep the serum level between 20 and 50 mg/mL.
SUPPLIED: Capsules 50 mg, 100 mg; elixir 18.5 mg/5 mL; suppositories 30 mg, 60 mg, 120 mg, 200 mg; injection 50 mg/mL.
NOTES: Drug can cause respiratory depression. May produce profound hypotension when used aggressively intravenously for cerebral edema. Tolerance to sedative-hypnotic effect acquired within 1–2 weeks. Reduce dose in patients with severe hepatic impairment.

Pentosan Polysulfate Sodium (Elmiron)

INDICATIONS: Relief of pain/discomfort associated with interstitial cystitis.
ACTIONS: Acts as buffer on bladder wall.
DOSAGE: 100 mg PO tid on empty stomach with water 1 hr before or 2 hr after meals.
SUPPLIED: Capsule 100 mg.
NOTES: Alopecia, diarrhea, nausea, and headaches have been reported.

Pentoxifylline (Trental)

INDICATIONS: Symptomatic management of peripheral vascular disease.
ACTIONS: Lowers blood cell viscosity by restoring erythrocyte flexibility.
DOSAGE: 400 mg PO tid with meals.
SUPPLIED: Tablets 400 mg.
NOTES: Treat for at least 8 weeks to see full effect; reduce dose to bid if GI or CNS effects occur.

Pergolide (Permax)

INDICATIONS: Parkinson's disease.
ACTIONS: Centrally active dopamine receptor agonist.
DOSAGE: Initial dose 0.05 mg PO tid, titrated every 2–3 days to desired effect; usual maintenance dose 2–3 mg/d in divided doses.
SUPPLIED: Tablets 0.05 mg, 0.25 mg, 1.0 mg.
NOTES: May cause hypotension during initiation of therapy.

Perindopril Erbumine (Aceon) [See Table 7–3, p 598]

Permethrin (Nix, Elimite)

INDICATIONS: Eradication of lice and scabies.
ACTIONS: Pediculicide.
DOSAGE: Saturate hair and scalp; allow to remain in the hair for 10 min before rinsing out.
SUPPLIED: Topical liquid 1%; cream 5%.

Perphenazine (Trilafon)

INDICATIONS: Psychotic disorders, intractable hiccups, severe nausea.
ACTIONS: Phenothiazine; blocks postsynaptic mesolimbic dopaminergic receptors in the brain.
DOSAGE: *Antipsychotic:* 4–16 mg PO tid; maximum 64 mg/d.
Hiccups: 5 mg IM Q 6 hr prn; OR 1 mg IV at not less than 1–2 mg/min intervals to a maximum of 5 mg.
SUPPLIED: Tablets 2 mg, 4 mg, 8 mg, 16 mg; oral concentrate 16 mg/5 mL; injection 5 mg/mL.

Phenazopyridine (Pyridium, Others)

INDICATIONS: Symptomatic relief of discomfort from lower urinary tract irritation.

ACTIONS: Local anesthetic on urinary tract mucosa.
DOSAGE: 100–200 mg PO tid for 2–3 days.
SUPPLIED: Tablets 95 mg, 100 mg, 200 mg.
NOTES: Side effects include GI disturbances. Drug causes red-orange discolorations to body secretions, which may stain clothing, contacts, etc. Adjust dosage in patients with renal impairment.

Phenelzine (Nardil)

INDICATIONS: Treatment of depression.
ACTIONS: Monoamine oxidase inhibitor.
DOSAGE: *Usual:* 15 mg tid.
Elderly: 15–60 mg per day in divided doses.
SUPPLIED: Tablets 15 mg.
NOTES: Drug may cause postural hypotension; it may take 2–4 weeks to see therapeutic effect. Instruct patient to avoid tyramine-containing foods.

Phenobarbital [C]

INDICATIONS: Management of seizure disorders, insomnia, anxiety.
ACTIONS: Barbiturate.
DOSAGE: *Sedative-hypnotic:* 30–120 mg PO or IM q day prn.
Anticonvulsant: Loading dose of 10–12 mg/kg in 3 divided doses; then 1–3 mg/kg/24 hr in divided doses bid–tid PO, IM, or IV.
SUPPLIED: Tablets 8 mg, 15 mg, 16 mg, 30 mg, 32 mg, 60 mg, 65 mg, 100 mg; elixir 15 mg/5 mL, 20 mg/5 mL; injection 30 mg/mL, 60 mg/mL, 65 mg/mL, 130 mg/mL.
NOTES: Tolerance develops to sedation; long half-life allows single daily dosing; follow levels as needed (see Table 7–16, p 613.

Phenylephrine (Neo-Synephrine)

INDICATIONS: Treatment of vascular failure in shock, hypersensitivity, or drug-induced hypotension; nasal congestion; mydriatic.
ACTIONS: Alpha-adrenergic agonist.
DOSAGE: *Mild to moderate hypotension:* 2–5 mg IM or SC elevates BP for 2 hr; 0.1–0.5 mg IV elevates BP for 15 min.
Severe hypotension or shock: Initiate continuous infusion at 100–180 μg/min; after BP is stabilized, maintenance rate of 40–60 μg/min.
Nasal congestion: 1–2 sprays into each nostril prn.
Ophthalmologic: 1 drop 15–30 min before examination.
SUPPLIED: Injection 10 mg/mL; nasal solution 0.125%, 0.16%, 0.25%, 0.5%, 1%; ophthalmic solution 0.12%, 2.5%, 10%.
NOTES: Promptly restore blood volume if loss has occurred. Use with extreme caution in patients with hyperthyroidism, bradycardia, partial heart block, myocardial disease, or severe arteriosclerosis. Use large veins for infusion to avoid extravasation; phentolamine 10 mg in 10–15 mL of NS may be injected locally as antidote for extravasation. Activity of drug is potentiated by oxytocin, monoamine oxidase inhibitors, and tricyclic antidepressants.

Phenytoin (Dilantin)

INDICATIONS: Management of seizure disorders.
ACTIONS: Inhibits seizure spread in the motor cortex.
DOSAGE: *Loading dose:* 15–20 mg/kg IV at a maximum infusion rate of 25 mg/min; OR orally in 400-mg doses at 4-hr intervals.
Maintenance: Initial dose 200 mg PO or IV bid or 300 mg Q HS; then follow serum concentrations.
SUPPLIED: Capsules 30 mg, 100 mg; chewable tablets 50 mg; oral suspension 30 mg/5 mL, 125 mg/5 mL; injection 50 mg/mL.
NOTES AND CAUTION: Be alert for cardiac depressant side effects, especially with IV administration; follow levels as needed (See Table 7–16, p 613). Nystagmus and ataxia are early

signs of toxicity; gum hyperplasia occurs with long-term use. Avoid use of oral suspension if possible because of erratic absorption. Avoid use of drug in pregnancy.

Physostigmine (Antilirium, Isopto Eserine) [See Table 7–12, pp 607-9]

INDICATIONS: Antidote for tricyclic antidepressant, atropine, and scopolamine overdose, glaucoma.

ACTIONS: Reversible cholinesterase inhibitor.

DOSAGE: 2 mg IV or IM every 20 min (ophthalmic dose).

SUPPLIED: Injection 1 mg/mL; ophthalmic ointment 0.25%.

NOTES: Rapid IV administration associated with convulsions. Drug has cholinergic side effects; may cause asystole.

Phytonadione (Vitamin K) (AquaMephyton, Others)

INDICATIONS: Coagulation disorders caused by faulty formation of factors II, VII, IX, and X; hyperalimentation.

ACTIONS: Supplementation; needed for the production of factors II, VII, IX, and X.

DOSAGE: *Anticoagulant-induced prothrombin deficiency:* 2.5–10.0 mg PO or IV slowly. *Hyperalimentation:* 10 mg IM or IV Q week.

SUPPLIED: Tablets 5 mg; injection 2 mg/mL, 10 mg/mL.

NOTES: With parenteral treatment, the first change in prothrombin is usually seen in 12–24 hr. Anaphylaxis can result from IV dosage; drug should therefore be administered *slowly* if IV route is used.

Pilocarpine (Isopto Carpine, Pilocar, Pilopine HS gel) [See Table 7–12, pp 607-9]

Pindolol (Visken) [See Table 7–7, pp 601-2]

Pioglitazone (Actos)

INDICATIONS: Management of Type 2 diabetes.

ACTIONS: Increases insulin sensitivity.

DOSAGE: 15–45 mg once daily.

SUPPLIED: Tablets 15 mg, 30 mg, 45 mg.

NOTES: Do not use in hepatic impairment.

Piperacillin (Pipracil) [See Table 7–6, p 600]

Piperacillin-Tazobactam (Zosyn) [See Table 7–6, p 600]

Pirbuterol (Maxair)

INDICATIONS: Prevention and treatment of reversible bronchospasm.

ACTIONS: $Beta_2$-adrenergic agonists.

DOSAGE: 2 inhalations Q 4–6 hr; maximum 12 inhalations/d.

SUPPLIED: Aerosol 0.2 mg/actuation.

Piroxicam (Feldene) [See Table 7–11, pp 605-6]

Plasma Protein Fraction (Plasmanate, Others)

INDICATIONS: Shock and hypotension.

ACTIONS: Plasma volume expansion.

DOSAGE: Initial dose 250–500 mL IV (not > 10 mL/min); subsequent infusions should depend on clinical response.

SUPPLIED: Injection 5%.

NOTES: Hypotension associated with rapid infusion. Preparation contains 130–160 mEq of sodium per liter. Do *not* use as a substitute for red blood cells.

Plicamycin (Mithracin)

INDICATIONS: Treatment of hypercalcemia of malignancy; disseminated embryonal cell carcinoma, or germ cell tumors of the testis.

ACTIONS: Antibiotic; binds to the outside of the DNA molecule, interrupting DNA-directed RNA synthesis, DNA intercalation.
DOSAGE: *Hypercalcemia:* 25 μg/kg/d IV on alternate days for 3–8 doses.
Cancer: Refer to specific protocol.
SUPPLIED: Injection.
NOTES: Toxicity includes thrombocytopenia and drug-induced deficiency of clotting factors II, V, VII, and X, resulting in bleeding and bruising. Adjust dosage in patients with renal or hepatic impairment.

Pneumococcal Vaccine, Polyvalent (Pneumovax-23)

INDICATIONS: Immunization against pneumococcal infections in patients predisposed to or at high risk of acquiring these infections; all people 65 years of age and older.
ACTIONS: Active immunization.
DOSAGE: 0.5 mL IM.
SUPPLIED: Injection 25 mg each of polysaccharide isolates per 0.5-mL dose.
NOTES: Do *not* vaccinate during immunosuppressive therapy.

Podophyllin (Podocon-25, Condylox Gel 0.5%, Condylox)

INDICATIONS: Topical therapy of benign growths: genital and perianal warts (condylomata acuminata), papillomas, fibroids.
ACTIONS: Direct anti-mitotic effect. Exact mechanism unknown.
DOSAGE: *Condylox gel and Condylox:* Apply 3 consecutive days per week for 4 weeks.
Podocon-25: Use sparingly and apply to the lesion. Leave on for 1–4 hours, then thoroughly wash off.
SUPPLIED: *Podocon-25:* Contains benzoin 15-mL bottles; *Condylox gel* 0.5%: 3.5 mL clear gel; *Condylox* solution 0.5%: 3.5 mL clear gel.
NOTES: Podocon-25 is applied only by the clinician and not to be dispensed to the patient. Contraindicated in pregnancy, diabetics, bleeding lesions, immunocompromised patients.

Polyethylene Glycol [Peg]–Electrolyte Solution (GoLYTELY, CoLYTE)

INDICATIONS: Bowel cleansing prior to examination or surgery.
ACTIONS: Osmotic cathartic.
DOSAGE: Have patient fast for 3–4 hr; then administer PO 240 mL of solution Q 10 min until patient has consumed 4 L.
SUPPLIED: Powder for reconstitution to 4 L in container.
NOTES: First bowel movement should occur in approximately 1 hr; solution may cause some cramping or nausea.

Polymyxin B and Hydrocortisone (Otobiotic Otic)

INDICATIONS: Superficial bacterial infections of external ear canal.
ACTIONS: Antibiotic anti-inflammatory combination.
DOSAGE: 4 ggts in ear/s tid–qid.
SUPPLIED: Solution: Polymyxin B 10,000 U/hydrocortisone 0.5%/mL.
NOTES: Useful in neomycin allergy.

Potassium Citrate (Urocit-K)

INDICATIONS: Alkalinization of urine, prevention of urinary stones (uric acid, calcium stones if hypocitraturic).
ACTIONS: Urinary alkalinizer.
DOSAGE: 10–20 mEq PO tid with meals, max 100 mEq/d.
SUPPLIED: Tablets 540 mg = 5 mEq, 1080 mg = 10 mEq.

Potassium Citrate and Citric Acid (Polycitra-K)

INDICATIONS: Alkalinization of urine, prevention of urinary stones (uric acid, calcium stones if hypocitraturic).
ACTIONS: Urinary alkalinizer.
DOSAGE: 10–20 mEq PO tid with meals, max 100 mEq/d.
SUPPLIED: Solution 10 mEq/5 mL; powder 30 mEq/packet.

Potassium Iodide (Lugol's Solution) (SSKI, Thyro-Block)

INDICATIONS: Thyroid crisis, reduction of vascularity before thyroid surgery, blocking thyroid uptake of radioactive isotopes of iodine, thinning of bronchial secretions, sporotrichosis.
ACTIONS: Iodine supplement.
DOSAGE: *Pre-op thyroidectomy:* 50–250 mg (1–5 drops SSKI; OR 2–6 drops of Lugol's sol) PO tid for 10 days prior to surgery.
Thyroid crisis: 300–500 mg (6–10 drops SSKI Q 8 hr).
Expectorant: 300–650 mg 2–3 × a day.
Sporotrichosis: 500 mg tid.
SUPPLIED: Tablets 130 mg; solution SSKI 1 g/mL; Lugol's solution, strong iodine 100 mg/mL; syrup 325 mg/5 mL.

Potassium Supplements (Kaon, Kaochlor, K-Lor, Slow-K, Micro-K, Klorvess, Others)

INDICATIONS: Prevention or treatment of hypokalemia (often related to diuretic use).
ACTIONS: Supplementation of potassium.
DOSAGE: 20–100 mEq/d PO divided q day–bid.
IV: 10–20 mEq/hr, max 40 mEq/hr and 150 mEq/d (monitor frequent potassium levels when using high-dose IV infusions). Infusion rate of 20 mEq/hr and greater require continuous cardiac monitoring to detect ECG signs of hypervolemia.
SUPPLIED: Sustained-release tablets 6.7 mEq, 8 mEq, 10 mEq, 20 mEq; sustained-release capsules 10 mEq; liquid 20 mEq/15 mL, 30 mEq/15 mL, 40 mEq/15 mL; powder packets 15 mEq, 20 mEq, 25 mEq; effervescent tablets (potassium bicarbonate) 20 mEq, 25 mEq, 50 mEq.
NOTES AND CAUTION: Potassium supplements can cause GI irritation. Powder and liquids must be mixed with a beverage (unsalted tomato juice, etc). Use cautiously in renal insufficiency, and along with NSAIDs, potassium-sparing diuretics, and ACE inhibitors. Chloride salt recommended in coexisting alkalosis; for coexisting acidosis use acetate, bicarbonate, citrate, or gluconate salt.

Pramipexole (Mirapex)

INDICATIONS: Treatment of Parkinson's disease.
ACTION: Dopamine agonist.
DOSAGE: 1.5–4.5 mg per day, beginning with 0.375 mg/d in 3 divided doses.
SUPPLIED: Tablets 0.125 mg, 0.25 mg, 1 mg, 1.5 mg.
NOTES: Dosage should be titrated slowly.

Pramoxine (Anusol Ointment, Proctofoam-NS, Others)

INDICATIONS: Relief of pain and itching from external and internal hemorrhoids and anorectal surgery; topical for burns and dermatosis.
ACTIONS: Topical anesthetic.
DOSAGE: Apply cream, ointment, gel, or spray freely to anal area Q 3–4 hr.
SUPPLIED: Foam (Proctofoam NS) 1% [OTC]; cream 1% [OTC]; ointment 1% [OTC]; lotion 1% [OTC]; gel 1% [OTC]; pads 1% [OTC]; spray 1% [OTC].

Pramoxine with Hydrocortisone (Enzone, Proctofoam-HC)

INDICATIONS: Relief of pain and itching from hemorrhoids.
ACTIONS: Topical anesthetic.
DOSAGE: Apply freely to anal area tid–qid.
SUPPLIED: *Cream:* Pramoxine hydrochloride 1% hydrocortisone acetate 0.5/1%; *Foam:* Pramoxine 1% hydrocortisone 1%; *Lotion:* Pramoxine 1% hydrocortisone 0.25/1/2.5%; pramoxine 2.5% and hydrocortisone 1%.

Pravastatin (Pravachol) [See Table 7–15, p 612]

Prazosin (Minipress)

INDICATIONS: Treatment of hypertension and congestive heart failure.

ACTIONS: Peripherally acting alpha-adrenergic blocker.
DOSAGE: 1 mg PO tid; may be increased to a total daily dose of up to 20 mg/d.
SUPPLIED: Capsules 1 mg, 2 mg, 5 mg.
NOTES: Prazosin may cause orthostatic hypotension, therefore the patient should take the first dose at bedtime; tolerance develops to this effect; tachyphylaxis may result.

Prednisolone [See Table 7–2, p 597]

Prednisolone (AK-PRED, Pred Forte) [See Table 7–12, pp 607-9]

Prednisone [See Table 7–2, p 597]

Probenecid (Benemid, Others)

INDICATIONS: Prevention of gout and hyperuricemia; prolong serum levels of penicillins or cephalosporins.
ACTIONS: Renal tubular blocking agent.
DOSAGE: *Gout*: 250 mg bid for 1 week; then 0.5 g PO bid. Can increase by 500 mg/month up to 2–3 g/d.
Increased antibiotic effect: 1–2 g PO 30 min prior to dose of antibiotic.
SUPPLIED: Tablets 500 mg.

Procainamide (Pronestyl, Procan)

INDICATIONS: Treatment of supraventricular and ventricular arrhythmias.
ACTIONS: Class 1a antiarrhythmic.
DOSAGE: *Emergency cardiac care:* See Section I, Chapter 9, Cardiopulmonary Arrest, V, p 46, and inside cover.
Chronic dosing: 50 mg/kg/d PO in divided doses Q 4–6 hr.
Maintenance: 15–50 mg/kg/24 hr PO divided Q 3–6 hr.
SUPPLIED: Tablets and capsules 250 mg, 375 mg, 500 mg; sustained-release tablets 250 mg, 500 mg, 750 mg, 1000 mg; injection 100 mg/mL, 500 mg/mL.
NOTES: Drug can cause hypotension and a lupus-like syndrome. Dosage must be adjusted with renal or hepatic impairment (see Table 7—16, p 613).

Procarbazine (Matulane)

INDICATIONS: Hodgkin's disease, non-Hodgkin's lymphoma, brain tumors.
ACTIONS: Alkylating agent; inhibition of DNA and RNA synthesis.
DOSAGE: Refer to specific protocol.
NOTES: Toxicity includes myelosuppression; hemolytic reactions (with glucose-6-phosphate dehydrogenase deficiency); nausea, vomiting, and diarrhea; a disulfiram-like reaction may occur. Cutaneous reactions may also occur. Constitutional symptoms, myalgia, and arthralgia may be seen. CNS effects may be related to the high concentrations of drug reached in CSF or because of monoamine oxidase inhibitor effects. Azoospermia and cessation of menses are common.

Prochlorperazine (Compazine)

INDICATIONS: Treatment of nausea and vomiting, agitation, psychotic disorders.
ACTIONS: Phenothiazine; blocks postsynaptic mesolimbic dopaminergic receptors in the brain.
DOSAGE: *Antiemetic:* 5–10 mg PO tid–qid; OR 25 mg PR bid; OR 5–10 mg deep IM Q 4–6 hr.
Antipsychotic: 10–20 mg IM in acute situations; OR 5–10 mg PO tid–qid for maintenance.
SUPPLIED: Tablets 5 mg, 10 mg, 25 mg; sustained-release capsules 10 mg, 15 mg, 30 mg; syrup 5 mg/5 mL; suppositories: 2.5 mg, 5 mg, 25 mg; injection 5 mg/mL.
NOTES: A much larger dose may be required for antipsychotic effect. Extrapyramidal side effects are common. Treat acute extrapyramidal reactions with diphenhydramine.

Promethazine (Phenergan)

INDICATIONS: Management of nausea and vomiting and motion sickness.
ACTIONS: Phenothiazine; blocks postsynaptic mesolimbic dopaminergic receptors in the brain.
DOSAGE: 12.5–50 mg PO, PR, or IM bid–qid prn.

SUPPLIED: Tablets 12.5 mg, 25 mg, 50 mg; syrup 6.25 mg/5 mL, 25 mg/5 mL; suppositories 12.5 mg, 25 mg, 50 mg; injection 25 mg/mL, 50 mg/mL.
NOTES: High incidence of drowsiness.

Propafenone (Rythmol)

INDICATIONS: Treatment of life-threatening ventricular arrhythmias.
ACTIONS: Class Ic antiarrhythmic.
DOSAGE: 150–300 mg PO Q 8 hr.
SUPPLIED: Tablets 150 mg, 225 mg, 300 mg.
NOTES: May cause dizziness, unusual taste, first-degree heart block, and prolongation of QRS and QT intervals.

Propantheline (Pro-Banthine)

INDICATIONS: Symptomatic treatment of small intestine hypermotility, spastic colon, ureteral spasm, bladder spasm, pylorospasm.
ACTIONS: Antimuscarinic agent.
DOSAGE: 15 mg PO AC and 30 mg PO HS.
SUPPLIED: Tablets 7.5 mg, 15 mg.
NOTES: Anticholinergic side effects such as dry mouth and blurred vision are common.

Propofol (Diprivan)

INDICATIONS: Induction or maintenance of anesthesia; continuous sedation in intubated patients.
ACTIONS: Sedative hypnotic; mechanism unknown.
DOSAGE: *Anesthesia:* 2–2.5 mg/kg induction; then 0.1–0.2 mg/kg/min continuous infusion. *ICU sedation:* 5–50 μg/kg/min continuous infusion.
SUPPLIED: Injection 10 mg/mL.
NOTES: 1 mL of propofol contains 0.1 g of fat. Drug may increase serum triglycerides when administered for extended periods.

Propoxyphene (Darvon) [C], Propoxyphene and Acetaminophen (Darvocet) [C], Propoxyphene and Aspirin (Darvon Compound-65, Darvon–N with Aspirin) [C]

INDICATIONS: Mild to moderate pain.
ACTIONS: Narcotic analgesic.
DOSAGE: 1–2 PO Q 4 hr prn.
SUPPLIED:

- Darvon (Propoxyphene HCl) capsule 65 mg.
- Darvon-N: Propoxyphene napsylate 100-mg tablet.
- Darvocet-N: Propoxyphene napsylate 50 mg/acetaminophen 325 mg.
- Darvocet-N 100: Propoxyphene napsylate 100 mg/acetaminophen 650 mg.
- Darvon Compound-65: Propoxyphene HCl 65-mg/aspirin 389-mg/caffeine 32-mg capsules.
- Darvon-N with aspirin: Propoxyphene napsylate 100 mg/aspirin 325 mg.

NOTES: Intentional overdose can be lethal.

Propranolol (Inderal) (Also see Table 7–7, pp 601-2]

INDICATIONS: Treatment of hypertension, angina, myocardial infarction, migraine headache prophylaxis, arrhythmias, and thyrotoxicosis.
ACTIONS: Competitively blocks beta-adrenergic receptors, β_1, β_2. Decreases conversion of T_4 to T_3.
DOSAGE:

- *Angina:* 80–320 mg PO q day divided bid–qid; OR 80-160 mg SR q day.
- *Arrhythmia:* 10–80 mg PO tid–qid; OR 1 mg IV slowly; repeat Q 5 min up to 5 mg.
- *HTN:* 40 mg PO bid; OR 60–80 mg SR q day; increase weekly to max 640 mg/d.
- *Hypertrophic subaortic stenosis:* 20–40 mg PO tid–qid.
- *MI:* 180–240 mg PO divided tid–qid.

- *Migraine headache prophylaxis:* 80 mg/d divided qid-tid; increase weekly to max 160–240 mg/d divided tid–qid; wean off if no response in 6 wk.
- *Pheochromocytoma:* 30–60 mg/d divided tid–qid.
- *Thyrotoxicosis:* 1–3 mg IV single dose; 10–40 mg PO Q 6 hr.
- *Tremor:* 40 mg PO bid; increase as needed to max 320 mg/d.

SUPPLIED: Tablets 10 mg, 20 mg, 40 mg, 60 mg, 80 mg, 90 mg; capsules SR 60 mg, 80 mg, 120 mg, 160 mg; solution oral 4 mg/mL, 8 mg/mL, 80 mg/mL; injection 1 mg/mL.
NOTES: Adjust dosage in patients with renal impairment.

Propylthiouracil (PTU)

INDICATIONS: Treatment of hyperthyroidism.
ACTIONS: Inhibits production of T_3 and T_4 and conversion of T_4 to T_3.
DOSAGE: Begin at 100 mg PO Q 8 hr (may need up to 1200 mg/d for control); after the patient is euthyroid (6–8 weeks), taper dose by ½ every 4–6 weeks to a maintenance dose of 50–150 mg/24 hr. Treatment can usually be discontinued in 2–3 years.
SUPPLIED: Tablets 50 mg.
NOTES: Follow up on the patient clinically; monitor thyroid function tests.

Protamine Sulfate

INDICATIONS: Reversal of heparin effect.
ACTIONS: Neutralizes heparin by forming a stable complex.
DOSAGE: Based on amount of heparin reversal desired; given slow IV; 1 mg will reverse approximately 100 U of heparin given in the preceding 3–4 hr, to a maximum dose of 50 mg.
SUPPLIED: Injection 10 mg/mL.
NOTES: Follow coagulation studies. Drug may have anticoagulant effect if given without heparin.

Pseudoephedrine (Sudafed, Novafed, Afrinol, Others)

INDICATIONS: Decongestant.
ACTIONS: Stimulates alpha-adrenergic receptors, resulting in vasoconstriction.
DOSAGE: 30–60 mg PO Q 6–8 hr; sustained-release capsules 120 mg PO Q 12 hr.
SUPPLIED: Tablets 30 mg, 60 mg; capsules 60 mg; sustained-release tablets 120 mg, 240 mg; sustained-release capsules 120 mg; liquid 7.5 mg/0.8 mL, 15 mg/5 mL, 30 mg/5 mL.
NOTES: Contraindicated in patients with poorly controlled hypertension or coronary artery disease and in patients taking monoamine oxidase inhibitors. Pseudoephedrine is an ingredient in many cough and cold preparations.

Psyllium (Metamucil, Serutan, Effer-Syllium)

INDICATIONS: Constipation, diverticular disease of the colon.
ACTIONS: Bulk laxative.
DOSAGE: 1 teaspoon (7 g) in a glass of water q day–tid.
SUPPLIED: Granules 4 g/tsp, 25 g/tsp; powder: 3.5 g/packet.
NOTES: Psyllium is one of the safest laxatives. Do not use if bowel obstruction is suspected. The effervescent form (Effer-Syllium) usually contains potassium and should be used with caution in patients with renal failure.

Pyrazinamide

INDICATIONS: Treatment of active tuberculosis.
ACTIONS: Bacteriostatic; mechanism unknown.
DOSAGE: 15–30 mg/kg/24 hr PO q day; maximum 2 g/d.
SUPPLIED: Tablets 500 mg.
NOTES: May cause hepatotoxicity; use in combination with other antituberculosis drugs. Consult *MMWR* for the latest recommendations on the treatment of tuberculosis. Dosage regimen differs for directly observed therapy; adjust dose for renal or hepatic impairment.

Pyridoxine (Vitamin B_6)

INDICATIONS: Treatment and prevention of vitamin B_6 deficiency.
ACTIONS: Supplementation of vitamin B_6.

DOSAGE: *Deficiency:* 10–20 mg PO q day.
Drug-induced neuritis: 100–200 mg/d; 25–100 mg/d prophylaxis.
SUPPLIED: Tablets 25 mg, 50 mg, 100 mg; injection 100 mg/mL.

Quazepam (Doral) [C]

INDICATIONS: Treatment of insomnia.
ACTIONS: Benzodiazepine.
DOSAGE: 7.5–15 mg PO Q HS prn.
SUPPLIED: Tablets 7.5 mg, 15 mg.
NOTES: Reduce dose in the elderly; do not discontinue abruptly.

Quetiapine (Seroquel)

INDICATIONS: Treatment of acute exacerbations of schizophrenia.
ACTIONS: Serotonin and dopamine antagonism.
DOSAGE: 150–750 mg per day; initiate at 25–100 mg 2–3 ×/d.
SUPPLIED: Tablets 25 mg, 100 mg, 200 mg.
NOTES: Dose must be slowly increased; adjust dose for hepatic and geriatric patients.

Quinapril (Accupril) [See Table 7–3, p 598]

Quinidine (Quinidex, Quinaglute)

INDICATIONS: Prevention of tachydysrhythmias.
ACTIONS: Class 1a antiarrhythmic.
DOSAGE: *Conversion of atrial fibrillation or flutter:* Use after digitalization, 200 mg Q 2–3 hr for 8 doses; then increase the daily dose to a maximum of 3–4 g or until normal rhythm.
SUPPLIED: *Sulfate:* tablets 200 mg, 300 mg; sustained-release tablets 300 mg.
Gluconate: Sustained-release tablets 324 mg; injection 80 mg/mL.
NOTES: Contraindicated in digitalis toxicity and AV block; follow serum levels if available (see Table 7–16, p 613). Extreme hypotension seen with IV administration. Sulfate salt contains 83% quinidine; gluconate salt contains 62% quinidine; dosage adjustment in renal impairment. Quinidine increases conduction through the AV node; must also use a drug to slow conduction through the AV node, such as digoxin, diltiazem, or a beta-blocker.

Quinupristin/Dalfopristin (Synercid)

INDICATIONS: Treatment of infections caused by vancomycin-resistant *Enterococcus faecium* (VREF); complicated skin and skin structure infections caused by *Staphylococcus aureus* and *Streptococcus pyogenes.*
ACTIONS: A streptogramin antimicrobial agent. Acts on the bacterial ribosome to inhibit protein synthesis.
DOSAGE: 7.5 mg/kg IV Q 8–12 hr (administer over 60 min).
SUPPLIED: 500 mg (150 mg quinupristin and 350 mg dalfopristin) per 10-mL vial.
NOTES: Significantly inhibits CYP3A4 isoenzymes. Use with caution when coadministered with drugs metabolized by this isoenzyme (eg, cyclosporin). May cause venous irritation, elevation in bilirubin, and arthralgias/myalgias. Administer through central line if possible; NOT compatible with saline or heparin; therefore, flush IV lines with dextrose.

Rabeprazole (Aciphex) [See Table 7–14, p 611]

Raloxifene (Evista)

INDICATIONS: Prevention of osteoporosis.
ACTIONS: Selective estrogen receptor modulator.
DOSAGE: 60 mg per day.
SUPPLIED: Tablets 60 mg.

Ramipril (Altace) [See Table 7–3, p 598]

Ranitidine (Zantac)

INDICATIONS: Duodenal ulcer, active benign ulcers, hypersecretory conditions, and gastroesophageal reflux disease (GERD).

ACTIONS: H_2-receptor antagonist.
DOSAGE: *Ulcer:* 150 mg PO bid, 300 mg PO Q HS, or 50 mg IV Q 6–8 hr; OR 400 mg IV/d continuous infusion; then maintenance of 150 mg PO Q HS.
Hypersecretion: 150 mg PO bid, up to 600 mg/d.
GERD: 300 mg PO bid; maintenance 300 mg PO Q HS.
SUPPLIED: Tablets 75 mg, 150 mg, 300 mg; syrup 15 mg/mL; injection 25 mg/mL.
NOTES: Reduce dose with renal failure; note that oral and parenteral doses are different.

Repaglinide (Prandin)

INDICATIONS: Management of Type 2 diabetes.
ACTIONS: Stimulates insulin release from pancreas.
DOSAGE: 0.5–4 mg AC.
SUPPLIED: Tablets 0.5 mg, 1 mg, 2 mg.

Reteplase (Retavase)

INDICATIONS: Post-acute myocardial infarction.
ACTIONS: Thrombolytic agent.
DOSAGE: 10 U IV over 2 min, 2nd dose 30 min later of 10 U IV over 2 min.
SUPPLIED: Injection 10.8 unit/2 mL.

Ribavirin (Virazole)

INDICATIONS: Treatment of hepatitis C (in combination with interferon alfa-2b).
ACTIONS: Unknown.
DOSAGE: *Hepatitis C:* 600 mg PO bid in combination with interferon alfa-2b (See Interferon Alpha-2B and Ribavirin combination, p 530).
SUPPLIED: Powder for aerosol 6 g; capsules 200 mg.
NOTES: Aerosolized by a SPAG generator; may accumulate on soft contact lenses. Monitor HCT/HGB frequently; give a pregnancy test monthly.

Rifabutin (Mycobutin)

INDICATIONS: Prevention of *Mycobacterium avium* complex infection in AIDS patients with a CD4 count < 100.
ACTIONS: Inhibits DNA-dependent RNA polymerase activity.
DOSAGE: 150–300 mg PO q day.
SUPPLIED: Capsules 150 mg.
NOTES: Has similar adverse effects and drug interactions as rifampin.

Rifampin (Rifadin)

INDICATIONS: Tuberculosis (treatment and prophylaxis). Prophylaxis for exposure to *N meningitidis and H influenzae.* Treatment of *S aureus* nasal carriers.
ACTIONS: Inhibits DNA-dependent RNA polymerase activity.
DOSAGE: *N meningitidis* and *H influenzae exposure/carrier:* 600 mg PO q day for 4 days. *S aureus nasal carrier dose:* 600 mg PO q day (times 5–10 days).
Tuberculosis: 600 mg PO or IV q day; OR twice weekly combination-therapy regimen.
SUPPLIED: Capsules 150 mg, 300 mg; injection 600 mg.
NOTES: Multiple drug interactions; causes orange-red discoloration of bodily secretions, including tears. Drug is never used as a single agent to treat active tuberculosis infections.

Rifapentine (Priftin)

INDICATIONS: Treatment of tuberculosis.
ACTIONS: Inhibits DNA-dependent RNA polymerase activity.
DOSAGE: *Intensive phase:* 600 mg PO twice weekly for 2 months; separate doses by 3 or more days.
Continuation phase: 600 mg once weekly.
SUPPLIED: Tablets 150 mg.
NOTES: Has similar adverse effects and drug interactions as rifampin.

Rimantadine (Flumadine)

INDICATIONS: Prophylaxis and treatment of influenza A virus infections.

ACTIONS: Antiviral agent.
DOSAGE: 100 mg PO bid.
SUPPLIED: Tablets 100 mg; syrup 50 mg/5 mL.
NOTES: Dosage adjustment in severe renal or hepatic impairment; initiate within 48 hr of symptom onset.

Rimexolone (Vexol Ophthalmic) [See Table 7–12, pp 607-9]

Risedronate (Actonel)

INDICATIONS: Prevention and treatment of postmenopausal osteoporosis; Paget's disease.
ACTIONS: Bisphosphonate; inhibits osteoclast-mediated bone resorption.
DOSAGE: *Usual:* 5 mg PO once daily with 6–8 oz of water.
Paget's disease: 30 mg q day for 2 months.
SUPPLIED: Tablets 5 mg, 30 mg.
NOTES: Have patient take risedronate 30 minutes before first food or drink of the day and maintain upright position for at least 30 minutes after administration. Drug has interaction with calcium supplements; may cause GI distress and arthralgia. Not recommended in moderate to severe renal impairment.

Risperidone (Risperdal)

INDICATIONS: Management of psychotic disorders.
ACTIONS: Benzisoxazole antipsychotic agent.
DOSAGE: 1–6 mg PO bid.
SUPPLIED: Tablets 1 mg, 2 mg, 3 mg, 4 mg.
NOTES: Use lower starting doses in elderly or in patients with renal or hepatic impairment or orthostatic hypotension. Extrapyramidal reactions are seen with higher doses.

Ritonavir (Norvir)

INDICATIONS: Treatment of HIV infection when therapy is warranted.
ACTIONS: Protease inhibitor; inhibits maturation of immature noninfectious virions to mature infectious virus.
DOSAGE: 600 mg PO bid; OR 400 mg PO bid in combination with saquinavir.
SUPPLIED: Capsules 100 mg; solution 80 mg/mL.
NOTES: Titrate dose over 1 week to avoid GI complications; should be taken with food. Ritonavir has many drug interactions; may cause perioral and peripheral paresthesias; store in refrigerator.

Rivastigmine (Exelon)

INDICATIONS: Treatment of mild to moderate dementia associated with Alzheimer's disease.
ACTIONS: Enhances cholinergic activity.
DOSAGE: 1.5 mg twice daily; increased to 6 mg twice daily, with dosage increases at 2-week intervals.
SUPPLIED: Capsules 1.5 mg, 3 mg, 4.5 mg, 6 mg; solution 2 mg/mL.
NOTES: Associated with significant GI adverse effects, many of which are dose-related.

Rizatriptan (Maxalt)

INDICATIONS: Treatment of acute migraine attacks.
ACTIONS: Serotonin 5-HT_1 receptor antagonist.
DOSAGE: 5–10 mg PO; may repeat once in 2 hr.
SUPPLIED: Tablets 5 mg, 10 mg; disintegrating tablets 5 mg, 10 mg.

Rocuronium (Zemuron)

INDICATIONS: Skeletal muscle relaxation during rapid-sequence intubation, surgery, or mechanical ventilation.
ACTIONS: Nondepolarizing neuromuscular blockade.
DOSAGE: *Rapid sequence intubation:* 0.6–1.2 mg/kg IV.
Continuous infusion: 4–16 μg/kg/min IV.
SUPPLIED: 10 mg/mL 5, 10 mL vials.

NOTES: Reduce dose in patients with hepatic impairment.

Rofecoxib (Vioxx) [See Table 7–11, pp 605-6]

Ropinirole (Requip)

INDICATIONS: Treatment of Parkinson's disease.
ACTIONS: Dopamine agonist.
DOSAGE: Initial dose 0.25 mg PO tid, with weekly dosage increases of 0.25 mg per dose, up to total daily dose of 3 mg.
SUPPLIED: Tablets 0.25 mg, 0.5 mg, 1 mg, 2 mg, 5 mg.
NOTES: Syncope or postural hypotension may result.

Rosiglitazone (Avandia)

INDICATIONS: Treatment of type 2 diabetes mellitus.
ACTIONS: Increase insulin sensitivity.
DOSAGE: 4–8 mg PO once daily or in 2 divided doses.
SUPPLIED: Tablets 2 mg, 4 mg, 8 mg.
NOTES: May be taken with or without meals; do not use in active liver disease.

Salmeterol (Serevent, Serevent Diskus)

INDICATIONS: Treatment of asthma and exercise-induced bronchospasm.
ACTIONS: Sympathomimetic bronchodilator.
DOSAGE: *Metered-dose inhaler:* 2 inhalations twice daily; *Diskus:* 1 inhalation bid.
SUPPLIED: Metered-dose inhaler 25 μg/spray; inhalation powder 50 μg/inhalation; not for relief of acute attacks.

Saquinavir (Invirase, Fortovase)

INDICATIONS: Treatment of HIV infection.
ACTIONS: HIV protease inhibitor.
DOSAGE: 1200 mg PO tid within 2 hr after a meal.
SUPPLIED: Capsules 200 mg.

Sargramostim [GM-CSF] (Prokine, Leukine)

INDICATIONS: Treatment of myeloid recovery following bone marrow transplantation or cancer chemotherapy.
ACTIONS: Activates mature granulocytes and macrophages.
DOSAGE: 250 $\mu g/m^2/d$ IV for 21 days (BMT).
SUPPLIED: Injection 250 μg, 500 μg.
NOTES: May cause bone pain.

Scopolamine, Transdermal (Transderm-Scop)

INDICATIONS: Prevention of nausea and vomiting associated with motion sickness.
ACTIONS: Anticholinergic, antiemetic.
DOSAGE: Apply 1 patch behind the ear every 3 days; 0.3–0.65 IM/IV/SC repeat prn Q 4–6 hr.
SUPPLIED: Patch 1.5 mg; injectable forms.
NOTES: May cause dry mouth, drowsiness, and blurred vision. Apply at least 4 hours before exposure.

Secobarbital (Seconal) [C]

INDICATIONS: Treatment of insomnia.
ACTIONS: Rapid-acting barbiturate.
DOSAGE: 100–200 mg IM Q HS prn.
SUPPLIED: Injection 50 mg/mL.
NOTES: Beware of respiratory depression; tolerance acquired within 1–2 weeks.

Selegiline (Eldepryl)

INDICATIONS: Parkinson's disease.
ACTIONS: Inhibits monoamine oxidase activity.

DOSAGE: 5 mg PO bid.
SUPPLIED: Tablets 5 mg.
NOTES: May cause nausea and dizziness.

Selenium Sulfide (Exsel Shampoo, Selsun Blue Shampoo, Selsun Shampoo)

INDICATIONS: Scalp seborrheic dermatitis, itching and flaking of the scalp due to dandruff; treatment of tinea versicolor.
ACTIONS: Anti-seborrheic.
DOSAGE: *Dandruff, seborrhea:* Massage 5–10 mL into wet scalp, leave on 2–3 minutes, rinse and repeat; use twice weekly, then once every 1–4 weeks prn.
Tinea versicolor: Apply daily for 7 days, 2.5% on area and lather with small amounts of water; leave on skin for 10 min, then rinse.
SUPPLIED: Shampoo 1%, 2.5%.

Sertraline (Zoloft)

INDICATIONS: Treatment of depression.
ACTIONS: Inhibits neuronal uptake of serotonin.
DOSAGE: 50–200 mg PO q day.
SUPPLIED: Tablets 25 mg, 50 mg, 100 mg.
NOTES: Can activate manic/hypomanic state; has caused weight loss in clinical trials. Use cautiously in patients with hepatic impairment. Can cause insomnia or hypersomnia and sexual dysfunction.

Sevelamer (Renagel)

INDICATIONS: Reduction of serum phosphorus in end-stage renal disease.
ACTIONS: Binds phosphate within intestinal lumen.
DOSAGE: 2–4 capsules PO tid with meals, with subsequent adjustment based on serum phosphorus.
SUPPLIED: Capsules 403 mg.
NOTES: Instruct patient not to open or chew capsules; may reduce fat-soluble vitamin absorption.

Sibutramine (Meridia) [C]

INDICATIONS: Management of obesity.
ACTIONS: Blocks uptake of norepinephrine, serotonin, and dopamine.
DOSAGE: 10 mg once daily, may titrate to 15 mg after 4 weeks.
SUPPLIED: Capsules 5 mg, 10 mg, 15 mg.
NOTES: Use with low-calorie diet; monitor blood pressure.

Sildenafil (Viagra)

INDICATIONS: Erectile dysfunction.
ACTIONS: Smooth muscle relaxation and increased inflow of blood to the corpus cavernosum; inhibits phosphodiesterase type 5 responsible for cGMP breakdown, resulting in increased cGMP activity.
DOSAGE: 25–100 mg 1 hr prior to attempted sexual activity; maximum dosing is once daily.
SUPPLIED: Tablets 25 mg, 50 mg, 100 mg.
NOTES: Contraindicated in patients taking nitrates of any form; adjust dose in persons > 65 years or with hepatic/severe renal impairment or potent CYP3A4 inhibitors. Drug may cause headache, blue haze visual disturbance, usually reversible. Cardiac ischemia and hypotension in the absence of nitrate use are debatable.

Silver Nitrate (Dey-Drop)

INDICATIONS: Removal of granulation tissue, warts, cauterization of wounds.
ACTIONS: Caustic antiseptic and astringent.
DOSAGE: Apply to moist surface 2–3 × a week for several weeks or until desired effect.
SUPPLIED: *Topical*: impregnated applicator sticks, 10% ointment, 10%, 25%, 50% solution.
NOTES: May stain tissue black, usually resolves.

Silver Sulfadiazine (Silvadene)

INDICATIONS: Prevention of sepsis in second- and third-degree burns.
ACTIONS: Bactericidal.
DOSAGE: Aseptically cover the affected area with 1/16-in. coating bid.
SUPPLIED: Cream 1%.
NOTES: Can have systemic absorption with extensive application.

Simethicone (Mylicon)

INDICATIONS: Symptomatic treatment of flatulence.
ACTIONS: Defoaming action.
DOSAGE: 40–125 mg PO after meals and HS prn.
SUPPLIED: Tablets 40 mg, 80 mg, 125 mg; capsules 125 mg; drops 40 mg/0.6 mL.

Simvastatin (Zocor) [See Table 7–15, p 612]

Sirolimus (Rapamune)

INDICATIONS: Prophylaxis of organ rejection.
ACTIONS: Inhibits T-lymphocyte activation.
DOSAGE: 2 mg PO per day.
SUPPLIED: Solution 1 mg/mL.
NOTES: Instruct patient to dilute drug in water or orange juice and do NOT drink grapefruit juice while on sirolimus. Drug should be taken 4 hours after cyclosporin. Adjust dosage in patients with hepatic impairment.

Sodium Bicarbonate

INDICATIONS: Alkalinization of urine, renal tubular acidosis (RTA), treatment of metabolic acidosis, hyperkalemia.
DOSAGE: *Emergency cardiac care:* Initiate adequate ventilation, 1 mEq/kg/dose IV; can repeat 0.5 mEq/kg in 10 min one time or based on acid/base status.
Metabolic acidosis: 2–5 mEq/kg IV over 8 hr and prn based on acid/base status.
Alkalinize urine: 4 g (48 mEq) PO, then 1–2 g Q 4 hr; adjust dose based on urine pH.
Chronic renal failure: 1–3 mEq/kg/d.
Distal RTA: 1 mEq/kg/d PO.
SUPPLIED: Injection 0.5 mEq/mL, 1 mEq/mL; tablets 325 mg, 650 mg.
NOTES: 1 g neutralizes 12 mEq of acid. Supplied as IV infusion, powder, and tablets 300 mg = 3.6 mEq; 325 mg = 3.8 mEq; 520 mg = 6.3 mEq; 600 mg = 7.3 mEq; 650 mg = 7.6 mEq. Avoid use of multiple ampoules; can cause hyperosmolar state.

Sodium Citrate (Bicitra)

INDICATIONS: Alkalinization of urine; dissolve uric acid and cysteine stones.
ACTIONS: Urinary alkalinizer.
DOSAGE: 2–6 teaspoonfuls (10–30 mL) diluted in 1–3 ounces of water PC and HS.
SUPPLIED: 15- or 30-mL unit dose: 16 (473 mL) or 4 (118 mL) fluid ounces.
NOTES: Should not be given to patients on aluminum-based antacids. Contraindicated in patients with severe renal impairment or sodium-restricted diets.

Sodium Phosphate (Visicol)

INDICATIONS: Bowel evacuation prior to colonoscopy.
ACTIONS: Hyperosmotic.
DOSAGE: 3 tablets with at least 8 ounces of clear liquid every 15 min for a total of 20 tablets the night before the procedure; 3–5 hours before the colonoscopy, repeat the process.
SUPPLIED: Tablets 2 g.
NOTES AND CAUTION: Use caution in patients with renal impairment or electrolyte disturbances. Contraindicated in congestive heart failure, ascites, unstable angina, gastric retention, ileus, bowel perforation, colitis, hypomotility; associated with QT prolongation.

Sodium Polystyrene Sulfonate (Kayexalate)

INDICATIONS: Treatment of hyperkalemia.

ACTIONS: Sodium and potassium ion exchange resin.
DOSAGE: 15–60 g PO; OR 30–60 g PR Q 6 hr based on serum K^+.
SUPPLIED: Powder; suspension 15 g/60 mL sorbitol.
NOTES: Can cause hypernatremia; given with an agent such as sorbitol to promote movement through the bowel.

Sorbitol

INDICATIONS: Constipation.
ACTIONS: Laxative.
DOSAGE: 30–60 mL of a 20–70% solution prn.
SUPPLIED: Liquid 70%.

Sotalol (Betapace)

INDICATIONS: Treatment of ventricular arrhythmias.
ACTIONS: Beta-adrenergic blocking agent.
DOSAGE: 80 mg PO bid; may be increased to 240–320 mg/d.
SUPPLIED: Tablets 80 mg, 120 mg, 160 mg, 240 mg.
NOTES: Dosage should be adjusted for renal insufficiency.

Sparfloxacin (Zagam)

INDICATIONS: Community-acquired pneumonia, acute exacerbations of chronic bronchitis.
ACTIONS: Fluoroquinolone antibiotic inhibits DNA gyrase.
DOSAGE: 2 tablets (400 mg) PO day 1, followed by 1 tablet q day for days 2–10.
SUPPLIED: Tablets 200 mg.
NOTES AND CAUTION: CNS stimulation, photosensitivity; caution in renal dysfunction.

Spironolactone (Aldactone)

INDICATIONS: Treatment of hyperaldosteronism, essential hypertension, and edematous states (congestive heart failure, cirrhosis).
ACTIONS: Aldosterone antagonist; potassium-sparing diuretic.
DOSAGE: 25–400 mg PO q day.
SUPPLIED: Tablets 25 mg, 50 mg, 100 mg.
NOTES: Drug can cause hyperkalemia and gynecomastia. Diuretic of choice for cirrhotic edema and ascites. In patients with NYHA Class III or Class IV congestive heart failure, spironolactone 25–50 mg/d has been shown to decrease mortality and improve function.

SSKI (See Potassium Iodide, p 563]

Stavudine (Zerit)

INDICATIONS: Treatment of adults with advanced HIV disease.
ACTIONS: Reverse-transcriptase inhibitor.
DOSAGE: Persons > 60 kg: 40 mg bid; persons < 60 kg: 30 mg bid.
SUPPLIED: Capsules 15 mg, 20 mg, 30 mg, 40 mg; solution 1 mg/mL.
NOTES: May cause peripheral neuropathy. Not a cure for HIV. Adjust dosage in patients with renal impairment.

Steroids, Systemic (See also Table 7–2, p 597]

INDICATIONS:

- Endocrine disorders (adrenal insufficiency)
- Rheumatoid disorders
- Collagen-vascular diseases
- Dermatologic diseases
- Allergic states
- Edematous states (cerebral, nephrotic syndrome)
- Immunosuppression for transplantation
- Hypercalcemia
- Malignancies (breast, lymphomas)

- Preoperatively (in any patient who has been on steroids in the previous year, known hypoadrenalism, pre-op for adrenalectomy)
- Injection into joints/tissue

ACTIONS: Glucocorticoid.
DOSAGE: Varies with use and institutional protocols. Some commonly used doses are listed here:

- *Adrenal insufficiency, acute* (*Addisonian crisis*): Hydrocortisone 100 mg IV Q 6 hr; then 300 mg/d divided Q 6 hr; convert to 50 mg PO Q 8 hr × 4–6 doses, taper to 30–50 mg/d divided bid.
- *Adrenal insufficiency, chronic (physiologic replacement):* May need mineralocorticoid supplementation such as DOCA. Hydrocortisone 20 mg PO Q am, 10 mg PO Q pm; cortisone 0.5–0.75 mg/kg/d divided bid; cortisone 0.25–0.35 mg/kg IM q day; dexamethasone: 0.03–0.15 mg/kg/d; OR 0.6–0.75 mg/m^2/d in divided Q 6–12 hr PO, IM, IV.
- *Asthma, acute:* Prednisolone 1–2 mg/kg/d; OR prednisone 1–2 mg/kg/d divided q day for up to 5 days; prednisolone 2–4 mg/kg/d IV divided tid.
- *Extubation/airway edema:* Dexamethasone 0.5–1 mg/kg/d IM/IV divided 6 H, start beginning 24 hours prior to extubation; continue 4 additional doses.
- *Immunosuppressive/anti-inflammatory:* Hydrocortisone: 15–240 mg PO, IM, IV Q 12 hr; methylprednisolone: 4–48 mg/d PO, taper to lowest effective dose; methylprednisolone sodium succinate 10–80 mg IM q day. Prednisone or prednisolone 5–60 mg/d PO, divided q day–qid.
- *Rheumatic disease: Intra-articular*: hydrocortisone acetate 25–37.5 mg large joint; 10–25 mg small joint; methylprednisolone acetate 20–80 mg large joint, 4–10 mg small joint.

Intra-bursal: Hydrocortisone acetate 25–37.5 mg. Intra-ganglia: hydrocortisone acetate 25–37.5 mg.

Tendon sheath: Hydrocortisone acetate 5–12.5 mg.

Perioperative steroid coverage: Hydrocortisone 100 mg IV night before surgery, 1 hour pre-op, intraoperatively, and 4, 8, and 12 hours postoperatively; POD No. 1 100 mg IV Q 6 hr; POD No. 2 100 mg IV Q 8 hr; POD No. 3 100 mg IV Q 12 hr; POD No. 4 50 mg IV Q 12 hr; POD No. 5 25 mg IV Q 12 hr; then, resume prior oral dosing if chronic use or discontinue if only perioperative coverage required.

- *Cerebral edema:* Dexamethasone 10 mg IV; then 4 mg IV Q 4–6 hr.

NOTES: See Table 7–2, p 597. All steroids can cause hyperglycemia, "steroid psychosis," adrenal suppression. *Never* acutely stop steroids, especially if patient has been receiving chronic treatment; taper dose. Hydrocortisone succinate is administered systemically, acetate form intra-articularly.

Streptokinase (Streptase, Kabikinase)

INDICATIONS: Coronary artery thrombosis, acute massive pulmonary embolism, deep vein thrombosis, and some occluded vascular grafts.
ACTIONS: Activates plasminogen to plasmin that degrades fibrin.
DOSAGE: *Pulmonary embolus:* Loading dose of 250,000 IU IV through a peripheral vein over 30 min; then 100,000 IU/hr IV for 24–72 hr.

Coronary artery thrombosis: 1.5 million U IV over 60 min.

Deep vein thrombosis or arterial embolism: Load as with pulmonary embolus, then 100,000 IU/hr for 72 hr.

SUPPLIED: Powder for injection 250,000 IU, 600,000 IU, 750,000 IU, 1,500,000 IU.
NOTES: If maintenance infusion is not adequate to maintain thrombin clotting time 2–5 × control, refer to the package insert, *PDR,* or the *AHFS Drug Information* for adjustments. Antibodies remain 3–6 months following dose.

Streptomycin

INDICATIONS: Treatment of tuberculosis or serious *Enterococcus* infections.
ACTIONS: Aminoglycoside; interferes with protein synthesis.

DOSAGE: 1–4 g/d IM in 1–2 divided doses (endocarditis); TB 15 mg/kg/d.
SUPPLIED: Injection 400 mg/mL.
NOTES: Increased incidence of vestibular toxicity; adjust dose in renal impairment.

Streptozocin (Zanosar)

INDICATIONS: Pancreatic islet cell tumors and carcinoid tumors.
ACTIONS: DNA-DNA (interstrand) cross-linking; DNA, RNA, and protein synthesis inhibitor.
DOSAGE: Refer to specific protocol.
NOTES: Toxicity includes nausea and vomiting and duodenal ulcers; myelosuppression is rare (20%) and mild; nephrotoxicity (proteinuria and azotemia often heralded by hypophosphatemia) can be dose-limiting. Hypo- or hyperglycemia may occur; phlebitis and pain at the site of injection may also occur. Use with caution/adjust dose in renal impairment.

Succimer (Chemet)

INDICATIONS: Treatment of lead poisoning.
ACTIONS: Heavy metal chelating agent.
DOSAGE: Based on weight, persons > 45 kg: 500 mg PO. Give the above dose Q 8 hr for 5 days, Q 12 hr for 14 days.
SUPPLIED: Capsules 100 mg.
NOTES: May cause a rash; patients should drink a lot of fluids.

Succinylcholine (Anectine, Quelicin, Sucostrin)

INDICATIONS: Adjunct to general anesthesia to facilitate endotracheal intubation and to induce skeletal muscle relaxation during surgery or mechanically supported ventilation.
ACTIONS: Depolarizing neuromuscular blocking agent.
DOSAGE: 0.6 mg/kg IV over 10–30 sec, followed by 0.04–0.07 mg/kg as needed to maintain muscle relaxation.
SUPPLIED: Injection 20 mg/mL, 50 mg/mL, 100 mg/mL; powder for injection 100 mg, 500 mg, 1 g per vial.
NOTES AND CAUTION: Drug may precipitate malignant hyperthermia; respiratory depression or prolonged apnea may occur. Succinylcholine has many drug interactions potentiating its activity; monitor patient for cardiovascular effects. Use only freshly prepared solutions; decrease dosage in severe liver disease.

Sucralfate (Carafate)

INDICATIONS: Treatment of duodenal and gastric ulcers.
ACTIONS: Forms ulcer-adherent complex that protects it against acid, pepsin, and bile acid.
DOSAGE: 1 g PO qid, 1 hr prior to meals and HS.
SUPPLIED: Tablets 1 g; suspension 1 g/10 mL.
NOTES: Treatment should be continued for 4–8 weeks unless healing is demonstrated by x-ray or endoscopy. Constipation is the most frequent side effect.

Sulfacetamide (Bleph-10, Cetamide, Sodium Sulamyd) [See Table 7–12, pp 607-9]

Sulfacetamide and Prednisolone (Blephamide, Others) (Also See Table 7–12, pp 607-9]

INDICATIONS: Steroid-responsive inflammatory ocular conditions with infection or a risk of infection.
ACTIONS: Antibiotic and anti-inflammatory.
DOSAGE: Have patient apply ointment to lower conjunctival sac q day–qid; solution 1–3 gtts 2–3 hours while awake.
SUPPLIED: *Ointment:* sulfacetamide 10%/prednisolone 0.5%; Sulfacetamide 10%/prednisolone 0.2%; Sulfacetamide 10%/prednisolone 0.25%; *Suspension:* Sulfacetamide 10%/prednisolone 0.25%; Sulfacetamide 10%/prednisolone 0.5%; Sulfacetamide sodium 10%/prednisolone 0.2%; Sulfacetamide 10% and prednisolone 0.25%.
NOTES: Ophthalmic suspension can be used as an otic agent.

Sulfasalazine (Azulfidine)

INDICATIONS: Ulcerative colitis.
ACTIONS: Sulfonamide; actions not clear.
DOSAGE: Initial dose 1 g tid–qid; increase to a maximum of 8 g/d in 3–4 divided doses; maintenance 500 mg PO qid.
SUPPLIED: Tablets 500 mg; enteric-coated tablets 500 mg; oral suspension 250 mg/5 mL.
NOTES: Can cause severe GI upset; discolors urine.

Sulfinpyrazone (Anturane)

INDICATIONS: Acute and chronic gout.
ACTIONS: Inhibits renal tubular absorption of uric acid.
DOSAGE: 100–200 mg PO bid for 1 week, then increase as needed to maintenance of 200–400 mg bid.
SUPPLIED: Tablets 100 mg; capsules 200 mg.
NOTES: Avoid in patients with renal impairment. Instruct patient to take with food or antacids, take with plenty of fluids; avoid salicylates.

Sulindac (Clinoril) [See Table 7–11, pp 605-6]

Sumatriptan (Imitrex)

INDICATIONS: Acute treatment of migraine attacks.
ACTIONS: Vascular serotonin receptor agonist.
DOSAGE: *Injection:* 6 mg SC as a single dose; may repeat in 1 hr, to a maximum of 12 mg/24 hr.
Oral: 25 mg, repeat in 2 hr, 100 mg/dose max oral dose. Daily maximum 300 mg.
Nasal spray: 1 single spray into 1 nostril, may repeat in 2 hours, maximum 40 mg/24 hr.
SUPPLIED: Injection 12 mg/mL; tablets 25 mg, 50 mg; nasal spray 5 mg, 20 mg.
NOTES: May cause pain and bruising at the injection site; avoid in patients with angina, ischemic heart disease, uncontrolled hypertension, recent ergot administration.

Tacrine (Cognex)

INDICATIONS: Treatment of mild to moderate dementia.
ACTIONS: Cholinesterase inhibitor.
DOSAGE: 10–40 mg PO qid, up to 160 mg/d.
SUPPLIED: Capsules 10 mg, 20 mg, 30 mg, 40 mg.
NOTES: Drug may cause elevations in transaminases; liver function tests should be monitored regularly. Separate doses from food.

Tacrolimus (FK 506) (Prograf)

INDICATIONS: Prophylaxis of organ rejection.
ACTIONS: Macrolide immunosuppressant.
DOSAGE: *IV:* 0.05–0.1 mg/kg/d as continuous infusion.
PO: 0.15–0.3 mg/kg/d divided into 2 doses.
SUPPLIED: Capsules 1 mg, 5 mg; injection 5 mg/mL.
NOTES: Drug may cause neurotoxicity and nephrotoxicity; use lower doses in patients with renal impairment. May need to reduce dose in hepatic impairment. Monitor serum drug levels; see Table 7–16, p 613.

Tamoxifen (Nolvadex)

INDICATIONS: Breast cancer (postmenopausal, estrogen receptor positive), endometrial cancer, melanoma, reduction of breast cancer in high-risk women.
ACTIONS: Nonsteroidal antiestrogen; mixed agonist/antagonist effect.
DOSAGE: 20–40 mg/d (typically 10 mg bid or 20 mg q day).
SUPPLIED: Tablets 10 mg, 20 mg.
NOTES: Toxicity includes menopausal symptoms (hot flashes, nausea, and vomiting) in premenopausal patients. Vaginal bleeding and menstrual irregularities may occur. Skin rash, pruritus vulvae, dizziness, headache, and peripheral edema may occur. Acute flare of bone

metastasis pain and hypercalcemia may occur. With high doses, retinopathy reported. Increases the risk of pregnancy in sexually active premenopausal women by inducing ovulation.

Tamsulosin (Flomax)

INDICATIONS: Benign prostatic hyperplasia.
ACTIONS: Antagonist of alpha receptors in the prostate.
DOSAGE: 0.4 mg q day.
SUPPLIED: Capsules 0.4 mg.
NOTES: Instruct patient not to crush, chew, or open capsule.

Tazarotene (Tazorac)

INDICATIONS: Facial acne vulgaris; stable plaque psoriasis up to 20% body surface area.
ACTIONS: Keratolytic.
DOSAGE: *Acne:* Cleanse face, and dry, apply thin film q day at night on acne lesions. *Psoriasis:* Apply q day at night.
SUPPLIED: Gel 0.05, 0.1%.

Telmisartan (Micardis) [See Table 7–4, p 599]

Temazepam (Restoril) [C]

INDICATIONS: Treatment of insomnia.
ACTIONS: Benzodiazepine.
DOSAGE: 15–30 mg PO Q HS prn.
SUPPLIED: Capsules 7.5 mg, 15 mg, 30 mg.
NOTES: Reduce dose in the elderly.

Tenecteplase (TNKase)

INDICATIONS: Reduction of mortality associated with acute myocardial infarction.
ACTIONS: Thrombolytic; tissue plasminogen activator.
DOSAGE: 30–50 mg; see table below.

Weight (kg)	TNKase (mg)	Volume TNKase*(mL)
< 60	30	6
≥ 60 to < 70	35	7
≥ 70 to < 80	40	8
≥ 80 to < 90	45	9
≥ 90	50	10

*From one vial of reconstituted TNKase.

SUPPLIED: Injection 50 mg, reconstituted with 10 mL sterile water.
NOTES: Contraindicated in patients with a history of stroke, intracranial/intraspinal surgery, or internal bleeding or trauma within the past 2 months.

Teniposide (VM-26, Vumon)

INDICATIONS: Small cell lung cancer, Kaposi's sarcoma, non-Hodgkin's lymphoma.
ACTIONS: Topoisomerase II inhibitor, interfering with strand passage and DNA ligase activities of topoisomerase II. Cell cycle-specific activity at S, early G_2 phase.
DOSAGE: Refer to specific protocol.
NOTES: Toxicity includes myelosuppression (especially leukopenia and thrombocytopenia), hypotension, chemical phlebitis, skin rashes, hypertension, hypersensitivity reactions (urticaria, flushing, rashes, or hypotension), and secondary leukemia. Adjust dose in significant renal impairment; consider adjustment in hepatic impairment.

Terazosin (Hytrin)

INDICATIONS: Treatment of benign prostatic hyperplasia and hypertension.
ACTIONS: Alpha-1 blocker (blood vessel and bladder neck/prostate).
DOSAGE: Initial dose 1 mg PO HS; titrate to a maximum of 20 mg PO Q HS.
SUPPLIED: Tablets 1 mg, 2 mg, 5 mg, 10 mg; capsules 1 mg, 2 mg, 5 mg, 10 mg.
NOTES: Hypotension and syncope following first dose; dizziness, weakness, nasal congestion, peripheral edema are common. Drug should be used with thiazide diuretic for hypertension.

Terbinafine (Lamisil)

INDICATIONS: Onychomycosis, athlete's foot.
ACTIONS: Inhibits squalene epoxidase resulting in fungal death.
DOSAGE: *Oral:* 250 mg PO once daily for 6–12 weeks.
Topical: apply to affected area.
SUPPLIED: Tablet 250 mg; cream: 1%.
NOTES: Full clinical effect may take months due to need for new nail growth; no occlusive dressings; dosage adjustment in renal impairment.

Terbutaline (Brethine, Bricanyl)

INDICATIONS: Reversible bronchospasm (asthma, chronic obstructive pulmonary disease).
ACTIONS: Sympathomimetic.
DOSAGE: *Bronchodilator, oral dose:* 2.5–5 mg PO qid; OR 0.25 mg SC; may repeat in 15 min (maximum 0.5 mg in 4 hr).
Metered-dose inhaler: 2 inhalations Q 4–6 hr.
SUPPLIED: Tablets 2.5 mg, 5 mg; injection 1 mg/mL; metered-dose inhaler.
NOTES: Use cautiously with diabetes, hypertension, hyperthyroidism; high doses may precipitate beta-$_1$-adrenergic effects.

Terconazole (Terazol 7)

INDICATIONS: Vaginal fungal infections.
ACTIONS: Topical antifungal.
DOSAGE: 1 applicatorful or 1 suppository intravaginally Q HS for 7 days.
SUPPLIED: Vaginal cream 0.4%, vaginal suppository 80 mg.

Tetanus Immune Globulin

INDICATIONS: Passive immunization against tetanus for any person with a suspected contaminated wound and unknown immunization status.
ACTIONS: Passive immunization.
DOSAGE: 250–500 U IM (higher doses if delay in initiation of therapy).
SUPPLIED: Injection 250-U vial or syringe.
NOTES: May begin active immunization series at different injection site if required.

Tetanus Toxoid

INDICATIONS: Protection against tetanus.
ACTIONS: Active immunization.
DOSAGE: *Fluid:* 3 doses of 0.5 mL IM or SC at 4- to 8-week intervals, with a 4th dose at 6–12 months and a booster every 10 years.
Adsorbed: 0.5 mL IM at 4–8 weeks and 6–12 months and then a booster every 5–10 years.
SUPPLIED: Injection: Tetanus toxoid, fluid, 4–5 Lf units/0.5 mL; tetanus toxoid, adsorbed, 5 Lf units/0.5 mL, 10 Lf units/0.5 mL.

Tetracycline (Achromycin V, Sumycin)

INDICATIONS: Broad-spectrum antibiotic treatment against *Staphylococcus, Streptococcus, Chlamydia, Rickettsia,* and *Mycoplasma.*
ACTIONS: Bacteriostatic; inhibits protein synthesis.
DOSAGE: 250–500 mg PO bid–qid.
SUPPLIED: Capsules 100 mg, 250 mg, 500 mg; tablets 250 mg, 500 mg; oral suspension 250 mg/5 mL.
NOTES: *Do not* use in pregnancy. *Do not* use in patients with impaired renal function. *Do not* use with antacids or milk products (See Doxycycline, p 508).

Thalidomide (Thalomid)

INDICATIONS: Graft-versus-host disease, aphthous ulceration in HIV-positive patients, erythema nodosum leprosum.
ACTIONS: Inhibits neutrophil chemotaxis, decreases monocyte phagocytosis.
DOSAGE: *GVHD:* 100–1600 mg PO q day.
Stomatitis: 200 mg bid for 5 days, then 200 mg q day for up to 8 weeks.

SUPPLIED: Limited distribution through Boston University.
NOTES: Pregnancy category X.

Theophylline (Theolair, Theo-Dur, Somophyllin, Others)

INDICATIONS: Asthma, bronchospasm.
ACTIONS: Relaxes smooth muscle of the bronchi and pulmonary blood vessels, stimulates CNS respiratory drive, increases diaphragmatic contraction.
DOSAGE: 900 mg PO divided Q 6 hr; sustained-release products may be divided Q 8–12 hr × (Maintenance).
SUPPLIED: Elixir 80 mg/15 mL, 150 mg/15 mL; liquid 80 mg/15 mL, 160 mg/15 mL; capsules 100 mg, 200 mg, 250 mg; tablets 100 mg, 125 mg, 200 mg, 225 mg, 250 mg, 300 mg; sustained-release capsules 50 mg, 75 mg, 100 mg, 125 mg, 200 mg, 250 mg, 260 mg, 300 mg; sustained-release tablets 100 mg, 200 mg, 250 mg, 300 mg, 400 mg, 450 mg, 500 mg.
NOTES: See drug levels in Table 7–16, p 613. Theophylline has many drug interactions; side effects include nausea, vomiting, tachycardia, and seizures.

Thiamine (Vitamin B_1)

INDICATIONS: Thiamine deficiency (beriberi); alcoholic neuritis; Wernicke's encephalopathy.
ACTIONS: Dietary supplementation.
DOSAGE: *Deficiency:* 100 mg IM q day for 2 weeks; then 5–10 mg PO q day for 1 month.
Wernicke's encephalopathy: 100 mg IV in a single dose, then 100 mg IV or IM q day for 2 weeks.
SUPPLIED: Tablets 5 mg, 10 mg, 25 mg, 50 mg, 100 mg, 500 mg; injection 100, 200 mg/mL.
NOTES: IV thiamine administration associated with anaphylactic reaction; **must be given slowly IV.**

Thiethylperazine (Torecan)

INDICATIONS: Nausea and vomiting.
ACTIONS: Antidopaminergic antiemetic.
DOSAGE: 10 mg PO, PR, or IM q day–tid.
SUPPLIED: Tablets 10 mg; suppositories: 10 mg; injection 5 mg/mL.
NOTES: Extrapyramidal reactions may occur.

6-Thioguanine (6-TG) (Tabloid)

INDICATIONS: Acute myelogenous leukemia, acute lymphocytic leukemia, chronic myelogenous leukemia.
ACTIONS: Purine-based antimetabolite (substitutes for natural purines interfering with nucleotide synthesis).
DOSAGE: Refer to specific protocol.
NOTES: Toxicity includes myelosuppression (especially leukopenia and thrombocytopenia), nausea and vomiting, anorexia, stomatitis, and diarrhea. Hepatotoxicity occurs rarely; dosage adjustment in renal or hepatic impairment.

Thioridazine (Mellaril)

INDICATIONS: Psychotic disorders; short-term treatment of depression, agitation, organic brain syndrome.
ACTIONS: Phenothiazine antipsychotic.
DOSAGE: Initial dose 50–100 mg PO tid; maintenance 200–800 mg/24 hr PO in 2–4 divided doses.
SUPPLIED: Tablets 10 mg, 15 mg, 25 mg, 50 mg, 100 mg, 150 mg, 200 mg; oral concentrate 30 mg/mL, 100 mg/mL; oral suspension 25 mg/5 mL, 100 mg/5 mL.
NOTES: Low incidence of extrapyramidal effects; may cause ventricular arrhythmias.

Thio-Tepa (Thioplex)

INDICATIONS: Hodgkin's and non-Hodgkin's lymphomas, leukemia, breast cancer, ovarian cancer, bladder cancer (intravenous and intravesical therapy), preparative regimens for allogeneic and autologous bone marrow transplantation (ABMT) in high doses.
ACTIONS: Polyfunctional alkylating agent.
DOSAGE: Refer to specific protocol.

NOTES: Toxicity includes myelosuppression, nausea, vomiting, dizziness, headache, allergy, and paresthesias.

Thiothixene (Navane)

INDICATIONS: Psychotic disorders.
ACTIONS: Antipsychotic.
DOSAGE: *Mild to moderate psychosis:* 2 mg PO tid, up to 20-30 mg/d.
Severe psychosis: 5 mg PO bid; increase to a maximum of 60 mg/24 hr prn.
IM use: 16–20 mg/24 hr divided bid–qid; maximum 30 mg/d.
SUPPLIED: Capsules 1 mg, 2 mg, 5 mg, 10 mg, 20 mg; oral concentrate 5 mg/mL; injection 2 mg/mL, 5 mg/mL.
NOTES: Drowsiness and extrapyramidal side effects most common.

Tiagabine (Gabitril)

INDICATIONS: Adjunctive therapy in treatment of partial seizures.
ACTIONS: Inhibition of GABA.
DOSAGE: Initial 4 mg once daily, increase by 4 mg during 2nd week; may keep increasing by 4–8 mg/d until clinical response is achieved; maximum dose 56 mg/d.
SUPPLIED: Tablets 4 mg, 12 mg, 16 mg, 20 mg.
NOTES: Use gradual withdrawal; used in combination with other anticonvulsants.

Ticarcillin (Ticar) [See Table 7–6, p 600]

Ticarcillin/Potassium Clavulanate (Timentin) [See Table 7–6, p 600]

Ticlopidine (Ticlid)

INDICATIONS: Reduces the risk of thrombotic stroke.
ACTIONS: Platelet aggregation inhibitor.
DOSAGE: 250 mg PO bid.
SUPPLIED: Tablets 250 mg.
NOTES: Instruct patient to take with food. Drug may cause neutropenia. Monitor CBC Q 2 weeks for the first 3 months of therapy; monitor LFTs.

Timolol (Blocadren) [See Table 7–7, pp 601-2]

Timolol, Ophthalmic (Timoptic) [See Table 7–12, pp 607-9]

Tinzaparin (Innohep)

INDICATIONS: Prophylaxis and treatment of deep venous thrombosis.
ACTIONS: Low molecular weight heparin.
DOSAGE: *Prophylaxis:* 3500 IU SC q day and 2 hours preoperatively.
Treatment: 175 IU/kg SC × 6 days or until patient has reached target INR on warfarin.
SUPPLIED: 20,000 IU/2 mL vial.
NOTES: Reports of priapism, GI/GU bleeding, transient LFT elevations. Drug contains benzyl alcohol. Use with caution in renal impairment.

Tioconazole (Vagistat)

INDICATIONS: Vaginal fungal infections.
ACTIONS: Topical antifungal.
DOSAGE: 1 applicatorful intravaginally at bedtime (single dose).
SUPPLIED: Vaginal ointment 6.5%.

Tirofiban (Aggrastat)

INDICATIONS: Management of acute coronary syndrome.
ACTIONS: Glycoprotein IIb/IIIa inhibitor.
DOSAGE: Initial 0.4 μg/kg/min for 30 min, followed by 0.1 μg/kg/min.
SUPPLIED: Injection 50 μg/mL, 250 μg/mL.
NOTES: Adjust dose in patients with renal insufficiency; use in combination with heparin.

Tobramycin (Nebcin)

INDICATIONS: Serious gram-negative infections, especially *Pseudomonas*.
ACTIONS: Aminoglycoside; inhibits protein synthesis.
DOSAGE: 1–2.5 mg/kg/dose IV Q 8–24 hr (see Tables 7–18 and 7–20, pp 614, 616-17).
SUPPLIED: Injection 10 mg/mL, 40 mg/mL.
NOTES: Drug is nephrotoxic and ototoxic. Decrease dose with renal insufficiency; monitor creatinine clearance and serum concentrations for dosage adjustments (see Table 7–17, p 613, Table 7–18, p 614, Table 7–19, p 615, and Table 7–20, pp 616-17).

Tobramycin Ophthalmic (AK TOB, Tobrex) [See Table 7–12, pp 607-9]

Tobramycin and Dexamethasone Ophthalmic (Tobradex) [See Table 7–12, pp 607-9]

Tolazamide (Tolinase) [See Table 7–13, p 610]

Tolazoline (Priscoline)

INDICATIONS: Treatment of peripheral vasospastic disorders.
ACTIONS: Competitively blocks alpha-adrenergic receptors.
DOSAGE: 10–50 mg IM/IV/SC qid.
SUPPLIED: Injection 25 mg/mL.

Tolbutamide (Orinase) [See Table 7–13, p 610]

Tolcapone (Tasmar)

INDICATIONS: Adjunct to carbidopa/levodopa in Parkinson's disease.
ACTIONS: Catechol-*o*-methyltransferase inhibitor slows metabolism of levodopa.
DOSAGE: 100 mg PO with first daily dose of levodopa/carbidopa, followed by doses 6 and 12 hours later.
SUPPLIED: Tablets 100 mg, 200 mg.
NOTES AND CAUTIONS: Reduce dose in patients with severe renal failure. *Do not* use in active liver disease; do not administer with nonselective MAO inhibitors.

Tolmetin (Tolectin) [See Table 7–11, pp 605-6]

Tolnaftate (Tinactin)

INDICATIONS: Tinea pedis, tinea cruris, tinea corporis, tinea manuum, tinea versicolor.
ACTIONS: Topical antifungal.
DOSAGE: Apply to area bid for 2–4 weeks.
SUPPLIED: All OTC: 1% liquid, 1% gel, 1% powder, 1% cream, 1% solution.

Tolterodine (Detrol)

INDICATIONS: Overactive bladder with symptoms of urinary frequency, urgency, or urge incontinence.
ACTIONS: Competitive muscarinic antagonist.
DOSAGE: 2 mg PO bid; may only require 1 mg bid; decrease to 1 mg bid with concomitant use of CYP3A4 inhibitors.
SUPPLIED: Tablets 1 mg, 2 mg.
NOTES: Use with caution in patients with renal impairment; patients may experience blurred vision.

Topiramate (Topamax)

INDICATIONS: Treatment of partial-onset seizures.
ACTIONS: Anticonvulsant.
DOSAGE: Total dose 400 mg per day. See product information for 8-week titration schedule.
SUPPLIED: Tablets 25 mg, 100 mg, 200 mg; capsule sprinkles 15 mg, 25 mg, 50 mg.
NOTES: May precipitate kidney stones; adjust dosage in patients with renal impairment. Acute myopia associated with secondary angle closure glaucoma has been reported. Discontinue topiramate to reverse symptoms.

Topotecan (Hycamtin)

INDICATIONS: Ovarian cancer (cisplatin-refractory), small cell lung cancer, and non-Hodgkin's lymphoma.
ACTIONS: Topoisomerase I inhibitor; interferes with DNA synthesis.
DOSAGE: Refer to specific protocol.
NOTES: Toxicities include myelosuppression, nausea and vomiting, diarrhea, drug fever, and skin rash. Dose reduction required for renal dysfunction.

Torsemide (Demadex)

INDICATIONS: Edema, hypertension, congestive heart failure, and hepatic cirrhosis.
ACTIONS: Loop diuretic; inhibits reabsorption of sodium and chloride in the ascending loop of Henle and distal tubule.
DOSAGE: 5–20 mg PO or IV once daily.
SUPPLIED: Tablets 5 mg, 10 mg, 20 mg, 100 mg; injection 10 mg/mL.

Tramadol (Ultram)

INDICATIONS: Management of moderate to severe pain.
ACTIONS: Centrally acting analgesic.
DOSAGE: 50–100 mg PO Q 4–6 hr prn, not to exceed 400 mg/d.
SUPPLIED: Tablets 50 mg.
NOTES: Lowers seizure threshold; tolerance or dependence may develop.

Trandolapril (Mavik) [See Table 7–3, p 598]

Trastuzumab (Herceptin)

INDICATIONS: Treatment of metastatic breast cancer tumors that overexpress the HER2/neu protein.
ACTIONS: Monoclonal antibody binds to the human epidermal growth factor receptor 2 protein (HER 2); mediates cellular cytotoxicity.
DOSAGE: Refer to specific protocol.
NOTES: Infusion-related reactions should be minimized with acetaminophen, diphenhydramine, and meperidine. Congestive heart failure has been reported.

Trazodone (Desyrel)

INDICATIONS: Treatment of depression.
ACTIONS: Antidepressant; inhibits reuptake of serotonin and norepinephrine.
DOSAGE: Adults and adolescents: 50–150 mg PO q day–qid; maximum 600 mg/d.
SUPPLIED: Tablets 50 mg, 100 mg, 150 mg, 300 mg.
NOTES: May take 1–2 weeks for symptomatic improvement. Drug has anticholinergic side effects.

Tretinoin, Topical [Retinoic Acid] (Retin-A, Avita)

INDICATIONS: Acne vulgaris, sun damaged skin, some skin cancers.
ACTIONS: Exfoliant retinoic acid derivative.
DOSAGE: Apply q day at bed time; if irritation develops, decrease frequency.
SUPPLIED: Cream 0.025%; 0.05%; 0.1%; Gel 0.01%, 0.025%, 0.1%; liquid 0.05%.
NOTES: Avoid sunlight.

Triamcinolone (Aristocort, Aristospan, Kenalog) [See Table 7–2, p 597]

Triamcinolone (Azmacort)

INDICATIONS: Chronic treatment of asthma.
ACTIONS: Topical steroid.
DOSAGE: Two inhalations tid–qid or 4 inhalations bid.
SUPPLIED: Inhaler: 100 µg/metered spray.
NOTES: May cause oral candidiasis; instruct patients to rinse their mouth after use; not for acute asthma.

Triamcinolone and Nystatin (Mycolog-II)

INDICATIONS: Cutaneous candidiasis.
ACTIONS: Antifungal and anti-inflammatory.
DOSAGE: Apply lightly to area twice a day; maximum 25 days.
SUPPLIED: Cream and ointment 15 mg, 30 mg, 60 mg, 120 mg.

Triamterene (Dyrenium)

INDICATIONS: Edema associated with congestive heart failure, cirrhosis.
ACTIONS: Potassium-sparing diuretic.
DOSAGE: 100–300 mg/24 hr PO divided q day–bid.
SUPPLIED: Capsules 50 mg, 100 mg.
NOTES: Can cause hyperkalemia, blood dyscrasias, liver damage, and other reactions. Adjust dosage in patients with renal or hepatic impairment.

Triazolam (Halcion) [C]

INDICATIONS: Short-term management of insomnia.
ACTIONS: Benzodiazepine.
DOSAGE: 0.125–0.25 mg PO Q HS prn.
SUPPLIED: Tablets 0.125 mg, 0.25 mg.
NOTES: Additive CNS depression with alcohol and other CNS depressants; reduce dose/avoid in cirrhosis.

Triethanolamine (Cerumenex)

INDICATIONS: Cerumen removal.
ACTIONS: Cerumenolytic agent.
DOSAGE: Fill the ear canal and insert the cotton plug; irrigate with water after 15 min; repeat as needed.
SUPPLIED: Solution 6 mL, 12 mL.

Trifluoperazine (Stelazine)

INDICATIONS: Management of psychotic disorders.
ACTIONS: Phenothiazine; blocks postsynaptic mesolimbic dopaminergic receptors in the brain.
DOSAGE: 2–10 mg PO bid.
SUPPLIED: Tablets 1 mg, 2 mg, 5 mg, 10 mg; oral concentrate 10 mg/mL; injection 2 mg/mL.
NOTES: Decrease dosage in elderly and debilitated patients; oral concentrate must be diluted to 60 mL or more prior to administration. Drug requires several weeks for onset of effects.

Trifluridine (Viroptic)

INDICATIONS: Herpes simplex keratitis and conjunctivitis.
ACTIONS: Antiviral.
DOSAGE: 1 drop Q 2 hr (max 9 drops per day); decrease to 1 drop Q 4 hr after healing begins; treat up to 14 days.
SUPPLIED: 1% solution.

Trihexyphenidyl (Artane)

INDICATIONS: Management of Parkinson's disease.
ACTIONS: Blocks excess acetylcholine at cerebral synapses.
DOSAGE: 2–5 mg PO q day–qid.
SUPPLIED: Tablets 2 mg, 5 mg; sustained-release capsules 5 mg; elixir 2 mg/5 mL.
NOTES: Contraindicated in narrow-angle glaucoma.

Trimethobenzamide (Tigan)

INDICATIONS: Treatment of nausea and vomiting.
ACTIONS: Inhibits medullary chemoreceptor trigger zone.
DOSAGE: 250 mg PO or 200 mg PR or IM tid–qid prn.
SUPPLIED: Capsules 100 mg, 250 mg; suppositories 100 mg, 200 mg; injection 100 mg/mL.
NOTES: In the presence of viral infections, may mask emesis or mimic CNS effects of Reye's syndrome; may cause parkinsonian-like syndrome.

Trimethoprim (Trimpex, Proloprim)

INDICATIONS: Urinary tract infections due to susceptible gram-positive and gram-negative organisms; often used for suppression of urinary tract infections.
ACTIONS: Inhibits dihydrofolate reductase.
DOSAGE: 100 mg PO bid; OR 200 mg PO q day.
SUPPLIED: Tablets 100 mg, 200 mg; oral solution: 50 mg/5 mL.
NOTES: Reduce dose in renal failure.

Trimethoprim-Sulfamethoxazole (CO-Trimoxazole, Bactrim, Septra)

INDICATIONS: Urinary tract infections, otitis media, sinusitis, bronchitis, and *Shigella, P carinii,* and *Nocardia* infections.
ACTIONS: Dual effect of sulfamethoxazole (SMX)-inhibiting synthesis of dihydrofolic acid and trimethoprim (TMP)-inhibiting dihydrofolate reductase to cause impaired protein synthesis.
DOSAGE: *Usual:* 1 double-strength (DS) tablet PO bid or 5–20 mg/kg/24 hr (based on TMP component) IV in 3–4 divided doses.
P carinii: 15–20 mg/kg/d IV or PO (TMP component) in 4 divided doses.
Nocardia: 10–15 mg/kg/d IV or PO (TMP component) in 4 divided doses.
SUPPLIED: Regular tablets 80 mg of TMP and 400 mg of SMX; double-strength tablets 160 mg of TMP and 800 mg of SMX; oral suspension: 40 mg of TMP and 200 mg of SMX per 5 mL; injection 80 mg of TMP and 400 mg of SMX per 5 mL.
NOTES: Synergistic combination; reduce dosage in renal failure; maintain adequate hydration.

Trimetrexate (Neutrexin)

INDICATIONS: Treatment of moderate to severe *P carinii* pneumonia.
ACTIONS: Inhibits dihydrofolate reductase.
DOSAGE: 45 mg/m^2 IV Q 24 hr for 21 days.
SUPPLIED: Injection.
NOTES: Must be administered with leucovorin 20 mg/m^2 IV Q 6 hr for 24 days. Use cytotoxic precautions; infuse over 60 minutes; reduce dose in patients with hepatic impairment.

Trovafloxacin (Trovan)

INDICATIONS: Life-threatening infections including pneumonia, complicated intra-abdominal, gynecologic/pelvic, or skin infections.
ACTIONS: Fluoroquinolone antibiotic inhibits DNA gyrase.
DOSAGE: 200 mg/d; dosage reduction in hepatic impairment.
SUPPLIED: Injection 5 mg/mL in 40 and 60 mL; tablets 100, 200 mg.
NOTES: Use restricted to hospitals; hepatotoxicity led to restricted availability.

Urokinase (Abbokinase)

INDICATIONS: Pulmonary embolism, deep venous thrombosis, restore patency to IV catheters.
ACTIONS: Converts plasminogen to plasmin that causes clot lysis.
DOSAGE: *Systemic effect:* 4400 IU/kg IV over 10 min, followed by 4400–6000 IU/kg/hr for 12 hr.
Restore catheter patency: Inject 5000 IU into catheter and gently aspirate.
SUPPLIED: Powder for injection 5000 IU/mL, 250,000 IU vial.
NOTES: Do not use systemically within 10 days of surgery, delivery, or organ biopsy.

Valacyclovir (Valtrex)

INDICATIONS: Treatment of herpes zoster; genital herpes.
ACTIONS: Prodrug of acyclovir, inhibits viral DNA replication.
DOSAGE: *Herpes zoster:* 1 g PO tid × 7 days.
Genital herpes treatment: 500 mg bid × 5 days.
Genital herpes prophylaxis: 500–1000 mg q day.
SUPPLIED: Caplets 500 mg.
NOTES: Dosage adjustment in patients with renal impairment.

Valproic Acid and Divalproex (Depakene, Depakote)

INDICATIONS: Management of epilepsy, mania, and prophylaxis of migraines.
ACTIONS: Anticonvulsant; increases the availability of gamma-aminobutyric acid (GABA).
DOSAGE: *Seizures:* 30–60 mg/kg/24 hr PO divided tid (after initiation of 10–15 mg/d).
Mania: 750 mg in three divided doses, increased to a maximum of 60 mg/kg/d.
Migraines: 250 mg bid, increased to 1000 mg/d.
SUPPLIED: *Valproic acid:* capsules 250 mg; syrup 250 mg/5 mL. *Divalproex:* Tablets enteric-coated 125 mg, 250 mg, 500 mg; capsules 125 mg. *Injection:* 100 mg/mL.
NOTES: Monitor liver function and follow serum levels (see Table 7–16, p 613). Concurrent use of phenobarbital and phenytoin may alter serum levels of these agents. Reduce dose in patients with hepatic impairment.

Valrubicin (Valstar)

INDICATIONS: Intravesical treatment of BCG-refractory bladder carcinoma-in-situ when immediate cystectomy would be associated with unacceptable morbidity or mortality.
ACTIONS: Semisynthetic doxorubicin analogue; cytotoxic.
DOSAGE: Refer to specific protocol.
NOTES AND CAUTIONS: Dilute 800 mg in approximately 75 mL normal saline. Minimal systemic absorption with intact bladder. Do *not* use within 1–2 weeks of biopsy as systemic absorption can cause myelosuppression. Can cause local bladder symptoms; contraindicated with bladder capacity of < 75 mL or active UTI.

Valsartan (Diovan) [See Table 7–4, p 599]

Vancomycin (Vancocin, Vancoled)

INDICATIONS: Serious infections caused by methicillin-resistant staphylococci and ampicillin-resistant enterococcal infections and in enterococcal endocarditis in combination with aminoglycosides in penicillin-allergic patients; oral treatment for *C difficile* pseudomembranous colitis.
ACTIONS: Inhibits cell wall synthesis.
DOSAGE: *Usual:* 1 g IV Q 12 hr.
Clostridium difficile *colitis:* 125–500 mg PO Q 6 hr.
SUPPLIED: Capsules 125 mg, 250 mg; powder for oral solution; powder for injection 500 mg, 1000 mg, 10 g per vial.
NOTES: Drug is ototoxic and nephrotoxic; not absorbed orally. Oral dose provides local effect in gut only; IV dose must be given slowly over 1 hr to prevent "red-neck syndrome." Adjust dose in patients with renal failure (for drug levels, see Table 7–17, p 613).

Varicella Virus Vaccine (Varivax)

INDICATIONS: Prevention of varicella (chickenpox) infection.
ACTIONS: Active immunization.
DOSAGE: 0.5 mL SC, repeated in 4–8 weeks.
SUPPLIED: Powder for injection.
NOTES AND CAUTIONS: Live virus. Do *not* administer to immunocompromised patients. Drug may cause mild varicella infection.

Vasopressin (Antidiuretic Hormone) (Pitressin)

INDICATIONS: Treatment of diabetes insipidus; postoperative abdominal distension; severe GI bleeding.
ACTIONS: Posterior pituitary hormone, potent GI vasoconstrictor.
DOSAGE: *Diabetes insipidus:* 2.5–10 U SC or IM tid–qid; OR 1.5–5.0 U IM every 1–3 days of the tannate.
GI hemorrhage: 0.2–0.4 U/min.
SUPPLIED: Injection 20 U/mL.
NOTES: Should be used with caution with any vascular disease.

Vecuronium (Norcuron)

INDICATIONS: Skeletal muscle relaxation during surgery or mechanical ventilation.

ACTIONS: Nondepolarizing neuromuscular blocker.
DOSAGE: 0.08–0.1 mg/kg IV bolus; maintenance of 0.010–0.015 mg/kg after 25–40 min followed with additional doses every 12–15 min.
SUPPLIED: Powder for injection 10 mg.
NOTES: Drug interactions leading to an increased effect of vecuronium include aminoglycosides, tetracycline, and succinylcholine; less cardiac effects than with pancuronium.

Venlafaxine (Effexor)

INDICATIONS: Treatment of depression.
ACTIONS: Potentiation of neurotransmitter activity in the CNS.
DOSAGE: 75–375 mg/d divided into 2–3 equal doses; *XR:* 37.5–75 mg q day, increase by 75 mg/d Q 4–7 days to a max dose of 225 mg/d.
SUPPLIED: Tablets 25 mg, 37.5 mg, 50 mg, 75 mg, 100 mg; extended release capsules 37.5 mg, 75 mg, 150 mg.
NOTES: Dosage adjustment in patients with renal or hepatic impairment.

Verapamil (Calan, Isoptin)

INDICATIONS: Treatment of angina, essential hypertension, arrhythmias, and migraine headache prophylaxis.
ACTIONS: Calcium channel blocker.
DOSAGE: *Arrhythmias (SVT)*: 5–10 mg IV over 2 min followed by 10 mg in 15–30 min **if tolerated** but **not** responding to the initial dose.

Angina: 80–120 mg PO tid, up to 480 mg/24 hr.

Hypertension: 80–180 mg PO tid; OR sustained-release tablet 120–240 mg PO q day to 240 mg bid.

Migraine headache prophylaxis: 180–240 mg q day to 240 mg bid.

SUPPLIED: Tablets 40 mg, 80 mg, 120 mg; sustained-release tablets 120 mg, 180 mg, 240 mg; sustained-release capsules 120 mg, 180 mg, 240 mg, 360 mg; injection 5 mg/2 mL.
NOTES: Use caution with elderly patients; reduce dose in patients with renal or hepatic failure. Constipation is a common side effect.

Vinblastine (Velban, Velbe)

INDICATIONS: Hodgkin's and non-Hodgkin's lymphomas, mycosis fungoides, testicular cancer, choriocarcinoma, breast cancer, histiocytosis X, non-small cell lung cancer, AIDS-related Kaposi's sarcoma, renal cell carcinoma.
ACTIONS: Inhibits microtubule assembly through binding to tubulin.
DOSAGE: Refer to specific protocol.
NOTES: Toxicity includes myelosuppression (especially leukopenia), nausea and vomiting (rarely), constipation, neurotoxicity (similar to that listed for vincristine but less frequent), alopecia, rash. Myalgia and tumor pain are common. Adjust dosage in patients with hepatic impairment.

Vincristine (Oncovin, Vincasar PFS)

INDICATIONS: Acute lymphocytic leukemia, breast carcinoma, sarcoma (including Ewing's and rhabdomyosarcoma), Wilms' tumor, Hodgkin's and non-Hodgkin's lymphomas, neuroblastoma, small cell lung cancer, multiple myeloma.
ACTIONS: Promotes disassembly of mitotic spindle, causing metaphase arrest.
DOSAGE: Refer to specific protocol.
NOTES: Toxicity includes neurotoxicity commonly dose-limited, jaw pain (trigeminal neuralgia), fever, fatigue and anorexia, constipation and paralytic ileus; bladder atony is reported. No significant myelosuppression is observed with standard doses. Soft tissue necrosis may occur with extravasation; adjust dosage in patients with hepatic impairment.

Vinorelbine (Navelbine)

INDICATIONS: Non-small cell lung cancer (single agent or with cisplatin), breast cancer.
ACTIONS: Inhibits polymerization of microtubules, impairing mitotic spindle formation, semisynthetic vinca alkaloid.

DOSAGE: Refer to specific protocol.
NOTES: Toxicity includes myelosuppression (especially leukopenia), mild GI effects, and infrequent neurotoxicity (6–29%), constipation and paresthesias (rarely). Tissue damage can result from extravasation. Adjust dosage adjustment in patients with hepatic impairment.

Vitamin B_1 (See Thiamine, p 579)

Vitamin B_6 (See Pyridoxine, p 566)

Vitamin B_{12} (See Cyanocobalamin, p 498)

Vitamin K (See Phytonadione, p 561)

Warfarin (Coumadin)

INDICATIONS: Prophylaxis and treatment of pulmonary embolism and venous thrombosis, atrial fibrillation with embolization, other postoperative indications.
ACTIONS: Inhibits vitamin K–dependent production of clotting factors in the order VII–IX–X–II.
DOSAGE: *Usual:* Individualize dose to keep international normalized ratio (INR) 2.0–3.0 for most indications.

For mechanical heart valves: Desired INR is 2.5–3.5.

ACCP guidelines: Recommend initiation with 5 mg, unless rapid attainment of therapeutic INR is necessary, then use 7.5–10 mg. In the elderly or if a bleeding risk is present, reduce dosing. *Maintenance:* 2–10 mg PO, IV, or IM q day; follow daily INR during initial phase to guide dosage change, then Q 1–4 weeks when INR is stable.
SUPPLIED: Tablets 1 mg, 2 mg, 2.5 mg, 3 mg, 4 mg, 5 mg, 6 mg, 7.5 mg, 10 mg; injection.
NOTES: INR is now the preferred test rather than PT. Check INR periodically on maintenance dose; beware of bleeding caused by over-anticoagulation (PT > 3 × control or INR > 5.0–6.0). To rapidly correct over-coumadinization, use vitamin K or fresh-frozen plasma or both. Drug is highly teratogenic; do *not* use in pregnancy. Caution patients on taking warfarin with other medications, especially aspirin. **Common warfarin drug interactions: Potentiated by:** acetaminophen, alcohol (with liver disease), amiodarone, cimetidine, ciprofloxacin, co-trimoxazole, erythromycin, fluconazole, isoniazid, itraconazole, metronidazole, omeprazole, phenytoin, propranolol, quinidine, tetracycline **Inhibited by:** barbiturates, carbamazepine, chlordiazepoxide, cholestyramine, dicloxacillin, nafcillin, rifampin, sucralfate, food high in vitamin K. If patients are on warfarin and require an IM injection, would give injection SC if the injection can be so administered.

Zafirlukast (Accolate)

INDICATIONS: Prophylaxis and chronic treatment of asthma.
ACTIONS: Selective and competitive inhibitor of leukotriene D4 and E4.
DOSAGE: 20 mg bid.
SUPPLIED: Tablet 20 mg.
NOTES: Not for acute exacerbations of asthma. Contraindicated in nursing women. Increases anticoagulant effect of warfarin.

Zalcitabine (Hivid)

INDICATIONS: Management of patients with HIV infection who are intolerant to zidovudine and didanosine.
ACTIONS: Antiretroviral agent.
DOSAGE: 0.75 mg PO tid.
SUPPLIED: Tablets 0.375 mg, 0.75 mg.
NOTES: May be used in combination with zidovudine; may cause peripheral neuropathy; dosage adjustment in patients with renal impairment.

Zaleplon (Sonata)

INDICATIONS: Insomnia.
ACTIONS: A non-benzodiazepine sedative hypnotic; a pyrazolopyrimidine.

DOSAGE: 5–20 mg Q HS prn.
SUPPLIED: Capsules 5 mg, 10 mg.

Zanamivir (Relenza)

INDICATIONS: Treatment of influenza.
ACTIONS: Inhibits viral neuraminidase.
DOSAGE: 2 inhalations (10 mg) twice daily for 5 days.
SUPPLIED: Powder for inhalation 5 mg.
NOTES: Administered via a Diskhaler; initiate within 48 hours of symptom onset. Do not use in pulmonary disease.

Zidovudine (Retrovir)

INDICATIONS: Management of patients with HIV infections.
ACTIONS: Inhibits reverse transcriptase.
DOSAGE: *Usual:* 200 mg PO tid; OR 300 mg PO bid; OR 1–2 mg/kg/dose IV Q 4 hr.
Pregnancy: 100 mg PO 5 × per day until the start of labor, then during labor 2 mg/kg over 1 hr followed by 1 mg/kg/hr until clamping of the umbilical cord.
SUPPLIED: Capsules 100 mg; tablets 300 mg; syrup 50 mg/5 mL; injection 10 mg/mL.
NOTES: Not a cure for HIV infections. Drug has hematologic toxicity; dosage adjustment in patients with renal impairment.

Zidovudine and Lamivudine (Combivir)

INDICATIONS: Management of patients with HIV infections.
ACTIONS: Combination inhibitors of reverse transcriptase.
DOSAGE: 1 tablet bid.
SUPPLIED: Capsules zidovudine 300 mg/lamivudine 150 mg.
NOTES: An alternative to reduce the number of capsules for combination therapy with the two agents.

Zileuton (Zyflo)

INDICATIONS: Prophylaxis and chronic treatment of asthma.
ACTIONS: Inhibitor of 5-lipoxygenase.
DOSAGE: 600 mg qid.
SUPPLIED: Tablet 600 mg.
NOTES: MUST take on a regular basis. Drug does not treat acute exacerbation. May cause hepatotoxicity. Monitor ALT every month for the first 3 months of therapy, then Q 2–3 months for 9 months, then periodically thereafter; CYP1A2 and CYP3A4 inhibitor.

Zolmitriptan (Zomig)

INDICATIONS: Acute treatment of migraine.
ACTION: Selective agonist of serotonin to cause vasoconstriction.
DOSAGE: Initial 2.5 mg, may repeat after 2 hr to a maximum of 10 mg in 24 hr.
NOTES: Use with caution in patients with hepatic impairment. Do not use in pregnant patients.

Zolpidem (Ambien) [C]

INDICATIONS: Short-term treatment of insomnia.
ACTIONS: Hypnotic agent.
DOSAGE: 5–10 mg PO Q HS prn.
SUPPLIED: Tablets 5 mg, 10 mg.

Zonisamide (Zonegran)

INDICATIONS: Partial seizures.
ACTIONS: Anticonvulsant.
DOSAGE: Initial 100 mg once daily; may be increased to 400 mg per day.
SUPPLIED: Capsules 100 mg.
NOTES: Contraindicated in persons with hypersensitivity to sulfonamides.

3. MINERALS: INDICATIONS/EFFECTS, RDA/DOSAGE, SIGNS/SYMPTOMS OF DEFICIENCY AND TOXICITY, AND OTHER

Calcium (See also p 489)

INDICATIONS/EFFECTS: Strengthens bones and teeth, used as adjunct with osteoporosis medications to promote bone rebuilding. May decrease blood pressure, aids premenstrual symptoms (pain, cramping, mood swings).
RDA/DOSAGE: Age 50 & under: 1000 mg daily. Age 51+: 1200 mg. Postmenopausal women not taking estrogen and men > 65 years: 1500 mg daily. Men and postmenopausal women taking estrogen (50–65 years): 1000 mg daily.
S/SX OF DEFICIENCY: Osteoporosis (over time) leading to increased risk of fractures and breaks.
S/SX OF TOXICITY: (> 2500 mg/d): Constipation, anorexia, dry mouth, nausea, polyuria, renal calculi.
OTHER: Avoid calcium sources from dolomite, oyster shell, and bone meal as they may contain heavy metal contamination (lead, arsenic). Caffeine and cigarette smoking may reduce calcium absorption. Hyperthyroidism, diabetes mellitus, use of corticosteroids, and use of loop diuretics all either reduce calcium absorption or increase excretion. Calcium supplementation should be strongly considered in these cases. Vitamin D/calcium combination decreases fracture rate and increases absorption in elderly.

Chromium

INDICATIONS/EFFECTS: Required for normal glucose metabolism (trace element).
RDA/DOSAGE: 50–200 μg.
S/SX OF DEFICIENCY: Rare, may cause development of adult diabetes mellitus and atherosclerosis, peripheral neuropathy.
S/SX OF TOXICITY: Irritation of GI (nausea, vomiting, ulcers), renal damage and eczema/dermatitis from occupational exposure.
OTHER: Balanced diet fulfills RDA.

Copper

INDICATIONS/EFFECTS: Bone formation, hematopoiesis, enzyme component.
RDA/DOSAGE: Balanced diet meets daily requirements.
S/SX OF DEFICIENCY: Anemia in malnourished children.
S/SX OF TOXICITY: Self-limiting nausea, vomiting, diarrhea (usually caused by occupational exposure).

Iron (See also p 531)

INDICATIONS/EFFECTS: Energy transfer and carrying oxygen, prevention of microcytic anemia.
RDA/DOSAGE: Adult females 10–15 mg daily (30 mg if pregnant), males 10 mg daily.
S/SX OF DEFICIENCY: Microcytic, hypochromic anemia; fatigue, breathlessness, pallor, dizziness, headache.
S/SX OF TOXICITY (> 75 MG/D): Nausea, diarrhea, abdominal pain, anorexia.
OTHER: Iron may decrease the absorption of other minerals when given concomitantly. In addition, it has numerous drug interactions and should not be given at the same time as other prescribed medications (eg, antacids, tetracycline). Concern exists in males of the risk of hemochromatosis when supplementing iron; in middle-aged men this can increase the risk of heart disease and hepatic disease. Iron is the most common cause of pediatric poisonings in the home. It is available in numerous salt forms with differing elemental iron content:

Iron Salt	Elemental Iron
Fumarate	33%
Gluconate	12%
Sulfate	20–30%

Magnesium (See also pp 538-9)

INDICATIONS/EFFECTS: Strengthens bones and teeth, reduces neurologic irritability in patients at risk for seizures (ie, eclampsia), may reduce premenstrual symptoms (headache, fluid retention, mood changes), maintains normal sinus rhythm.
RDA/DOSAGE: 200–400 mg (1 g = 82.3 mEq).
S/SX OF DEFICIENCY: Weakness, confusion, tingling, muscle contractions, cramps.
S/SX OF TOXICITY (> 350 MG/D): Diarrhea, nausea, drowsiness, lethargy, sweating, slurred speech.

Selenium

INDICATIONS/EFFECTS: Decreases risk of heart disease (antioxidant), essential for normal function of immune system and thyroid gland.
RDA/DOSAGE: Women: 55 µg; Men: 70 µg.
S/SX OF DEFICIENCY: Rare, due to TPN or GI malabsorptive diseases; can cause cardiomyopathy.
S/SX OF TOXICITY (> 400 MG/D): "Selenosis": GI upset, hair loss, white-blotchy nails, mild nerve damage.
OTHER: Balanced diet meets RDA requirements (dietary source: plant foods).

Zinc

INDICATIONS/EFFECTS: Supplementation strengthens immune system if patient is zinc deficient, may prevent macular degeneration, may improve cognition. Zinc supports normal growth and development during pregnancy, childhood, and adolescence.
RDA/DOSAGE: Females: 12 mg, Males: 10 mg.
S/SX OF DEFICIENCY: Impaired night vision, immune function, taste; also poor appetite, poor growth, delayed wound healing, anemia, hyperpigmentation, hepatosplenomegaly.
S/SX OF TOXICITY (> 100–450 MG/D): Altered iron function, reduced immune function, lowered HDL levels, GI intolerance, anemia, copper deficiency.
OTHER: High calcium intake (> 1400 mg/d) reduces zinc absorption, requiring increased zinc intake of 18 mg/d.

4. NATURAL PRODUCTS: USES, DOSE, CAUTIONS, ADVERSE EFFECTS, AND DRUG INTERACTIONS

Black Cohosh

USES: Manages symptoms of menopause (especially hot flashes) as well as premenstrual syndrome, hypercholesterolemia, and peripheral arterial disease; has anti-inflammatory and sedative effects.
DOSE: 40–200 mg daily.
CAUTIONS: Overdose can cause nausea, vomiting, dizziness, nervous system and visual disturbances, bradycardia, and (possibly) seizures. Contraindicated in pregnancy (associated with miscarriage, premature birth).
ADVERSE EFFECTS: Nausea, dizziness, visual changes, migraine, increased sweating, hypotension.
DRUG INTERACTIONS: May further reduce lipids and/or blood pressure when used with prescription medications.

Chamomile

USES: Antispasmodic, sedative, anti-inflammatory, astringent, antibacterial.
DOSE: 10–15 g daily (taken as 3 g dried flower heads tid–qid between meals; can steep in 250 mL hot water).
CAUTIONS: Avoid use if allergic to chrysanthemums, ragweed, asters (family *Compositae*).
ADVERSE EFFECTS: Contact dermatitis, hypersensitivity reaction (allergy, anaphylaxis) if allergic to ragweed.
DRUG INTERACTIONS: Monitor anticoagulant levels due to additive anticoagulant effects. Additive with other medications that cause sedation (benzodiazepines). Chamomile can cause

delayed gastric absorption of medications if concomitantly administered, due to altered GI motility.

Dong Quai (*Angelica polymorpha, sinensis*)

USES: Uterine stimulant; regulates menstrual flow; is an anti-inflammatory, vasodilator, CNS stimulant, immunosuppressant, analgesic, antipyretic, antiasthmatic.
DOSE: 9–12 g tablet bid.
CAUTIONS: Avoid in pregnancy and lactation.
ADVERSE EFFECTS: Diarrhea, photosensitivity, skin cancer.
DRUG INTERACTIONS: Blood-thinning agents (increases INR in patients on warfarin).

Echinacea (*Echinacea purpurea*)

USES: Immune system stimulant; prevention/treatment of colds, flu; as supportive therapy for colds and chronic infections of the respiratory tract and lower urinary tract.
DOSE: 6–9 mL expressed juice or 2–5 g dried root.
CAUTIONS: Should not be used in progressive systemic or immune diseases, such as tuberculosis, collagen-vascular disorders, and multiple sclerosis. May interfere with immunosuppressive therapy. Echinacea is not recommended for use during pregnancy; should not be used for longer than 8 consecutive weeks due to possible immunosuppression.
ADVERSE EFFECTS: Nausea; may cause dermatitis in sensitive patients.
DRUG INTERACTIONS: Avoid use with anabolic steroids, amiodarone, methotrexate, corticosteroids, cyclosporin.

Ephedra/Ma Huang

USES: Stimulant, aid in weight loss, aid in bronchial dilation.
DOSE: USE NOT RECOMMENDED DUE TO REPORTED DEATHS. (> 100 mg/d can be life-threatening).
CAUTIONS: Adverse cardiac events, seizures, and death; avoid if patient has diabetes, hypertension, glaucoma, or thyroid disorders.
ADVERSE EFFECTS: Nervousness, headache, insomnia, palpitations, vomiting, hyperglycemia.
DRUG INTERACTIONS: Interacts with digoxin, antihypertensives, antidepressants, diabetic medications.

Feverfew (*Tanacetum parthenium*)

USES: Prophylaxis and treatment of migraine; fever; menstrual disorders; arthritis; toothache; insect bites.
DOSE: 125 mg of dried leaf (containing at least 0.2% of parthenolide).
CAUTIONS: Not recommended during pregnancy.
ADVERSE EFFECTS: Occasional mouth ulceration or gastric disturbance, swollen lips, abdominal pain; long-term adverse effects are unknown.
DRUG INTERACTIONS: Aspirin and warfarin (inhibits arachidonic acid, inhibits platelet-collagen binding in clotting cascade).

Garlic (*Allium sativum*)

USES: Antioxidant; used for hyperlipidemia and hypertension; used as anti-infective (antibacterial, antifungal).
DOSE: 400–1200 mg dried garlic powder (2–5 mg of allicin).
CAUTIONS: Do *not* use in pregnancy due to abortifacient properties.
ADVERSE EFFECTS: Increased serum insulin levels, decreased serum lipid and cholesterol levels, anemia, burning sensation in mouth, nausea/vomiting, diarrhea.
DRUG INTERACTIONS: Warfarin and aspirin (inhibits platelet aggregation). Additive effect with antidiabetic agents may lead to hypoglycemia.

Ginger (*Zingiber officinale*)

USES: Prevention of motion sickness, nausea and vomiting, post-op/anesthesia, and early pregnancy; dyspepsia.
DOSE: 1–4 g rhizome or 0.5–2 g of powdered drug daily.

CAUTIONS: Ginger is to be used only after consultation with a physician in a patient with gallstones; excessive amounts may cause CNS depression and may interfere with cardiac function or anticoagulant activity.
ADVERSE EFFECTS: Heartburn.
DRUG INTERACTIONS: Excessive consumption of ginger (dosage not stated) may interfere with cardiac, antidiabetic, or anticoagulant therapy (inhibits platelet aggregation).

Ginkgo Biloba

USES: Memory deficits, dementia, anxiety, improvement of distance and pain-free walking in peripheral occlusive vessel disease, vertigo, tinnitus, asthma/bronchospasm, antioxidant uses, premenstrual dysphoric disorder (especially breast tenderness), impotence, SSRI-induced sexual dysfunction.
DOSE: 60–80 mg standardized dry extract bid–tid.
CAUTIONS: Risk of bleeding due to antagonism of platelet activating factor (PAF) is a concern, especially if patient is on concomitant antiplatelet agents.
ADVERSE EFFECTS: GI upset, headaches, dizziness, heart palpitations.
DRUG INTERACTIONS: Aspirin, other salicylates, warfarin.

Ginseng

USES: "Energy booster," stress reduction, enhancement of brain activity and physical endurance (adaptogenic), antioxidant, aid in glucose control.
DOSE: 1–2 g of root or 100–300 mg of extract (standardized to contain 7% ginsenosides) tid.
CAUTIONS: Use with caution in patients with cardiac disorders, diabetes, hypotension, hypertension, mania, and schizophrenia, and in patients receiving corticosteroids. Avoid during pregnancy.
ADVERSE EFFECTS: Controversial "ginseng abuse syndrome" (nervousness, excitation, headache, insomnia) reported in high doses; palpitations, vaginal bleeding, breast nodules, hypoglycemia.
DRUG INTERACTIONS: Warfarin, antidepressants (augmented stimulant effect), caffeine (augmented stimulant effect), antidiabetic agents (additive hypoglycemic effect).

Glucosamine Sulfate (a.k.a. chitosamine) and Chondroitin Sulfate

USES: Osteoarthritis (glucosamine is the rate-limiting step in glycosaminoglycan biosynthesis and promotes cartilage rebuilding; chondroitin is a biological polymer that acts as the flexible connecting matrix between protein filaments in cartilage and draws fluid and nutrients into joint, "shock absorption" creating).
DOSE: Glucosamine 500 PO tid, chondroitin 400 mg tid.
CAUTIONS: None known.
ADVERSE EFFECTS: None known; because these agents are concentrated in cartilage, the theory is that they are unlikely to produce toxic or teratogenic effects.
DRUG INTERACTIONS: Glucosamine—none known, chondroitin—monitor anticoagulant therapy.

Kava Kava (Kava Kava Root Extract, *Piper methysticum*)

USES: Reduction of anxiety, stress, and restlessness; sedative effect.
DOSE: Standardized extract (70% kavalactones) 100 mg 2–3 × daily.
CAUTIONS: Endogenous depression. Not recommended during pregnancy and lactation. Extended use may result in yellow discoloration of skin, hair, and nails, which signals need for discontinuation.
ADVERSE EFFECTS: Mild gastrointestinal disturbances; in rare cases, allergic skin reactions can occur; may increase cholesterol; may cause rash and/or vision changes, red eyes, puffy face, muscle weakness.
DRUG INTERACTIONS: Avoid using with other sedatives, alcohol, or stimulants. Potentiation of effectiveness is possible for substances acting on the CNS, such as alcohol, barbiturates, and other psychopharmacological agents.

Melatonin

USES: Insomnia, jet lag, use as antioxidant, use as immunostimulant.

DOSE: 1–3 mg 20 minutes prior to bedtime (controlled-release: administer 2 hours prior to bedtime).
CAUTIONS: Use synthetic rather than product derived from animal pineal gland; avoid if patient has autoimmune disease or AIDS/HIV or is a teenager or woman trying to get pregnant.
ADVERSE EFFECTS: "Heavy head," headache, depression.
DRUG INTERACTIONS: Beta blockers, corticosteroids, NSAIDs, benzodiazepines.

Saw Palmetto (*Serenoa repens*)

USES: Treatment of benign prostatic hypertrophy (BPH) stages 1 and 2 (inhibits testosterone-5-alpha-reductase), increases sperm production, increases breast size (estrogenic), increases sexual vigor.
DOSE: 320 mg q day.
CAUTIONS: Due to its hormonal effects, should be avoided in pregnancy, during lactation, and in women of childbearing years.
ADVERSE EFFECTS: Mild GI upset, mild headache. Large amounts may cause diarrhea.
DRUG INTERACTIONS: May increase iron absorption; may increase effects of estrogen replacement.

St. John's Wort (*Hypericum perforatum*)

USES: Mild to moderate depression and anxiety, gastritis, insomnia, vitiligo; use as anti-inflammatory; use as immune stimulant/anti-HIV/antiviral.
DOSE: 2–4 g of herb or 0.2–1.0 mg of total hypericin in standardized extract preparations daily. Commonly available preparations: 300 mg PO tid (0.3% hypericin).
CAUTIONS: Excessive doses may potentiate existing MAO inhibitor therapy, and may cause an allergic reaction. Not recommended for use during pregnancy.
ADVERSE EFFECTS: Photosensitivity, dry mouth, dizziness, constipation, confusion.
DRUG INTERACTIONS: Should not be used at the same time as prescription antidepressants, especially MAO inhibitors. More recently reported interactions include decrease in efficacy of cyclosporin (with resultant organ rejection), digoxin (with congestive heart failure exacerbation), protease inhibitors, theophylline, and oral contraceptives. Potent cytochrome P-450 3A4 enzyme inducer.
OTHER: Potency of St. John's wort can vary widely from one product and batch to another based on harvesting and extraction techniques. St. John's wort may result in fluctuating mood when taken chronically.

Valerian (*Valeriana officinalis*)

USES: Use as anti-anxiety agent, use as sedative, restlessness, dysmenorrhea.
DOSE: 2–3 g extract q day–bid.
CAUTIONS: None known.
ADVERSE EFFECTS: Sedation, hangover effect, headache, cardiac disturbances, and GI upset.
DRUG INTERACTIONS: Use with caution when taking other sedating agents; alcohol or prescription sedatives may cause drowsiness that could impair function.

Yohimbine (*Pausinystalia yohimbe*)

USES: To improve sexual vigor (impotence).
DOSE: 5 mg tid (should only be used under direction of physician).
CAUTIONS: May exacerbate schizophrenia or mania (if patient is predisposed). Alpha-2 adrenergic antagonism causes hypotension, abdominal distress, and weakness at high doses (overdose can be fatal); salivation, dilated pupils, irregular heartbeat.
ADVERSE EFFECTS: Anxiety, tremors, dizziness, high blood pressure, increased heart rate. Do not use in patients with renal/hepatic diseases.
DRUG INTERACTIONS: Do not combine with antidepressants, especially MAOIs or similar agents.

Unsafe Herbs

Agent	Toxicities
Aconite	Salivation, nausea/vomiting, blurred vision, cardiac arrhythmias
Calamus	Possible carcinogenicity
Chaparral	Hepatotoxicity, possible carcinogenicity

"Chinese herbal mixtures"	May contain Ma huang or other dangerous herbs
Coltsfoot	Hepatotoxicity, possible carcinogenicity
Comfrey	Hepatotoxicity, carcinogenicity
Juniper	High allergy potential, diarrhea, seizures, nephrotoxicity
Licorice	Large daily amounts (> 30 g) over months can result in hypokalemia, sodium/fluid retention with resultant hypertension, myoglobinuria, and hyporeflexia
Life root	Hepatotoxicity, liver cancer
Ma-huang/ephedra	Elevated BP, MI, stroke, psychosis
Pokeweed	Severe GI cramping, nausea, diarrhea, vomiting, labored breathing, hypotension, seizures
Sassafras	Vomiting, stupor, hallucinations, dermatitis, abortion, hypothermia, liver cancer
Yohimbine	Hypotension, abdominal distress, CNS stimulation (including mania and psychosis in predisposed individuals)

5. VITAMINS: INDICATIONS/EFFECTS, RDA/DOSAGE, SIGNS/SYMPTOMS OF DEFICIENCY AND TOXICITY, AND OTHER

Vitamin A

INDICATIONS/EFFECTS: *General:* Healthy skin and vision, resistance to infection, bone and sperm development. *Pregnancy:* Maintains healthy fetus and prevents neural tube defects, may decrease maternal transmission of AIDS to fetus.

RDA/DOSAGE: *Males:* 1000 μg/d (5000 IU) (900μg/d per IOM report*). *Females:* 800 μg/d (4000 IU) (700 μg/d*) *Food and Nutrition Board, Institute of Medicine, the National Academies, 2001. www.iom.edu

S/SX OF DEFICIENCY: (Vitamin A deficiency is rare.) Anemia, night blindness, diarrhea, renal calculi, tooth decay, flaking skin.

S/SX OF TOXICITY: > 3000 μg/d (= 10,000 IU) can result in fatigue, night sweats, GI upset, headache, dry skin, alopecia, pruritus, and hepatotoxicity; in pregnancy can result in birth defects (head, heart, brain, spinal column).

OTHER: Should avoid vitamin A supplements if patient smokes or drinks > 2 drinks/d.

Folate (Folic Acid, Pteroylglutamic Acid) (See also p 519)

INDICATIONS/EFFECTS: *General:* Prevention of stroke, heart disease (via decreased homocysteine levels), dementia, cancer (antioxidant effect). *Pregnancy:* Prevention of neural tube defects.

RDA/DOSAGE: *To prevent deficiency:* Males: 200 μg, Females: 180 μg; *To promote health and prevent chronic disease:* 400 μg daily; *Women of childbearing age:* 400 μg daily to reduce the risk of spina bifida and other neural tube defects to the fetus.

S/SX OF DEFICIENCY: Megaloblastic and macrocytic anemia, glossitis; risk of deficiency increased on methotrexate.

S/SX OF TOXICITY: Few (irritability, nausea), but doses of > 1000 μg/d can mask B_{12} deficiency.

OTHER: Enhances the metabolism of phenytoin.

Thiamine (Vitamin B_1) (See also p 579)

INDICATIONS/EFFECTS: Carbohydrate metabolism, myocardial function.

RDA/DOSAGE: Males: 1.5 mg. Females: 1.1 mg.

S/SX OF DEFICIENCY: Most likely to occur in chronic alcoholics and/or those with poor nutritional intake (eg, cachectic elderly in nursing home); peripheral neuropathy, nystagmus, confusion, ataxia, high output heart failure. Early stages of deficiency known as Wernicke's encephalopathy, which is reversible, may progress to Korsakoff's psychosis, which is not. Dose to treat encephalopathy: 100 mg IV, then 50–100 mg IM/IV until normal diet resumed.

S/SX OF TOXICITY: Unknown.

Vitamin B_6 (Pyridoxine) (See also p 566)

INDICATIONS/EFFECTS: Reduces the severity/risk of depression, PMS, hypertension, carpal tunnel syndrome, morning sickness. May help reduce cardiovascular disease by effects on homocysteine levels.

RDA/DOSAGE: Under age 50: 1.3 mg. Age 50+: males 1.7 mg, females 1.5 mg.

S/SX OF DEFICIENCY: Microcytic anemia, glossitis, cheilosis, irritability, muscle fasciculations, dermatitis, neuritis, seizures, renal calculi.

S/SX OF TOXICITY: (> 2 G/D) Ataxia, distal paresthesias, muscle weakness, nerve damage.

OTHER: May reduce the effect of levodopa in Parkinson's disease; avoid use in these patients. Often prescribed concomitantly with isoniazid, cycloserine, or penicillamine to prevent CNS adverse effects (pyridoxine dose 10–50 mg/d).

Vitamin B_{12} (Cyanocobatamin) (See also p 498)

INDICATIONS/EFFECTS: Prevents anemia, promotes healthy nerve conduction, decreases homocysteine accumulation, delays progression from HIV-positive status to AIDS.

RDA/DOSAGE: 2.4 μg (patients over age 50 may not absorb B_{12} as well as PO; should take 100 μg/d PO or 100–1000 μg/mo IM if over 50 and also taking folate).

S/SX OF DEFICIENCY: Fatigue, nerve damage/neuropathy, dementia, depression, confusion, pernicious anemia (lack of intrinsic factor), megaloblastic anemia, glossitis, paralysis.

S/SX OF TOXICITY: (> 100 MG/D) Diarrhea.

OTHER: Avoid megadoses of vitamin C due to destruction of vitamin B_{12}. Contraindicated in hereditary optic nerve atrophy; potassium levels may fall rapidly when replacing B_{12} at high doses. Increased B_{12} requirements: pregnancy, hyperthyroidism. Increased B_{12} excretion: alcoholics. Need B_{12} supplement in strict vegans (no egg/milk intake) if they are not eating fortified cereals.

Vitamin C (Ascorbic Acid)

INDICATIONS/EFFECTS: Antioxidant, healthy gums, assists in collagen formation, improves iron absorption, may improve wound healing, may shorten duration of a viral upper respiratory infection.

RDA/DOSAGE*: Males: 90 mg. Females: 75 mg. Smokers: add 35 mg. *Food and Nutrition Board, Institute of Medicine, the National Academies, 2000. www.iom.edu

S/SX OF DEFICIENCY: Anemia, hemorrhage, muscle weakness, gum disease (scurvy), delayed wound healing, skin changes including perifollicular hyperkeratotic papules and hemorrhage and purpura.

S/SX OF TOXICITY: (> 2000 mg/d): Abdominal cramps, nausea, diarrhea, nosebleeds. May increase risk of renal calculi and exacerbate hemochromatosis; interferes with the absorption of vitamin B_{12}.

Vitamin D (See also p 489)

INDICATIONS/EFFECTS: Assists in calcium and phosphorus absorption; may reduce risks of colon and breast cancer.

RDA/DOSAGE: Under age 50, 200 IU. Age 50–70, 400 IU. Over age 70, 600 IU (may have difficulty with absorption).

S/SX OF DEFICIENCY: Osteomalacia, increased risk of fractures (especially in postmenopausal women), muscle spasms.

S/SX OF TOXICITY (> 1000 IU/D): Nausea, headache, fatigue, heart irregularities, anorexia, metallic taste, increased calcium levels with subsequent renal disease.

OTHER: Requires UV light to convert to active forms (sufficient amount of sun exposure: 5–15 minutes, 2–3 × a week).

Vitamin E

INDICATIONS/EFFECTS: Cardioprotective (decreases LDL oxidation, anticoagulant, 40% reduction in CHD on 100 IU q day × 2 years), immunostimulant, protects against cataracts, slows progression of Alzheimer's disease, reduces premenstrual symptoms.

RDA/DOSAGE: 15 mg/33 IU (although many studies use 100–400 IU q day–qid for prevention of CV/CNS disease).
S/SX OF DEFICIENCY: Deficiency more likely on low-fat diet; may need to supplement; erythrocyte hemolysis.
S/SX OF TOXICITY (> 1000 IU/D): Can result in bleeding (inhibits platelet aggregation), this effect may occur at lower doses on warfarin. Also fatigue, headache, nausea, diarrhea, flatulence, blurred vision, dermatitis.
OTHER: Discontinue use before surgery due to its effects on platelet aggregation and tendon healing.

Vitamin K (See also p 566)

INDICATIONS/EFFECTS: Enhances production of clotting factors, healthy bone formation.
RDA/DOSAGE: 65–80 μg (1 μg/kg).
S/SX OF DEFICIENCY: Rare, but more likely to occur in hospitalized patients, newborn infants, those on tube feedings, and/or those on antibiotics, especially sulfas; bruising, bleeding.
S/SX OF TOXICITY: Usually not toxic in older children/adults.
OTHER: Blocks pharmacologic effects of warfarin (as a supplement and in dietary intake).

REFERENCES

Anonymous: *Dietary Reference Intakes: Applications in Dietary Assessment.* National Academy Press; 2000.

Anonymous: *Review of Natural Products,* Facts & Comparisons, Inc.; 2001.

Foster S, Tyler VE, eds: *Tyler's Honest Herbal: A Sensible Guide to the Use of Herbs and Related Remedies.* 4th ed. Haworth Press; 1999.

Fowler JB, German TC: The essence of herbal products for the hospital pharmacist. Pharmacy Practice News 2001;1:28.

Kava R: Vitamins and Minerals: Does the Epidemiologic Evidence Justify General Supplementation? American Council on Science and Health monograph (www.acsh.org);2000.

Pray S: *Diet for a Healthy Lifestyle.* Monograph. University of Kentucky College of Pharmacy; 2000.

Robbers JE, Tyler VE: *Tyler's Herbs of Choice: The Therapeutic Use of Phytomedicinals.* Haworth Press; 1999.

Internet Sites: www.fda.gov, www.herbalgram.org, www.herbs.org, www.nih.gov, www.drkoop.com, www.webmd.com, www.medscape.com

6. TABLES

TABLE 7–1. INSULINS.

Type of Insulin	Onset (hr)	Peak (hr)	Duration (hr)	Compatible to Mix With
■ Rapid-acting				
Aspart (Novolog)	0.25	0.5–1.5	3–5	All
Lispro (Humalog)	0.25	0.5–1.5	3–4	All
Regular Iletin II	0.5–1	5–10	6–8	All
Humulin R	0.5–1	5–10	6–8	All
Novolin R	0.5–1	5–10	6–8	All
■ Intermediate-acting				
NPH Iletin II	1–1.5	4–6	24	Regular
Humulin N	1–1.5	4–6	24	Regular
Novolin N	1–1.5	4–6	24	Regular
Lente Iletin II	1–2.5	7.5	24	Regular, Semilente
■ Long-acting				
Humulin U	4–8	10–30	36	Regular
Ultralente	4–8	10–30	36	Regular
Insulin Glargine (Lantus)	1–1.5	Peakless	24	Do not mix with other insulins
■ Combinations				
Humulin 70/30	0.5	4–8	24	
Novolin 70/30	0.5	4–8	24	

TABLE 7–2. COMPARISON OF GLUCOCORTICOIDS.

Drug (Trade)	Equivalent Dose (mg)	Anti-inflammatory Potency	Mineralocorticoid Potency
■ Short-Acting			
Cortisone (Cortone)	25	0.8	2
Hydrocortisone (Cortef)	20	1	2
■ Intermediate-Acting			
Methylprednisolone (Medrol)	4	5	0
Prednisone (Deltasone)	5	4	1
Prednisolone (Delta-Cortef)	5	4	1
Triamcinolone	4	5	0
■ Long-Acting			
Betamethasone (Celestone)	0.6–0.75	20–30	0
Dexamethasone (Decadron)	0.75	20–30	0

TABLE 7–3. ANGIOTENSIN-CONVERTING ENZYME INHIBITORS.[1]

Drug (Trade)	Hypertension	Heart Failure	Left Ventricular Dysfunction
Benazepril (Lotensin)	10–40 mg/d divided q day–bid		
Captopril (Capoten)	25–50 mg bid–tid	6.25–25 mg tid	Titrate to 50 mg tid
Enalapril (Vasotec)	5–40 mg/d divided q day–bid	2.5–10 mg bid	Titrate to 10 mg bid
Fosinopril (Monopril)	10–40 mg q day	10–40 mg q day	
Lisinopril (Prinivil, Zestril)	10–40 mg q day	5–20 mg q day	
Moexipril (Univasc)	7.5–30 mg/d divided q day–bid		
Perindopril (Aceon)	4–16 mg/d	4 mg/d	
Quinapril (Accupril)	10–80 mg q day	5–20 mg bid	
Ramipril (Altace)	2.5–20 mg/d divided q day–bid	1.25–5 mg bid	
Trandolapril (Mavik)	2–8 mg/d	1 mg/d	

[1]*Notes:*

1. Pro-drugs (metabolized to active agent): Benazepril, Enalapril, Fosinopril, Moexipril, Perindopril, Quinapril, Ramipril, Trandolapril.
2. Persistent, nonproductive cough has occurred with the use of *all* ACE inhibitors. Cough typically resolves within 1–4 days after therapy is discontinued. Angiotensin-II receptor antagonists (see Table 7–4) are less frequently associated with cough.
3. Co-administration of ACE inhibitors with potassium preparations may result in elevated serum potassium concentrations.
4. Strictly contraindicated in pregnancy. Women of child-bearing age should be warned regarding risk of teratogenicity and use of ACE inhibitors.

TABLE 7–4. ANGIOTENSIN RECEPTOR ANTAGONISTS.

Drug (Trade)	Daily Dosage Range	Renal Dysfunction	Product Availability (mg)
Candesartan (Atacand)	8–32 mg q day	No adjustment necessary	Tablets 4, 8, 16, 32
Eprosartan (Teveten)	400–800 mg q day	No adjustment necessary	Tablets 400, 600
Irbesartan (Avapro)	140–300 mg q day	No adjustment necessary	Tablets 75, 150, 300
Irbesartan/ Hydrochlorothiazide (Avalide)	1–2 tablets q day	HCTZ not recommended in severe impairment	Tablets Irbesartan 150/HCTZ 12.5 Irbesartan 300/HCTZ 12.5
Losartan (Cozaar)	25–100 mg q day or bid	No adjustment necessary	Tablets 25, 50
Losartan/ Hydrochlorothiazide (Hyzaar)	50/12.5 mg 1–2 q day 100 mg/25 mg q day	HCTZ not recommended in severe impairment	Tablets Losartan 50/HCTZ 12.5 Losartan 100/HCTZ 25
Telmisartan (Micardis)	20–80 mg q day	No adjustment necessary	Tablets 40, 80
Valsartan (Diovan)	80–320 mg q day	Decrease dose if $Cl_{cr} < 10$ mL/min	Capsules 80, 160
Valsartan/ Hydrochlorothiazide (Diovan HCT)	1–2 capsules q day	HCTZ not recommended in severe impairement	Tablets Valsartan 80/HCTZ 12.5 Valsartan 160/HCTZ 12.5

TABLE 7–5. ANTISTAPHYLOCCOCCAL PENICILLINS.[1, 2]

Drug (Brand)	Dosage	Dosing Interval	Suplied	Notes
Oxacillin (Bactocill)	1–2 g	4–6 hr	Injection	
Nafcillin (Nafcil, Unipen)	1–2 g	4–6 hr	Injection	No dosage adjustments for renal function
Cloxacillin (Cloxapen, Tegopen)	250–500 mg	6 hr	Oral	Administer on an empty stomach
Dicloxacillin (Dynapen, Dycill)	250–500 mg	6 hr	Oral	Administer on an empty stomach

[1]***Indications:*** Treatment of infections caused by susceptible strains of *Staphylococcus* and *Streptococcus.*
[2]***Actions:*** Bactericidal: Inhibits cell wall synthesis.

TABLE 7–6. EXTENDED-SPECTRUM PENICILLINS.[1–3]

Drug (Brand)	Dose	Dosing Interval	mEq Na^+ Per Gram	Notes
Ticarcillin (Ticar)	3 g	4–6 hr	5.2	May cause hypokalemia/ sodium overload, acquired platelet dysfunction with the potential for bleeding to occur
Ticarcillin-clavulanate (Timentin)	3.1 g	4–6 hr	4.75	Clavulanate is a beta-lactamase inhibitor
Mezlocillin (Mezlin)	3 g	4–6 hr	1.85	Activity against *Entero-bacteriaceae*
Piperacillin (Pipracil)	3 g	4–6 hr	1.85	Best activity against *Pseudomonas*
Piperacillin-tazobactam (Zosyn)	3.375 g	6 hr		Tazobactam is a beta-lactamase inhibitor (Does not improve activity against *Pseudomonas* when compared to pipera-cillin without tazobactam)

[1]***Indications:*** Treatment of infections caused by susceptible gram-negative bacteria (including *Klebsiella, Proteus, E coli, Enterobacter, P aeruginosa, Serratia*) involving the skin, bone and joints, respiratory tract, urinary tract, abdomen, and vascular system.
[2]***Actions:*** Bactericidal, inhibits cell wall synthesis.
[3]***Notes:*** These agents are often used in combination with an aminoglycoside to treat *P aeruginosa* and in neuropenic patients with a fever. Dosage adjustment necessary in renal impairment.

TABLE 7–7. BETA-ADRENERGIC BLOCKING AGENTS.[1–4]

Drug (Trade)	Receptor	Angina	Hypertension	Myocardial Infarction	Congestive Heart Failure
Acebutolol (Sectral)	B_1, ISA		200–400 mg bid		
Atenolol (Tenormin)	B_1	50–100 mg q day	50–100 mg q day	5 mg IV × 2 doses, then 50 mg PO bid	
Betaxolol (Kerlone)	B_1		10–20 mg q day		
Bisoprolol (Zebeta))	B_1		5–10 mg q day		
Carteolol (Cartrol)	B_1, B_2, ISA		2.5–5 mg q day		
Carvedilol (Coreg)	B_1, B_2, α		6.25–25 mg bid		3.125–25 bid
Esmolol (Brevibloc)	(See p 511)				
Labetalol (Trandate, Normodyne)	B_1, B_2, α_1		100–400 mg bid		
Metoprolol (Lopressor, Toprol XL)	B_1	50–100 mg bid	100–450 mg q day	5 mg IV × 3 doses, then 50 mg PO Q 6 hr × 48 hr, then 100 mg PO bid	6.25–50 mg bid **or** 12.5–200 mg XL q day
Nadolol (Corgard)	B_1, B_2	40–80 mg q day	40–80 mg q day		
Penbutolol (Levatol)	B_1, B_2, ISA		20–40 mg q day		
Pindolol (Visken)	B_1, B_2, ISA		5–10 mg bid		

(*continued*)

TABLE 7–7. BETA-ADRENERGIC BLOCKING AGENTS (*continued*).

Drug (Trade)	Receptor	Angina	Hypertension	Myocardial Infarction	Congestive Heart Failure
Propranolol (Inderal)	B_1, B_2,	160 mg SR q day	120–160 mg SR q day	60 mg tid–qid	
Sotalol (Betapace)	(See p 573)				
Timolol (Blocadren)	B_1, B_2		10–20 mg bid	10 mg bid	

Notes: ISA = intrinsic sympathomimetic activity.

Other Uses:
- Cardiac Arrhythmias: Various agents and doses
- Migraine Prophylaxis: Atenolol 50–100 mg/d **or** Nadolol 40–80 mg/d **or** [1]Propranolol 80–240 mg/d
- Essential Tremor: Propranolol 40 mg bid; maximal dose 320 mg/d
- Adjunctive Therapy: Pheochromocytoma (after alpha-adrenergic drugs are added); Hyperthyroidism (propranolol); Rebleeding of esophageal varices in cirrhotic patients and alcohol withdrawal (atenolol)

[1]FDA-approved indication.

Precautions:

[1] Use with caution in diabetic patients. May blunt symptoms/signs of acute hypoglycemia; nonselective agents may potentiate insulin-induced hypoglycemia. Beta-blockade also reduces the release of insulin in response to hyperglycemia.

[2] May increase serum lipid concentrations. May not be as pronounced with agents having intrinsic sympathomimetic activity.

[3] Use with caution in patients with congestive heart failure (decreased myocardial contractility) and chronic obstructive pulmonary diseases (potential blockade of B_2 receptors).

[4] When discontinuing chronically administered beta-blockers, particularly in patients with ischemic heart disease, reduce dose gradually, especially with agents with a short half-life (propranolol, metoprolol).

TABLE 7–8. FIRST-GENERATION CEPHALOSPORINS.[1–3]

Drug (Brand)	Dose	Dosing Interval	Supplied	Notes
Cefadroxil (Duricef, Ultracef)	500 mg–1 g	12–24 hr	Capsules, tablets	
Cefazolin (Ancef, Kefzol)	1–2 g	8 hr	Injection	For surgical prophylaxis most widely used antibiotic
Cephalexin (Keflex)	250–500 mg	qid	Capsules, tablets	
Cephalothin (Keflin)	1–2 g	6 hr	Injection	
Cephapirin (Cefadyl)	1–2 g	6 hr	Injection	
Cephradine (Velosef)	250–500 mg 1 g	qid 6 hr	Capsules Injection	

[1]***Indications:*** Treatment of infections caused by susceptible strains of *Streptococcus, Staphylococcus, E coli, Proteus, and Klebsiella* involving the skin, bone and joints, upper and lower respiratory tract, and urinary tract.
[2]***Actions:*** Bactericidal: inhibits cell wall synthesis.
[3]***Dosage adjustments:*** Necessary in renal impairment.

TABLE 7–9. SECOND-GENERATION CEPHALOSPORINS.[1–3]

Drug (Brand)	Dose	Dosing Interval	Supplied	Notes
Cefaclor (Ceclor)	250–500 mg	8 hr	Capsules Tablets	
Cefamandole (Mandol)	1–2 g	4–6 hr	Injection	
Cefmetazole (Zefazone)	1–2 g	8 hr	Injection	Activity against anaerobes
Cefonicid (Monocid)	1–2 g	24 hr	Injection	
Cefotetan (Cefotan)	1–2 g	12 hr	Injection	Activity against anaerobes
Cefoxitin (Mefoxin)	1–2 g	6 hr	Injection	Best activity against anaerobes
Cefprozil (Cefzil)	250–500 mg	q day–bid	Tablets	Use higher doses for otitis and pneumonia
Cefuroxime (Zinacef, Ceftin)	750 mg–1.5 g 250–500 mg	8 hr bid	Injection Tablets	Ceftin should be taken with food
Loracarbef (Lorabid)	200–400 mg	bid	Capsules	Similar to cefaclor

[1]***Indications:*** Treatment of infections caused by susceptible bacteria involving the upper and lower respiratory tract, skin, bone, urinary tract, abdomen, and female reproductive system.
[2]***Actions:*** Bactericidal; inhibits cell wall synthesis.
[3]***Notes:*** More active than 1st-generation agents against *H influenzae, E coli, Klebsiella* species, and *P mirabilis*. Risk of hypoprothrombinemia or bleeding has been associated with cephalosporins containing a N-methylthiotetrazole (NMTT) side chain. These agents include cefotetan, cefmetazole, and cefoperazone (3rd-generation). Administration of vitamin K will prevent clinical bleeding associated with these drugs for patients with vitamin K deficiency.

Dosage adjustment necessary in renal impairment.

TABLE 7–10. THIRD- AND FOURTH-GENERATION CEPHALOSPORINS.[1–3]

Drug (Brand)	Dose	Interval	Supplied	Notes
Cefdinir (Omnicef)	300–600 mg	12–24 hr	Capsules	
Cefepime[4] (Maxipime)	1–2 g	12 hr	Injection	
Cefixime (Suprax)	200–400 mg	12–24 hr	Tablets, suspension	Use suspension for otitis media
Cefoperazone (Cefobid)	1–2 g	12 hr	Injection	See Footnote 3, Table 7–9
Cefotaxime (Claforan)	1–2 g	4–8 hr	Injection	Crosses the blood-brain barrier
Cefpodoxime (Vantin)	200–400 mg	12 hr	Tablets	Drug interations with agents increasing the gastric pH
Ceftazidime (Fortaz, Ceptaz) Tazidime, Tazicef)	1–2 g	8 hr	Injection	Best activity against *Pseudomonas*. Crosses the blood-brain barrier.
Ceftibuten (Cedax)	400 mg	12 hr	Capsule	Take on an empty stomach
Ceftizoxime (Cefizox)	1–2 g	8–12 hr	Injection	
Ceftriaxone (Rocephin)	1–2 g	12–24 hr	Injection	Treatment of choice for gonorrhea. Crosses the blood-brain barrier.

[1]***Indications:*** Treatment of infections caused by susceptible bacteria involving the respiratory tract, skin, bone and joints, and urinary tract; treatment of meningitis, febrile neutropenia, and septicemia.
[2]***Actions:*** Bactericidal; inhibits cell wall synthesis.
[3]***Notes:*** Less active against gram-positive cocci than 1st- and 2nd-generation agents. Increased activity against gram-negative aerobes (*Enterobacteriaceae* including *Enterobacter* and *Serratia*) due to increased stability to beta-lactamases. May be used in combination with an aminoglycoside. Dosage adjustment necessary in renal impairment.
[4]***Notes:*** 4th-generation cephalosporin.

TABLE 7–11. NONSTEROIDAL ANTI-INFLAMMATORY DRUGS.[1]

Drug (Trade)	Arthritis	Analgesia	Dysmenorrhea	Maximum Daily Dose (MG)
■ **Salicylates**[2]				
Diflunisal[3] (Dolobid)	500 mg bid–tid	500 mg bid–tid		1500
■ **Acetic acids**[2]				
Diclofenac (Cataflam, Voltaren)	50–75 mg bid–tid	50 mg tid	50 mg tid	200
Etodolac (Lodine)	200–400 mg bid–tid	200–400 mg Q 6–8 hr		1200
Indomethacin (Indocin)	25–50 mg bid–tid			200 **or** SR 150
Ketorolac (Toradol)		IV/IM 15–30 mg Q 6 hr; PO 10 mg Q 6 hr		IV: 120; PO: 40; do not use for more than 5 days
Nabumetone (Relafen)	1000–2000 mg/d divided q day–bid			2000
Sulindac (Clinoril)	150–200 mg bid			400
Tolmetin (Tolectin)	200–600 mg tid			2000
■ **Oxicams**[2]				
Piroxicam (Feldene)	10–20 mg q day			20

(*continued*)

TABLE 7–11. NONSTEROIDAL ANTI-INFLAMMATORY DRUGS (*continued*).

Drug (Trade)	Arthritis	Analgesia	Dysmenorrhea	Maximum Daily Dose (MG)
■ **Propionic acids**[2]				
Fenoprofen (Nalfon)	300–600 mg tid–qid	200 mg Q 4–6 hr		3200
Flurbiprofen (Ansaid)	50–100 mg bid–qid			300
Ibuprofen (Advil, Motrin)	400–800 mg tid–qid	400 mg Q 4–6 hr	400 mg Q 4 hr	3200
Ketoprofen (Orudis)	50–75 mg tid–qid	25–50 mg Q 6–8 hr		300
Meloxicam[4, 6] (Mobic)	7.5–15 mg q day			
Naproxen (Naprosyn)	250–500 mg bid	250 mg Q 6–8 hr	250 mg Q 6–8 hr	1500
Naproxen sodium (Aleve, Anaprox)	275–550 mg bid	275 mg Q 6–8 hr	275 mg Q 6–8 hr	1375
Oxaprozin (Daypro)	600–1200 mg q day			1200
■ **Selctive COX-2 Inhibitors**				
Celecoxib[5, 6] (Celebrex)	100 mg bid or 200 mg q day (osteoarthritis) 100–200 mg bid (rheumatoid arthritis)			400
Rofecoxib[6] (Vioxx)	12.5–25 mg q day	50 mg q day × 5 days	50 mg q day × 5 days	50

Notes:

1 Can cause renal insufficiency/failure, especially in the elderly. **Do not** take in the third trimester of pregnancy.

2 Chronic use can cause gastrointestinal bleeding from gastroduodenal ulceration. Inhibits platelet aggregation except for meloxicam.

3 First dose 1000 mg, then 500 mg bid–tid.

4 Inhibits COX-2 more than COX-1.

5 Dosage for familial adenomatous polyposis is 400 mg bid.

6 Does not inhibit platelet aggregation.

TABLE 7–12. OPHTHALMIC AGENTS.

Drug (Trade)	Strength (%)	Dosing Schedule
AGENTS FOR GLAUCOMA		
Alpha-$_2$ Adrenergic Agonists		
Brimonidine (Alphagan)	0.2	1 gtt tid
Apraclonidine (Iopidine)	0.5, 1.0	1–2 gtts tid (0.5%), 1 gtt 1 hr prior to surgery (1.0%)
Dipivefrin (Propine)	0.1	1 gtt Q 12 hr
Beta-Blockers		
Betaxolol (Betoptic-S, Betoptic)	0.25, 05	1 gtt bid
Levobunolol (Betagan Liquifilm)	0.25, 0.5	1 gtt q day–bid
Metipranolol (OptiPranolol)	0.3	1 gtt bid
Timolol[1] (Timoptic)	0.25, 0.5	1 gtt q day–bid
Carteolol (Ocupress)	1.0	1 gtt bid
Levobetaxolol (Betaxon)	0.5	1 gtt bid
Carbonic Anhydrase Inhibitors		
Brinzolamide (Azopt)	1.0	1 gtt tid
Dorzolamide (Trusopt)	2.0	1 gtt tid
Miotics, Cholinesterase Inhibitors		
Carbachol (Isopto Carbachol)	0.75–3	1–2 gtts tid
Physostigmine (Isopto Eserine)	0.25, 0.5	2 gtts up to qid
Demecarium (Humorsol)	0.125, 0.25	1–2 gtts twice weekly, up to 1–2 gtts bid
Echothiophate iodine (Phospholine iodide)	0.03, 0.06, 0.125, 0.25	1 gtt bid
Pilocarpine (Isopto Carpine, Pilocar)	0.25–10	1–2 gtts up to 6 × per day
(Pilopine HS gel)	4.0	0.5 inch Q HS

(*continued*)

TABLE 7–12. OPTHALMIC AGENTS (*continued*).

Drug (Trade)	Strength (%)	Dosing Schedule
Prostaglandin Agonists		
Latanoprost[2] (Xalatan)	0.005	1 gtt Q HS
Combination Agents		
Dorzolamide and Timolol (Cosopt)	2/0.5	1 gtt bid
ANTIBIOTICS		
Bacitracin (See p 484)		
Chloramphenicol (AK-Chlor)	oint/sol	1–2 gtts or 0.5 inch Q 3–4 hr
Ciprofloxacin (Ciloxan)	solution	1–2 gtts 4–6 × per day
Erythromycin (AK-Mycin, Ilotycin)	ointment	0.5 inch 2–8 × per day
Gentamicin (Garamycin)	oint/sol	1–2 gtts or 0.5 inch 2–3 × per day, up to Q 3–4 hr
Neomycin, Polymyxin B, Hydrocortisone 1% (Cortisporin)	sus	1–2 gtts Q 3–4 hr
Sulfacetamide Sodium (Sodium Sulamyd, Bleph 10)	10–30% oint/sol	1–2 gtts Q 1–3 hr or 0.5 inch q day–qid
Tobramycin (Tobrex)	oint/sol	1–2 gtts or 0.5 inch 2–3 × per day, up to Q 3–4 hr
ANTI-INFLAMMATORY		
NSAIDs		
Diclofenac (Voltaren)	0.1	
Flurbiprofen (Ocufen)	0.03	1 gtt qid (post-op inflammation following cataract surgery)
Ketorolac (Acular)	0.5	1 gtt Q 4 hr × 3 days (ocular inflammation) 1 gtt qid (relieves itching due to seasonal allergic conjunctivitis)

Corticosteroids		
Dexamethasone (AK-Dex, others)	0.05 (oint), 0.1 (sol)	1–2 gtts or 0.5 inch tid–qid
Fluorometholone (FML, Flarex)	0.1	1–2 gtts bid–qid
Prednisolone (AK-Pred, Pred Forte)	0.12, 0.125, 1.0	1–2 gtts Q 1 hr day, Q 2 night until response, then 1 gtt Q 4 hr
Rimexolone (Vexol)	1	1–2 gtts Q 1 hr to qid
Decongestant/Anti-allergy		
Ketotifen[3] (Zaditor)	0.025	1 gtt bid–tid
Levocabastine (Livostin)	0.05	1 gtt qid
Lodoxamide (Alomide)	0.1	1–2 gtts qid
Naphazoline and Antazoline (Albalon-A)	0.05/0.5	1–2 gtts tid–qid
Naphazoline and Pheniramine Acetate (Naphcon A)	0.025/0.3	1–2 gtts tid–qid
Mast Cell Stabilizers		
Nedocromil sodium (Alocril)	2%	1–2 gtts bid
Pemirolast potassium (Alamast)	0.1%	1–2 gtts qid
COMBINATION AGENTS (also see Glaucoma)		
Gentamicin and Prednisolone (Pred-G)	Oint/sol	0.5 inch bid–tid (oint), 1–2 gtts Q 2–4 hr up to Q 2 hr (sol)
Neomycin & Dexamethasone (Dex-Neo-Dex)	Oint/sol	0.5 inch tid–qid (oint), 1–2 gtts Q 3–4 hr (sol)
Neomycin, Polymyxin, Hydrocortisone (Cortisporin)	Oint/sol	0.5 inch Q day–qid (oint), 1–2 gtts bid–qid
Neomycin, Polymyxin, & Dexamethasone (Maxitrol)	Oint/sol	0.5 inch tid–qid (oint), 1–2 gtts Q 4–6 hr (sol)
Neomycin, Polymyxin, & Prednisolone (Poly-Pred)	Oint/sol	0.5 inch tid–qid (oint), 1–2 gtts Q 4–6 hr (sol)
Sulfacetamide & Prednisolone (Blephamide)	Oint/sol	0.5 inch Q day—qid (oint), 1–3 gtts Q 2–3 hr

Notes:

[1] Systemic absorption may cause bradycardia.
[2] May darken light irides.
[3] Wait at least 10 minutes before putting in contact lens.

TABLE 7–13. SULFONYLUREA AGENTS.[1, 2]

Drug (Trade)	Duration of Activity (hr)	Equivalent Dose (mg)	Dosing Schedule
■ First-generation			
Acetohexamide (Dymelor)	24	500	250–1500 mg q day
Chlorpropamide (Diabinese)	≥ 60	250	100–500 mg q day
Tolazamide (Tolinase)	12–24	250	100–500 mg q day
Tolbutamide (Orinase)	6–12	1000	500–1000 mg bid
■ Second-generation			
Glipizide[3] (Glucotrol, Glucotrol-XL)	10–16	10	5–15 mg q day–bid
Glyburide non-micronized[4] (DiaBeta, Micronase)	24	5	1.25–10 mg q day–bid
Glyburide micronized[4] (Glynase)	24	3	1.5–6 mg q day–bid
Glimepiride (Amaryl)	24	2	1–4 mg q day 8 mg q day[5]

[1]***Indications:*** Management of non-insulin-dependent diabetes mellitus (NIDDM).
[2]***Actions:*** Stimulates the release of insulin from the pancreas; increase insulin sensitivity at peripheral sites; reduces glucose output from the liver.
[3]***Glipizide:*** Give approximately 30 minutes before a meal. Divide total daily doses when doses exceed 15 mg. Maximum daily recommended daily dose is 40 mg.
[4]***Glyburide:*** Administer with first main meal. Maximum recommended daily dose non-micronized, 20 mg; micronized, 12 mg.
[5]Given with the first main meal in patients receiving low-dose insulin.

TABLE 7–14. PROTON PUMP INHIBITORS.[1–3]

	Duodenal Ulcer	Gastric Ulcer	Hypersecretory Conditions	GERD		*H pylori* Eradication
				Healing	Maintenance	
Esomeprazole (Nexium)[2] –Delayed-release capsules: 20, 40 mg				20–40 mg q day × 4–8 wks	20 mg q day	40 mg q day; Amoxicillin 1 g bid, & Clarithromycin 500 mg bid × 10 days
Lansoprazole (Prevacid) –Delayed-release capsules: 15, 30 mg	15 mg q day × 4 wks	30 mg q day × 8 wks	60 mg q day up to 90 mg bid (divide doses > 120 mg/d	15–30 mg q day × 8 wks	15 mg q day	30 mg bid; Amoxicillin 1 g bid; & Clarithromycin 500 mg bid × 14 days
Omeprazole (Prilosec) –Delayed-release capsules: 10, 20, 40 mg	20 mg q day × 4–8 wks	40 mg q day × 4–8 wks	60 mg q day up to 120 mg tid (divide doses > 80 mg/d)	20–40 mg q day × 4–8 wks	20 mg q day	20 mg bid; Amoxicillin 1 g bid & Clarithromycin 500 mg bid × 10 days **OR** 40 mg q day & Clarithromycin 500 mg tid × 14 days
Pantoprazole (Protonix)[3] –Delayed-release tablet: 40 mg				40 mg × 8 wks		
Rabeprazole (Aciphex) –Delayed-release tablet: 20 mg	20 mg q day × 4 wks	60 mg q day	20 mg × 4–8 wks	20 mg q day		

Notes:

[1] All products are delayed-release formulations. Swallow whole—do not crush or chew.

[2] If patient has dificulty swallowing the capsule, open delayed-release capsule and mix the pellets inside the capsule in 1 tablespoon of applesauce. Swallow immediately—do not chew or crush pellets.

[3] Pantoprazole is now available in an IV formulation.

TABLE 7–15. HMG-CoA REDUCTASE INHIBITORS.[1–3]

	Dose	Comparative Dosages	Hydrophilic/ Lipophilic	Metabolism	LFT Monitoring
Atorvastatin (Lipitor) Tablet: 10, 20, 40, 80 mg	10–80 mg q day	5 mg	Lipophilic	P450 3A4	Baseline or elevation of dose, 12 wks, semiannually
Fluvastatin (Lescol) Capsule: 20, 40 mg	20–80 mg q day	20 mg	Lipophilic	P450 2C9	Baseline or elevation of dose, 12 wks, semiannually
Lovastatin (Mevacor) Tablet: 10, 20, 40 mg	10–80 mg q day	20 mg	Lipophilic	P450 3A4	Baseline or elevation of Dose, 6 wks, 12 wks, semiannually
Pravastatin (Pravachol) Tablet: 10, 20, 40 mg	10–40 mg q day	20 mg	Hydrophilic	Not extensively metabolized	Baseline or elevation of dose, 12 wks
Simvastatin (Zocor) Tablet: 10, 20, 40, 80 mg	10–80 mg q day	10 mg	Lipophilic	P450 3A4	Baseline or elevation of dose, semiannually

Notes:

1. Pregnancy category X.
2. Maximum response occurs in 4–6 weeks.
3. Counsel patients to report unexplained muscle pain, tenderness or weakness due to risk of myopathy, or jaundice and abdominal pain due to the risk of hepatic injury.

TABLE 7–16. NON-ANTIBIOTIC DRUG LEVELS.[1]

Drug	Therapeutic Level	Toxic Level
Carbamazepine	8.0–12.0 μg/mL	> 15.0 μg/mL
Digoxin	0.8–2.0 ng/mL	> 2.0 ng/mL
Ethanol		> 80–100 mg/100 mL (legally intoxicated) 100–200 mg/100 mL (labile) 150–300 mg/100 mL (confusion) 250–400 mg/100 mL (stupor) 350–500 mg/100 mL (coma) > 450 mg/100 mL (death)
Ethosuximide	40–100 μg/mL	> 150 μg/mL
Lidocaine	1.5–6.5 μg/mL	> 6.5 μg/mL
Lithium	0.6–1.2 mmol/L	> 2.0 mmol/L
Phenobarbital	15.0–40.0 μg/mL	> 45.0 μg/mL
Phenytoin (total)	10.0–20.0 μg/mL	> 20.0 μg/mL
Phenytoin (free)	1–2 μg/mL	> 2.0 μg/mL
Procainamide	4.0–10.0 μg/mL	> 16.0 μg/mL
N-acetylprocainamide (NAPA-active metabolite of procainamide)	5.0–30.0 μg/mL	> 40.0 μg/mL
Quinidine	3.0–5.0 μg/mL	> 7 μg/mL
Salicylate	20–30 μg/mL	40–50 μg/mL
Tacrolimus	5–15 ng/mL	
Theophylline	5–15 μg/mL	> 20.0 μg/mL
Valproic acid	50–100 μg/mL	> 150 μg/mL

Note: Each lab may have its own set of values that vary slightly from those given.
[1]*Modified and reproduced with permission from Gomella LG, ed.* Clinician's Pocket Reference. *9th ed. McGraw-Hill; 2002.*

TABLE 7–17. THERAPEUTIC DRUG LEVELS: ANTIBIOTICS.[1]

Antibiotic	Trough (μg/mL) Maintain Below Upper Limit)	Peak (μg/mL)
Amikacin	5.0–7.5	25–35
Gentamicin	1.0–2.0	5–8
Gentamicin (24-hour dosing with normal renal function)	1.0–2.0	> 10
Tobramycin	1.0–2.0	5–8
Tobramycin (24-hour dosing with normal renal function)	1.0–2.0	> 10
Vancomycin	5.0–10.0	20–40

[1]*Modified and reproduced with permission from Gomella LG, ed.* Clinician's Pocket Reference. *9th ed. McGraw-Hill; 2002.*

TABLE 7–18. AMINOGLYCOSIDE DOSING IN ADULTS: EVERY 8- OR 12-HOUR DOSING[1] (FOR Q DAY DOSING OF GENTAMICIN AND TOBRAMYCIN SEE PAGES 616 AND 617, RESPECTIVELY).

1. Select the loading dose:
   Gentamicin 1.5–2.0 mg/kg
   Tobramycin 1.5–2.0 mg/kg
   Amikacin 5.0–7.5 mg/kg
2. Calculate the estimated creatinine clearance (CrCl) based on serum creatinine (SCr), age, and weight (kg); OR order a formal creatinine clearance, if time permits.

   $$\text{CrCl for male} = \frac{(140 - \text{age} \times \text{weight in kg})}{(\text{ScCr} \times 72)} \times 100.$$

   CrCl for female = 0.85 × (CrCl male)
3. By using Table 7–19, p XXX, you can now select the maintenance dose (as a percentage of the chosen loading dose) most appropriate for the patient's renal function based on CrCl and dosing interval. Shaded areas are the percentages and intervals suggested for any given creatinine clearance. For patients over 60 years old, it is recommended to give the dose no more frequently than every 12 hours.
4. Empiric dosing, as above, is used to begin therapy. Serum levels (see Table 7–17, p 613) should be monitored and adjustments made in the dosing based on the drug levels for optimal therapy.

Note: See Table 7–17, p 613, for the trough and peak levels of the aminoglycosides gentamicin, tobramycin, and amikacin. Peak levels should be drawn 30 minutes after the dose is completely infused; trough levels should be drawn 30 minutes prior to dose. As a general rule, draw the peak and trough around the fourth maintenance dose. Therapy can be initiated with the recommended guidelines. **These calculations are not valid for netilmicin.**

[1]*Modified and reproduced with permission from Gomella LG, ed.* Clinician's Pocket Reference. *9th ed. McGraw-Hill; 2002.*

TABLE 7–19. AMINOGLYCOSIDE DOSING: PERCENTAGE OF LOADING DOSE REQUIRED FOR DOSAGE INTERVAL SELECTED.[1]

Creatinine Clearance (mL/min)	Dosing Interval (hr)		
	8	12	24
90	90%	—	—
80	88	—	—
70	84	—	—
60	79	91%	—
50	74	87	—
40	66	80	—
30	57	72	92%
25	51	66	88
20	45	59	83
15	37	50	75
10	29	40	64
7	24	33	55
5	20	28	48
2	14	20	35
0	9	13	25

Note: Shaded areas indicate suggested dosage intervals.

[1] *Reproduced with permission from Hull JH, Sarubbi FA: Gentamicin serum concentrations: Pharmacokinetic predictions.* Ann Intern Med *1976;85:183–189.*

TABLE 7–20. AMINOGLYCOSIDE DOSING: ONCE-DAILY DOSING OF GENTAMICIN AND TOBRAMYCIN (*NOT* AMIKACIN).[1]

Several studies suggest that larger doses of aminoglycosides given once daily are just as effective, and less toxic, than conventional dosing given three times a day. Once-daily dosing of gentamicin and tobramycin regimens takes advantage of concentration-dependent killing through the optimization of peak concentration/MIC rations. In addition, there are potential cost savings for nursing, pharmacy, and laboratory personnel.

Inclusion Criteria: All patients ordered aminoglycosides for prophylaxis, empiric therapy, or documented infection. (Aminoglycosides are usually indicated as synergistic or adjunctive therapy with other antibiotics as double coverage for gram-negative infections.)

Exclusion Criteria:

1. Patients with ascites
2. Patients with burns on > 20% of body surface
3. Pregnant patients
4. Patients receiving dialysis
5. Patients with gram-positive bacterial endocarditis
6. Pediatric patients

Initial Dose: Doses will be based on **DOSING BODY WEIGHT**, ideal body weight plus 40% of estimated adipose tissue mass (*see Dosing Guidelines*). Patients with estimated $Cl_{cr} \geq 40$ mL/min/1.73 m^2 will receive initial gentamicin dose of 7 mg/kg-DBW, infused over 30 minutes. Patients with estimated creatinine clearances < 40 mL/min/1.73 m^2 will receive an initial gentamicin dose of 3 mg/kg, infused over 30 minutes.

Monitoring: Two random concentrations will be obtained to monitor. Once-daily dosing of gentamicin and tobramycin:

The ***1st random*** concentration will be drawn ***4 hours**** after completion of the ***1st*** dose. The average 4-hour random sample, with a 7 mg/kg dose will be ~ 13–15 mg/L 4 hours after a 30-minute infusion. ***Note:*** *The Therapeutic Drug Monitoring Lab should be notified that the expected gentamicin/tobramycin level will be greater than 10 mg/L.*

The ***2nd random*** concentration will be drawn ***12 hours*** after completion of the ***1st*** dose.

The rationale for the 4-hour sample versus a "peak" is to determine the serum concentration after the distribution phase. A study (Jennings HJ, Davis GA, June 2000) was conducted at the University of Kentucky Medical Center that demonstrated a prolonged distribution phase following a 7 mg/kg dose in trauma surgery patients.

Subsequent Doses: Scr/BUN should be measured at baseline and 2 times per week thereafter. Subsequent doses will be the same as the initial dose, but the dosing intervals will be adjusted to achieve troughs ***less than or equal to 1 mg/L.*** Appropriate dosing intervals include every 24, 36, or 48 hours.

If the serum concentration following a 7 mg/kg dose requires > 48 hours to decline to 1 mg/L, then 3 mg/kg or conventional dosing may be warranted. Some patients may have a prolonged "drug-free" period that may warrant conventional dosing to maintain concentrations. Patients should not receive a single dose of 7 mg/kg more frequently than every 24 hours until more studies are available.

(*continued*)

TABLE 7–20. AMINOGLYCOSIDE DOSING: ONCE-DAILY DOSING OF GENTAMICIN AND TOBRAMYCIN (*NOT* AMIKACIN) (*continued*).

INITIAL DOSING GUIDELINES FOR ADULTS:

1. Estimate Creatinine Clearance (Cl_{cr}) using Actual Body Weight (ABW) for nonobese patients; in obese patients (> *125% IBW*) use Dosing Body Weight (see below for equation).

$$\text{Males} \quad Cl_{cr} = \frac{(140 - \text{Age}) \times \text{ABW}}{72 \times \text{Scr}} \qquad \text{Females} \quad Cl_{cr} = Cl_{cr} \times 0.85$$

2. Estimate Body Surface Area (BSA) using the Mosteller equation:

$$\text{BSA}(\text{m}^2) = \frac{\sqrt{\text{Ht(cm)} \times \text{Wt (kg)}}}{60}$$ **(Mosteller; *N Engl J Med* 1987;317:109**

3. Calculate Standardized Creatinine Clearance:

$$Cl_{cr(Std)} = Cl_{cr} \times \frac{1.73\text{m}^2}{\text{BSA}}$$

4. Determine Ideal Body Weight (IBW).

$$\text{IBW (kg)} = 50\ \text{(kg)} + (2.3\ \text{(kg)} \times \text{ea. inch over 5 ft})\ \text{male}$$
$$= 45\ \text{(kg)} + (2.3\ \text{(kg)} \times \text{ea. inch over 5 ft})\ \text{female}$$

5. Calculate Dosing Body Weight (DBW):

$$\text{DBW} = \text{IBW} + 0.4\,(\text{ABW} - \text{IBW})$$
(*If ABW < IBW, then DBW = ABW*)

6. Calculate the patient's dose based on Dosing Body Weight:
   a) **If Clcr(std) ≥ 40 mL/min/1.73 m^2, then give 7 mg/kg – DBW.**
   b) **If Clcr(std) < 40 mL/min/1.73 m^2, then give 3 mg/kg – DBW.**

Dilute dose in 100 mL of either 5% Dextrose or Normal Saline and infuse over 30 minutes.

Order two random concentrations at **4 and 12 hours** after the end of 1st dose. *Notify lab of the patient's name to allow for proper dilution of sample.*

[1] *Modified and reproduced with permission from Davis GA:* Clinical Pharmacokinetics Service Policy and Procedural Manual. *23rd ed. University of Kentucky Medical Center; 2000.*

Appendix

CONTENTS

Item	Description	Page
Table A–1	Fahrenheit/centigrade temperature conversion	618
Table A–2	Pounds/kilograms weight conversion	619
Table A–3	Glasgow Coma Scale	619
Figure A–1	Calculating body surface area	620
Table A–4	Endocarditis prophylaxis	621
Table A–5	Specimen tubes for venipuncture	622

TABLE A–1. FAHRENHEIT/CENTIGRADE TEMPERATURE CONVERSION.[1]

°F	°C	°C	°F
95.0	35.0	35.0	95.0
96.0	35.5	35.5	95.9
97.0	36.1	36.0	95.8
98.0	36.6	36.5	97.7
98.6	37.0	37.0	98.6
99.0	37.2	37.5	99.5
100.0	37.7	38.0	100.4
101.0	38.3	38.5	101.3
102.0	38.8	39.0	102.2
103.0	39.4	39.5	103.1
104.0	40.0	40.0	104.0
105.0	40.5	40.5	104.9
106.0	41.1	41.0	105.8
°C = (°F – 32) × 5/9		°F = (°C × 95) ÷ 32	

[1]*Modified and Reproduced with permission from Gomella LG, ed. Clinician's Pocket Reference. 9th ed. McGraw-Hill; 2002.*

TABLE A–2. POUNDS/KILOGRAMS WEIGHT CONVERSION.[1]

lb	kg	kg	lb
1	0.5	1	2.2
2	0.9	2	4.4
4	1.8	3	6.6
6	2.7	4	8.8
8	3.6	5	11.0
10	4.5	6	13.2
20	9.1	8	17.6
30	13.6	10	22.0
40	18.2	20	44.0
50	22.7	30	66.0
60	27.3	40	88.0
70	31.8	50	110.0
80	36.4	60	132.0
90	40.9	70	154.0
100	45.4	80	176.0
150	68.2	90	198.0
200	90.8	100	220.0
kg = lb × 0.454		lb = kg × 2.2	

[1]*Reproduced with permission from Gomella LG, ed. Clinician's Pocket Reference. 9th ed. McGraw-Hill; 2002.*

TABLE A–3. GLASGOW COMA SCALE.[1]

Parameter	Response		Score
Eyes	Open	Spontaneously	4
		To verbal command	3
		To pain	2
		No response	1
Best motor response	To verbal command	Obeys	6
	To painful stimulus	Localizes pain	5
		Flexion-withdrawal	4
		Decorticate (flex)	3
		Decerebrate (extend)	2
		No response	1
Best verbal response		Oriented, converses	5
		Disoriented, converses	4
		Inappropriate responses	3
		Incomprehensible sounds	2
		No response	1

Note: The Glasgow Coma Scale (EMV Scale) is a fairly reliable and objective way to monitor changes in levels of consciousness. It is based on eye opening, motor responses, and verbal responses (EMV). A person's EMV score is based on the total of the three different responses. The score ranges from 3 (lowest) to 15 (highest).
[1]*Modified and reproduced with permission from Gomella LG, ed.* Clinician's Pocket Reference. *9th ed. McGraw-Hill; 2002.*

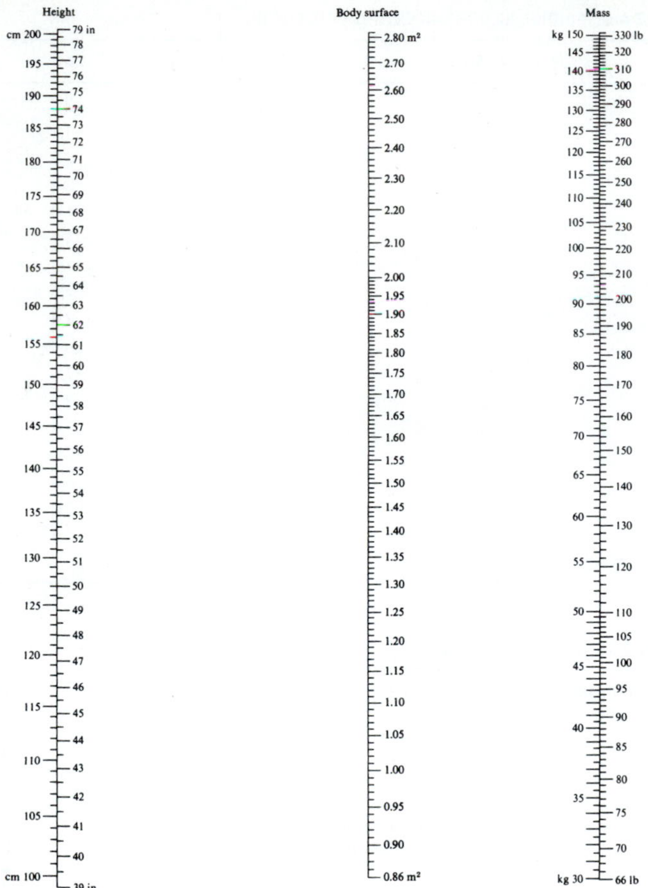

Figure A–1. Calculating body surface area. To determine the body surface of an adult, use a straightedge to connect height and mass. The point of intersection in the body surface line gives the body surface area in meters squared (m^2). (Reproduced with permission from Lentner C, ed. *Geigy Scientific Tables.* Vol 1. 8th ed. Basel: CIBA-Geigy;1981:227.

TABLE A–4. ENDOCARDITIS PROPHYLAXIS.[1,2,3]

Agent	Regimen
■ Dental and upper respiratory procedures[3]	
Oral	
Amoxicillin[4]	2 g PO 1 hr before procedure
Penicillin allergy:	
Clindamycin	600 mg PO 1 hr before procedure
OR	
Cephalexin[5] OR Cefadroxil[5]	2 g PO 1 hr before procedure
OR	
Azithromycin or Clarithromycin	500 mg PO 1 hr before procedure
Parenteral	
Ampicillin	2 g IV or IM 30 min before procedure
Penicillin allergy:	
Clindamycin	600 mg IV within 30 min before procedure
OR	
Cefazolin[5]	1 g IV or IM within 30 min before procedure
■ Gastrointestinal and genitourinary procedures[3]	
Oral	
Amoxicillin[4]	2 g PO 1 hr before procedure
Parenteral[6]	
Ampicillin	2 g IV or 1 M within 30 min before procedure
plus/minus	
Gentamicin	1.5 mg/kg (120 mg maximum dose) IV or IM 30 min before procedure
Penicillin allergy:[6]	
Vancomycin	1 g IV infused *slowly over 1 hr* beginning 1 hr before procedure
plus/minus	
Gentamicin	1.5 mg/kg (120 maximum dose) IV or IM 30 min before procedure

[1] *Modified and reproduced with permission from* Med Lett *1999;41:80.*

[2] For patients with previous endocarditis, valvular heart disease, prosthetic heart valves, or complex cyanotic congenital heart disease (eg, tetralogy of Fallot), the risk is considered high. The risk is also considered high enough to treat in patients with other forms of congenital heart disease (but not uncomplicated secundum atrial septal defect), acquired valvular disease (eg, rheumatic heart disease), hypertrophic cardiomyopathy, and mitral valve prolapse with regurgitation or thickened valve leaflets. Viridans streptococci are the most likely cause of bacterial endocarditis after dental or upper respiratory procedures; enterococci are the most common cause of endocarditis after gastrointestinal or genitourinary procedures.

[3] For a review of the risk of bacteremia and endocarditis with various procedures, see Dajani AS, Taubert KA, Wilson W et al: Prevention of bacterial endocarditis: Recommendations by the American Heart Association. *JAMA* 1997;277:1794; and Durack DT: Prophylaxis of infective endocarditis. In: Mandell GL, Bennet JE, Dolin R, eds. *Principles and Practice of Infectious Diseases.* 5th ed. Churchill Livingstone; 2000:917. Among dental procedures, tooth extraction and gingival surgery (including implant placement) are thought to have the highest risk for bacterial endocarditis (Durack DT: Antibiotics for prevention of endocarditis during dentistry: Time to scale back? *Ann Intern Med* 1998;129:829.

[4] Amoxicillin is recommended because of its excellent bioavailability and good activity against streptococci and enterococci.

[5] Not recommended for patients with a history of immediate-type allergic reaction to penicillin (eg, urticaria, angioedema, anaphylaxis).

[6] Gentamicin should be added for patients with a high risk for bacterial endocarditis (see footnote 1). High-risk patients given parenteral ampicillin before the procedure should receive a dose of ampicillin 1 g IV or IM or a dose of amoxicillin 1 g PO 6 hours after the first dose.

TABLE A–5. SPECIMEN TUBES FOR VENIPUNCTURE.[1]

Tube Color	Additives	General Use
Red	None	Clot tube to collect serum for chemistry, cross-matching, serology
Red and black (hot pink)	Silicone gel for rapid clot	As above, but not for osmolality or blood bank work
Blue	Sodium citrate (binds calcium)	Coagulation studies (best kept on ice, not for fibrin split products)
Blue/yellow label		Fibrin split products
Royal blue		Heavy metals, arsenic
Purple	Disodium EDTA (binds calcium)	Hematology, not for lipid profiles
Green	Sodium heparin	Ammonia, cortisol, ionized calcium (best kept on ice)
Green/glass beads		LE prep
Gray	Sodium fluoride	Lactic acid
Yellow	Transport medium	Blood cultures

Note: Individual labs may vary slightly from these listings.

[1] *Reproduced with permission from Gomella LG, Lefor AT:* Surgery On Call. *3rd ed. McGraw-Hill; 2001.*

Subject Index

NOTE: Page numbers in **boldface** type indicate a major discussion. A *t* following a page number indicates tabular material, and an *f* following a page number indicates a figure. Drugs are listed under their generic names. When a drug trade name is listed, the reader is referred to the generic name.

A
A-K Beta. *See* Levobunolol
A wave, cannon
 in bradycardia, 41–42
 in tachycardia, 328
Abacavir, 470
Abbokinase. *See* Urokinase
Abciximab, 470
 for myocardial infarction, 65
Abdomen, examination of
 in abdominal pain, 4–5
 in acidosis, 15
 in alcohol withdrawal/delirium tremens, 93
 in alkalosis, 22
 in anemia, 30
 in coagulopathy, 69
 in coma/acute mental status changes, 79
 in constipation, 82, 84
 in diarrhea, 101
 in dysuria, 119
 in fever, 130
 in HIV-positive patient, 138
 Foley catheter problems and, 142
 in hematemesis/melena, 159
 in hematochezia, 164
 in hematuria, 168
 in hemoptysis, 173
 in hypercalcemia, 177
 in hyperglycemia, 181
 in hypokalemia, 208
 in hypomagnesemia, 212
 in hyponatremia, 218
 in hypotension, 226
 in hypothermia, 231
 in jaundice, 243
 in leukocytosis, 253
 in leukopenia, 258
 in nausea and vomiting, 264
 in oliguria/anuria, 270
 in overdose, 278
 pain management and, 288
 in polycythemia, 293
 in pruritus, 300
 in shock, 226
 in tachycardia, 328
 in thrombocytopenia, 336
 in ventilator patient with high peak pressures, 457
Abdominal compartment syndrome, high peak pressures and, 457
Abdominal computed tomography
 in constipation, 85
 in hypotension/shock, 227
 in polycythemia, 294
 in thrombocytopenia, 337
Abdominal migraine, 4
Abdominal pain, **1–9**
 characteristics/location of, 1–2
 diarrhea and, 2, 98
 differential diagnosis/causes of, 2–4, 3*t*
 extra-abdominal disease causing, 4
 hematuria and, 2, 6, 166
 imaging/clinical studies in, 6–7
 urgent surgery and, 8*t*
 initial evaluation of, 1–2
 intra-abdominal disease causing, 2–3, 3*t*
 jaundice and, 242
 laboratory findings/data in, 5–6
 management of, 7–8, 8*t*
 nausea and vomiting and, 2, 262
 oliguria/anuria and, 267, 271
 physical examination/findings in, 4–5, 5*t*, 288
 urgent surgery and, 8*t*
 in special populations, 4
 surgery for, 8, 8*t*
Abdominal plain films (KUB)
 in abdominal pain, 6
 in constipation, 84
 in fever, 131
 in hematuria, 169
 in hypercalcemia, 178
 in nausea and vomiting, 265
 in overdose, 279
Abdominal surgery
 diarrhea and, 100
 hematuria after, 166
 leukocytosis and, 252
Abdominal trauma, leukocytosis and, 252
Abelcet. *See* Amphotericin B lipid complex
ABG. *See* Arterial blood gases
ABO incompatibility, transfusion reaction and, 339
Absolute neutrophil count, 255
AC (assist control) ventilation, 445
Acanthocytes (burr cells), 378
Acarbose, 470
 for hyperglycemia, 183
Accelerated hypertension, 196
 management of, 198
Accelerated idioventricular rhythm, 327
Accessory muscles of breathing, use of in dyspnea, 113
Accolate. *See* Zafirlukast
Accupril. *See* Quinapril
Accutane. *See* Isotretinoin
ACE inhibitors (angiotensin-converting enzyme inhibitors), 598*t*
Acebutolol, 601*t*
Aceon. *See* Perindopril
Acetaminophen, 289, 471
 for alcohol withdrawal/delirium tremens, 96
 with butalbital and caffeine, 471
 with codeine, 290, 471
 with hydrocodone, 525
 with hydrocodone/chlorpheniramine/phenylephrine/caffeine, 526
 with isometheptene and dichloralphenazone, for

Acetaminophen, *(cont)*
migraine headache, 150
overdose/toxicity of, 276
antidote for, 282
with oxycodone, 290, 556
in pain management, 289
with propoxyphene, 565
Acetazolamide, 471
Acetic acid derivatives, as nonsteroidal anti-inflammatory drugs, 605*t*
Acetoacetate, in hyperglycemia, 182
Acetohexamide, 610*t*
Acetretin, 470–471
Acetylcysteine/*N*-acetylcysteine, 471–472
for acetaminophen overdose/toxicity, 282
N-Acetylprocainamide (NAPA), therapeutic/toxic levels of, 613*t*
Achromycin V. *See* Tetracycline
Acid aspiration, 36
Acid-fast organisms, pulmonary disease in HIV-positive patient and, 136–137
Acid-fast stain, **345**
Acidemia, 9. *See also* Acidosis
coma/acute mental status changes and, 74
differential diagnosis/causes of, 11–15
pacemaker failure to capture and, 284
Acidosis, **9–18**
cardiopulmonary arrest and, 45, 46
characteristics of, 9–11, 350*t*
coma/acute mental status changes and, 74
compensation in, 11, 350*t*
differential diagnosis/causes of, 11–15
hyperkalemia and, 187
hypophosphatemia and, 221
imaging/clinical studies in, 16
initial evaluation of, 9–11
laboratory findings/data in, 15–16
management of, 16–18
nausea and vomiting and, 263
pacemaker failure to capture and, 284
physical examination/findings in, 15
Aciphex. *See* Rabeprazole
Aconite, toxicity of, 593
Acoustic neuromas, dizziness/vertigo and, 106
Acova. *See* Argatroban
Acquired immunodeficiency syndrome (AIDS). *See* HIV infection/AIDS
Acromegaly, hypercalcemia and, 176
ACTH (adrenocorticotropic hormone), **345**
ectopic/excess production of
hypokalemia and, 207
leukocytosis and, 253
ACTH (Cortrosyn) stimulation test, **345**
in hyponatremia, 218
in hypothermia, 231–232
Actidose. *See* Charcoal, activated
Actimmune. *See* Interferon gamma-1b
Actiq. *See* Fentanyl, transmucosal system
Activase. *See* Alteplase
Activated charcoal, 492
for overdose, 280
Actonel. *See* Risedronate
Actos. *See* Pioglitazone
Acular. *See* Ketorolac, ophthalmic
Acute abdomen. *See* Abdominal pain
Acute lung injury, mechanical ventilation for, 442
Acute respiratory distress syndrome (ARDS)
dyspnea and, 112
high peak pressures in ventilator patient and, 456
hypoxemia in ventilator patient and, 451
mechanical ventilation for, 442
Acute tubular necrosis
dopamine for, 273
hypernatremia and, 191
oliguria/anuria/acute renal failure and, 268, 273
urinary indices in, 386*t*
Acyclovir, 472
ADA (American Diabetes Association) diet, 184
Adalat/Adalat CC. *See* Nifedipine
Adapin. *See* Doxepin
Addisonian crisis
coma/acute mental status changes and, 75
management of, 134, 229
Addison's disease
diarrhea in, 99
hyponatremia and, 216
nausea and vomiting and, 264
Adenocard. *See* Adenosine
Adenosine, 472
for tachycardia, 330
Adrenal gland disorders. *See also* Adrenal insufficiency
ACTH/ACTH stimulation tests in evaluation of, **345**
coma/acute mental status changes and, 75
Adrenal insufficiency
hypercalcemia and, 176
hyperkalemia and, 188
hyponatremia and, 214
hypothermia and, 230
nausea and vomiting and, 263
Adrenalin. *See* Epinephrine
Adrenocorticotropic hormone (ACTH), **345**
ectopic/excess production of
hypokalemia and, 207
leukocytosis and, 253
Adrenocorticotropic hormone (ACTH/Cortrosyn) stimulation test, **345**
in hyponatremia, 218
in hypothermia, 231–232
Adrenogenital syndrome, hypokalemia and, 208
Adriamycin. *See* Doxorubicin
Adrucil. *See* Fluorouracil
Advil. *See* Ibuprofen
AeroBid. *See* Flunisolide
AFP. *See* Alpha-fetoprotein
Afrinol. *See* Pseudoephedrine
Afterload reduction, for pulmonary edema, 344
Agenerase. *See* Amprenavir
Aggrastat. *See* Tirofiban
Aggrenox. *See* Dipyridamole, with aspirin
Agitation, in ventilator patient, **447–450**
high peak pressures and, 456–457
AHF. *See* Antihemophilic factor
AIDS. *See* HIV infection/AIDS
Air trapping, agitation in ventilator patient and, 448
Airway obstruction
anaphylaxis and, 25
aspiration and, 37
cardiopulmonary arrest and, 44
respiratory acidosis and, 12
Airway pressure release ventilation (APRV), 445–446
for high peak pressures in ventilator patient, 458

Airway status/management
in alcohol withdrawal/delirium tremens, 91
cardiopulmonary arrest and, 44
hemoptysis and, 174
AIVR. *See* Accelerated idioventricular rhythm
AK-Chlor. *See* Chloramphenicol, ophthalmic
AK-Dex Ophthalmic. *See* Dexamethasone, ophthalmic
AK-Mycin. *See* Erythromycin, ophthalmic
AK-Neo-Dex Ophthalmic. *See* Neomycin, with dexamethasone, ophthalmic
AK-Poly Bac Ophthalmic. *See* Bacitracin, with polymyxin B, ophthalmic
AK-Pred. *See* Prednisolone, ophthalmic
AK-Spore HC Ophthalmic. *See* Bacitracin, with polymyxin B and neomycin and hydrocortisone, ophthalmic
AK-Spore Ophthalmic. *See* Bacitracin, with polymyxin B and neomycin, ophthalmic
AK-Tob. *See* Tobramycin, ophthalmic
AK-Tracin Ophthalmic. *See* Bacitracin, ophthalmic
Alamast. *See* Pemirolast
Alanine aminotransferase (ALT/SGPT), **346–347**
in jaundice, 243
in nausea and vomiting, 265
pain management and, 289
Albalon-A. *See* Naphazoline, with antazoline
Albumin
in diarrhea, 101
electrophoresis values for, 374*f*, 375*t*
in hypercalcemia, 177, 178
in hypocalcemia, 200
in hypophosphatemia, 222
serum calcium affected by, 177, 199, 200
serum levels of, **345**
therapeutic, 472
urine levels of, **346**
Albumin gradient, ascitic fluid, 421*t*
Albuminar. *See* Albumin, therapeutic
Albutein. *See* Albumin, therapeutic
Albuterol, 472
for bronchospasm, 344
for dyspnea in asthma, 116
hypokalemia and, 207
with ipratropium, 472–473
Alcohol use/abuse
coma/acute mental status changes and, 73, 74
gastrointestinal bleeding and hematemesis/melena, 158
hematochezia, 162
hypertension and, 195
hypoglycemia and, 203
hypomagnesemia and, 211
hypophosphatemia and, 94, 96, 221
insomnia and, 234, 235
jaundice and, 242, 245
leukopenia and, 256
metabolic acidosis and, 16
nausea and vomiting and, 262
seizures and, 91, 309, 314
toxic levels and, 613*t*
withdrawal and, **90–97**. *See also* Alcohol withdrawal
Alcohol withdrawal, **90–97**. *See also* Alcohol use/abuse
differential diagnosis of delirium and, 91–93
hypertension and, 195
imaging/clinical studies in, 94–95
initial evaluation in, 90–91
laboratory findings/data in, 94
management of, 95–96
physical examination/findings in, 93–94
seizures and, 91, 309, 314
Alcoholic ketoacidosis, 13, 17
Alcoholic liver disease, jaundice and, 242, 245
Alcoholism. *See* Alcohol use/abuse
Aldactone. *See* Spironolactone
Aldara. *See* Imiquimod cream, 5%
Aldaztazide. *See* Hydrochlorothiazide, with spironolactone
Aldesleukin, 473
Aldomet. *See* Methyldopa
Aldosterone levels, **346**
in hyperkalemia, 189
Aldosteronism
hypernatremia and, 192
hypertension and, 195
hypokalemia and, 207
hypomagnesemia and, 211
metabolic alkalosis and, 22
Alendronate, 473
Aleve. *See* Naproxen sodium
Alka-Mints. *See* Calcium carbonate
Alkalemia, 18–19. *See also* Alkalosis
coma/acute mental status changes and, 74
differential diagnosis/causes of, 20–22
Alkaline phosphatase, **346**
in abdominal pain, 6
in hypercalcemia, 177
in jaundice, 243
leukocyte. *See* Leukocyte alkaline phosphatase (LAP) score
in nausea and vomiting, 265
pain management and, 289
Alkalinization of urine, in overdose management, 282
Alkalosis, **18–24**
cardiopulmonary arrest and, 45
characteristics of, 18–20, 350*t*
coma/acute mental status changes and, 74
compensation in, 19–20, 350*t*
differential diagnosis/causes of, 20–22
hypokalemia and, 206
hypophosphatemia and, 222
imaging/clinical studies in, 23
initial evaluation of, 18–20
laboratory findings/data in, 22–23
management of, 23–24
physical examination/findings in, 22
pseudorespiratory, 12, 21
Alkeran. *See* Melphalan
Alkylating agents, for polycythemia vera, 295
Allegra. *See* Fexofenadine
Allen test, 391
arterial line placement and, 390
arterial puncture and, 391
Allergic reactions
pruritus in, 298
wheezing and, 342
management of, 344
Allium sativum (garlic), 591
Allopurinol, 473
Alocril. *See* Nedocromil, ophthalmic
Alomide. *See* Lodoxamide
Aloprim. *See* Allopurinol
Alpha$_2$-adrenergic agonists, for glaucoma, 607*t*

Alpha$_1$-antitrypsin deficiency, protein electrophoresis in, 374*f*
Alpha-fetoprotein (AFP), **346**
Alpha$_1$-globulin, electrophoresis values for, 374*f*, 375*t*
Alpha$_2$-globulin, electrophoresis values for, 374*f*, 375*t*
Alpha$_1$ protease inhibitor, 473
Alphagan. *See* Brimonidine
Alport's syndrome, hematuria in, 167
Alprazolam, 473–474
Alprostadil
 intracavernosal, 474
 urethral suppository, 474
ALT (alanine aminotransferase/SGPT), **346–347**
 in jaundice, 243
 in nausea and vomiting, 265
 pain management and, 289
Altace. *See* Ramipril
Alteplase, recombinant (t-PA), 474
Altered mental status. *See* Mental status
Altered visual input, disequilibrium and, 107
Alternagel. *See* Aluminum hydroxide
Alternative therapies. *See also* Natural products
 for insomnia, 237
Altretamine, 474
Alum. *See* Ammonium aluminum sulfate
Aluminum carbonate, 474
Aluminum hydroxide, 474–475
 with magnesium carbonate, 475
 with magnesium hydroxide, 475
 with magnesium hydroxide and simethicone, 475
 with magnesium trisilicate, 475
Aluminum sulfate, ammonium, 477
Alupent. *See* Metaproterenol
Alveolar filling, hypoxemia in ventilator patient caused by, 451
Alveolar hemorrhage, diffuse, management of, 175
Alveolar hypoventilation
 pO_2 in, 370
 polycythemia and, 292
Amantadine, 475
Amaryl. *See* Glimepiride
Ambien. *See* Zolpidem
Ambisome. *See* Amphotericin B liposomal
Ambu bag
 for cardiopulmonary resuscitation, 44
 for evaluating high peak ventilator pressures, 458
Amcil. *See* Ampicillin
Amerge. *See* Naratriptan
American Diabetes Association (ADA) diet, 184
Amicar. *See* Aminocaproic acid
Amifostine, 475–476
Amikacin, 476
 dosing guidelines for, 614*t*
 therapeutic levels of, 613*t*
Amikin. *See* Amikacin
Amiloride, 476
 with hydrochlorothiazide, 525
Aminocaproic acid, 476
Amino-Cerv pH 5.5 cream, 476
Aminoglutethimide, 476
Aminoglycosides, dosing guidelines for, 614*t*, 615*t*, 616–617*t*
Aminophylline, 476–477
Aminotransferases. *See* Alanine aminotransferase; Aspartate aminotransferase
Amiodarone, 477
 for tachycardia, 330–331
 for ventricular fibrillation, 47
 for ventricular tachycardia
 stable, 47, 49
 unstable, 49
Amitriptyline, 477
 for insomnia, 237
 in pain management, 291
Amlodipine, 477
Ammonia, **347**
Ammonium aluminum sulfate, 477
Ammonium chloride, for metabolic alkalosis, 23
Ammonium hydroxide and lactic acid (ammonium lactate), 533
Amoxapine, 477–478
Amoxicillin, 478
 with clavulanic acid, 478
 for endocarditis prophylaxis, 621*t*
Amoxil. *See* Amoxicillin
Amphetamines
 delirium and, 93
 hypertension and, 194, 195
Amphojel. *See* Aluminum hydroxide
Amphotec. *See* Amphotericin B cholesteryl
Amphotericin B, 478
Amphotericin B cholesteryl, 478
Amphotericin B lipid complex, 478
Amphotericin B liposomal, 479
Ampicillin, 479
 for endocarditis prophylaxis, 621*t*
Ampicillin-sulbactam, 479
Amprenavir, 479
Amylase, **347**
 in abdominal pain, 6
 in hypercalcemia, 178
 in hyperglycemia, 182
 in jaundice, 244
 in nausea and vomiting, 265
ANA. *See* Antinuclear antibodies
Anagrelide, for polycythemia vera, 295
Analgesia, 289–291, 462*t*. *See also specific agent*
 patient-controlled, 291
 spinal, 291
Anaphylactic shock, 24. *See also* Shock
 epinephrine for, 26, 228–229, 510
 management of, 228–229
Anaphylactoid reaction, to gamma-globulin transfusion, 440
Anaphylaxis/anaphylactic reaction, **24–27**
 epinephrine for, 26, 228–229, 510
 pruritus in, 297
Anaprox. *See* Naproxen sodium
Anaspaz. *See* Hyoscyamine
Anastrozole, 479
ANC. *See* Absolute neutrophil count
ANCA. *See* Anti-neutrophil cytoplasmic antibodies
Ancef. *See* Cefazolin
Ancobon. *See* Flucytosine
Anectine. *See* Succinylcholine
Anemia, **27–33**. *See also specific type*
 aplastic, leukopenia and, 257
 blood transfusions for, 32, **437–438**
 of chronic disease, 28, 29, 29*t*, 33
 differential diagnosis/causes of, 29–30, 29*t*
 initial evaluation of, 28
 laboratory findings/data in, 31–32

management of, 32–33
in hypoxemic ventilator patient, 453
physical examination/findings in, 30–31
Anestacon topical. *See* Lidocaine
Aneurysm
cerebral, rupture of, headache and, 146
thoracic, cough and, 87
Angelica polymorpha, sinensis (dong quai), 591
Anger, insomnia and, 236
Angina pectoris, 57, 58. *See also* Chest pain
falls and, 124
heart murmur and, 152, 157
hypertension and, 196
Angiocath, insertion of, 411–412, 413*f*
for paracentesis, 420
Angiodysplasia, hematochezia and, 163
Angiography. *See also specific type*
CT, in hemoptysis, 174
in dyspnea, 115
in hematochezia, 165
in hemoptysis, 174
in hypotension/shock, 227
Angiomatosis, bacillary, in HIV-positive patient, 137
Angiomax. *See* Bivalirudin
Angiotensin-converting enzyme (ACE) inhibitors, 598*t*
cough associated with, 86–87
Angiotensin receptor antagonists, 599*t*
Anion gap, **347**
acidosis and, 12–15, 347
elevated, 13–15
evaluation and, 14–15
normal, 12–13
alkalosis and, 22
calculation of, 12
in hyperglycemia, 182
Anisocytosis, 377
Anistreplase, 479
Ankle, arthrocentesis of, 394, 395*f*
Anorexia, in HIV-positive patient, fever and, 135
Anorexia nervosa, leukopenia and, 256, 257
Anoscopy, in hematochezia, 164
Anoxic encephalopathy, coma/acute mental status changes and, 77
Ansaid. *See* Flurbiprofen
Antabuse. *See* Disulfiram
Antacids, 462*t*. *See also specific agent*
calcium carbonate, metabolic alkalosis and, 22
diarrhea caused by, 99
for gastritis/esophagitis, 66
hypophosphatemia and, 221
Antazoline, with naphazoline, 609*t*
Anthraderm. *See* Anthralin
Anthralin, 479–480
Anti-allergy preparations, ophthalmic, 609*t*
Antianxiety agents, 462*t*. *See also specific agent*
Antiarrhythmics, 462*t*. *See also specific agent*
Antibiotics, 462–463*t*. *See also specific agent*
for aspiration, 39
for diarrhea, 103–104
diarrhea associated with, 99
for endocarditis prophylaxis, 621*t*
for fever, 132
hypokalemia and, 208
ophthalmic, 608*t*. *See also specific agent*
therapeutic levels of, 613*t*
Anticardiolipin antibodies, 349
Anticholinergic agents
for dizziness/vertigo, 110
overdose/toxicity of, 275
antidote for, 281
delirium and, 93
Anticoagulant antibodies, bleeding and, 68
Anticoagulants, 463*t*. *See also specific agent*
headache and, 144
hematuria and, 166
hemoptysis and, 172
Anticonvulsants, 463*t*. *See also specific agent*
hypocalcemia and, 199
levels of, seizures and, 308–309, 312
in pain management, 291
Antidepressants, 463*t*. *See also specific agent*
for chronic tension-type headache, 149
for insomnia, 237
overdose/toxicity of, antidote for, 281
in pain management, 291
Antidiabetic agents, 463–464*t*. *See also specific agent and* Hypoglycemic agents
Antidiarrheal agents, 103, 464*t*. *See also specific agent*
Antidiuretic hormone, 585. *See also* Vasopressin
syndrome of inappropriate secretion of (SIADH)
coma/acute mental status changes and, 76
hyponatremia and, 215, 217
management of, 219–220
Antidotes, 281–282, 464*t*. *See also specific agent*
Antiemetics, 265–266, 464*t*. *See also specific agent*
Antifungal agents, 464*t*. *See also specific agent*
Antigas agents, 462*t*. *See also specific agent*
Anti-GBM antibody. *See* Anti-glomerular basement membrane (anti-GBM) antibody
Antiglobulin testing, direct, post-transfusion, 340
Anti-glomerular basement membrane (anti-GBM) antibody, in hemoptysis, 173
Antigout agents, 464*t*. *See also specific agent*
Anti-HAV, 364*t*, 365
Anti-HBc, 364*t*, 365
Anti-HBe, 364*t*, 365
Anti-HBs, 364*t*, 365
Anti-HCV, 364*t*, 365
Anti-HCV RIBA, 364*t*, 365
Anti-HDV, 364*t*, 365
Antihemophilic factor (factor VIII) therapy, 71, 440, 480
Antihistamines, 464*t*. *See also specific agent*
for anaphylaxis, 26–27
for dizziness/vertigo, 110
for insomnia, 237
for pruritus, 302
Antihistone antibodies, 348
Antihyperlipidemics, 464*t*. *See also specific agent*
Antihypertensives, 197–198, 464–465*t*. *See also specific agent*
diarrhea caused by, 100
for hypertensive emergency, 197–198
overdose/toxicity of, 276
Anti-inflammatory drugs, 462*t*. *See also specific agent*
nonsteroidal. *See* Nonster-

Anti-inflammatory drugs, *(cont)*
oidal anti-inflammatory drugs
Antilirium. *See* Physostigmine
Antimicrosomal antibodies, 348
Antimitochondrial antibodies, 348
Antimotility drugs, 103
Antineoplastic agents, 465*t*. *See also specific agent*
cancer pain and, 288
hematuria and, 166–167
leukopenia and, 256
thrombocytopenia and, management of, 338
Anti-neutrophil cytoplasmic antibodies (ANCA), **347–348**
in hemoptysis, 173
Antinuclear antibodies (ANA), **348**
in arthritis, 249
in leukopenia, 258
in thrombocytopenia, 336
Antiparkinsonism agents, 465*t*. *See also specific agent*
Antiphospholipid antibodies, 349
Antiplatelet agents, for polycythemia vera, 295
Anti-PM-1 antibodies, 348
Antipsychotic agents, 465*t*. *See also specific agent*
Antipyretic agents, 132, 462*t*. *See also specific agent*
for alcohol withdrawal/delirium tremens, 96
Antipyrine and benzocaine, 485
Antiretroviral agents, fever caused by, 136
Antiribonucleoproteins (anti-RNP), 348
Antiseizure agents (anticonvulsants), 463*t*. *See also specific agent*
hypocalcemia and, 199
levels of, seizures and, 308–309, 312
in pain management, 291
Anti-Sm antibodies, 348
Anti-smooth muscle antibodies, 348
Anti-SS antibodies, 348
Antistaphylococcal penicillins, 600*t*
Antithymocyte globulin (ATG), 480
Antithyroid/thyroid agents, 469*t*
α_1-Antitrypsin deficiency, protein electrophoresis in, 374*f*
Antitussive agents, 465–466*t*. *See also specific agent*
Antivert. *See* Meclizine
Antiviral agents, 466*t*. *See also specific agent*
Antizol. *See* Fomepizole
Anturane. *See* Sulfinpyrazone
Anuria, **266–274**. *See also* Oliguria
definition of, 266
Anus, pruritus affecting, 297
Anusol/Anusol-HC, 480, 526, 563
Anxiety
insomnia and, 236
respiratory alkalosis and, 21
syncope and, 317
Anzemet. *See* Dolasetron
Aorta, coarctation of, hypertension and, 195
Aortic dissection
chest pain and, 59, 62, 65
heart murmur and, 152
hypertension and, 196, 198
management of, 65, 198
oliguria/anuria/acute renal failure and, 268
syncope and, 318
Aortic insufficiency, heart murmur and, 152, 154
Aortic stenosis
heart murmur in, 153, 154
syncope and, 318
thrombocytopenia and, 335, 336
Aortoenteric fistula
hematemesis/melena and, 159, 161
management of, 161
Aphonia, in aspiration, 36
Aphthous ulcers, in diarrhea, 101
Apical impulse, in hypertension, 196
Aplastic anemia, leukopenia and, 257
Apnea, sleep, polycythemia and, 292
Apneustic breathing, in coma/acute mental status changes, 78
Appendicitis, nausea and vomiting and, 262
Apraclonidine, 607*t*
Apresoline. *See* Hydralazine
Aprotinin, 480
APRV (airway pressure release ventilation), 445–446
for high peak pressures in ventilator patient, 458
AquaMephyton. *See* Phytonadione
Ara-C (cytarabine), 499
Arava. *See* Leflunomide
Ardeparin, 480
ARDS (acute respiratory distress syndrome)
dyspnea and, 112
high peak pressures in ventilator patient and, 456
hypoxemia in ventilator patient and, 451
mechanical ventilation for, 442
Aredia. *See* Pamidronate
Argatroban, 481
Arginine hydrochloride
hyperkalemia and, 187
for metabolic alkalosis, 23
Arginine vasopressin, deamino-8-D (DDAVP), for von Willebrand's disease, 71
Arimidex. *See* Anastrozole
Aristocort. *See* Triamcinolone
Aristospan. *See* Triamcinolone
Arms. *See also* Extremities
pruritus affecting, 296
Aromasin. *See* Exemestane
Arrhythmias/dysrhythmias
acidosis and, 9
alkalosis and, 19
central venous line problems and, 53
dyspnea and, 113
falls and, 124
heart murmurs and, 153
in hyperkalemia, 186, 189
in hypokalemia, 206
in hypomagnesemia, 210, 211
in hypothermia, 232
irregular pulse caused by, **238–241**
in overdose, management of, 280
pulmonary artery catheterization and, 428
sinus, 239
syncope and, 318
Artane. *See* Trihexyphenidyl
Arterial blood gases, 350*t*
in abdominal pain, 6
in acidosis, 9, 10, 350*t*
in alcohol withdrawal/delirium tremens, 94
in alkalosis, 19, 20, 350*t*
in aspiration, 38
in cardiopulmonary arrest, 46

in chest pain, 62, 64
in coma/acute mental status changes, 80, 94
in cough, 88
in dyspnea, 114
in fever, in HIV-positive patient, 139
in heart murmur, 156
in hemoptysis, 173
in hypercalcemia, 177
in hyperglycemia, 182
in hyperkalemia, 189
in hypokalemia, 209
in hypophosphatemia, 222
in hypotension, 226
in hypothermia, 232
in irregular pulse, 240
laboratory reference/normal values for, 350*t*
in leukocytosis, 254
in nausea and vomiting, 265
in overdose, 278
in pacemaker complications, 286
in polycythemia, 294
pulmonary artery catheter problems and, 305
sample collection for, **391–392**
in seizures, 312
in shock, 226
in tachycardia, 328
in ventilator patient, 447–448
agitation and, 449
high peak pressures and, 456, 457
hypercarbia and, 454, 455
hypoxemia and, 450, 452
in wheezing, 343
Arterial line, **390–391**
for monitoring patient with heart murmur, 157
problems with, **34–36**
Arterial puncture, **391–392**
Arteriography
in abdominal pain, 7
in oliguria/anuria, 271
Arteriovenous malformation, hemoptysis and, 172
Arteritis, temporal, headache and, 145
Arthritis, 245–250
falls and, 124
imaging/clinical studies in, 250
juvenile rheumatoid, 248
laboratory findings/data in, 248–250
management of, 250
monarticular, 246–247
physical examination/findings in, 248
polyarticular, 247–248
psoriatic, 247
reactive, 246
rheumatoid, 248
septic, 246, 249, 250
Arthrocentesis
in arthritis, 248–249
diagnostic and therapeutic, **391–394**, 394*f*, 395*f*
Artificial tears, 481
Asacol. *See* Mesalamine
Ascaris lumbricoides, pruritus caused by, 299
Ascitic fluid, testing, 421*t*. *See also* Paracentesis
Ascorbic acid (vitamin C), 595
ASD. *See* Atrial septal defect
Asendin. *See* Amoxapine
L-Asparaginase, 481
Aspart, 597*t*
Aspartate aminotransferase (AST/SGOT), **349**
in jaundice, 243
in nausea and vomiting, 265
pain management and, 289
Aspergillus fungus ball (mycetoma), hemoptysis and, 171
Aspiration, **36–39**
acid, 36
bronchospasm and, 342
cardiopulmonary arrest and, 45
cough and, 87
dyspnea and, 112
foreign body, 37
stridor and, 201
wheezing and, 342
particulate, 36
in ventilator patient
agitation and, 449
hypoxemia and, 451
wheezing and, 342
Aspirin, 289, 481
for alcohol withdrawal/delirium tremens, 96
anemia and, 28
with butalbital, 481
with butalbital/caffeine/codeine, 481–482
with codeine, 482
with dipyridamole, 506
with hydrocodone, 525
for myocardial infarction, 64, 116
with oxycodone, 290, 556
in pain management, 289
platelet function affected by, 68
for polycythemia vera, 295
with propoxyphene, 565
Reye's encephalopathy and, 76
Assist control (AC) ventilation, 445
AST (aspartate aminotransferase/SGOT), **349**
in jaundice, 243
in nausea and vomiting, 265
pain management and, 289
Astelin. *See* Azelastine
Asthma
cardiac, 342
childhood, reactivation of, 342
cough and, 87, 89
dyspnea and, 112, 115–116
epinephrine for, 510
"factitious," 342
management of, 89, 115–116, 344
respiratory acidosis and, 11
respiratory alkalosis and, 21
Asystole, management of, 50–51, 50–51*f*
Atacand. *See* Candesartan
Atarax. *See* Hydroxyzine
Ataxia, coma/acute mental status changes and, 73
Ataxic breathing, in coma/acute mental status changes, 78
Atelectasis, hypoxemia in ventilator patient caused by, 451, 453
Atenolol, 601*t*
for alcohol withdrawal/delirium tremens, 96
ATG/ATGAM. *See* Antithymocyte globulin
Ativan. *See* Lorazepam
Atorvastatin, 612*t*
Atovaquone, 482
Atracurium, 482
Atrial fibrillation, 239, 325
in coma/acute mental status changes, 79
dyspnea and, 113
hemoptysis and, 172
in hypothermia, 232
syncope and, 318
Atrial flutter, 239, 324–325
syncope and, 318
Atrial myxoma
heart murmur in, 153, 155
syncope and, 318
Atrial premature contractions, 238–239
Atrial pressure, abnormalities

Atrial pressure, *(cont)*
of, pulmonary artery catheter measurements in, 429*t*
Atrial septal defect (ASD), heart murmur in, 153, 155
Atrial tachycardia
multifocal, 326
paroxysmal
with block, 325
syncope and, 318
Atrioventricular (AV) junctional tachycardia, automatic, 325–326
Atrioventricular (AV) nodal reentry tachycardia, 326
Atrioventricular (AV) node blocks, 41, 239–240. *See also specific type and* Heart block
paroxysmal atrial tachycardia and, 325
syncope and, 318
Atrioventricular (AV) reciprocating tachycardia (Wolff-Parkinson-White syndrome), 326
management of, 332
syncope and, 318
Atrophic vaginitis
dysuria and, 118
management of, 121
Atropine, 482
for asystole, 50–51
for bradycardia, 43
with diphenoxylate, 103, 505
with hyoscyamine/scopolamine/phenobarbital, 527
for organophosphate and carbamate toxicity, 282
Atrovent. *See* Ipratropium
Audiometry, in dizziness/vertigo, 109
Auditory canal, external, examination of, in dizziness/vertigo, 107
Auer rods, 389
Augmentin. *See* Amoxicillin, with clavulanic acid
Aura
migraine headache and, 145
seizures and, 308, 316
Auralgan. *See* Benzocaine and antipyrine
Australia antigen. *See* Hepatitis B surface antigen
Autoantibodies, 348
bleeding and, 68
Autoimmune disease
anemia and, 28
hemoptysis and, 172
Automatic atrioventricular junctional tachycardia, 325–326
Automatic supraventricular tachycardias, 325–326
Autonomic hyperactivity, in alcohol withdrawal/delirium tremens, 90
Autonomic insufficiency, syncope and, 317
Autonomic neuropathy, constipation and, 84
Auto-PEEP
agitation in ventilator patient and, 448
high peak pressures and, 456, 457
AV node blocks. *See* Atrioventricular (AV) node blocks
Avandia. *See* Rosiglitazone
Avapro. *See* Irbesartan
Avelox. *See* Moxifloxacin
Aventyl. *See* Nortriptyline
Avilide. *See* Irbesartan, with hydrochlorothiazide
Avita. *See* Tretinoin (retinoic acid), topical
Avlosulfon. *See* Dapsone
Axid. *See* Nizatidine
Azactam. *See* Aztreonam
Azathioprine, 482
Azelastine, 482–483
Azithromycin, 483
for endocarditis prophylaxis, 621*t*
Azmacort. *See* Triamcinolone, inhalation
Azopt. *See* Brinzolamide
Azotemia, prerenal, urinary indices in, 386*t*
AZT. *See* Zidovudine
Aztreonam, 483
Azulfidine. *See* Sulfasalazine

B

B & O Supprettes. *See* Belladonna and opium suppositories
B_{12}. *See* Vitamin B_{12}
Babinski reflex, in seizures, 312
Baciguent. *See* Bacitracin, topical
Bacillary angiomatosis, in HIV-positive patient, 137
Bacillus Calmette-Guérin, 483
Bacillus cereus, diarrhea caused by, 98
Bacitracin
ophthalmic, 484, 608*t*
with polymyxin B
ophthalmic, 484
topical, 483
with polymyxin B and neomycin
ophthalmic, 484
topical, 483
with polymyxin B and neomycin and hydrocortisone
ophthalmic, 484
topical, 483
with polymyxin B and neomycin and lidocaine, topical, 483
topical, 483
Back, examination of, in seizures, 311
Baclofen, 483
Bacteremia, heart murmur and, 152
Bacterial infection. *See also* Infection
diarrhea and, 98
leukocytosis and, 252
leukopenia and, 255
meningitis, cerebrospinal fluid findings in, 419*t*
pneumonia, in HIV-positive patient, 136
Bacterial overgrowth, diarrhea and, 100
Bacterial vaginosis
dysuria and, 118
management of, 121
Bacteriuria, 119
Bactocill. *See* Oxacillin
Bactrim. *See* Trimethoprim-sulfamethoxazole
Bactroban. *See* Mupirocin
Balsalazide disodium, 484
Banded (stab) neutrophils, **387**
laboratory reference/normal values for, 354*t*, 387
Barbiturate withdrawal, 91
Barium
hypokalemia caused by, 206
retained, constipation caused by, 83
Barium enema
in constipation, 85
in diarrhea, 102
Barotrauma, from mechanical ventilation, pneumothorax and, 59
Bartonella (Rochalimaea) henselae, bacillary angiomatosis caused by, in HIV-positive patient, 137

Bartter's syndrome
hypokalemia and, 208
hypomagnesemia and, 211
metabolic alkalosis and, 22
Basaljel. *See* Aluminum carbonate
Base deficit, **349**, 350*t*
Base excess, **349**, 350*t*
in acidosis, 9
in alkalosis, 19
Basilar artery insufficiency, syncope and, 318
Basilic vein, median, for central venous catheterization, 406–407
Basiliximab, 484
Basophilic stippling, 377
Basophils, **388**
laboratory reference/normal values for, 354*t*, 388
Bayer Aspirin. *See* Aspirin
BCNU. *See* Carmustine
BE. *See* Base excess
Becaplormin, 484
Beclomethasone
nasal inhaler, 484
oral metered-dose inhaler, 484–485
Beclovent inhaler. *See* Beclomethasone, oral metered-dose inhaler
Beconase. *See* Beclomethasone, nasal inhaler
Bed rest, prolonged, hypercalcemia and, 176
Beer potomania, hyponatremia and, 217
Belladonna and opium suppositories, 485
Benadryl. *See* Diphenhydramine
Benazepril, 598*t*
Bence–Jones protein, urine, **350**, 373, 374*f*
Benemid. *See* Probenecid
Benign positional vertigo, 105, 105–106
Bentyl. *See* Dicyclomine
Benylin Dm. *See* Dextromethorphan
Benzocaine and antipyrine, 485
Benzodiazepines. *See also specific agent*
for alcohol withdrawal/delirium tremens, 95, 96
for dizziness/vertigo, 110
for insomnia, 237
overdose/toxicity of, antidote for, 281
Benzonatate, 485
Benztropine, 485
for extrapyramidal side effects of antiemetics, 265, 266
Bepridil, 485
Bernard-Soulier syndrome, 68
Beta-adrenergic blocking agents, 601–602*t*
for alcohol withdrawal/delirium tremens, 96
cessation of, rebound hypertension and, 194
for glaucoma, 607*t*
for myocardial infarction, 64, 157
overdose/toxicity of, antidote for, 281
for tachycardia, 331
Beta-globulin, electrophoresis values for, 374*f*, 375*t*
Beta-thalassemia. *See* Thalassemia
Betagan Liquifilm. *See* Levobunolol
Betamethasone, 597*t*
with clotrimazole, 497
Betapace. *See* Sotalol
Betaseron. *See* Interferon beta-1b
Betaxolol, 601*t*
ophthalmic, 607*t*
Betaxon. *See* Levobetaxolol
Bethanechol, 485–486
Betoptic/Betoptic-S, . *See* Betaxolol, ophthalmic
Bexarotene, 486
Biaxin. *See* Clarithromycin
Bicalutamide, 486
Bicarbonate. *See also* Bicarbonate therapy
in body fluids, 436*t*
gastrointestinal loss of, acidosis and, 12–13
in hyperglycemia, 182
in hypophosphatemia, 222
renal loss of, acidosis and, 13
serum levels of, **350–351**, 350*t*
in acidosis, 9–10, 10–11, 350–351, 350*t*
in alkalosis, 19, 350–351, 350*t*
laboratory reference/normal values for, 350, 350*t*
Bicarbonate therapy (sodium bicarbonate), 572
for diabetic ketoacidosis, 185
for hyperkalemia, 189
hypernatremia and, 192
for metabolic acidosis, 17
for overdose, 281
Bicillin. *See* Penicillin G, benzathine
Bicitra. *See* Sodium citrate
BICNU. *See* Carmustine
Bidirectional positive airway pressure (BiPAP), 443
extubation to, 460
for pulmonary edema, 344
for stridor, 344
Bile, composition/daily production of, 436*t*
Bile salt deficiency, hypocalcemia and., 199
Biliary cirrhosis
primary, jaundice and, 242
pruritus in, 298
Biliary colic, 2
chest pain and, 60
jaundice and, 242
nausea and vomiting and, 262
Biliary obstruction
acute, jaundice and, 242
pruritus and, 299
Biliary surgery, jaundice and, 242
Biliary tract disorders, abdominal pain and, 3*t*
Bilirubin, **351**
in abdominal pain, 6
in hypophosphatemia, 222
in jaundice, 243–244
in nausea and vomiting, 265
urine, **383**
Biofeedback, for chronic tension-type headache, 149
BiPAP (bidirectional positive airway pressure), 443
extubation to, 460
for pulmonary edema, 344
for stridor, 344
Birth control pills (oral contraceptives), 554
Bisacodyl, 85*t*, 486
Bismuth subsalicylate, 103, 486
Bisoprolol, 601*t*
Bisphosphonates, for hypercalcemia, 179
Bitolterol, 486
Bivalirudin, 486
Black cohosh, 590
Bladder catheterization, **394–397**
dysuria after catheter removal and, 117
hematuria and, 166
problems with catheter and, **141–143**

Bladder disruption, Foley catheter problems and, 142
Bladder distension, Foley catheter problems and, 141, 142
Bladder irrigation, neomycin-polymyxin for, 549
Bladder outlet obstruction
 management of, 273
 oliguria/anuria and, 267, 273
Bladder spasms
 Foley catheter problems and, 142, 143
 management of, 143
Bleeding/blood loss, **66–72**
 abdominal pain and, 5*t*
 anemia and, 28, 32
 blood transfusions for, 437
 cardiopulmonary arrest and, 45
 differential diagnosis/causes of, 67–68
 imaging/clinical studies in, 70
 initial evaluation of, 67
 laboratory findings/data in, 69–70, 69*t*
 management of, 70–73
 physical examination/findings in, 68–69
 syncope and, 317
 in thrombocytopenia, 333
 management of, 337
 in transfusion reaction, 339
Bleeding scan, technetium-labeled
 in hematemesis/melena, 160
 in hematochezia, 165
Bleeding time, **351**
 in coagulopathy, 70
Blenoxane. *See* Bleomycin sulfate
Bleomycin sulfate, 487
Bleph-10. *See* Sulfacetamide
Blephamide. *See* Sulfacetamide, with prednisolone
Blocadren. *See* Timolol
Blood
 in cerebrospinal fluid, 418
 disorders of, hematuria and, 167
 in pleural fluid, 433*t*
 in stool, testing for, **379**
 in anemia, 30
 in constipation, 84
 in diarrhea, 102
 in urine, **383**. *See also* Hematuria
 Foley catheter problems and, 141, 141–142
Blood/serum chemistry. *See also specific test*
 in coma/acute mental status changes, 80
 in oliguria/anuria, 266, 270
Blood component therapy, **437–441**. *See also* Transfusion reaction; Transfusions
 for anemia, 32, **437–438**
 for disseminated intravascular coagulation (DIC), 71
 plasma component therapy, **439–440**
 platelet transfusions, **438–439**
 red blood cell transfusions, **437**
Blood culture
 in arthritis, 249
 central venous line problems and, 55
 in coma/acute mental status changes, 80
 in dysuria, 119
 in fever, 130
 in HIV-positive patient, 139
 in heart murmur, 156
 in hypothermia, 232
 in leukopenia, 258
 pulmonary artery catheter problems and, 305
Blood gas sampling kit, 391
Blood gas values, 350*t*. *See also* Arterial blood gases; Mixed venous blood gases; Venous blood gases
Blood loss. *See* Bleeding/blood loss
Blood pressure. *See also* Hypertension; Hypotension
 arterial monitoring of, **390–391**
 problems with, **34–36**
 in bradycardia, 39
 in coagulopathy, 67, 68–69
 in coma/acute mental status changes, 77–78
 in dizziness, 104
 in heart murmur, 153
 in hematemesis/melena, 158, 159
 in hematochezia, 163
 in hyperglycemia, 181
 in hypotension, 224
 irregular pulse and, 238
 manual assessment of, arterial line problems and, 34–35
 in oliguria/anuria, 269
 pacemaker complications and, 285
 in shock, 224
Blood pressure support. *See* Vasopressors
Blood replacement. *See* Transfusions
Blood smear. *See* Peripheral blood smear
Blood urea nitrogen (BUN), **351–352**
 in abdominal pain, 6
 in delirium, 94
 in fever, in HIV-positive patient, 139
 Foley catheter problems and, 142
 in hematemesis/melena, 160
 in hematochezia, 164
 in hematuria, 169
 in hemoptysis, 173
 in hypercalcemia, 177
 in hyperglycemia, 182
 in hyperkalemia, 189
 in hypertension, 197
 in hypocalcemia, 200
 in hypoglycemia, 204
 in hypothermia, 231
 in nausea and vomiting, 264
 in oliguria/anuria, 266, 270
 in overdose, 279
 in pruritus, 301
 in syncope, 319
 in thrombocytopenia, 336
Blood urea nitrogen/creatinine ratio, **352**
 in hematemesis/melena, 160
 in hematochezia, 164
 in oliguria/anuria, 270
Blue top tubes, 622*t*
Blue/yellow label tubes, 622*t*
Body fluids, composition/daily production of, 436*t*
Body surface area, calculating, 620*f*
Body temperature, 129. *See also* Fever; Hyperthermia; Hypothermia
 in coma/acute mental status changes, 76, 78
 in heart murmur, 153
 in hypophosphatemia, 221
 in hypothermia, 231
 in oliguria/anuria, 269
 in overdose, 277
Bone, tumor invasion of
 hypercalcemia and, 176
 pain caused by, 288
Bone films
 in hypercalcemia, 178

in hypocalcemia, 201
in hypophosphatemia, 222
Bone marrow aspiration/biopsy, **397–399**
in coagulopathy, 70
in leukocytosis, 254
in leukopenia, 259
in pruritus, 302
in thrombocytopenia, 336–337
Bone marrow failure, leukopenia and, 256–257, 260
Bone marrow infiltration
leukopenia and, 257
thrombocytopenia and, 334
Bone resorption, decreased, hypocalcemia and, 200
Bone scan
in fever, 131
in hypercalcemia, 178
Bowel bypass/resection
arthritis and, 247
hypomagnesemia and, 211
diarrhea and, 100
Bowel ischemia/strangulation
abdominal pain and, 1, 5*t*
diarrhea and, 99
Bowel obstruction
abdominal pain and, 2, 3, 5*t*
constipation and, 82, 83
Bowel resection. *See* Bowel bypass/resection
Bowel sounds
in fever, 130
in hematemesis/melena, 159
in hematochezia, 164
BPV. *See* Benign positional vertigo
Bradyarrhythmias. *See also* Bradycardia
dyspnea and, 113
falls and, 124
Bradycardia, **39–44**
atrioventricular (AV) node blocks and, 41
in chest pain, 61
in coma/acute mental status changes, 78
differential diagnosis/causes of, 40–41
dyspnea and, 113
falls and, 124, 125
in hypotension, 224
initial evaluation of, 39–40
laboratory findings/data in, 42
management of, 42–43
in nausea and vomiting, 261
pacemaker complications and, 283
physical examination/findings in, 41–42
in shock, 224
sinus, 40, 113, 318
syncope and, 316, 318
Bradypnea
in acidosis, 9
in coma/acute mental status changes, 78
Brain abscess, delirium and, 92
Brain imaging
in dizziness/vertigo, 109
in seizures, 313
Brain stem evoked audiometry, in dizziness/vertigo, 109
Brain stem tumor, dizziness/vertigo and, 106
Brain tumor
coma/acute mental status changes and, 73, 76, 82
headache and, 146
in HIV-positive patient, 138
nausea and vomiting and, 263
Breast, male, examination of, in jaundice, 243
Breath odor, in diabetic ketoacidosis, 181
Breath sounds
in chest pain, 61
in cough, 88
in dyspnea, 114
in fever, 130
in hypotension/shock, 225
in nausea and vomiting, 264
in oliguria/anuria, 270
in syncope, 319
in tachycardia, 328
in ventilator patient
agitation and, 449
high peak pressures and, 457, 458
hypercarbia and, 455
hypoxemia and, 452
Breathlessness. *See also* Dyspnea
psychogenic, 113
Brethine. *See* Terbutaline
Brevibloc. *See* Esmolol
Bricanyl. *See* Terbutaline
Brimonidine, 607*t*
Brinzolamide, 607*t*
Broad casts, in urine, microscopic appearance of, 385
Bromocriptine, 487
Bronchi, obstructed, hypoxemia in ventilator patient caused by, 451
Bronchial adenoma, hemoptysis and, 171
Bronchial breath sounds, in cough, 88
Bronchial provocation testing
in cough, 88–89
in dyspnea, 115
Bronchial tear, hemoptysis and, 172
Bronchiectasis, hemoptysis and, 171
Bronchitis
cough and, 87, 89
dyspnea and, 115–116
hemoptysis and, 171
management of, 89, 115–116
Bronchodilators, 466*t*. *See also specific agent*
for anaphylaxis, 26
for aspiration, 39
for asthma, 89
for hypoxemic ventilator patient, 453
respiratory and nasal inhalants, 468*t*
Bronchogenic carcinoma. *See also* Lung cancer
cough and, 87
hemoptysis and, 171, 174
management of, 174
Bronchoprovocation testing
in cough, 88–89
in dyspnea, 115
Bronchoscopy
for aspiration, 39
in cough, 88
fever and, 128
in hemoptysis, 174
in HIV-positive patient, 140
Bronchospasm. *See also* Wheezing
acute, 342
cough and, 87
management of, 344
in ventilator patient
hypercarbia and, 454
hypoxemia and, 451
Brontex. *See* Guaifenesin, with codeine
Brudzinski's sign, in coma/acute mental status changes, 79
Bucladin-S Softabs. *See* Buclizine
Buclizine, 487
Budesonide, 487
Bulimia, hypokalemia and, 207
Bullous diseases, pruritus in, 298
Bumetanide, 487
for oliguria/anuria/acute renal failure, 272
Bumex. *See* Bumetanide
Buminate. *See* Albumin, therapeutic

BUN. *See* Blood urea nitrogen
Bundle branch block, right (RBBB), pulmonary artery catheterization and, 428
Bupivacaine, 487
Buprenex. *See* Buprenorphine
Buprenorphine, 487–488
Bupropion, 488
Burns
 hypernatremia and, 191
 thrombocytopenia and, 335
Burr cells (acanthocytes), 378
Buspar. *See* Buspirone
Buspirone, 488
Busulfan, 488
Butalbital
 with acetaminophen and caffeine, 471
 with aspirin, 481
 with aspirin/caffeine/codeine, 481–482
Butorphanol, 488
"Butterfly" needle, for intravenous access, 412, 414*f*
Butyrophenones, for nausea and vomiting, 265
Bypass surgery, intestinal
 arthritis and, 247
 hypomagnesemia and, 211
 diarrhea and, 100

C

C-ANCA. *See* Cytoplasmic-staining ANCA
C-peptide, **357–358**
 in hypoglycemia, 204
C-reactive protein (CRP), **358**
 in arthritis, 249
 in constipation, 84
 in diarrhea, 101
C3, **356**
C4, **356**
Cable systems, for pulmonary artery catheter, problems related to, 304
Cachexia
 coma/acute mental status changes and, 78
 diarrhea and, 100
Cafergot. *See* Ergotamine tartrate
Caffeine
 with acetaminophen and butalbital, 471
 with hydrocodone/chlorpheniramine/phenylephrine/acetaminophen, 526
 insomnia and, 234, 235
Calamus, toxicity of, 593
Calan. *See* Verapamil
Calcipotriene, 488
Calcitonin, **352**, 488–489
 for hypercalcemia, 179
Calcitriol, 489
 for hypocalcemia, 201
Calcium, 589
 in constipation, 84
 in diarrhea, 101
 disorders of balance of. *See also* Hypercalcemia; Hypocalcemia
 coma/acute mental status changes and, 74, 94
 delirium and, 94
 exogenous, hypercalcemia and, 176
 in hyperglycemia, 182
 for hyperkalemia, 189
 in hypomagnesemia, 212
 in hypophosphatemia, 222
 loss/displacement of, in hypocalcemia, 200
 in pruritus, 301
 serum, **352**
 albumin levels and, 177, 199, 200
 in hypercalcemia, 175, 177
 in hypocalcemia, 199, 200
 pain management and, 289
 supplementary, for hypocalcemia, 201
 urine, **352–353**
Calcium acetate, 489
Calcium carbonate, 489
 for hypocalcemia, 201
Calcium channel blockers, overdose/toxicity of, antidote for, 281
Calcium chloride
 for calcium channel blocker overdose/toxicity, 281
 for hypocalcemia, 201
Calcium citrate, for hypocalcemia, 201
Calcium gluceptate, for hypocalcemia, 201
Calcium gluconate, for hypocalcemia, 201
Calcium hydroxyapatite crystals, in arthritis, 247, 249
Calcium lactate, for hypocalcemia, 201
Calcium pyrophosphate dihydrate crystals, in arthritis, 249
Calcium salts, 489
Calphron. *See* Calcium acetate
Camptosar. *See* Irinotecan
Campylobacter, diarrhea caused by, 98
 in HIV infection/AIDS, 100, 137
 management of, 104
Cancer
 dysuria in men and, 118
 fever and, 128
 gastrointestinal
 hematemesis/melena and, 159
 hematochezia and, 163
 in HIV-positive patient, fever and, 138
 hypercalcemia and, 175, 176
 hypoglycemia and, 204
 leukocytosis and, 252
 pain management in, 287–291
 pericarditis and, 59
 pruritus and, 299
 renal, hematuria and, 167, 168, 170
 seizures and, 309
 syndrome of inappropriate antidiuretic hormone secretion (SIADH) and, 217
Cancer chemotherapy agents (antineoplastic agents), 465*t*. *See also specific agent*
 hematuria and, 166–167
 leukopenia and, 256
 pain and, 288
 thrombocytopenia and, management of, 338
Candesartan, 599*t*
Candida esophagitis, in HIV-positive patient, 137
Candida vaginitis
 dysuria and, 118
 management of, 121
 pruritus and, 297, 298
Cannon "A" waves
 in bradycardia, 41–42
 in tachycardia, 328
Capecitabine, 489
Capoten. *See* Captopril
Capsaicin, 490
Capsin. *See* Capsaicin
Captopril, 598*t*
 for pulmonary edema, 344
Capture (pacemaker), failure of, 283–284, 284*f*
 management of, 286
Carafate. *See* Sucralfate
Carbachol, 607*t*
Carbamate toxicity, antidote for, 282
Carbamazepine, 490
 for alcohol withdrawal/delirium tremens, 96

therapeutic/toxic levels of, 613*t*
Carbidopa/levodopa, 490
Carbon dioxide. *See also* $PaCO_2/pCO_2$
increased production of, in hypercarbic ventilator patient, 454
Carbon monoxide poisoning, 276
Carbonic anhydrase inhibitors, for glaucoma, 607*t*
Carboplatin, 490
Carboxyhemoglobin, **353**
polycythemia and, 292, 294
Carcinoembryonic antigen (CEA), **353**
Carcinoid, pruritus in, 298
Carcinoid syndrome, diarrhea and, 99
Cardene. *See* Nicardipine
Cardiac asthma, 342
Cardiac disease. *See* Heart disease
Cardiac enzymes, in chest pain, 62
Cardiac examination. *See* Heart, examination of
Cardiac failure. *See* Congestive heart failure
Cardiac index, pulmonary artery catheter measurement of, 428*t*
Cardiac level shunt, hypoxemia in ventilator patient caused by, 451
Cardiac medications, 466*t*. *See also specific agent*
cardiopulmonary arrest and, 44
diarrhea caused by, 99
Cardiac monitoring, in cardiopulmonary arrest, 46
Cardiac murmurs. *See* Heart murmurs
Cardiac output (CO)
low
coma/acute mental status changes and, 82, 93
delirium and, 93
in hypoxemic ventilator patient, correction of, 454
pulmonary artery catheter measurement of, 426, 428*t*
inaccurate/poorly reproducible, 306–307
in shock, 423*t*
Cardiac shock. *See* Cardiogenic shock; Shock
Cardiac syncope, 316, 318, 321
coma/acute mental status changes and, 82
management of, 322
Cardiac/pericardial tamponade
cardiopulmonary arrest and, 45
dyspnea and, 112
pulseless electrical activity and, 51
syncope and, 318
Cardiac troponins. *See* Troponin I; Troponin T
Cardiogenic pulmonary edema
hemoptysis and, 172
in ventilator patient
high peak pressures and, 456
hypoxemia and, 451, 453
wheezing and, 342
Cardiogenic shock, 225. *See also* Shock
management of, 229
pulmonary artery catheter monitoring in, 423*t*
syncope and, 318
Cardiomyopathy, hypertrophic, heart murmur in, 153, 155
Cardiopulmonary arrest, **44–53**
differential diagnosis/causes of, 45
imaging/clinical studies in, 46
initial evaluation in, 44–45
laboratory findings/data in, 46
management of, 46–53
in asystole, 50–51, 50–51*f*
in pulseless electrical activity (PEA), 51–53, 52–53*f*
in sustained ventricular tachycardia with no palpable pulse, 47, 48–49*f*
in ventricular fibrillation, 46–47, 48–49*f*
in ventricular tachycardia with palpable pulse, 47–49
physical examination/findings in, 45–46
Cardiopulmonary bypass, leukopenia and, 257
Cardiopulmonary examination. *See* Cardiovascular examination; Heart, examination of; Lungs, examination of
Cardiopulmonary exercise testing
in dyspnea, 115
in syncope, 321
Cardiopulmonary resuscitation (CPR), 44, 46. *See also* Cardiopulmonary arrest, management of
in ventricular fibrillation, 46–47
Cardiovascular agents, 466*t*. *See also specific agent*
cardiopulmonary arrest and, 44
diarrhea caused by, 99
Cardiovascular disorders. *See also* Heart disease
falls and, 124
polycythemia and, 442
Cardiovascular examination. *See also* Heart, examination of
in heart murmur, 154–155
in hyperkalemia, 189
in hypokalemia, 208
in insomnia, 236
in overdose, 278
pacemaker complications and, 285
Cardioversion, electrical (defibrillation)
for tachyarrhythmias, 329–330
for ventricular fibrillation, 46–47
for ventricular tachycardia, 329–330
stable, 47, 49
unstable, 49
Cardizem. *See* Diltiazem
Cardura. *See* Doxazosin
Carisoprodol, 490
Carmustine, 490
Carotene, serum, in leukopenia, 258
Carotid artery dissection, headache and, 147
Carotid sinus hypersensitivity/carotid sinus syndrome
falls and, 124
pre-syncope and, 107
syncope and, 317, 318, 322
Carotid sinus massage, for supraventricular tachycardia, 330
Carotid upstroke, decreased, in heart murmur, 154
Carteolol, 601*t*
ophthalmic, 607*t*
Cartrol. *See* Carteolol
Carvedilol, 601*t*
Casodex. *See* Bicalutamide
Casts, in urine
in hematuria, 167, 168
microscopic appearance of, 385

Cataflam. *See* Diclofenac
Catapres. *See* Clonidine, oral
Catapres TTS. *See* Clonidine, transdermal
Catatonia, 77
Catecholamines
fractionated, **353**, 354*t*
urine, unconjugated, **354**
Cathartics, 466*t*. *See also specific agent*
Catheter/catheterization. *See also specific type*
arterial, **390–391**
problems with, **34–36**
bladder (urinary/Foley), **394–397**
dysuria after removal and, 117
hematuria and, 166
problems and, **141–143**
central venous, **399–407**, 403*f*
culture of tip of, 55, 131
problems associated with, **53–57**
fever in patient with, 127
intravenous, 411–412, 413*f*, 414*f*
pacemaker, malposition of, pacemaker complications and, 283, 287
pulmonary artery, **421–429**, 423*t*, 424*f*, 427*f*, 428*t*, 429*t*
culture of tip of, 305
problems with, **303–307**
Catheter-over-needle assembly, insertion of, 411–412, 413*f*
for pulseless electrical activity, 51
Caverject. *See* Alprostadil, intracavernosal
CBC. *See* Complete blood count
CCNU. *See* Lomustine
CD4 count, in HIV-positive patient, fever and, 135
CEA. *See* Carcinoembryonic antigen
Ceclor. *See* Cefaclor
Cedax. *See* Ceftibuten
CeeNU. *See* Lomustine
Cefaclor, 603*t*
Cefadroxil, 603*t*
for endocarditis prophylaxis, 621*t*
Cefadyl. *See* Cephapirin
Cefamandole, 603*t*
Cefazolin, 603*t*
for endocarditis prophylaxis, 621*t*
Cefdinir, 604*t*
Cefepime, 604*t*
Cefixime, 604*t*
Cefizox. *See* Ceftizoxime
Cefmetazole, 603*t*
Cefobid. *See* Cefoperazone
Cefonicid, 603*t*
Cefoperazone, 604*t*
Cefotan. *See* Cefotetan
Cefotaxime, 604*t*
Cefotetan, 603*t*
Cefoxitin, 603*t*
Cefpodoxime, 604*t*
Cefprozil, 603*t*
Ceftazidime, 604*t*
Ceftibuten, 604*t*
Ceftin. *See* Cefuroxime
Ceftizoxime, 604*t*
Ceftriaxone, 604*t*
Cefuroxime, 603*t*
Cefzil. *See* Cefprozil
Celebrex. *See* Celecoxib
Celecoxib, 606*t*
for arthritis, 250
Celestone. *See* Betamethasone
Celexa. *See* Citalopram
Celiac axis compression syndrome, abdominal pain and, 4
Celiac sprue, diarrhea and, 100
Cellcept. *See* Mycophenolate mofetil
Cenestin. *See* Estrogens, conjugated, synthetic
Centigrade/Fahrenheit temperature conversion chart, 618*t*
Central diabetes insipidus
hypernatremia and, 191, 192, 193, 194
management of, 194
water deprivation/vasopressin test in diagnosis of, 193
Central nervous system
disorders of. *See also* Neurologic disorders
coma/acute mental status changes and, 73
infection, 76, 92
tumors, 73, 76, 82
delirium and, 92
hyponatremia and, 215
hypothermia and, 230–231
respiratory acidosis and, 12
respiratory alkalosis and, 20–21
syndrome of inappropriate antidiuretic hormone secretion (SIADH) and, 217
tumors
coma/acute mental status changes and, 73, 76, 82
dizziness/vertigo and, 106
nausea/vomiting and, 263
imaging studies of. *See* Neuroimaging
Central venous catheterization, **399–407**, 403*f*. *See also* Central venous line
approaches for, 400–407
femoral vein, 405–406
left internal jugular vein, 402
median basilic vein, 406–407
right internal jugular vein, 400–402
subclavian vein (left/right), 402–405, 403*f*
contraindications for, 399
indications for, 399
materials for, 399–400
problems associated with, **53–57**
pulmonary artery catheterization and, 425
complications related to, 428
Central venous line. *See also* Central venous pressure (CVP) monitoring
clotted, 54, 55
culture of tip of, 55, 131
infected, 54, 56, 131
fever and, 131
insertion of. *See* Central venous catheterization
kinked, 54, 56
misdirected, 54, 55–56
problems with, **53–57**
thrombosis and, 54, 55, 56
Central venous pressure (CVP) monitoring
in oliguria/anuria/acute renal failure, 271
pulmonary artery catheter for, in shock, 423*t*
waveform appearance and, 53
Cephalexin, 603*t*
for endocarditis prophylaxis, 621*t*
Cephalosporins
first-generation, 603*t*
second-generation, 603*t*
third- and fourth-generation, 604*t*
Cephalothin, 603*t*
Cephapirin, 603*t*
Cephradine, 603*t*

Cephulac. *See* Lactulose
Ceptaz. *See* Ceftazidime
Cerebellar disease
assessment of, in dizziness/vertigo, 108
disequilibrium and, 107
Cerebellar hemangioblastomas, polycythemia and, 292
Cerebellar tumor, dizziness/vertigo and, 106
Cerebellopontine-angle tumors, dizziness/vertigo and, 106
Cerebral aneurysm rupture, headache and, 146
Cerebral infarction, coma/acute mental status changes and, 77
Cerebral salt wasting, hyponatremia and, 216
Cerebral vascular accident. *See* Cerebrovascular accident
Cerebrospinal fluid
collection of, 417–418. *See also* Lumbar puncture
differential diagnosis of, 419*t*
normal characteristics of, 419*t*
Cerebrovascular accident (stroke)
aspiration and, 38–39
coma/acute mental status changes and, 77
constipation and, 84
falls and, 124
headache and, 145
hypertension and, 196
hypothermia and, 230
respiratory acidosis and, 12
respiratory alkalosis and, 21
seizures and, 309
Cerebrovascular disease
dizziness/vertigo in, 106
headache and, 145
Cerebyx. *See* Fosphenytoin
Cerubidine. *See* Daunorubicin
Cerumenex. *See* Triethanolamine
Cervical culture, in abdominal pain, 6
Cervical x-rays, in overdose, 279
Cetamide. *See* Sulfacetamide
Cetirizine, 491
Cevimeline, 491–492
CH50, **356**
Chamomile, 590–591
Chaparral, toxicity of, 593
Charcoal, activated, 492
for overdose, 280
Chemet. *See* Succimer
Chemical exposure. *See* Drugs/toxins; Environmental exposures
Chemotherapy. *See* Cancer chemotherapy
Chest
abnormalities of
alkalosis and, 22
respiratory acidosis and, 12
examination of
in alcohol withdrawal/delirium tremens, 93
in chest pain, 61
in coma/acute mental status changes, 79
in hematemesis/melena, 159
in hemoptysis, 172
in hypercalcemia, 177
in hypotension, 225
in nausea and vomiting, 264
pain management and, 288
in pruritus, 300
in shock, 225
in syncope, 319
in tachycardia, 328
in transfusion reaction, 340
in ventilator patient
agitation and, 449
high peak pressures and, 457
hypercarbia and, 455
hypoxemia and, 452
in wheezing, 343
Chest compressions, in cardiopulmonary resuscitation, 44
Chest computed tomography, in hemoptysis, 174
Chest pain, **57–66**
alkalosis and, 19
cardiac causes of, 58–59
characteristics/location of, 57–58
differential diagnosis/causes of, 58–60
gastrointestinal causes of, 60
heart murmur and, 152
hemoptysis and, 171
hypertension and, 61, 196
imaging/clinical studies in, 63
initial evaluation of, 57–58
laboratory findings/data in, 62
management of, 63–66
musculoskeletal, 60
physical examination/findings in, 60–62
pulmonary artery catheter problems and, 304
pulmonary causes of, 59–60
vascular causes of, 59
Chest tube, for pneumothorax, 66
high peak ventilator pressures and, 458
hypoxemic ventilator patient and, 453
Chest x-ray
in abdominal pain, 6–7
in alcohol withdrawal/delirium tremens, 94
in anaphylaxis, 26
in aspiration, 38
in cardiopulmonary arrest, 46
in central venous line problems, 55
in chest pain, 63, 64
in coagulopathy, 70
in coma/acute mental status changes, 81
in cough, 88
in dyspnea, 114
in fever, 131
in HIV-positive patient, 139
in heart murmur, 156
in hemoptysis, 173
in hypercalcemia, 178
in hyperglycemia, 182
in hypertension, 197
in hyponatremia, 218
in hypophosphatemia, 222
in hypotension, 227
in hypothermia, 232
in leukocytosis, 254
in leukopenia, 259
in oliguria/anuria, 271
in overdose, 279
in pacemaker complications, 285
in pruritus, 301
pulmonary artery catheter problems and, 305, 306
in respiratory acidosis, 16
in seizures, 313
in shock, 227
in ventilator patient
agitation and, 450
high peak pressures and, 457
hypercarbia and, 455
hypoxemia and, 452
setup and, 446
Cheyne-Stokes respiration, in coma/acute mental status changes, 78
"Chinese herbal mixtures," toxicity of, 594
Chitosamine (glucosamine sulfate) and chondroitin sulfate, 592
Chlamydia trachomatis
ligase chain reaction for, for

Chlamydia trachomatis, (cont)
urine, 120, **368**
urethritis caused by
dysuria in men and, 118
dysuria in women and, 118
management of, 121
Chlor-Trimeton. *See* Chlorpheniramine
Chloral hydrate, for insomnia, 237
Chlorambucil, 492
Chloramphenicol, 492
ophthalmic, 608*t*
Chlordiazepoxide, 492
for alcohol withdrawal, 95
Chloride, **355**
in acidosis, 15
in alkalosis, 21, 23
in body fluids, 436*t*
serum, **355**
urine, **355**, 386
in hypokalemia, 209
Chloride-responsive metabolic alkalosis, 21, 23, 24
Chloride-unresponsive metabolic alkalosis, 22, 23, 24
Chloromycetin. *See* Chloramphenicol
Chloromycetin Ophthalmic. *See* Chloramphenicol, ophthalmic
Chlorothiazide, 492
for oliguria/anuria/acute renal failure, 272
Chlorpheniramine, 492
with hydrocodone/phenylephrine/acetaminophen/caffeine, 526
Chlorpromazine, 493
for nausea and vomiting, 265
Chlorpropamide, 610*t*
Chlorthalidone, 493
Chlorzoxazone, 493
Cholangiogram, percutaneous transhepatic, in jaundice, 244
Cholangiopancreatography, endoscopic retrograde (ERCP), in jaundice, 244
Cholangitis, jaundice and, 242, 244–245
Cholecalciferol (vitamin D_3), 493
Cholecystectomy, diarrhea and, 100
Cholecystitis, management of, 134
Cholestasis
jaundice and, 245
postoperative, jaundice and, 243
of pregnancy, pruritus in, 299, 302
Cholestatic hepatitis, in HIV-positive patient, 137
Cholesterol, **355–360**
Cholestyramine, 493
Cholinergic agents
diarrhea caused by, 100
overdose/toxicity of, 275–276
Cholinesterase inhibitors, for glaucoma, 607*t*
Chondroitin sulfate and glucosamine sulfate (chitosamine), 592
Chordae tendinae rupture, heart murmur and, 152
Chromium, 589
Chronic disease
anemia of, 28, 29, 29*t*, 33
pruritus in, 297
Chronic obstructive airway disease, dyspnea and, 112
Chronic obstructive pulmonary disease (COPD)
management of, 344
mechanical ventilation for, 442
polycythemia and, 292
Chronulac. *See* Lactulose
Chvostek's sign, 200
delirium and, 93
in hypocalcemia, 200
in hypomagnesemia, 212
CI. *See* Cardiac index
Cibacalcin. *See* Calcitonin
Ciclopirox, 493
Cidofovir, 493–494
CIE. *See* Counterimmunoelectrophoresis
Cigarette smoking
cough and, 87
hematemesis/melena and, 158
hemoptysis and, 171
insomnia and, 234, 235
Cilostazol, 494
Ciloxan. *See* Ciprofloxacin, ophthalmic
Cimetidine, 494
for anaphylaxis, 26–27
for gastritis/esophagitis, 66
Cipro. *See* Ciprofloxacin
Cipro HC Otic. *See* Ciprofloxacin, otic
Ciprofloxacin, 494
ophthalmic, 608*t*
otic, 494
Cirrhosis
biliary
jaundice and, 242
pruritus in, 298
coma/acute mental status changes and, 75
hyponatremia and, 214, 217, 220
jaundice and, 242
leukopenia and, 256
management of, 220
oliguria/anuria/acute renal failure and, 268
respiratory alkalosis and, 21
Cisplatin, 494
Citalopram, 495
CK. *See* Creatine phosphokinase/creatine kinase
CK-BB, 358
CK-MB, 358
CK-MM, 358
Cladribine, 495
Claforan. *See* Cefotaxime
Clarithromycin, 495
for endocarditis prophylaxis, 621*t*
Clavulanic acid/clavulanate
amoxicillin with, 478
ticarcillin with, 600*t*
Clay ingestion, hypokalemia and, 207
Clemastine fumarate, 495
Cleocin/Cleocin-T. *See* Clindamycin
Clindamycin, 495
for endocarditis prophylaxis, 621*t*
Clinoril. *See* Sulindac
Clofazimine, 495
Clomycin. *See* Bacitracin, with polymyxin B and neomycin and lidocaine, topical
Clonazepam, 496
Clonidine
for accelerated hypertension, 198
for alcohol withdrawal/delirium tremens, 96
cessation of, rebound hypertension and, 194
oral, 496
transdermal, 496
Clonus, in coma/acute mental status changes, 79
Clopidogrel, 496
Clopra. *See* Metoclopramide
Clorazepate, 496
Clostridium, diarrhea caused by, 98
antibiotic use and, 99
management of, 103
testing for, 102

Clostridium difficile toxin testing, 102
in HIV-positive patient, 139
Clotrimazole, 496–497
with betamethasone, 497
Clotting. *See also under Coagulation*
central venous line malfunction and, 54, 55
disorders of, 67, 68. *See also* Bleeding/blood loss; Coagulopathy
Foley catheter problems and, 141, 141–142
Cloxacillin, 600*t*
Cloxapen. *See* Cloxacillin
Clozapine, 497
Clozaril. *See* Clozapine
Clubbing
in cough, 88
in dyspnea, 114
in heart murmur, 155
in hyponatremia, 218
in polycythemia, 293
in wheezing, 343
Cluster headaches, 145
management of, 150–151
CMV-IVIG. *See* Cytomegalovirus immune globulin
CO. *See* Cardiac output
CO_2. *See* Carbon dioxide
Coagulation/clotting
central venous line malfunction and, 54, 55
disorders of, 67, 68. *See also* Bleeding/blood loss; Coagulopathy
Foley catheter problems and, 141, 141–142
Coagulation factors, deficiency of, 68
Coagulation studies. *See also* Partial thromboplastin time; Prothrombin time
in coma/acute mental status changes, 80
Foley catheter problems and, 142
in hematuria, 168
in thrombocytopenia, 336
Coagulopathy, **66–72**. *See also specific disorder and* Bleeding/blood loss
differential diagnosis/causes of, 67–68
hematuria and, 167, 170
imaging/clinical studies in, 70
initial evaluation of, 67
laboratory findings/data in, 69–70, 69*t*
management of, 70–72, 170
physical examination/findings in, 68–69
Coarctation of aorta, hypertension and, 195
Cobalamin (vitamin B_{12}), **349**, 595
deficiency of, 29–30, 31, 32–33, 349
coma/acute mental status changes and, 75
in leukocytosis, 254
in leukopenia, 258
in polycythemia vera, 292, 294
supplementary, 498, 595
Cocaine, 497
delirium and, 93
hypertension and, 194, 195
Codeine, 497
with acetaminophen, 290, 471
for cough suppression, 90
with guaifenesin, 523
Coffee-ground emesis. *See* Hematemesis
Cogentin. *See* Benztropine
Cognex. *See* Tacrine
Cohosh, black, 590
Colace (docusate sodium). *See* Docusate calcium/potassium/sodium
Colazal. *See* Balsalazide
Colchicine, 497
diarrhea caused by, 99
Cold agglutinins, **356**
Colesevelam, 497
Colestid. *See* Colestipol
Colestipol, 497–498
Colic
biliary, 2
chest pain and, 60
jaundice and, 242
nausea and vomiting and, 262
gallbladder, chest pain in, 57
intestinal, 2. *See also* Abdominal pain
Colistin
with neomycin and hydrocortisone, otic, 548–549
with neomycin and hydrocortisone and thonzonium, otic, 548–549
Colitis
ischemic, hematochezia and, 163
pseudomembranous, 99
Collagen-vascular/connective tissue diseases
antinuclear antibody tests in, 348
arthritis and, 246, 247, 248, 249–250
fever and, 128
pericarditis and, 59
thrombocytopenia and, 67
Colon
carcinoma of, diarrhea and, 99
obstruction of. *See also* Intestinal obstruction
nausea and vomiting and, 262
Colonoscopy
in constipation, 85
in diarrhea, 102
in hematemesis/melena, 160
in hematochezia, 164
hyponatremia after, 215, 217
Coltsfoot, toxicity of, 594
CoLYTE. *See* Polyethylene glycol (Peg)–electrolyte solution
Coma, **72–82**. *See also* Mental status
body temperature alteration and, 76
differential diagnosis/causes of, 73–77
drugs/toxins causing, 72, 74, 81
endocrine causes of, 75
exogenous causes of, 74, 81
fluid/electrolyte status and, 74–75
hypernatremia and, 74, 75, 190
infections causing, 76, 82
initial evaluation of, 72–73
intracranial hemorrhage causing, 77, 82
laboratory findings/data in, 80–81
management of, 81–82
metabolic causes of, 74–76, 81
organ failure and, 75
physical examination/findings in, 77–80
psychiatric causes of, 76–77
time course of mental status changes and, 72
in trauma patient, 73, 73–74
tumors causing, 76, 82
in vitamin deficiency states, 75–76
Coma scale (Glasgow), 80, 619*t*
Combivent. *See* Albuterol, with ipratropium

Combivir. *See* Zidovudine (AZT), with lamivudine
Comfrey, toxicity of, 594
Common cold, cough and, 87
Community-acquired pneumonia, management of, 89, 132–133
Compazine. *See* Prochlorperazine
Compensation
in metabolic acidosis, 11, 350*t*
in metabolic alkalosis, 20, 350*t*
in respiratory acidosis, 11, 350*t*
in respiratory alkalosis, 20, 350*t*
Complement C3, **356**
Complement C4, **356**
Complement CH50 (total), **356**
Complete blood count (CBC), **354**. *See also* Hemogram
in alcohol withdrawal/delirium tremens, 94
in arthritis, 248
in cardiopulmonary arrest, 46
central venous line problems and, 55
in coagulopathy, 69
in coma/acute mental status changes, 80, 94
in constipation, 84
in diarrhea, 101
in dizziness/vertigo, 109
in dysuria, 119
in falls, 126
in fever, 130
in HIV-positive patient, 138–139
in headache, 148
in heart murmur, 156
in hematemesis/melena, 160
in hematochezia, 164
in hemoptysis, 173
in hyperglycemia, 182
in hypertension, 197
in hypoglycemia, 204
in hypophosphatemia, 222
in hypotension, 226
in hypothermia, 231
laboratory reference/normal values for, **354**, 354*t*
in leukopenia, 258
in nausea and vomiting, 264
pain management and, 289
in seizures, 312
in shock, 226
in syncope, 319
in ventilator patient
high peak pressures and, 457
hypercarbia and, 455
in wheezing, 343
Complete (third-degree) atrioventricular block, 41
cardiopulmonary arrest and, 45
dyspnea and, 113
ECG/rhythm strip in, 42
syncope and, 318
Computed tomography (CT)
in abdominal pain, 7
in alcohol withdrawal/delirium tremens, 94
in chest pain, 63
in coagulopathy, 70
in coma/acute mental status changes, 81
in constipation, 85
in falls, 126
in fever, 131
in headache, 148
in hemoptysis, 174
in hypertension, 197
in hyponatremia, 218
in hypotension, 227
in jaundice, 244
in leukocytosis, 254
in oliguria/anuria, 271
in overdose, 279
in polycythemia, 294
in respiratory acidosis, 16
in seizures, 313
in shock, 227
in thrombocytopenia, 337
Comtan. *See* Entacapone
Comvax. *See Haemophilus B* conjugate vaccine
Concussion, coma/acute mental status changes and, 74
Conduction abnormalities, in hypothermia, 232
Condylox/Condylox Gel 0.5%. *See* Podophyllin
Confusion. *See also* Delirium
in alcohol withdrawal/delirium tremens, 90, 93
after seizure, 311
Congenital heart disease, murmurs in, 151, 153
Congestive heart failure
cough and, 87
dyspnea and, 112, 116
falls and, 125
heart murmur and, 152
hypertension and, 196
hyponatremia and, 214, 217, 220
management of, 116, 220
oliguria/anuria/acute renal failure and, 268
Conjunctival petechiae, in coma/acute mental status changes, 78
Connective tissue/collagen-vascular disorders
antinuclear antibodies in, 348
arthritis and, 246, 247, 248, 249–250
fever and, 128
pericarditis and, 59
thrombocytopenia and, 67
Consciousness. *See also* Coma
assessment of, in overdose, 274–275
impairment of, aspiration and, 37
Constipation, **82–86**
Contact dermatitis, pruritus in, 296, 297, 298, 302
Continuous positive airway pressure (CPAP), 443, 445
for pulmonary edema, 344
for stridor, 344
for ventilator weaning, 459–460
Contraception/sexual protection, dysuria and, 117
Contraceptives, oral, 554
Contrast bowel studies, in abdominal pain, 7
Contusion, brain, coma/acute mental status changes and, 74
Conversion disorder, syncope and, 317
Convulsive syncope, 316
Coombs' test
direct, **357**
in anemia, 31–32, 33
indirect, **357**
in anemia, 31–32, 33
COPD. *See* Chronic obstructive pulmonary disease
Copper, 589
Cordarone. *See* Amiodarone
Core rewarming, 233
Core temperature. *See also* Body temperature
in hypothermia, 231
Coreg. *See* Carvedilol
Corgard. *See* Nadolol
Corlopam. *See* Fenoldopam
Coronary artery disease. *See also* Heart disease
heart murmur and, 152
Corrigan's pulse, 154

Cortef. *See* Hydrocortisone
Corticosteroids. *See also* Glucocorticoids; Steroids
 comparison of, 597*t*
 for hypercalcemia, 179
 ophthalmic, 609*t*
 in pain management, 291
Cortifoam rectal. *See* Hydrocortisone, rectal
Cortisol, **357**
 ACTH stimulation test in evaluation of, 345
 dexamethasone suppression test in evaluation of, 359–360
 in hyponatremia, 218
Cortisone, 597*t*
Cortisporin
 ophthalmic, 484, 549, 608*t*, 609*t*
 otic, 498, 548–549, 549
 topical, 483
Cortone. *See* Cortisone
Cortrosyn stimulation test. *See* Cosyntropin (Cortrosyn) stimulation test
Corvert. *See* Ibutilide
Corynebacterium minutissimum, erythrasma caused by, pruritus and, 297, 298
Cosmegen. *See* Dactinomycin
Cosopt. *See* Dorzolamide, with timolol
Costochondritis
 chest pain and, 60, 66
 management of, 66
Cosyntropin (Cortrosyn) stimulation test, **345**
 in hyponatremia, 218
 in hypothermia, 231–232
Cotazyme. *See* Pancreatin/pancrelipase
Co-trimoxazole. *See* Trimethoprim-sulfamethoxazole
Cough, **86–90**
 abdominal pain and, 2
 hemoptysis and, 171
 hyponatremia and, 215
 management of, 89–90
 syncope and, 323
Cough suppression, 89–90
 in hemoptysis, 174
Cough syncope, 317
Coumadin. *See* Warfarin
Counterimmunoelectrophoresis (CIE), **357**
Courvoisier's sign, in jaundice, 243
COX-2 Inhibitors, 606*t*
 for arthritis, 250
Cozaar. *See* Losartan
CPAP (continuous positive airway pressure), 443, 445
 for pulmonary edema, 344
 for stridor, 344
 for ventilator weaning, 459–460
CPK. *See* Creatine phosphokinase
CPPD. *See* Calcium pyrophosphate dihydrate crystals
CPR. *See* Cardiopulmonary resuscitation
Crackles
 in chest pain, 61
 in cough, 88
 in hyponatremia, 218
Cranial nerves, evaluation of function of
 in dizziness/vertigo, 108
 in seizures, 311–312
Creatine phosphokinase/creatine kinase
 in chest pain evaluation, 62
 in coma/acute mental status changes, 80–81
 in hyperkalemia, 189
 in hypophosphatemia, 222
 in hypotension, 226
 isoenzymes of, 358
 in chest pain evaluation, 62
 in hypotension, 226
 in overdose, 278
 in seizures, 312
Creatinine
 in abdominal pain, 6
 in arthritis, 249
 in delirium, 94
 in fever, in HIV-positive patient, 139
 Foley catheter problems and, 142
 in hematemesis/melena, 160
 in hematochezia, 164
 in hematuria, 169
 in hemoptysis, 173
 in hypercalcemia, 177
 in hyperglycemia, 182
 in hyperkalemia, 189
 in hypertension, 197
 in hypocalcemia, 200
 in hypoglycemia, 204
 in hyponatremia, 218
 in hypothermia, 231
 in nausea and vomiting, 264
 in overdose, 279
 in pruritus, 301
 ratio of to blood urea nitrogen. *See* Blood urea nitrogen/creatinine ratio
 serum, **359**
 in oliguria/anuria/acute renal failure, 266, 270, 386*t*
 in thrombocytopenia, 336
 urine, **359**
 in oliguria/anuria/acute renal failure, 270, 386*t*
Creatinine clearance, **358–359**
Creon. *See* Pancreatin/pancrelipase
Crescent sign, in mycetoma, 171
Crixivan. *See* Indinavir
Crohn's disease
 constipation and, 83
 diarrhea and, 99
 hematochezia and, 163
Cromolyn sodium, 498
Cross-match. *See* Type and cross-match
CRP. *See* C-reactive protein
Cryocrit, **359**
Cryoprecipitate, transfusion of, 439–440
 for von Willebrand's disease, 71
Cryptococcal antigen test, serum, in HIV-positive patient, 139
Cryptococcal meningitis, in HIV-positive patient, 137
 management of, 140
Cryptosporidium, diarrhea caused by, 98
 in HIV infection/AIDS, 98, 100, 137
Crystalloid solutions
 composition of, 435*t*
 for oliguria/anuria/acute renal failure, 273
Crystals
 joint fluid, in arthritis, 247, 249
 in urine, microscopic appearance of, 384
CT. *See* Computed tomography
Culdocentesis, in hypotension/shock, 227
Cultures. *See also specific type*
 in arthritis, 249
 catheter tip
 of central venous line, 55, 131
 of pulmonary artery catheter, 305
 in hyperglycemia, 182
 in hyponatremia, 218
 in hypotension/shock, 227
 in leukocytosis, 254

Cushing's reflex, 40
  coma/acute mental status changes and, 78
Cushing's syndrome/disease
  coma/acute mental status changes and, 75, 76
  dexamethasone suppression test in diagnosis of, 359–360
  hypernatremia and, 192
  hypertension and, 195
  hypokalemia and, 207
  metabolic alkalosis and, 22
Cutaneous T-cell lymphoma, pruritus in, 298
CVP. *See* Central venous pressure
CXR. *See* Chest x-ray
Cyanocobalamin, 498, 595. *See also* Vitamin B_{12}
Cyanosis
  in anaphylaxis, 26
  in aspiration, 36, 37
  dyspnea and, 111
  in polycythemia, 293
  in ventilator patient
  agitation and, 449, 450
  high peak pressures and, 457
  hypoxemia and, 452
Cyclic AMP, urinary, in hypocalcemia, 200
Cyclic neutropenia, 256, 257
Cyclobenzaprine, 498
Cyclophosphamide, 498–499
  hematuria and, 166–167
Cyclosporine, 499
Cycrin. *See* Medroxyprogesterone
Cyproheptadine, 499
  for pruritus, 302
Cystitis, 117, 118. *See also* Dysuria; Urinary tract infection
  hematuria and, 168
  hemorrhagic, 170
  management of, 121
Cystogram, retrograde, in hematuria, 169
Cytadren. *See* Aminoglutethimide
Cytarabine (Ara-C), 499
Cytarabine liposome, 499
Cytogam. *See* Cytomegalovirus immune globulin
Cytomegalovirus immune globulin (CMV-IVIG), 499
Cytomegalovirus (CMV)-negative products, transfusion of, 438
Cytomegalovirus retinitis, in HIV-positive patient, 136
  management of, 140
Cytomel. *See* Liothyronine
Cytoplasmic-staining ANCA (C-ANCA), 348
Cytosar-U. *See* Cytarabine
Cytospaz. *See* Hyoscyamine
Cytotec. *See* Misoprostol
Cytotoxic therapy
  contraindications to in secondary polycythemia, 295
  for polycythemia vera, 295
Cytovene. *See* Ganciclovir
Cytoxan. *See* Cyclophosphamide

D

D-dimer assay
  in coagulopathy, 70
  in thrombocytopenia, 336
Dacarbazine (DTIC), 499
Daclizumab, 500
Dactinomycin, 500
Dalfopristin/quinupristin, 500, 567
Dalgan. *See* Dezocine
Dalmane. *See* Flurazepam
Dalteparin, 500
  for myocardial infarction, 64
Danaparoid, 500
Dantrium. *See* Dantrolene
Dantrolene, 500–501
Dapsone, 501
Darvocet. *See* Propoxyphene, with acetaminophen
Darvon. *See* Propoxyphene
Darvon Compound-65. *See* Propoxyphene, with aspirin
Darvon–N with aspirin. *See* Propoxyphene, with aspirin
Daunomycin. *See* Daunorubicin
Daunorubicin, 501
Daypro. *See* Oxaprozin
Daytime sleep pattern, insomnia and, 234
DDAVP. *See* Deamino-8-D-arginine vasopressin; Desmopressin
ddC. *See* Zalcitabine
ddI (didanosine), 504
Deamino-8-D-arginine vasopressin (DDAVP), for von Willebrand's disease, 71
Decadron. *See* Dexamethasone
Decadron Ophthalmic. *See* Dexamethasone, ophthalmic
Decerebrate posturing, 78
Declomycin. *See* Demeclocycline
Decompression, for pneumothorax, 66
Decongestants, 465–466*t*. *See also specific agent*
  ophthalmic, 609*t*
Decontamination, for overdose/toxic exposure, 280–281
Decorticate posturing, 78
Deep tendon reflexes, in hyponatremia, 218
Deferoxamine, for iron overdose/toxicity, 282
Defibrillation (electrical cardioversion)
  for tachyarrhythmias, 329–330
  for ventricular fibrillation, 46–47
  for ventricular tachycardia, 329–330
  stable, 47, 49
  unstable, 49
Dehydration
  constipation and, 83
  fever and, 132
  hypernatremia and, 190, 191
  syncope and, 317
Delavirdine, 501
Delirium
  in alcohol withdrawal. *See* Delirium tremens
  differential diagnosis of, 91–93
  insomnia and, 234, 235
  perioperative, 73
Delirium tremens (DTs), **90–97**
  differential diagnosis of, 91–93
  imaging/clinical studies in, 94–95
  initial evaluation of, 90–91
  laboratory findings/data in, 94
  management of, 95–96
  physical examination/findings in, 93–94
Delta-Cortef. *See* Prednisolone
Delta D. *See* Cholecalciferol
Deltasone. *See* Prednisone
Demadex. *See* Torsemide
Demecarium, 607*t*
Demeclocycline, 501
Dementia
  coma/acute mental status changes and, 77

falls and, 123, 124, 125
insomnia and, 234
Demerol. *See* Meperidine
Denavir. *See* Penciclovir
Dental disease, headache and, 146
Dental Panorex, in leukopenia, 259
Dental procedures, endocarditis prophylaxis for, 621*t*
Dentition
disease involving, headache and, 146
examination of, in headache, 147
Deoxyribonucleoprotein (DNP) antibodies, 348
Depakene. *See* Valproic acid
Depakote. *See* Divalproex
Depo Provera. *See* Medroxyprogesterone
Depocyt. *See* Cytarabine liposome
Depression
coma/acute mental status changes and, 77
falls and, 125
insomnia and, 236
syncope and, 317
Dermatitis, pruritus in, 296, 297, 298
Dermatologic agents, 466–467*t*. *See also specific agent*
Dermatomyositis, pruritus in, 298
DES (diethylstilbestrol), 504
Desipramine, 501
for insomnia, 237
Desmopressin (DDAVP), 501–502
Desyrel. *See* Trazodone
Detrol. *See* Tolterodine
Dex-Neo-Dex. *See* Neomycin, with dexamethasone, ophthalmic
Dexacort Phosphate Turbinaire. *See* Dexamethasone, nasal
Dexamethasone, 597*t*
for coma/acute mental status changes in CNS tumor, 82
nasal, 502
ophthalmic, 609*t*
with neomycin, 609*t*
with neomycin and polymyxin B, 609*t*
Dexamethasone suppression test, **359–360**
Dexferrum. *See* Iron dextran
Dexpanthenol, 502
Dexrazoxane, 502
Dextran 40, 502
Dextromethorphan, 90, 502–503
with guaifenesin, 523
Dextrose
for coma/acute mental status changes, 81
in crystalloid solutions, 435*t*
daily maintenance requirements for, 435
for hyperkalemia, 189
for hyperosmolar/hyperglycemia nonketotic syndrome, 184
for hypoglycemia, 205
for seizures, 314
Dey-Drop. *See* Silver nitrate
Dezocine, 503
DiaBeta. *See* Glyburide
Diabetes insipidus
hypernatremia and, 191, 192, 193, 194
management of, 194
water deprivation/vasopressin test in diagnosis of, 193
Diabetes mellitus, 180
diarrhea in, 99
falls and, 123, 124–125
gestational, 180
hemoglobin A_{1C} (glycohemoglobin) in, 362
hyperglycemia and, 180
hypernatremia and, 191, 194
hypoglycemia and, 202
hypomagnesemia and, 211
hyponatremia and, 215, 215–216
jaundice and, 242
management of, 185–186, 194. *See also* Insulin; Sulfonylureas
syncope and, 317
type 1 (juvenile/insulin-dependent), 180
type 2 (adult-onset/non–insulin-dependent), 180
management of, 183–184
Diabetic ketoacidosis, 13, 17, 180
fruity breath odor in, 181
hypoglycemia and, 202
hypophosphatemia and, 221, 222
Kussmaul respirations in, 180, 181
management of, 185
Diabinese. *See* Chlorpropamide
Dialose (docusate potassium). *See* Docusate calcium/potassium/sodium
Dialysate, hypertonic, hypernatremia and, 192
Dialysis
for hypercalcemia, 179
for hyperkalemia, 190
for oliguria/anuria/acute renal failure, 274
Diamox. *See* Acetazolamide
Diaphoresis. *See also* Sweat
in hypoglycemia, 202, 204
in hypomagnesemia, 211
Diaphragm (contraceptive), dysuria associated with use of, 117
Diarrhea, **97–104**
abdominal pain and, 2, 98
acute, 97
bloody, 97
chronic, 97
differential diagnosis/causes of, 98–100
electrolyte composition of, 436*t*
in HIV-positive patient, 100, 137
parasitic, 98, 100, 137
hypernatremia and, 192
hypokalemia and, 206, 207
hypomagnesemia and, 211
hyponatremia and, 214
hypophosphatemia and, 221
imaging/clinical studies in, 102
infectious, 98
inflammatory, 99
initial evaluation of, 97–98
laboratory findings/data in, 101–102
management of, 102–104
metabolic alkalosis and, 21
physical examination/findings in, 100–101
stool volume and, 98
Diastolic pressure, pulmonary artery catheter measurement of, 428*t*
Diazepam, 503
for alcohol withdrawal/delirium tremens, 95, 96
for dizziness/vertigo, 110
for seizures, 314
Diazoxide, 503
Dibucaine, 503
DIC. *See* Disseminated intravascular coagulation
Dichloralphenazone, with isometheptene and aceta

Dichloralphenazone, *(cont)*
minophen, for migraine headache, 150
Diclofenac, 605*t*
ophthalmic, 608*t*
Dicloxacillin, 600*t*
Dicyclomine, 503–504
Didanosine (ddI), 504
Didronel. *See* Etidronate
Diet
in diabetes management, 184
in diarrhea management, 103
Diethylstilbestrol (DES), 504
Differential count, **387–388**
in alcohol withdrawal/delirium tremens, 94
in arthritis, 248
central venous line problems and, 55
in coma/acute mental status changes, 80, 94
in diarrhea, 101
in dysuria, 119
in fever, 130
in HIV-positive patient, 138–139
in heart murmur, 156
in hypophosphatemia, 222
laboratory reference/normal values for, 354*t*, 387–388
in leukopenia, 258
in nausea and vomiting, 264
pleural fluid, 433*t*
in pruritus, 300–301
in seizures, 312
in ventilator patient
high peak pressures and, 457
hypercarbia and, 455
Diffuse alveolar hemorrhage, management of, 175
Diflucan. *See* Fluconazole
Diflunisal, 605*t*
Digibind. *See* Digoxin immune Fab
Digital clubbing
in cough, 88
in dyspnea, 114
in heart murmur, 155
in hyponatremia, 218
in polycythemia, 293
in wheezing, 343
Digital disimpaction, for constipation, 86
Digitalis. *See also* Digoxin
overdose/toxicity of, 43
coma/acute mental status changes and, 81
hyperkalemia and, 187
irregular pulse and, 240
Digitalis delirium, 81
Digoxin, 504. *See also* Digitalis
bradycardia and, 42, 43
cardiopulmonary arrest and, 45
diarrhea caused by, 99
overdose/toxicity of, 43, 276, 613*t*
antidote for, 282
hypokalemia and, 209
paroxysmal atrial tachycardia with block and, 325
for tachycardia, 331
therapeutic levels of, 613*t*
Digoxin immune Fab, 504
for digitalis overdose/toxicity, 43, 282, 504
Dihydroergotamine, for migraine headache, 149
Dihydrohydroxycodeinone (oxycodone), 555–556
with acetaminophen, 556
with aspirin, 556
Dihydrotachysterol, for hypocalcemia, 201
1,25-Dihydroxy-vitamin D_3. *See* Calcitriol
Dihydroxyaluminum sodium carbonate, 504
Dilacor. *See* Diltiazem
Dilantin. *See* Phenytoin
Dilaudid. *See* Hydromorphone
Diltiazem, 505
for tachycardia, 331
Dilutional hyponatremia, 215–216
Dimenhydrinate, 505
for dizziness/vertigo, 110
Dimethyl sulfoxide (DMSO), 505
Diovan. *See* Valsartan
Diovan HCT. *See* Valsartan, with hydrochlorothiazide
Dipentum. *See* Olsalazine
Diphenhydramine, 505
for anaphylaxis, 26–27
for cough suppression, 90
for dizziness/vertigo, 110
for extrapyramidal side effects of antiemetics, 265, 266
for insomnia, 237
for pruritus, 302
Diphenoxylate with atropine, 103, 505
2,3-Diphosphoglyceric acid, deficiency of, polycythemia and, 292
Dipivefrin, 607*t*
Diprivan. *See* Propofol
Dipyridamole, 505
with aspirin, 506
for polycythemia vera, 295
Direct antiglobulin testing, posttransfusion, 340
Direct Fick, for cardiac output, 307
Dirithromycin, 506
Disequilibrium, 107
management of, 110
Disimpaction, for constipation, 86
Disopyramide, 506
Disorientation
in alcohol withdrawal/delirium tremens, 93
falls and, 125
Disseminated intravascular coagulation (DIC), 67, 68
hemoptysis and, 172
management of, 71–72
oliguria/anuria/acute renal failure and, 268
Distal renal tubular acidosis, 13, 16
Distributive shock. *See also* Shock
pulmonary artery catheter monitoring in, 423*t*
Disulfiram, 506
Ditropan/Ditropan XL. *See* Oxybutynin
Diulo. *See* Metolazone
Diuresis
osmotic, hyponatremia and, 216
in overdose management, 282
postobstructive, 273
hypernatremia and, 191
Diuretics, 467*t*. *See also specific agent*
hypercalcemia and, 176, 178–179
hypernatremia and, 191
hypokalemia and, 207
hyponatremia and, 214, 216
hypophosphatemia and, 221
metabolic alkalosis and, 21
for oliguria/anuria/acute renal failure, 272
Diuril. *See* Chlorothiazide
Divalproex, 585. *See also* Valproic acid
Diverticular disease, hematochezia and, 163
Diverticulitis, nausea and vomiting and, 262
Dizziness, **104–110**
differential diagnosis/causes of, 105–107
falls and, 123

imaging/clinical studies in, 109
initial evaluation of, 104–105
laboratory findings/data in, 109
management of, 109–110
physical examination/findings in, 107–108
physical tests in evaluation of, 108–109
DKA. *See* Diabetic ketoacidosis
DMSO (dimethyl sulfoxide), 505
DNA
double-stranded, antibodies to, 348
hepatitis B, 364*t*, 365
DNP antibodies, 348
Dobbhoff tube, 410
Dobutamine, 506
for hemodynamic support in patient with heart murmur, 157
Dobutrex. *See* Dobutamine
Docetaxel, 506
Docusate calcium/potassium/sodium, 85*t*, 506–507
Dofetilide, 507
Döhle bodies, 389
in leukocytosis, 254
in leukopenia, 258
Dolasetron, 507
Doll's eyes, in coma/acute mental status changes, 80
Dolobid. *See* Diflunisal
Dolophine. *See* Methadone
Dong quai *(Angelica polymorpha, sinensis),* 591
Donnatal. *See* Hyoscyamine, with atropine/scopolamine/phenobarbital
Dopamine, 507–508
for bradycardia, 43
for hemodynamic support in patient with heart murmur, 157
for oliguria/anuria/acute renal failure, 273
serum/urine levels of, laboratory reference/normal values for, 354*t*
Dopastat. *See* Dopamine
Doppler ultrasound
in central venous line problems, 55
in oliguria/anuria/acute renal failure, 271
Doral. *See* Quazepam
Dornase alfa, 508
Dorzolamide, 608*t*
with timolol, 608*t*
Doss (docusate sodium). *See* Docusate calcium/potassium/sodium
Double-stranded DNA antibodies, 348
Dovonex. *See* Calcipotriene
Down's syndrome, leukocytosis and, 253
Doxazosin, 508
Doxepin, 508
topical, 508
Doxorubicin, 508
Doxycycline, 508–509
Dramamine. *See* Dimenhydrinate
Dressler's syndrome, 58
Dronabinol, 509
"Drop attacks," 318
Droperidol, 509
for nausea and vomiting, 265
Droxia. *See* Hydroxyurea
Drug interactions, hypoglycemia and, 203
Drug screen. *See* Toxicology screening
Drugs of abuse. *See* Substance abuse
Drugs/toxins. *See also* Overdoses; Substance abuse
acidosis and
metabolic, 13–14
respiratory, 12
acute renal failure and, 267, 268
agitation in ventilator patient and, 449
alcohol withdrawal/delirium tremens and, 91, 93
alkalosis and, 19
metabolic, 21, 22
respiratory, 20
anaphylaxis and, 24–25
anemia and, 28
bronchospasm and, 342
cardiopulmonary arrest and, 44–45, 45
coma and, 72, 74, 80, 81
constipation and, 82, 83
delirium and, 93
diarrhea and, 99–100
disequilibrium and, 107
dizziness and, 104–105, 106, 109
falls and, 123, 125, 126
fever and, 127, 129, 134
in HIV-positive patient, 136
hematemesis and, 158
hematochezia and, 162
hematuria and, 167
hemoptysis and, 172
hypercalcemia and, 175, 176
hypercarbia in ventilator patient and, 455
hyperglycemia and, 181
hyperkalemia and, 186
hypernatremia and, 190
hypertension and, 194, 195
hypoglycemia and, 202, 203
hypokalemia and, 206, 207
hypomagnesemia and, 211
hyponatremia and, 214
hypotension and, 224
hypothermia and, 230
hypoxemia in ventilator patient and, 451
insomnia and, 235
irregular pulse and, 238, 240
jaundice and, 243
leukocytosis and, 251, 252, 253
leukopenia and, 255, 256, 257, 260
melena and, 158
mental status changes and, 72, 74, 80, 81
Mobitz type I (Wenckebach) second-degree AV block and, 41
nausea and vomiting and, 263
oliguria/anuria and, 267, 268
pacemaker failure to capture and, 284
platelet function and, 68
pruritus and, 297, 299
screening for. *See* Toxicology screening
seizures and, 309–310, 310
shock and, 224
sinus bradycardia and, 40
syncope and, 316–317, 317
syndrome of inappropriate antidiuretic hormone secretion (SIADH) and, 217
tachycardia and, 323
thrombocytopenia and, 67, 333, 334, 334–335, 335
wheezing and, 342
Dry skin (xerosis), pruritus and, 298, 302
DTIC (dacarbazine), 499
Dulcolax. *See* Bisacodyl
Duodenum, fluids produced by, composition/daily production of, 436*t*
Duplex Doppler. *See* Doppler ultrasound

Duragesic. *See* Fentanyl, transdermal
Duramorph. *See* Morphine
Duricef. *See* Cefadroxil
Duvoid. *See* Bethanechol
Dyazide. *See* Hydrochlorothiazide, with triamterene
Dycill. *See* Dicloxacillin
Dymelor. *See* Acetohexamide
Dynabac. *See* Dirithromycin
DynaCirc. *See* Isradipine
Dynapen. *See* Dicloxacillin
Dyrenium. *See* Triamterene
Dyspnea, **111–116**
 cardiac causes of, 112–113
 in cough, 86
 definition of, 111
 differential diagnosis/causes of, 111–113
 imaging/clinical studies in, 114–115
 initial evaluation of, 111
 laboratory findings/data in, 114
 management of, 115–116
 neuromuscular diseases and, 113
 physical examination/findings in, 113–114
 psychogenic causes of, 113
 pulmonary causes of, 111–112
Dysrhythmias. *See* Arrhythmias
Dysuria, **117–122**
 differential diagnosis/causes of, 117–118
 imaging/clinical studies in, 120
 initial evaluation of, 117
 laboratory findings/data in, 119–120
 management of, 120–122
 in men, 118
 physical examination/findings in, 119
 in women, 117–118

E

E. coli, diarrhea caused by, 98
E-Mycin. *See* Erythromycin
Ear
 disorders of, cough and, 87
 examination of. *See also* HEENT examination
 in coma/acute mental status changes, 79
 in cough, 87
 in dizziness/vertigo, 107
 in headache, 147
Eating, reactive hypoglycemia and, 203
Eating/drinking habits, insomnia and, 234
ECG/rhythm strip. *See* Electrocardiogram (ECG)/rhythm strip
Echinacea *(Echinacea purpurea)*, 591
Echocardiogram
 in chest pain, 63
 in dizziness/vertigo, 109
 in dyspnea, 115
 in fever, 131
 in heart murmur, 156
 in hypotension/shock, 227
 in oliguria/anuria, 271
 in pericarditis, 66
 in polycythemia, 294
 in syncope, 321
Echothiophate iodide, 607*t*
Econazole, 509
Ecstasy (MDMA), toxicity of, 276–277
Ectopy
 acidosis and, 9
 alkalosis and, 19
Eczema, pruritus in, 296, 297, 298, 302
Edecrin. *See* Ethacrynic acid
Edema, in hypercarbic ventilator patient, 455
Edex. *See* Alprostadil, intracavernosal
Edrophonium, 509
EDTA, for lead overdose/toxicity, 282
EEG. *See* Electroencephalogram
Efavirenz, 509
Effer-Syllium. *See* Psyllium
Effexor. *See* Venlafaxine
Efudex. *See* Fluorouracil, topical
EGD. *See* Upper GI endoscopy
Egophony, in cough, 88
Elavil. *See* Amitriptyline
Eldepryl. *See* Selegiline
Elderly patients
 abdominal pain in, 4
 falls in, causes of, 123–125
 infections in, coma/acute mental status changes and, 76
Electrical cardioversion (defibrillation)
 for tachyarrhythmias, 329–330
 for ventricular fibrillation, 46–47
 for ventricular tachycardia, 329–330
 stable, 47, 49
 unstable, 49
Electrocardiogram (ECG)/rhythm strip
 in abdominal pain, 7
 in alcohol withdrawal/delirium tremens, 94
 in anaphylaxis, 26
 in bradycardia, 42
 in cardiopulmonary arrest, 46
 in chest pain, 63
 in coma/acute mental status changes, 81
 in dizziness/vertigo, 109
 in dyspnea, 114–115
 in falls, 126
 in heart murmur, 156
 in hemoptysis, 174
 in hypercalcemia, 178
 in hyperglycemia, 182
 in hyperkalemia, 186, 189
 in hypertension, 197
 in hypocalcemia, 200
 in hypotension, 227
 in hypothermia, 232
 in hypoxemic ventilator patient, 452
 in irregular pulse, 240–242
 in nausea and vomiting, 265
 in oliguria/anuria, 271
 in overdose, 279
 in pacemaker complications, 285–286
 in seizures, 313
 in shock, 227
 in syncope, 319, 321, 321–322
 in tachycardia, 329
Electrodes, pacemaker
 checking pacing threshold of, 286
 pacemaker complications and, 283–284, 286
Electroencephalogram (EEG)
 in alcohol withdrawal/delirium tremens, 95
 in coma/acute mental status changes, 81
 in dizziness/vertigo, 109
 in hypophosphatemia, 222
 in seizures, 313
Electrolyte imbalance. *See also specific type and* Electrolyte studies
 agitation in ventilator patient caused by, 449
 in alcohol withdrawal/delirium tremens, 94
 management of, 95–96
 cardiopulmonary arrest and, 45

coma/acute mental status changes and, 74, 94
falls and, 124
nausea and vomiting and, 263
Electrolyte studies. *See also* Electrolyte imbalance; Electrolytes
in abdominal pain, 6
in acidosis, 15–16
in agitated ventilator patient, 450
in alcohol withdrawal/delirium tremens, 94
in alkalosis, 22
in bradycardia, 42
in cardiopulmonary arrest, 46
in constipation, 84
in diarrhea, 101
in dizziness/vertigo, 109
in dyspnea, 114
in falls, 126
in fever, in HIV-positive patient, 139
in heart murmur, 156
in hyperglycemia, 182
in hyperkalemia, 189
in hypertension, 197
in hypocalcemia, 200
in hypoglycemia, 204
in hypokalemia, 208
in hypomagnesemia, 212
in hyponatremia, 218
in hypophosphatemia, 222
in hypotension, 226
in irregular pulse, 240
in leukocytosis, 254
in nausea and vomiting, 264
in overdose, 279
in pacemaker complications, 286
in seizures, 312
in shock, 226
in syncope, 319
in tachycardia, 328
Electrolytes, **435**, 435*t*, 436*t*. *See also* Electrolyte studies; Electrolyte imbalance; Fluid management
in body fluids, 436*t*
urinary, **385–386**
in oliguria/anuria/acute renal failure, 270
Electromyography, in respiratory acidosis, 16
Electronystamogram (ENG), in dizziness/vertigo, 109
Electrophoresis
hemoglobin, in anemia, 29*t*
protein, **373**, 374*f*, 375*t*
Electrophysiologic testing, in syncope, 321
Elimite. *See* Permethrin
ELISA (enzyme-linked immunosorbent assay), for HIV antibody, 366
Ellence. *See* Epirubicin
Elmiron. *See* Pentosan polysulfate sodium
Elspar. *See* L-Asparaginase
Embolectomy, for pulmonary embolism, 66
Embolism
hematuria and, 118
oliguria/anuria/acute renal failure and, 268
pulmonary. *See* Pulmonary embolism
EMCYT. *See* Estramustine phosphate
Emesis. *See* Nausea and vomiting
EMG. *See* Electromyography
Eminase. *See* Anistreplase
EMLA. *See* Lidocaine, with prilocaine
Emotional stimuli, leukocytosis and, 252
Empirin Nos. 2–4. *See* Aspirin, with codeine
EMV scale (Glasgow coma scale), 80, 619*t*
E-Mycin. *See* Erythromycin
Enalapril, 598*t*
for pulmonary edema, 344
Enalaprilat, for hypertensive emergency, 198
Enbrel. *See* Etanercept
Encephalitis
delirium and, 92
in HIV-positive patient, 137
Encephalopathy
anoxic, coma/acute mental status changes and, 77
hepatic, coma/acute mental status changes and, 75
hypertensive, 195
coma/acute mental status changes and, 77, 92, 195
delirium and, 92, 93
metabolic, falls and, 125
Reye's, coma/acute mental status changes and, 76
Wernicke's, 92
coma/acute mental status changes and, 75, 92
hypothermia and, 230–231
Endocarditis
arthritis and, 247
in HIV-positive patient, 137
management of, 157
Endocarditis prophylaxis, 621*t*
Endocrine disorders
coma/acute mental status changes and, 75, 92
constipation and, 83
delirium and, 92
diarrhea and, 99, 101
hypercalcemia and, 176
hypoglycemia and, 203
Endolymphatic shunts, for dizziness/vertigo, 110
Endoscopic retrograde cholangiopancreatography (ERCP), in jaundice, 244
Endoscopy
in abdominal pain, 7
urgent surgery and, 8*t*
in nausea and vomiting, 265
upper GI
in hematemesis/melena, 160
in hematochezia, 164
Endotracheal intubation, **407–410**, 409*f*, 444. *See also* Endotracheal tube; Mechanical ventilation
in hemoptysis, 174
in overdose, 279
for stridor, 344
Endotracheal tube (ETT), 408, 444. *See also* Endotracheal intubation; Mechanical ventilation
displacement/leak/plugging of
agitation and, 449, 450
high peak pressures and, 456, 457, 457–458, 458
hypercarbia and, 454, 455
hypoxemia and, 451, 452
removal of
care after, 460
requirements for, 458
timing of, 460
weaning techniques for, 458–459
Enema
barium
in constipation, 85
in diarrhea, 102
for constipation, 85, 85*t*
ENG. *See* Electronystamogram
Engerix-B. *See* Hepatitis B vaccine
Enoxaparin, 509
for myocardial infarction, 64
Entacapone, 510
Entamoeba histolytica, diarrhea caused by, 98
Enterobius vermicularis, pruritus caused by, 297, 299
Entriflex tube, 410

Entuss-D. *See* Hydrocodone, with pseudoephedrine
Environmental exposures
coma/acute mental status changes and, 73, 74
hypothermia and, 230, 232
Environmental hazards, falls and, 123
Enzone. *See* Pramoxine, with hydrocortisone
Enzyme-linked immunosorbent assay (ELISA), for HIV antibody, 366
Eosinophilia, 254
Eosinophilic gastroenteritis, diarrhea and, 100
Eosinophils, **388**
laboratory reference/normal values for, 354*t*, 388
EP testing. *See* Electrophysiologic testing
Ephedra (Ma huang), 591
hypertension and, 195
toxicity of, 591, 594
Ephedrine, 510
hypertension and, 195
Epidural hematoma, coma/acute mental status changes and, 73
Epidural opioids, 291
Epiglottitis, stridor and, 201
Epileptic seizures, **308–315**. *See also* Seizures
Epinephrine, 510
for anaphylaxis/anaphylactic shock, 26, 228–229, 510
for asthma, 510
for asystole, 50
for bradycardia, 43
in cardiopulmonary resuscitation, 47
for dyspnea in asthma, 116
for pulseless electrical activity, 51
racemic, for stridor, 344
serum/urine levels of, laboratory reference/normal values for, 354*t*
for ventricular fibrillation, 47
EpiPen, 27
Epirubicin, 510
Episodic tension-type headache, 144
management of, 148–149
Epithelial casts, in urine, microscopic appearance of, 385
Epithelial cells, in urine, microscopic appearance of, 384
Epivir/Epivir-HBV. *See* Lamivudine
EPO. *See* Erythropoietin
Epoetin alfa, 510
Epogen. *See* Epoetin alfa
Epoprostenol, 510
Eprosartan, 599*t*
Eptifibatide, 511
for myocardial infarction, 65
Equinil. *See* Meprobamate
ERCP. *See* Endoscopic retrograde cholangiopancreatography
Ergamisol. *See* Levamisole
Ergocalciferol, for hypocalcemia, 201
Ergot alkaloids, for migraine headache, 149
Ergotamine tartrate, for migraine headache, 149
Erythrasma, pruritus in, 297, 298
Erythrocin. *See* Erythromycin
Erythrocyte sedimentation rate (ESR), **378–379**
in arthritis, 249
in constipation, 84
in diarrhea, 101
in headache, 148
Erythromycin, 511
ophthalmic, 608*t*
Erythropoietin (EPO), **360**
in polycythemia, 294
therapeutic (epoetin alfa), 510
Escherichia coli, diarrhea caused by, 98
Esgic. *See* Acetaminophen, with butalbital and caffeine
Esidrix. *See* Hydrochlorothiazide
Eskalith. *See* Lithium
Esmolol, 511
for aortic dissection, 65
for tachycardia, 331
Esomeprazole, 611*t*
Esophageal dysfunction, aspiration and, 37
Esophageal spasm, chest pain and, 57, 60
Esophageal varices
hematemesis/melena and, 158, 159, 161
management of, 161
Sengstaken-Blakemore tube for, 410
Esophagitis
chest pain and, 57, 66
in HIV-positive patient, 137
management of, 66, 161
ESR. *See* Sedimentation test
Essential hyponatremia, 216
Estazolam, 511
for insomnia, 237
Esterified estrogens, 511
with methyltestosterone, 512
Estinyl. *See* Ethinyl estradiol
Estrace. *See* Estradiol
Estracyte. *See* Estramustine phosphate
Estraderm. *See* Estradiol, transdermal
Estradiol, 512
ethinyl, 513
with norethindrone, 552
transdermal, 512
Estramustine phosphate, 512
Estratab. *See* Esterified estrogens
Estratest. *See* Esterified estrogens, with methyltestosterone
Estrogens, 467*t*. *See also specific agent*
conjugated, 512
with methylprogesterone, 512–513
with methyltestosterone, 513
synthetic, 512
esterified, 511
with methyltestosterone, 512
hypertension and, 195
Etanercept, 513
Ethacrynic acid, 513
Ethambutol, 513
Ethanol, for methanol and ethylene glycol toxicity, 18, 282
Ethanol use/abuse
coma/acute mental status changes and, 73, 74
gastrointestinal bleeding and hematemesis/melena, 158
hematochezia and, 162
hypertension and, 195
hypoglycemia and, 203
hypomagnesemia and, 211
hypophosphatemia and, 94, 96, 221
insomnia and, 234, 235
jaundice and, 242, 245
leukopenia and, 256
metabolic acidosis and, 16
nausea and vomiting and, 262
toxic levels and, 613*t*
withdrawal and, **90–97**. *See also* Alcohol withdrawal
Ethinyl estradiol, 513
with norethindrone, 552
Ethnic background, leukopenia and, 256, 257
Ethosuximide, 513
therapeutic/toxic levels of, 613*t*

Ethylene glycol
metabolic acidosis caused by, 13, 16, 18
overdose/toxicity of, antidote for, 282
Ethyol. *See* Amifostine
Etidronate, 513
for hypercalcemia, 179
Etodolac, 605*t*
Etoposide, 514
ETT. *See* Endotracheal tube
Eulexin. *See* Flutamide
Euvolemic hyponatremia, 217
management of, 219–220
Event monitor/recorder
in dizziness/vertigo, 109
in syncope, 321–322
Evista. *See* Raloxifene
Evoxac. *See* Cevimeline
Ewald tube, 410
Excretory urography (IV pyelography)
in dysuria, 120
in hematuria, 169
Exelon. *See* Rivastigmine
Exemestane, 514
Exercise, hematuria caused by, 168
Exercise testing
in dyspnea, 115
in syncope, 321
Exertional syncope, 315
Expectorants, 90, 465–466*t*. *See also specific agent*
Exposure. *See* Environmental exposures
Exsel Shampoo. *See* Selenium sulfide
Extensor plantar reflex, in coma/acute mental status changes, 80
External auditory canal, examination of, in dizziness/vertigo, 107
Extracardiac obstructive shock. *See also* Shock
pulmonary artery catheter monitoring in, 423*t*
Extremities, examination of
central venous line problems and, 54
in chest pain, 62
in coagulopathy, 69
in cough, 88
in dyspnea, 114
in falls, 125
in fever, 130
in HIV-positive patient, 138
in heart murmur, 155
in hemoptysis, 173
in hyperglycemia, 181
in hyponatremia, 218
in hypotension, 226
in oliguria/anuria, 270
pain management and, 289
in polycythemia, 293
in seizures, 311
in shock, 226
in tachycardia, 328
in ventilator patient
agitation and, 449
high peak pressures and, 457
hypercarbia and, 455
hypoxemia and, 452
in wheezing, 343
Extubation
care after, 460
requirements for, 458
timing of, 460
weaning techniques for, 458–459
Exudate, pleural, 433*t*
Eye movements
in alcohol withdrawal/delirium tremens, 93
in coma/acute mental status changes, 79, 93
Eyes
decontamination of, 281
disorders of
headache and, 145
in HIV infection/AIDS, 136
examination of. *See also* HEENT examination
in alcohol withdrawal/delirium tremens, 93
in arthritis, 248
in coma/acute mental status changes, 78–79, 93
in dizziness/vertigo, 108
in headache, 147
in hematemesis/melena, 159
in hypertension, 196

F

Facial weakness, seizures and, 311–312
"Factitious asthma," 342
Factitious fever, 129
Factitious hematuria, 168
Factitious hyperkalemia, 187
Factitious hypoglycemia, 203
Factor VII, for vitamin K deficiency/liver disease, 72
Factor VIII deficiency (hemophilia A), 68
management of, 71, 440, 480
Factor VIII (antihemophilic factor) therapy, 71, 440, 480
Factor IX deficiency (hemophilia B), 68
management of, 71
Factor IX concentrate, 71
Fahrenheit/centigrade temperature conversion chart, 618*t*
Failure to capture (pacemaker), 283–284, 284*f*
management of, 286
Failure to sense (pacemaker), 284–285, 284*f*
management of, 287
Falls, **122–127**
differential diagnosis/causes of, 123–125
imaging/clinical studies in, 126
initial evaluation and, 122–123
laboratory findings/data in, 125–126
management of, 126
physical examination/findings in, 125
prevention of, 126
Famciclovir, 514
Familial hypocalciuric hypercalcemia, 175, 177
Familial (racial) neutropenia, 256, 257
Familial periodic paralysis, hypokalemia and, 206
Famotidine, 514
for gastritis/esophagitis, 66
Famvir. *See* Famciclovir
Fasting, hypoglycemia and, 203
Fat, fecal
in diarrhea, 101
in hypocalcemia, 200
Fatigue, in HIV-positive patient, fever and, 135
Fatty casts, in urine, microscopic appearance of, 385
FDP. *See* Fibrin degradation products
Febrile transfusion reaction, self-limiting, 339–340
management of, 341
Fecal fat
in diarrhea, 101
in hypocalcemia, 200
Fecal impaction
constipation and, management of, 86
diarrhea and, 100
Fecal leukocytes, testing for, **379**
in diarrhea, 102
in HIV-positive patient, 139

Feeding tubes, 410, 411
Feet. *See also* Extremities
pruritus affecting, 297
Feldene. *See* Piroxicam
Felodipine, 514
Felty's syndrome, 256, 257
Female genitalia, examination of. *See* Gynecologic examination
Females, bladder catheterization in, 396
Femara. *See* Letrozole
FemHRT. *See* Norethindrone acetate/ethinyl estradiol
Feminone. *See* Ethinyl estradiol
Femoral artery, for arterial puncture, 391
Femoral vein, for central venous catheterization, 405–406
FE_{Na}. *See* Fractional excreted sodium
Fenofibrate, 514
Fenoldopam, 515
Fenoprofen, 606*t*
Fentanyl, 515
transdermal, 515
transmucosal system, 515
Fentanyl Oralet. *See* Fentanyl, transmucosal system
Fergon. *See* Ferrous gluconate
Ferric gluconate complex, 515
Ferritin levels, **360**
in anemia, 29*t*, 31
Ferrlecit. *See* Ferric gluconate complex
Ferrous gluconate, 515
Ferrous sulfate, 515
for anemia, 32, 515
Fever, **127–135**
abdominal pain and, 1
in Addisonian crisis, 134
in alcohol withdrawal/delirium tremens, 93
in alkalosis, 22
arthritis and, 246
central venous line problems and, 53, 54, 131
in chest pain, 61
in cholecystitis, 134
in coma/acute mental status changes, 72, 78
in cough, 87
cyclic, leukopenia and, 256
in diarrhea, 97
differential diagnosis/causes of, 128–129
in HIV-positive patient, 136–138
drug-induced, 127, 129, 134
in HIV-positive patient, 136
in dyspnea, 113
factitious (self-induced), 129
headache and, 144, 147
in heart murmur, 153
hematuria and, 166
in hemoptysis, 172
in HIV-positive patient, **135–141**
in hyperglycemia, 180
hypernatremia and, 191, 192
hypotension and, 132, 224
imaging/clinical studies in, 131
in HIV-positive patient, 139–140
initial evaluation of, 127–128, 132
in HIV-positive patient, 135
IV catheter infection and, 132
in jaundice, 242
laboratory findings/data in, 130–131
in HIV-positive patient, 138–139
in leukocytosis, 253
leukopenia and, 255, 257
management of, 259–260
in malignant neuroleptic syndrome, 134
management of, 132–134
in HIV-positive patient, 140
in leukopenia, 259–260
in meningitis, 134
in nausea and vomiting, 261
neutropenia and, 133–134
in oliguria/anuria, 269
pain management and, 288
physical examination/findings in, 129–130
in HIV-positive patient, 138
in pneumonia, 132–133
in polycythemia, 293
pulmonary artery catheter problems and, 304, 305
in shock, 224
tachycardia and, 323
thyroid storm and, 134
in transfusion reaction, 338, 339, 339–340
of unknown origin, 129
Feverfew *(Tanacetum parthenium),* 591
Fexofenadine, 516
Fiberglass dermatitis, 298
Fiberoptic bronchoscopy. *See* Bronchoscopy
Fibrillation
atrial, 239, 325
in coma/acute mental status changes, 79
dyspnea and, 113
in hypothermia, 232
syncope and, 318
ventricular, 327–328
in hypothermia, 232
management of, 46–47, 48–49*f*
Fibrin degradation products/fibrin split products, **360**
in coagulopathy, 70
in transfusion reaction, 340
Fibrinogen, **360–361**
in coagulopathy, 70
pleural fluid, 433*t*
in thrombocytopenia, 336
in transfusion reaction, 340
Fibromuscular dysplasia, hypertension and, 195
Fibrosis, at pacemaker electrode, failure to capture and, 284
Fick method, for cardiac output, 307
Filgrastim (G-CSF), 516
leukocytosis and, 251
for leukopenia, 260
Finasteride, 516
FiO_2 (inspired fraction of oxygen)
adjusting for ventilator patient, 447
high peak pressures and, 458
hypoxemia and, 453
ratio of to PaO_2 (P/F ratio), in respiratory failure, mechanical ventilation and, 442
ventilator set up and, 445
Fioricet. *See* Acetaminophen, with butalbital and caffeine
Fiorinal. *See* Aspirin, with butalbital
Fiorinal with codeine. *See* Aspirin, with butalbital/caffeine/codeine
Fistulae, gastrointestinal, hypernatremia and, 192
Fitz-Hugh–Curtis syndrome, abdominal pain and, 4
FK 506 (tacrolimus), 576
therapeutic levels of, 613*t*
Flagyl. *See* Metronidazole
Flamp. *See* Fludarabine phosphate
Flank pain, oliguria/anuria and, 267
Flarex. *See* Fluorometholone
Flatus, constipation and, 82

Flavoxate, 516
Flecainide, 516
Fleet enema, 85*t*
for hypophosphatemia, 223
Fleet Phospho-Soda, for hypophosphatemia, 223
Flexeril. *See* Cyclobenzaprine
Flolan. *See* Epoprostenol
Flomax. *See* Tamsulosin
Flonase. *See* Fluticasone, nasal
Florinef. *See* Fludrocortisone acetate
Flovent/Flovent Rotadisk. *See* Fluticasone, oral
Flow murmur, 152, 154
Floxin. *See* Ofloxacin
Floxuridine (FUDR), 516
Fluconazole, 517
Flucytosine, 517
Fludara. *See* Fludarabine phosphate
Fludarabine phosphate, 517
Fludrocortisone acetate, 517
Fluid challenge, for pulseless electrical activity, 51
Fluid and electrolyte disorders. *See also* Electrolyte imbalance
coma/acute mental status changes and, 74–75
Fluid loss
hyponatremia and, 216
hypovolemic shock and, 225
Fluid management, **435**, 435*t*, 436*t*
abdominal pain and, 8
alcohol withdrawal/delirium tremens and, 95
daily maintenance requirements and, 435
diabetic ketoacidosis and, 185
diarrhea and, 103
hematemesis/melena and, 161
hematochezia and, 165
hypernatremia and, 191
hyponatremia and, 219–220
hypovolemic shock and, 228
inadequate, oliguria/anuria/acute renal failure and, 268
intravenous cannulation/catheterization for, 411–412, 413*f*, 414*f*
oliguria/anuria/acute renal failure and, 273, 274
Fluid status
constipation and, 83
falls and, 124
hypernatremia and, 190
Fluids, body, composition/daily production of, 436*t*
Fluids and electrolytes, **435**, 435*t*, 436*t*. *See also* Fluid management; Electrolytes
Flumadine. *See* Rimantadine
Flumazenil, 281, 517
Flunisolide, 517
Fluogen. *See* Influenza vaccine
Fluorescent treponemal antibody absorbed (FTA-ABS) test, **361**
Fluorometholone, ophthalmic, 609*t*
Fluorouracil, 518
topical, 518
Fluoxetine, 518
Fluoxymesterone, 518
Fluphenazine, 518
Flurazepam, 518–519
for insomnia, 237
Flurbiprofen, 606*t*
ophthalmic, 608*t*
Flushield. *See* Influenza vaccine
Flushing syndromes, anaphylaxis and, 25
Flutamide, 519
Fluticasone
nasal, 519
oral, 519
Flutter, atrial, 239, 324–325
syncope and, 318
"Flutter waves," 325
Fluvastatin, 612*t*
Fluvirin. *See* Influenza vaccine
Fluvoxamine, 519
Fluzone. *See* Influenza vaccine
FML. *See* Fluorometholone
Folate/folic acid, 594
deficiency of, 29–30, 31, 32
in leukopenia, 258
red blood cell, **360–361**
serum (folic acid), **361**
supplementary, 519
Folex. *See* Methotrexate
Foley balloon, inability to deflate, 142, 143
Foley catheter
hematuria and, 166
in hypotension/shock, 227
improperly positioned, 142
insertion of, **394–397**
dysuria after removal and, 117
irrigating, 143
obstructed, 141–142
in oliguria/anuria, 271–272
problems with, **141–143**
Folic acid. *See* Folate
Folliculitis, pruritus in, 296, 298
Fomepizole, 519–520
for methanol and ethylene glycol toxicity, 282
Fomivirsen, 520
Food, reactive hypoglycemia and, 203
Foreign body
aspirated, 37
stridor and, 201
wheezing and, 342
retained, hemoptysis and, 172
Fortaz. *See* Ceftazidime
Fortovase. *See* Saquinavir
Fosamax. *See* Alendronate
Foscarnet, 520
Foscavir. *See* Foscarnet
Fosfomycin, 520
Fosinopril, 598*t*
Fosphenytoin, 520
for seizures, 314
Fourth heart sound. *See* Heart sounds
Fractional excreted sodium, in oliguria/anuria/acute renal failure, 270, 386*t*
Fragmin. *See* Dalteparin
Free hemoglobin, in transfusion reaction, 340
Fremitus, tactile, in cough, 88
Fresh-frozen plasma, transfusion of, 439
for disseminated intravascular coagulation (DIC), 71
for vitamin K deficiency/liver disease, 72
for von Willebrand's disease, 71
Friction rub, in chest pain
pericardial, 61
pleural, 61
Frozen stored red blood cells (RBCs), transfusion of, 438
FTA-ABS (fluorescent treponemal antibody absorbed) test, **361**
5-FU. *See* Fluorouracil
FUDR (floxuridine), 516
Functional (paralytic) ileus
abdominal pain and, 5*t*
nausea and vomiting and, 262
Fundus, ocular
in coma/acute mental status changes, 78–79
in dizziness/vertigo, 108
in heart murmur, 155
in hyperglycemia, 181
Fungal infection. *See also* Infection

Fungal infection, *(cont)*
leukocytosis and, 252
serologic tests for, **361**
Fungal meningitis, cerebrospinal fluid findings in, 419*t*
Fungizone. *See* Amphotericin B
Fungus ball (mycetoma), hemoptysis and, 171
FUO. *See* Fever, of unknown origin
Furadantin. *See* Nitrofurantoin
Furosemide, 520
for congestive heart failure, 116
for hypercalcemia, 178–179
for hyponatremia, 219
for oliguria/anuria/acute renal failure, 272
for pulmonary edema, 344
Fusion beat, 327

G

G-CSF (filgrastim), 516
leukocytosis and, 251
for leukopenia, 260
G-Mycitin. *See* Gentamicin
Gabapentin, 520–521
Gabitril. *See* Tiagabine
Gallbladder colic, chest pain and, 57
Gallium nitrate, 521
Gallop, in bradycardia, 42
Gamimmune N. *See* Immune globulin, intravenous
Gamma-globulins
electrophoresis values for, 374*f*, 375*t*
transfusion of, 440
Gamma-glutamyltransferase/transpeptidase (GGT), **361**
alkaline phosphatase elevation and, 346
in jaundice, 243
pain management and, m, 289
Gamma hydroxybutyrate (GHB), toxicity of, 277
Gammar IV. *See* Immune globulin, intravenous
Gammopathy, polyclonal, protein electrophoresis in, 374*f*
Ganciclovir, 521
Ganite. *See* Gallium nitrate
Gap acidosis, 13–15
Garamycin. *See* Gentamicin
Garlic *(Allium sativum),* 591
Gastrectomy, hypocalcemia after, 199
Gastric contents, aspiration of, 36
Gastric decompression, for abdominal pain, 8
Gastric emptying scan, in nausea and vomiting, 265
Gastric juices, composition/daily production of, 436*t*
Gastric lavage
in hematemesis/melena, 160
in hematochezia, 164
Gastric outlet obstruction, nausea and vomiting and, 262
Gastric surgery, diarrhea and, 100
Gastrin, **362**
Gastrinomas, diarrhea and, 99
Gastritis
chest pain and, 60, 66
hemorrhagic
hematemesis/melena and, 159, 161
management of, 66, 161
Gastroenteritis
eosinophilic, diarrhea and, 100
nausea and vomiting and, 263
Gastroesophageal reflux
chest pain and, 60
cough and, 87, 89
management of, 89
Gastrointestinal agents, 467*t*. *See also specific agent*
Gastrointestinal bleeding. *See also* Rectal bleeding
anemia and, 28
hematemesis/melena, **158–162**
hematochezia, **162–166**
Gastrointestinal procedures, endocarditis prophylaxis for, 621*t*
Gastrointestinal system
bicarbonate loss through, acidosis and, 12–13
disorders of
abdominal pain and, 2–3, 3*t*
chest pain and, 60
constipation and, 83
hematemesis/melena and, 158
hematochezia and, 163
in HIV-positive patient, fever and, 137
leukopenia and, 255
potassium loss through, hypokalemia and, 206
sodium loss through
hypernatremia and, 191–192
hyponatremia and, 216
water loss through
hypernatremia and, 191–192
hyponatremia and, 216
Gastrointestinal tubes, **410–411**
Gastrointestinal tumors, constipation and, 83
Gatifloxacin, 521
Gaviscon/Gaviscon-2. *See* Aluminum hydroxide, with magnesium carbonate; Aluminum hydroxide, with magnesium trisilicate
G-CSF (filgrastim), 516
leukocytosis and, 251
for leukopenia, 260
Gemcitabine, 521
Gemfibrozil, 521
Gemtuzumab ozagamicin, 521–522
Gemzar. *See* Gemcitabine
Generator, pacemaker, pacemaker complications and, 283, 286
Genitalia, examination of. *See also* Gynecologic examination
in dysuria, 119
Foley catheter problems and, 142
Genitourinary examination
in fever, 130
in hematemesis/melena, 159
in jaundice, 243
in leukocytosis, 253
in oliguria/anuria, 270
in seizures, 311
in syncope, 319
Genitourinary procedures, endocarditis prophylaxis for, 621*t*
Genitourinary tract agents, 469*t*. *See also specific agent*
Genoptic. *See* Gentamicin, ophthalmic
Gentacidin. *See* Gentamicin, ophthalmic
Gentak. *See* Gentamicin, ophthalmic
Gentamicin, 522
dosing guidelines for, 614*t*, 615*t*, 616–617*t*
for endocarditis prophylaxis, 621*t*
ophthalmic, 608*t*
with prednisolone, 609*t*

therapeutic levels of, 613*t*
topical, 522
Gestational diabetes, 180
GGT. *See* Gamma-glutamyltransferase/transpeptidase
GHB (gamma hydroxybutyrate), toxicity of, 277
Giardia, diarrhea caused by, 98
Ginger *(Zingiber officinale),* 591–592
Ginkgo biloba, 592
Ginseng, 592
Glanzmann's thrombasthenia, 68
Glargine insulin, 597*t*. *See also* Insulin
Glasgow coma scale, 80, 619*t*
Glaucoma, agents for, 607–608*t*
Glimepiride, 610*t*
Glipizide, 610*t*
α_1-Globulin, electrophoresis values for, 374*f*, 375*t*
α_2-Globulin, electrophoresis values for, 374*f*, 375*t*
β-Globulin, electrophoresis values for, 374*f*, 375*t*
γ-Globulins, electrophoresis values for, 374*f*, 375*t*
Glomerular disease
hematuria and, 167, 168, 170
oliguria/anuria/acute renal failure and, 268
Glomerulonephritis
management of, 170
rapidly progressive, oliguria/anuria/acute renal failure and, 268
thrombocytopenia and, 335
Glossitis, in anemia, 30
Glossopharyngeal neuralgia, syncope and, 317
Glucagon, 522
for anaphylaxis, 27
for beta-blocker overdose/toxicity, 281
for calcium channel blocker overdose/toxicity, 281
for hypoglycemia, 205
Glucocorticoids, 597*t*. *See also* Corticosteroids; Steroids
for anaphylaxis, 27
hypernatremia and, 192
hyponatremia and, 217
Glucophage. *See* Metformin
Glucosamine sulfate (chitosamine) and chondroitin sulfate, 592
Glucose, **362**. *See also* Hyperglycemia; Hypoglycemia
in alcohol withdrawal/delirium tremens, 94
cerebrospinal fluid, 419*t*
in dizziness/vertigo, 109
exogenous, hyperglycemia and, 181
for hyperkalemia, 189
for hypoglycemia, 205
in hypomagnesemia, 212
in hypophosphatemia, 222
in hypothermia, 231
in metabolic gap acidosis, 16
in overdose, 278
pleural fluid, 433*t*
in pruritus, 301
in seizures, 312
serum
in hyperglycemia, 181
in hypoglycemia, 204
serum sodium and, 215, 215–216
in syncope, 319
urine, **384**
Glucose intolerance. *See also* Diabetes mellitus
pregnancy and, 180
Glucotrol/Glucotrol-XL. *See* Glipizide
Glutamic-oxaloacetic transferase, serum (SGOT). *See* AST
Glutamic-pyruvic transferase, serum (SGPT). *See* ALT
γ-Glutamyltransferase/transpeptidase (GGT), **361**
alkaline phosphatase elevation and, 346
in jaundice, 243
pain management and, 289
Glyburide
micronized, 610*t*
non-micronized, 610*t*
Glycerin suppositories, 85, 85*t*, 522
Glycohemoglobin (hemoglobin A_{1C}), **362**
Glycoprotein IIb/IIIa inhibitors
for myocardial infarction, 65
platelet function affected by, 68
Glycyrrhizic acid, in licorice, hypokalemia and, 208
Glynase. *See* Glyburide, micronized
Glyset. *See* Miglitol
GM-CSF (sargramostim), 570
leukocytosis and, 251
for leukopenia, 260
G-Mycitin. *See* Gentamicin
GoLYTELY. *See* Polyethylene glycol (Peg)–electrolyte solution
Gonococcal arthritis, 247, 250
Gonococcal urethritis
dysuria in men and, 118
management of, 121–122
Gonorrhea
pruritus in, 297
urine test for (ligase chain reaction), 120, **368**
Goodpasture's syndrome, hemoptysis and, 172
Goserelin, 522
Gout, arthritis and, 247, 249
Gram-negative bacteria, 362–363
Gram-positive bacteria, 362
Gram's stain, **362–363**
joint fluid, 249
sputum
in dyspnea, 114
in fever, 131
of untransfused blood, in transfusion reaction, 340
Granisetron, 522–523
Granular casts, in urine, microscopic appearance of, 385
Granulocyte colony-stimulating factor (G-CSF/filgrastim), 516
leukocytosis and, 251
for leukopenia, 260
Granulocyte-macrophage colony-stimulating factor (GM-CSF/sargramostim), 570
leukocytosis and, 251
for leukopenia, 260
Granulomatous disease
hypercalcemia and, 176
meningitis, cerebrospinal fluid findings in, 419*t*
Gray top tubes, 622*t*
Green top tubes, 622*t*
Groin, pruritus affecting, 297
Guaifenesin, 523
with codeine, 523
with dextromethorphan, 523
with hydrocodone, 525
Guanfacine, 523
Guillain-Barré syndrome, mechanical ventilation for, 443
Gynecologic disorders
abdominal pain and, 2, 3, 3*t*
in HIV-positive patient, fever and, 138
Gynecologic examination. *See also* Genitalia, examination of

Gynecologic examination, *(cont)*
abdominal pain and, 5
in dysuria, 119
in hematuria, 168
in hypotension/shock, 226
in leukocytosis, 253
in nausea and vomiting, 264

H

H-BIG. *See* Hepatitis B immune globulin
H_1 blockers. *See also* Antihistamines
for pruritus, 302
H_2 antagonists, for gastritis/esophagitis, 66
Habitrol. *See* Nicotine, transdermal
Haemophilus B conjugate vaccine, 523
Halcion. *See* Triazolam
Haldol. *See* Haloperidol
Hallpike-Dix (Nylen-Barany) maneuver, in dizziness/vertigo, 108
Hallucinations, in alcohol withdrawal/delirium tremens, 90, 93
Hallucinogens, overdose/toxicity of, 276
Haloperidol, 523
for alcohol withdrawal/delirium tremens, 96
for nausea and vomiting, 265
Halotestin. *See* Fluoxymesterone
Ham test, in leukopenia, 258
Hands. *See also* Extremities
pruritus affecting, 296
Haptoglobin, **363**
in anemia, 31
HAV (hepatitis A virus), antibody to (anti-HAV), 364*t*, 365
Havrix. *See* Hepatitis A vaccine
HBcAg (hepatitis B core antigen), antibody to (anti-HBc), 364*t*, 365
HBeAg (hepatitis B_e antigen), 364*t*, 365
antibody to, 364*t*, 365
H-BIG. *See* Hepatitis B immune globulin
HBsAg (hepatitis B surface antigen), 363, 364*t*
antibody to (anti-HBs), 364*t*, 365
HBV-DNA, 364*t*, 365
HCB beta subunit. *See* Human chorionic gonadotropin (HCG), serum
HCG. *See* Human chorionic gonadotropin
$HCO_3^!$. *See* Bicarbonate
HCV, antibody to (anti-HCV), 364*t*, 365
HCV-RNA, 364*t*, 365
HDL cholesterol. *See* High-density lipoprotein (HDL) cholesterol
HDV (hepatitis D virus), antibody to (anti-HDV), 364*t*, 365
Head, examination of. *See also* HEENT examination
in coma/acute mental status changes, 78
Head computed tomography
in alcohol withdrawal/delirium tremens, 94
in coma/acute mental status changes, 81
in falls, 126
in headache, 148
in hyponatremia, 218
in overdose, 279
in polycythemia, 294
Head trauma
coma/acute mental status changes and, 73, 73–74
in falls, patient observation and, 126
hypothermia and, 230
seizures and, 309
Head-up tilt table, in syncope, 322
Headache, **143–151**. *See also specific type*
coma/acute mental status changes and, 73
differential diagnosis/causes of, 144–147
in HIV-positive patient, fever and, 135
imaging/clinical studies in, 148
initial evaluation of, 143–144
laboratory findings/data in, 148
management of, 148–151
physical examination/findings in, 147–148
post-lumbar puncture, 418
Hearing loss, dizziness/vertigo and, 105, 107
Heart. *See also under Cardiac*
examination of. *See also* Cardiovascular examination
in abdominal pain, 4
in anemia, 30
in bradycardia, 42
in chest pain, 61–62
in coma/acute mental status changes, 79
in cough, 88
in dizziness/vertigo, 108
in dyspnea, 114
in fever, 130
in HIV-positive patient, 138
in heart murmur, 154–155
in hematochezia, 164
in hemoptysis, 172–173
in hyperglycemia, 181
in hyperkalemia, 189
in hypertension, 196
in hypokalemia, 208
in hypomagnesemia, 212
in hypotension, 225
in hypothermia, 231
in irregular pulse, 240
in leukocytosis, 253
in oliguria/anuria, 270
pacemaker complications and, 285
in polycythemia, 293
in seizures, 311
in shock, 225
in syncope, 319
in tachycardia, 328
in thrombocytopenia, 336
in ventilator patient
high peak pressures and, 457
hypercarbia and, 455
hypoxemia and, 452
in wheezing, 343
Heart block, 41
cardiopulmonary arrest and, 45
dyspnea and, 113
paroxysmal atrial tachycardia and, 325
pulmonary artery catheterization and, 428
second-degree atrioventricular, 239–240
Mobitz type I (Wenckebach), 41, 239–240
ECG/rhythm strip in, 42
Mobitz type II, 41, 239–240
ECG/rhythm strip in, 42
management of, 241
syncope and, 318
third-degree atrioventricular, 41
cardiopulmonary arrest and, 45
dyspnea and, 113

ECG/rhythm strip in, 42
syncope and, 318
Heart disease. *See also* Coronary artery disease
congenital, murmurs in, 151, 153
dyspnea and, 112–113
in HIV-positive patient, fever and, 137
insomnia and, 235
irregular pulse and, 238
pre-syncope and, 107
syncope and, 316, 318, 321
coma/acute mental status changes and, 82
Heart failure
cough and, 87
dyspnea and, 112, 116
falls and, 125
heart murmur and, 152
hypertension and, 196
hyponatremia and, 214, 217, 220
management of, 116, 220
oliguria/anuria/acute renal failure and, 268
Heart murmurs, **151–157**. *See also* Heart sounds
in anemia, 30
in bradycardia, 42
in chest pain, 62
differential diagnosis/causes of, 152–153
in dyspnea, 114
in fever, 130
in hemoptysis, 173
in hypotension, 225
in hypoxemic ventilator patient, 452
identification of, 154–155
imaging/clinical studies in, 156
initial evaluation of, 151–152
in irregular pulse, 240
laboratory findings/data in, 156
in leukocytosis, 253
management of, 156–157
noncardiac, 152
in oliguria/anuria, 270
physical examination/findings in, 153–155
in polycythemia, 293
in shock, 225
in tachycardia, 328
Heart rate/rhythm. *See also* Arrhythmias; Bradycardia; Tachycardia
in coma/acute mental status changes, 78
in dizziness, 104
in fever, 129–130
in heart murmur, 153
in hematochezia, 163
in hyponatremia, 217
irregular, **238–241**
in oliguria/anuria, 269
pacemaker complications and, 285
in syncope, 319
Heart sounds, 154. *See also* Heart murmurs
in bradycardia, 42
in chest pain, 61, 62
in cough, 88
in dyspnea, 114
in hemoptysis, 172–173
in hyperglycemia, 181
in hypertension, 196
in hyponatremia, 218
in hypotension, 225
in hypothermia, 231
in oliguria/anuria, 270
in polycythemia, 293
in shock, 225
in tachycardia, 328
in ventilator patient
high peak pressures and, 457
hypercarbia and, 455
hypoxemia and, 452
Heat stroke, hypophosphatemia and, 221
Heat therapy, for chronic tension-type headache, 149
Heavy metals, toxicity of, 276
HEENT examination
in acidosis, 15
in anaphylaxis, 25
in aspiration, 37
in chest pain, 61
in coma/acute mental status changes, 78–79
in diarrhea, 101
in falls, 125
in fever, 130
in HIV-positive patient, 138
in headache, 147
in hematochezia, 164
in hemoptysis, 172
in hypercalcemia, 177
in hyperglycemia, 181
in hypocalcemia, 200
in hypomagnesemia, 212
in hyponatremia, 218
in hypophosphatemia, 221
in leukopenia, 258
in nausea and vomiting, 264
in oliguria/anuria, 270
in overdose, 277
pain management and, 288
in polycythemia, 293
in pruritus, 300
in seizures, 311
in syncope, 319
in ventilator patient
agitation and, 449
high peak pressures and, 457
in wheezing, 343
Helicobacter antibodies, 66, **363**
Helmet cells (schistocytes), 378
Hemangioblastomas, cerebellar, polycythemia and, 292
Hemarthrosis, 246
in coagulopathy, 69
Hematemesis, **158–162**
abdominal pain and, 2
anemia and, 28
hematochezia and, 158, 163
volume of, 158
Hematochezia, **162–166**
anemia and, 28
establishing source of bleeding in, 165–166
hematemesis and, 158, 163
volume of, 162–163
Hematocrit
in abdominal pain, 6
in coagulopathy, 69
elevated, **291–296**. *See also* Polycythemia
in hematemesis/melena, 160
in hematochezia, 162
laboratory reference/normal values for, 354*t*
in polycythemia, 294
Hematologic disorders
cancer, hypercalcemia and, 176
hematuria and, 167
leukocytosis and, 251–252, 252
pruritus and, 299, 302
Hematologic studies, in abdominal pain, 6
Hematuria, **166–170**, 383
abdominal pain and, 2, 6, 166
anemia and, 28
dysuria and, 119
false, 168
oliguria/anuria and, 267, 270
Hemiparesis
coma/acute mental status changes and, 73
falls and, 124
Hemoccult test, **379**. *See also* Occult blood, in stool, testing for
in anemia, 30

Hemodialysis. *See also* Dialysis
for hyperkalemia, 190
leukopenia and, 257
for oliguria/anuria/acute renal failure, 274
for overdose, 282
Hemodynamic status
arterial line monitoring of, **390–391**
problems with, **34–36**
central venous line monitoring of, **399–407**, 403*f*
pulmonary artery catheter monitoring of, **421–429**, 423*t*, 424*f*, 427*f*, 428*t*, 429*t*
Hemofiltration, for overdose, 282
Hemoglobin
free, in transfusion reaction, 340
hereditary disorders of. *See also specific type*
anemia and, 28
high-oxygen-affinity, polycythemia and, 292, 294
laboratory reference/normal values for, 354*t*
oxygen affinity of, polycythemia and, 292, 294
urine, **383**
in transfusion reaction, 340
Hemoglobin A_{1C} (glycohemoglobin), **362**
Hemoglobin A_2, in anemia, 29*t*
Hemoglobin electrophoresis, in anemia, 29*t*
Hemoglobinopathy, hematuria and, 167
Hemoglobinuria
paroxysmal nocturnal
leukopenia and, 256, 257
thrombocytopenia and, 334
in transfusion reaction, 340
Hemogram. *See also* Complete blood count
in acidosis, 15
in aspiration, 38
in chest pain, 62
in cough, 88
in dyspnea, 114
in hematuria, 169
laboratory reference/normal values for, **354**, 354*t*
in pruritus, 300–301
in tachycardia, 329
in transfusion reaction, 340
Hemolysis, jaundice and, 242, 245
Hemolytic anemia, 33
Coombs' test in, 31–32
Hemolytic transfusion reaction, 339
delayed, 340
management of, 341
Hemophilia
abdominal pain in, 4
type A (factor VIII), 68
management of, 71, 440, 480
type B (factor IX), 68
management of, 71
Hemoptysis, **170–175**
differential diagnosis/causes of, 171–172
hyponatremia and, 215
imaging/clinical studies in, 173–174
initial evaluation of, 170–171
laboratory findings/data in, 173
management of, 174–175
physical examination/findings in, 172–173
pulmonary artery catheter problems and, 304
volume of, 171
Hemorrhage. *See also* Bleeding/blood loss
cardiopulmonary arrest and, 45
oliguria/anuria/acute renal failure and, 268
Hemorrhagic cystitis, hematuria and, 170
Hemorrhagic gastritis
hematemesis/melena and, 159, 161
management of, 161
Hemorrhagic shock, 224–225. *See also* Shock
metabolic acidosis caused by, 17
Hemorrhoids
constipation and, 83
hematochezia and, 163
pruritus and, 297
Hemosiderin, urine, in anemia, 31
Hemostasis, inadequate, 67. *See also* Bleeding/blood loss; Coagulopathy
Heparin, 523–524
for disseminated intravascular coagulation (DIC), 71–72
hyperkalemia and, 188
for myocardial infarction, 64
for pulmonary embolism, 65
thrombocytopenia and, 335
Hepatic encephalopathy, coma/acute mental status changes and, 75
Hepatic failure, nausea and vomiting and, 263
Hepatic porphyria, coma/acute mental status changes and, 76
Hepatic tumors, polycythemia and, 292
Hepatitis
chronic active, arthritis and, 247
fulminant, coma/acute mental status changes and, 75
in HIV-positive patient, 137
jaundice and, 242, 245
nausea and vomiting and, 262
pruritus and, 299
tests for, **363–365**, 364*t*
in jaundice, 244
in leukopenia, 258
Hepatitis A vaccine, 524
Hepatitis A virus (HAV), antibody to (anti-HAV), 364*t*, 365
Hepatitis B core antigen (HBcAg), antibody to (anti-HBc), 364*t*, 365
Hepatitis B_e antigen (HBeAg), 364*t*, 365
antibody to (anti-HBe), 364*t*, 365
Hepatitis B immune globulin, 524
Hepatitis B surface antigen (HBsAg), 363, 364*t*
antibody to (anti-HBs), 364*t*, 365
Hepatitis B vaccine, 524
Hepatitis B virus (HBV) DNA, 364*t*, 365
Hepatitis C virus (HCV), antibody to (anti-HCV), 364*t*, 365
Hepatitis C virus (HCV) RNA, 364*t*, 365
Hepatitis D virus (HDV), antibody to (anti-HDV), 364*t*, 365
Hepatobiliary disease
in HIV-positive patient, fever and, 137
hypocalcemia and, 199
Hepatocellular cholestasis, jaundice and, 245
Herald bleed, in aortoenteric fistula, 159
Herbs. *See also specific type and* Natural products
unsafe, 40*t*, 593–594

Herceptin. *See* Trastuzumab
Heroin withdrawal, 91
Hespan. *See* Hetastarch
Hetastarch, 524
Hexalen. *See* Altretamine
5-HIAA (5-hydroxyindoleacetic acid), 365
HIDA scan
in fever, 131
in jaundice, 244
in nausea and vomiting, 265
High-altitude acclimatization, polycythemia and, 292
High-density lipoprotein (HDL) cholesterol, **355–360**
High-dose dexamethasone suppression test, 360
High-oxygen-affinity hemoglobins, polycythemia and, 292
Hiprex. *See* Methenamine
Histamine, in anaphylaxis, 25
Histoplasma capsulatum antigen, urine, **365–366**
Histussin-D. *See* Hydrocodone, with pseudoephedrine
HIV infection/AIDS
abdominal pain and, 4
arthritis and, 247
diarrhea and, 100, 137
parasitic, 98, 100, 137
fever in patient with, **135–141**
differential diagnosis/causes of, 136–138
imaging/clinical studies in, 139–140
initial evaluation in, 135
laboratory findings/data in, 138–139
management of, 140
physical examination/findings in, 138
leukopenia and, 256
testing for, **366**
thrombocytopenia and, 335
Hivid. *See* Zalcitabine
HLA antibodies, from platelet transfusions, 70
HMG-CoA reductase inhibitors, 612*t*
Hollow viscus
cancer pain and, 288
perforation of
abdominal pain and, 2–3, 5*t*
nausea and vomiting and, 262
Holoxan. *See* Ifosfamide
Holter monitoring
in dizziness/vertigo, 109
in syncope, 321
Homatropine, with hydrocodone, 526
Homocysteine, **366**
Hookworm infection, pruritus in, 297, 298, 299
Hormone therapy/synthetic substitutes, 467*t*. *See also specific agent*
Horner's syndrome, in carotid artery dissection, 147
Howell-Jolly bodies, 377
Humalog. *See* Lispro
Human chorionic gonadotropin (HCG), serum (HCB beta subunit), **366**
in nausea and vomiting, 265
Human immunodeficiency virus (HIV) antibody test, **366**. *See also* HIV infection/AIDS
Humorsol. *See* Demecarium
Humulin, 597*t*
Hyaline casts, in urine, microscopic appearance of, 385
Hycamtin. *See* Topotecan
Hycodan. *See* Hydrocodone, with homatropine
Hycomine. *See* Hydrocodone, with chlorpheniramine/phenylephrine/acetaminophen/caffeine
Hycotuss Expectorant. *See* Hydrocodone, with guaifenesin
Hydralazine, 524–525
Hydrea. *See* Hydroxyurea
Hydrochlorothiazide, 525
with amiloride, 525
with diovan, 599*t*
with irbesartan, 599*t*
with losartan, 599*t*
with spironolactone, 525
with triamterene, 525
with valsartan, 599*t*
Hydrocodone
with acetaminophen, 525
with aspirin, 525
with chlorpheniramine/phenylephrine/acetaminophen/caffeine, 526
with guaifenesin, 525
with homatropine, 526
with ibuprofen, 526
with pseudoephedrine, 526
Hydrocortisone, 597*t*
with bacitracin and neomycin and polymyxin B, topical, 483
with neomycin and colistin, otic, 548–549
with neomycin and colistin and thonzonium, otic, 548–549
with neomycin and polymyxin B, ophthalmic, 549, 608*t*, 609*t*
with polymyxin B, 562
with pramoxine, 563
rectal, 526
HydroDIURIL. *See* Hydrochlorothiazide
Hydromorphone, 526
Hydroxyapatite crystals, in arthritis, 247, 249
5-Hydroxyindoleacetic acid (5-HIAA), 365
11-Hydroxylase deficiency, hypokalemia and, 208
17-Hydroxylase deficiency, hypokalemia and, 208
Hydroxyurea, 526
for polycythemia vera, 295, 296
Hydroxyzine, 527
for insomnia, 237
for pruritus, 302
Hygroton. *See* Chlorthalidone
Hyoscyamine, 527
with atropine/scopolamine/phenobarbital, 527
Hyperaldosteronism
hypernatremia and, 192
hypertension and, 195
hypokalemia and, 207
hypomagnesemia and, 211
metabolic alkalosis and, 22
Hyperammonemia, in coma/acute mental status changes, 80
Hyperamylasemia. *See* Amylase
Hypercalcemia, **175–179**
cancer and, 76, 175, 176
coma/acute mental status changes and, 74, 75, 94
metastatic disease and, 76
delirium and, 94
falls and, 124
familial hypocalciuric, 175, 177
hyperparathyroidism and, 175, 176
hypomagnesemia and, 211
oliguria/anuria/acute renal failure and, 268
Hypercalciuria, hypomagnesemia and, 211
Hypercapnia, correction of, al

Hypercapnia, *(cont)*
kalosis and, 21
Hypercarbia
mechanical ventilation for agitated patient and, 448
in neuromuscular disease, 442–443
in ventilator patient, **454–455**
Hypercarbic ventilatory failure, mechanical ventilation for, 442
Hyperdefecation, in hyperthyroidism, 99
Hyperglycemia, **180–186**
alcohol withdrawal/delirium tremens and, 94
coma/acute mental status changes and, 75, 92, 94
delirium and, 92
differential diagnosis/causes of, 180–181
falls and, 123
hypernatremia and, 191
hyponatremia and, 215, 216
imaging/clinical studies in, 182–183
initial evaluation of, 180
laboratory findings/data in, 181–182
management of, 183–186, 183*t*
physical examination/findings in, 181
spurious, 181
Hyperhep. *See* Hepatitis B immune globulin
Hypericum perforatum (St. John's wort), 593
Hyperkalemia, **186–190**
cardiopulmonary arrest and, 45
coma/acute mental status changes and, 74, 94
delirium and, 94
factitious, 187
in hyponatremia, 218
pacemaker failure to capture and, 284
Hyperkalemic periodic paralysis, 187
Hyperlipidemia
hyponatremia and, 215
in nephrotic syndrome, protein electrophoresis in, 374*f*
Hypermagnesemia, coma/acute mental status changes and, 74
Hypermetabolism, hypercarbia in ventilator patient caused by, 454
Hypernatremia, **190–194**
coma/acute mental status changes and, 74, 75, 190
correction of, 193–194
Hyperosmolality, hyperkalemia and, 187
Hyperosmolar/hyperglycemic nonketotic syndrome, management of, 184
Hyperparathyroidism
coma/acute mental status changes and, 75
hypercalcemia and, 175, 176
hypertension and, 196
hypophosphatemia and, 221
multiple endocrine neoplasia and, 175
Hyperphosphatemia, hypocalcemia and, 200
Hyperpnea, in coma/acute mental status changes, 78
Hyperproteinemia, hyponatremia and, 215
Hyperreflexia
in alcohol withdrawal/delirium tremens, 93
in coma/acute mental status changes, 79
Hyperreninemia, hypokalemia and, 208
Hyperresonance, in chest pain, 61
Hypersegmentation, white blood cell, 389
Hypersplenism, 257
platelet sequestration and, 335, 336
Hyperstat. *See* Diazoxide
Hypertension, **194–198**
accelerated, 196
management of, 198
acute renal failure and, 268, 269
in alcohol withdrawal/delirium tremens, 93
in chest pain, 61
in coma/acute mental status changes, 78
differential diagnosis/causes of, 195–196
essential, 195
headache and, 144
in heart murmur, 153
in hypercalcemia, 177
in hypoglycemia, 204
imaging/clinical studies in, 197
initial evaluation of, 194–195
laboratory findings/data in, 197
malignant, 196
management of, 197–198. *See also* Antihypertensives
in nausea and vomiting, 261
oliguria/anuria and, 268, 269
in overdose, management of, 280
physical examination/findings in, 196–197
in polycythemia, 293
pulmonary. *See* Pulmonary hypertension
rebound, 194
renovascular, 195
secondary, 195–196
Hypertensive crisis/emergency, 194
management of, 197–198
Hypertensive encephalopathy, 195
coma/acute mental status changes and, 77, 92, 195
delirium and, 92, 93
Hyperthermia
coma/acute mental status changes and, 76, 78
malignant, 128
Hyperthyroidism
coma/acute mental status changes and, 75, 92, 94
delirium and, 92, 94
falls and, 124
hypercalcemia and, 176
hyperdefecation in, 99
hypertension and, 195
hypokalemia and, 207
insomnia and, 235
Hypertonic hyponatremia, 215–216
Hypertonic saline, for hyponatremia, 219
Hypertrophic cardiomyopathy, heart murmur in, 153, 155
Hyperventilation
for coma/acute mental status changes in CNS tumor, 82
dizziness and, 107, 109
dyspnea and, 113
hypophosphatemia and, 221
in respiratory alkalosis, 20
syncope and, 318, 323
Hyperventilation maneuver, in dizziness/vertigo, 109
Hyperviscosity syndrome, coma/acute mental status changes and, 77
Hypervolemic hyponatremia, 217
management of, 220

Hypnotic medications, 468*t*. *See also specific agent and* Sedatives
insomnia and, 234, 235
overdose/toxicity of, 275
Hypoalbuminemia
calcium levels affected in, 177, 199, 200
hypomagnesemia and, 211
in nephrotic syndrome, protein electrophoresis in, 374*f*
protein electrophoresis in, 374*f*
Hypoaldosteronism, hyporeninemic, hyperkalemia and, 188
Hypocalcemia, **198–201**
coma/acute mental status changes and, 74, 75, 93, 94
delirium and, 93, 94
diarrhea and, 101
hypomagnesemia differentiated from, 211
Hypocalciuric hypercalcemia, familial, 175, 177
Hypoglycemia, **202–205**
alcohol withdrawal/delirium tremens and, 94
coma/acute mental status changes and, 75, 92, 94, 202, 204
delirium and, 92
factitious, 203
falls and, 124
hypothermia and, 230
reactive, 203
seizures and, 314
syncope and, 318
Hypoglycemic agents, 463–464*t*. *See also* Insulin
oral, 183
hypoglycemia and, 203
overdose/toxicity of, 276
Hypokalemia, **206–210**
in alcohol withdrawal/delirium tremens, 94, 95–96
cardiopulmonary arrest and, 45
coma/acute mental status changes and, 74, 94
falls and, 124
hypomagnesemia and, 208, 210, 211
hyponatremia and, 218
hypophosphatemia and, 221
management of, 95–96
tachycardia and, 328
Hypomagnesemia, **210–214**
in alcohol withdrawal/delirium tremens, 94, 96
cardiopulmonary arrest and, 45
coma/acute mental status changes and, 74, 94
falls and, 124
hypocalcemia and, 199, 201
hypokalemia and, 208, 210, 211
hypophosphatemia and, 221
management of, 96, 201
tachycardia and, 328
Hyponatremia, **214–220**
coma/acute mental status changes and, 74, 94, 218
delirium and, 94
differential diagnosis/causes of, 215–217
dilutional, 215–216
essential, 216
euvolemic, 217, 219–220
hypertonic, 215–216
hypervolemic, 217, 220
hypotonic, 216
hypovolemic, 216, 219
imaging/clinical studies in, 218
initial evaluation of, 214–215
laboratory findings/data in, 218
management of, 219–220
physical examination/findings in, 217–218
Hypoparathyroidism
coma/acute mental status changes and, 75
diarrhea in, 99
hypocalcemia and, 199
Hypoperfusion, pacemaker complications and, 283
Hypophosphatemia, **220–223**, 223*t*
alcoholism and, 221
withdrawal/delirium tremens and, 94, 96
management of, 96, 222–223, 223*t*
Hypopituitarism
coma/acute mental status changes and, 75
hyponatremia and, 217
hypothermia and, 230
Hyporeninemic hypoaldosteronism, hyperkalemia and, 188
Hypotension, **224–229**
in abdominal pain, 1
in acidosis, 9
in anemia, 30
in bradycardia, 39
in chest pain, 61
in coagulopathy, 68–69
in coma/acute mental status changes, 72, 77, 77–78
in diarrhea, 97, 100
differential diagnosis/causes of, 224–225
in dizziness, 104, 105
in dyspnea, 113
falls and, 123, 124, 125
in fever, 129, 132
in heart murmur, 153
in hematemesis/melena, 158, 159
in hematochezia, 162, 163
in hyperglycemia, 180, 181
in hypernatremia, 192–193
in hyponatremia, 217
imaging/clinical studies in, 227
initial evaluation of, 224
laboratory findings/data in, 226–227
in leukopenia, 257
management of, 227–229
in nausea and vomiting, 261, 263–264
oliguria/anuria and, 267, 269
in overdose, management of, 280
pacemaker complications and, 283
physical examination/findings in, 225–226
in pre-syncope, 106
syncope and, 316, 317, 322
tachycardia and, 323, 328
wheezing and, 341
Hypotensive shock, **224–229**. *See also* Shock
anaphylaxis and, 24
Hypothermia, **229–233**
coma/acute mental status changes and, 76, 78, 93
delirium and, 93
in leukocytosis, 253
rewarming from, cardiopulmonary arrest and, 45
Hypothyroidism
coma/acute mental status changes and, 75, 94
delirium and, 94
hypertension and, 195
hyponatremia and, 214, 217
nausea and vomiting and, 263
Hypotonic hyponatremia, 216
Hypoventilation
alveolar
pO_2 in, 370
polycythemia and, 292

Hypoventilation, *(cont)*
in respiratory acidosis, 11–12
in ventilator patient
agitation and, 448, 449
hypoxemia and, 451, 453
Hypovolemia,
oliguria/anuria/acute renal failure and, 267, 268
Hypovolemic hyponatremia, 216
management of, 219
Hypovolemic shock, 224–225. *See also* Shock
management of, 228
Hypoxemia
dyspnea and, 111
mechanical ventilation for, 442
pacemaker failure to capture and, 284
syncope and, 318
in ventilator patient, **450–454**
agitation and, 448
Hytrin. *See* Terazosin
Hyzaar. *See* Losartan, with hydrochlorothiazide

I

Ibuprofen, 289–290, 606*t*
with hydrocodone, 526
Ibutilide, 527
ICU psychosis, 77, 92
agitation in ventilator patient caused by, 449, 450
Idamycin. *See* Idarubicin
Idarubicin, 527
Idiopathic hypertrophic subaortic stenosis, syncope and, 318
Idiopathic thrombocytopenic purpura (ITP), 67, 334
management of, 71, 337
Idioventricular rhythm, accelerated, 327
Ifex. *See* Ifosfamide
Ifosfamide, 527
IgA, quantitative, laboratory reference/normal values for, 376
IgD, quantitative, laboratory reference/normal values for, 376
IgE, quantitative, laboratory reference/normal values for, 376
IgG, quantitative, laboratory reference/normal values for, 376
IgM
anti-HAV, 364*t*, 365
anti-HBc, 364*t*, 365
anti-HDV, 364*t*, 365
quantitative, laboratory reference/normal values for, 376
IL-2 (aldesleukin), 473
Iletin II, 597*t*
Ileum, fluids produced by, composition/daily production of, 436*t*
Ileus, paralytic
abdominal pain and, 5*t*
nausea and vomiting and, 262
Iliac crest, posterior, bone marrow aspiration and biopsy from, 397–399
Ilopan. *See* Dexpanthenol
Ilopan-Choline Oral. *See* Dexpanthenol
Ilosone. *See* Erythromycin
Ilotycin. *See* Erythromycin, ophthalmic
IMDUR. *See* Isosorbide mononitrate
Imipenem-cilastin, 527–528
Imipramine, 528
for insomnia, 237
Imiquimod cream, 5%, 528
Imitrex. *See* Sumatriptan
Immobilization, hypercalcemia and, 176
Immune globulin, intravenous, 528
for idiopathic thrombocytopenic purpura (ITP), 337
Immune-mediated disorders, thrombocytopenia and, 334–335
management of, 337
Immunocompromised host. *See also* HIV infection/AIDS
fever in, 127
irradiated platelets for, 70–71
parasitic diarrhea in, 98, 100, 137
Immunoglobulins. *See also specific type under Ig*
electrophoresis values for, 374*f*, 375*t*
quantitative analysis of, **376**
Immunosuppressive agents, 467*t*. *See also specific agent*
Imodium. *See* Loperamide
Impedance plethysmography, in central venous line problems, 55
Imuran. *See* Azathioprine
IMV (intermittent mandatory ventilation), 445
synchronized (SIMV), 445
for ventilator weaning, 459
Inamrinone, 528
Inapsine. *See* Droperidol
Incisions, examination of, in coagulopathy, 69
Indapamide, 528
Inderal. *See* Propranolol
Indinavir, 528–529
Indirect Fick, for cardiac output, 307
Indocin. *See* Indomethacin
Indomethacin, 605*t*
for pericarditis, 66
Infection. *See also* Sepsis
arthritis and, 246, 247
central nervous system
coma/acute mental status changes and, 76, 92
delirium and, 92
central venous line problems and, 54, 55, 56, 131
coma/acute mental status changes and, 76, 82
cough and, 89
diarrhea and, 98
falls and, 125
fever and, 128
hematuria and, 167
hypothermia and, 229–230, 230
leukocytosis and, 251, 252
leukopenia and, 255, 257
management of, 259–260
oliguria/anuria/acute renal failure and, 268
pericarditis and, 58
respiratory alkalosis and, 21
seizures and, 309
thrombocytopenia and, 335
Infed. *See* Iron dextran
Infergen. *See* Interferon alfacon-1
Infestation, pruritus caused by, 296, 297, 298
Infiltrative processes
leukopenia and, 257
thrombocytopenia and, 334
Inflammation/inflammatory disorders
anemia and, 28
arthritis and, 247, 248
diarrhea and, 99
gastrointestinal, constipation and, 83
leukocytosis and, 252
Inflammatory bowel disease
arthritis and, 246

constipation and, 83
diarrhea and, 99
hematochezia and, 163
Infliximab, 529
Influenza vaccine, 529
Ingestion overdose, decontamination for, 280
INH. *See* Isoniazid
Inhalants, respiratory and nasal, 468*t*. *See also specific agent and* Bronchodilators
Inhaled irritants, cough and, 87
Innohep. *See* Tinzaparin
Inocor. *See* Inamrinone
Inotropin. *See* Dopamine
INR. *See* International normalized ratio
Insomnia, **234–238**
alternative therapies for, 237
drugs in management of, 237
nonmedical management of, 237
rebound, 234
Inspired fraction of oxygen (FiO_2)
adjusting, for ventilator patient, 447
high peak pressures and, 458
hypoxemia and, 453
ratio of to PaO_2 (P/F ratio), in respiratory failure, mechanical ventilation and, 442
ventilator set up and, 445
Insulin, 529, 597*t*
for diabetic ketoacidosis, 185
for hyperkalemia, 189
for hyperosmolar/hyperglycemia nonketotic syndrome, 184
islet cell tumor producing, 203
overdose/toxicity of, 276
hypoglycemia and, 202, 203
serum, in hypoglycemia, 204
for type 2 diabetes, 183, 183*t*
Insulin Glargine, 597*t*
Insulinoma, hypoglycemia and, 203
Intake/output values, in hypernatremia, 190
Intal. *See* Cromolyn sodium
Integrilin. *See* Eptifibatide
Intensive care unit, admission to
hematemesis/melena and, 160–161, 163
hematochezia and, 163, 165
hemoptysis and, 171, 174
hypertensive emergency and, 197
Intensive care unit (ICU) psychosis, 77, 92
agitation in ventilator patient caused by, 449, 450
Interferon, for polycythemia vera, 295
Interferon alfa, 529
Interferon alfa-2B and ribavirin combination, 530
Interferon alfacon-1, 530
Interferon beta-1b, 530
Interferon gamma-1b, 530
Interleukin-2 (IL-2/aldesleukin), 473
Intermediate-acting insulins, 597*t*. *See also* Insulin
Intermittent mandatory ventilation (IMV), 445
synchronized (SIMV), 445
for ventilator weaning, 459
Internal jugular vein, for central venous catheterization
left, 402
right, 400–402
International normalized ratio (INR), **366–367**
Interstitial lung disease
cough and, 87
dyspnea and, 112
high peak pressures and, 456
respiratory alkalosis and, 21
Interstitial renal disease/interstitial nephritis
hematuria and, 167
oliguria/anuria/acute renal failure and, 268
Intestinal bypass surgery
arthritis and, 247
hypomagnesemia and, 211
diarrhea and, 100
Intestinal colic, 2. *See also* Abdominal pain
Intestinal ischemia, nausea and vomiting and, 262
Intestinal motility, decreased, nausea and vomiting and, 263
Intestinal obstruction
abdominal pain and, 2, 3, 5*t*
constipation and, 82, 83
nausea and vomiting and, 262
Intoxications. *See also* Drugs/toxins
delirium and, 93
Intracath, insertion of, 411–412, 413*f*
Intracranial hemorrhage
coma/acute mental status changes and, 77, 82, 92
delirium and, 92
headache and, 144, 146
Intracranial mass lesions
coma/acute mental status changes and, 73, 76, 82
headache and, 146
in HIV-positive patient, 138
nausea and vomiting and, 263
Intracranial pressure, increased
bradycardia and, 40, 43
nausea and vomiting and, 263
Intracranial surgery, hyponatremia after, 217
Intratubular renal obstruction, oliguria/anuria/acute renal failure and, 269
Intravenous cannulation/catheterization, 411–412, 413*f*, 414*f*
in chest pain patient, 63
in hematemesis/melena, 158
in hematochezia, 162
in hemoptysis, 174
in hypoglycemia, 202
infection and, management of, 132
for seizures, 314
Intravenous drug use. *See also* Substance abuse
jaundice and, 242
Intravenous fluids. *See* Fluid management
Intravenous immune globulin, 528
for idiopathic thrombocytopenic purpura (ITP), 337
Intravenous pyelography
in dysuria, 120
in hematuria, 169
in oliguria/anuria, 271
Intron A. *See* Interferon alfa
Intubation, **407–410**, 409*f*, 444. *See also* Endotracheal tube; Mechanical ventilation
in hemoptysis, 174
in overdose, 279
for stridor, 344
Invirase. *See* Saquinavir
Ionized calcium
in hypercalcemia, 177
in hypocalcemia, 199
Iopidine. *See* Apraclonidine
Ipecac syrup, 530
Ipratropium, 530–531
with albuterol, 472–473
Irbesartan, 599*t*
with hydrochlorothiazide, 599*t*
Irinotecan, 531
Iron binding capacity, total

Iron binding capacity, *(cont)* (TIBC), **367**
  in anemia, 29*t*, 31
Iron deficiency anemia, 29, 29*t*, 31, 32
  pruritus and, 299
Iron dextran, 531
Iron levels, **367**
  in anemia, 29, 29*t*, 31
  laboratory reference/normal values for, 367
Iron sucrose, 531
Iron therapy, 589
  for anemia, 32
  overdose/toxicity of, antidote for, 282
Irregular pulse, **238–241**. *See also* Arrhythmias; Bradycardia; Tachycardia
Irritable bowel syndrome, 100
Ischemia
  bowel
  abdominal pain and, 1, 5*t*
  diarrhea and, 99
  hematuria and, 167
  leukocytosis and, 252
  myocardial. *See also* Myocardial infarction
  dyspnea and, 112
  management of, 64–65
  renal, oliguria/anuria/acute renal failure and, 268
  tissue, cancer pain and, 288
Ischemic colitis, hematochezia and, 163
ISMO. *See* Isosorbide mononitrate
Isometheptene/dichloralphenazone/acetaminophen, for migraine headache, 150
Isoniazid (INH), 531
Isoproterenol, 532
Isoptin. *See* Verapamil
Isopto Carbachol. *See* Carbachol
Isopto Carpine. *See* Pilocarpine
Isopto Eserine. *See* Physostigmine
Isordil. *See* Isosorbide dinitrate
Isosorbide dinitrate, 532
Isosorbide mononitrate, 532
Isotretinoin (13-*cis* retinoic acid), 532
Isradipine, 532
Isuprel. *See* Isoproterenol
Itching. *See* Pruritus
ITP. *See* Idiopathic thrombocytopenic purpura
Itraconazole, 532
IV. *See* Intravenous cannulation/catheterization
IVIG (intravenous immune globulin), 528
IVP. *See* Intravenous pyelography

J

J wave, in hypothermia, 232
Jamshidi needle, for bone marrow aspiration and biopsy, 397
Jaundice, **242–245**
Jelco assembly, for paracentesis, 420
Joint fluid analysis. *See also* Arthrocentesis
  in arthritis, 248–249
Joint fluid drainage, in septic arthritis, 250
Joint swelling, **245–250**
  differential diagnosis/causes of, 246–248
  imaging/clinical studies in, 250
  initial evaluation of, 246
  laboratory findings/data in, 248–250
  management of, 250
  physical examination/findings in, 248
Joint x-rays, in arthritis, 250
Joints, examination of, in leukopenia, 258
JRA. *See* Juvenile rheumatoid arthritis
Jugular vein, for central venous catheterization
  left internal, 402
  right internal, 400–402
Jugular venous distention. *See also* Neck/neck veins, examination of
  in cardiopulmonary arrest, 46
  in cough, 88
  in dyspnea, 114
  in heart murmur, 154
  in hyponatremia, 218
  in hypotension/shock, 225
  in tachycardia, 328
Jugular venous pulsations, in bradycardia, 41–42
Junctional tachycardia, automatic atrioventricular, 325–326
Juniper, toxicity of, 594
Juvenile rheumatoid arthritis, 248

K

K-Lor. *See* Potassium, supplementary
Kabikinase. *See* Streptokinase
Kaletra. *See* Lopinavir/ritonavir
Kao-Spen. *See* Kaolin-pectin
Kaochlor. *See* Potassium, supplementary
Kaodene. *See* Kaolin-pectin
Kaolin-pectin, 532–533
Kaon. *See* Potassium, supplementary
Kapectolin. *See* Kaolin-pectin
Kava kava (kava kava root extract/*Piper methysticum*), 592
Kayexalate. *See* Sodium polystyrene
Keflex. *See* Cephalexin
Keflin. *See* Cephalothin
Keftab. *See* Cephalexin
Kefzol. *See* Cefazolin
Kenalog. *See* Triamcinolone
Keogh tube, 410
Keppra. *See* Levetiracetam
Kerlone. *See* Betaxolol
Kernig's sign
  in coma/acute mental status changes, 79
  in nausea and vomiting, 264
Ketamine, overdose/toxicity of, 277
Ketoacidosis
  alcoholic, 13, 17
  diabetic, 13, 17, 180
  management of, 185
  starvation, 13, 17
Ketoconazole, 533
17-Ketogenic steroids (17-KGS), **367**
Ketones
  in diabetic ketoacidosis, 181
  in hyperglycemia, 182
  in metabolic gap acidosis, 16
  urine, **384**
  in diabetic ketoacidosis, 185
Ketoprofen, 606*t*
Ketorolac, 605*t*
  ophthalmic, 608*t*
Ketosis. *See also* Ketoacidosis
  starvation, 13, 17
17-Ketosteroids (17-KS), **367**
Ketotifen, 609*t*
17-KGS. *See* 17-Ketogenic steroids
Kidney stones
  Foley catheter problems and, 142
  hematuria and, 168, 169–170
  management of, 169–170

Kidney transplant. *See* Renal transplant
Kidney/ureter/bladder (KUB) film. *See* Abdominal plain films
Kidneys. *See also under Renal*
 bicarbonate loss through, acidosis and, 13
 potassium loss through, hypokalemia and, 207
Kilograms/pounds weight conversion chart, 619*t*
Klonopin. *See* Clonazepam
K-Lor. *See* Potassium, supplementary
Klorvess. *See* Potassium, supplementary
Knee, arthrocentesis of, 393, 394*f*
KOH prep, **368**
 in pruritus, 301
Korsakoff's psychosis, coma/acute mental status changes and, 75
17-KS. *See* 17-Ketosteroids
KUB (kidney/ureter/bladder) film. *See* Abdominal plain films
Kussmaul respirations
 in coma/acute mental status changes, 78
 in diabetic ketoacidosis, 180, 181
Kussmaul's sign, in oliguria/anuria, 270
Kwashiorkor (protein calorie malnutrition), hypoglycemia and, 203
Kwell. *See* Lindane
Kyphoscoliosis, respiratory acidosis and, 12
Kytril. *See* Granisetron

L

L-asparaginase, 481
L-PAM. *See* Melphalan
Labetalol, 533, 601*t*
 for aortic dissection, 65
 for hypertensive emergency, 198
Laboratory diagnosis, **345–389**. *See also specific test and specific disorder*
Labyrinthectomy, for dizziness/vertigo, 110
Labyrinthitis, 106
 nausea and vomiting and, 263
LAC-Hydrin. *See* Lactic acid and ammonium hydroxide
Lactate dehydrogenase (LDH), **368**
 pleural fluid, 433*t*
 pleural fluid-to-serum ratio, 433*t*
Lactated Ringer's solution, composition of, 435*t*
Lactation, excessive, hypomagnesemia and, 211
Lactic acid and ammonium hydroxide (ammonium lactate), 533
Lactic acid (lactate) levels, **368**
 in metabolic gap acidosis, 16
Lactic acidosis, 13, 16
Lactinex granules. *See* Lactobacillus
Lactobacillus, 533
Lactose intolerance, diarrhea and, 100
Lactulose, 85*t*, 533
 diarrhea caused by, 99
Lamictal. *See* Lamotrigine
Lamisil. *See* Terbinafine
Lamivudine, 534
 with zidovudine, 588
Lamotrigine, 534
Lamprene. *See* Clofazimine
Lanorinal. *See* Aspirin, with butalbital
Lanoxicaps. *See* Digoxin
Lanoxin. *See* Digoxin
Lansoprazole, 611*t*
Lantus. *See* Insulin Glargine
LAP score. *See* Leukocyte alkaline phosphatase (LAP) score
Large bowel obstruction. *See also* Intestinal obstruction
 nausea and vomiting and, 262
Laryngeal tumor, stridor and, 201
Laryngospasm
 in hypocalcemia, prevention of, 201
 stridor and, 342
Larynx, disorders of, cough and, 87
Lasix. *See* Furosemide
Latanoprost, 608*t*
Laxative abuse, 98, 99
 hypocalcemia and, 199
Laxatives, 466*t*. *See also specific agent*
 for constipation, 85, 85*t*
 diarrhea caused by, 98, 99
LDH. *See* Lactate dehydrogenase
LDL cholesterol. *See* Low-density lipoprotein (LDL) cholesterol
Lead, overdose/toxicity of, antidote for, 282
Leads, pacemaker, failure to capture and, 283
Leflunomide, 534
Left internal jugular vein, for central venous catheterization, 402
Left ventricular function, impaired, premature ventricular contractions with, 241
Legs. *See also* Extremities
 pruritus affecting, 297
Leiomyomas, uterine, polycythemia and, 292
Lente Iletin II, 597*t*
Lepirudin, 534
Lescol. *See* Fluvastatin
Letrozole, 534
Leucovorin, 534
Leukemia
 hypokalemia and, 206
 leukopenia and, 256
 pruritus and, 299
Leukeran. *See* Chlorambucil
Leukine. *See* Sargramostim
Leukocyte alkaline phosphatase (LAP) score, **368**
 in leukocytosis, 254
 in leukopenia, 258
 in polycythemia vera, 292, 294
Leukocyte count. *See* White blood cell (WBC) count
Leukocyte esterase, urine, **384**
Leukocyte-poor red blood cells (RBCs), transfusion of, 437–438
Leukocytes. *See also under White blood cell*
 fecal, testing for, **379**
 in diarrhea, 102
 in HIV-positive patient, 139
 in urine, hematuria and, 168
Leukocytosis, **251–255**
 in chest pain, 62
 definition of, 252
 differential diagnosis/causes of, 252–253
 imaging/clinical studies in, 254
 initial evaluation of, 251–252
 laboratory findings/data in, 253–254
 management of, 255
 physical examination/findings in, 253
 in polycythemia vera, 292, 294

Leukopenia, **255–261**
bone marrow failure and, 256–257, 260
differential diagnosis/causes of, 256–257
imaging/clinical studies in, 259
initial evaluation of, 255–256
laboratory findings/data in, 258
management of, 259–261
physical examination/findings in, 257–258
Leuprolide, 534–535
Leustatin. *See* Cladribine
Levalbuterol, 535
Levamisole, 535
Levaquin. *See* Levofloxacin
Levatol. *See* Penbutolol
Level of consciousness. *See* Coma; Consciousness
Levetiracetam, 535
Levine tube, 410, 411
Levobetaxolol, 607*t*
Levobunolol, 607*t*
Levocabastine, ophthalmic, 609*t*
Levodopa/carbidopa, 490
Levofloxacin, 535
Levonorgestrel implant, 535
Levophed. *See* Norepinephrine
Levothyroxine, 535–536
Levsin. *See* Hyoscyamine
Librium. *See* Chlordiazepoxide
Lice (pediculosis), pruritus and, 296, 297, 298
Lichen planus, pruritus in, 297, 298
Lichen simplex, pruritus in, 297, 298
Licorice, toxicity of, 594
hypokalemia and, 208
Liddle's syndrome, hypokalemia and, 208
Lidocaine, 536
with bacitracin and neomycin and polymyxin B, topical, 483
for cluster headache, 150
intranasal, for migraine headache, 150
with prilocaine, 536
for tachycardia, 331–332
therapeutic/toxic levels of, 613*t*
for ventricular fibrillation, 47
for ventricular tachycardia
stable, 47, 49
unstable, 49
Life root, toxicity of, 594
Ligase chain reaction, for *Neisseria gonorrhoeae* and *Chlamydia trachomatis*, for urine, 120, **368**
Lightheadedness, 107. *See also* Dizziness
management of, 110
Lindane, 536
Linezolid, 536
Liothyronine, 536–537
Lipase, **368**
in abdominal pain, 6
in hypercalcemia, 178
in hyperglycemia, 182
in nausea and vomiting, 265
Lipitor. *See* Atorvastatin
Liqui-Char. *See* Charcoal, activated
Lisinopril, 598*t*
Lispro, 597*t*
Lithium, 537
overdose/toxicity of, 276, 613*t*
therapeutic levels of, 613*t*
Liver biopsy, in jaundice, 244
Liver disease
alcoholic, jaundice and, 242, 245
hypoglycemia and, 203
hypophosphatemia and, 221
pruritus in, 298–299
Liver disorders
abdominal pain and, 3, 3*t*
bleeding and, 68
management of, 72
coma/acute mental status changes and, 75
hematemesis/melena and, 158
hemoptysis and, 172
hypocalcemia and, 199
respiratory alkalosis and, 21
Liver enzymes, in hypophosphatemia, 222
Liver failure, nausea and vomiting and, 263
Liver function tests
in abdominal pain, 6
in alcohol withdrawal/delirium tremens, 94
in falls, 126
in fever, in HIV-positive patient, 139
in hematemesis/melena, 158
in hypoglycemia, 204
in hyponatremia, 218
in jaundice, 243–244
in leukocytosis, 254
in leukopenia, 258
in nausea and vomiting, 265
in overdose, 279
in pruritus, 301
in respiratory alkalosis, 22
in thrombocytopenia, 337
Liver scan, in thrombocytopenia, 337
Liver tumors, polycythemia and, 292
Livostin. *See* Levocabastine
Local anesthetic agents, 468*t*. *See also specific agent*
Locked-in syndrome, 77
Lodine. *See* Etodolac
Lodoxamide, 609*t*
Lomefloxacin, 537
Lomotil. *See* Diphenoxylate with atropine
Lomustine (CCNU), 537
Long-acting insulins, 597*t*. *See also* Insulin
Long-term loop ECG, in syncope, 321–322
Loniten. *See* Minoxidil
Loop diuretics. *See also* Furosemide
for oliguria/anuria/acute renal failure, 272
Loop ECG, long-term, in syncope, 321–322
Loperamide, 103, 537
Lopid. *See* Gemfibrozil
Lopinavir/ritonavir, 537
Lopressor. *See* Metoprolol
Loprox. *See* Ciclopirox
Lopurin. *See* Allopurinol
Lorabid. *See* Loracarbef
Loracarbef, 603*t*
Loratadine, 537–538
Lorazepam, 538
for alcohol withdrawal/delirium tremens, 95, 96
for seizures, 314
Lorcet. *See* Hydrocodone, with acetaminophen
Lortab ASA. *See* Hydrocodone, with aspirin
Losartan, 599*t*
with hydrochlorothiazide, 599*t*
Lotensin. *See* Benazepril
Lotrimin. *See* Clotrimazole
Lotrisone. *See* Clotrimazole, with betamethasone
Lovastatin, 612*t*
Lovenox. *See* Enoxaparin
Low-density lipoprotein (LDL) cholesterol, 355–356
Low-dose dexamethasone suppression test, 359–360
Low molecular weight heparin, for myocardial infarction, 64

Low systemic vascular resistance (SVR) shock. *See also* Shock
  pulmonary artery catheter monitoring in, 423*t*
Lower airway obstruction. *See also* Airway obstruction
  anaphylaxis and, 25
Lowsium. *See* Magaldrate
Lozol. *See* Indapamide
LP. *See* Lumbar puncture
L-PAM. *See* Melphalan
Lugol's solution (potassium iodide/SSKI), 563
Lumbar puncture, **412–418**, 416*f*, 419*t*
  in alcohol withdrawal/delirium tremens, 94
  in coma/acute mental status changes, 81
  complications of, 418
  contraindications for, 414
  in dizziness/vertigo, 109
  in fever, 131
  in HIV-positive patient, 139
  in headache, 148
  headache after, 418
  indications for, 412–414
  in leukopenia, 259
  procedure for, 414–418, 416*f*
  in seizures, 313
  traumatic, 418
Lung abscess, hemoptysis and, 171
Lung cancer
  cough and, 87
  hemoptysis and, 171, 174
  management of, 174
  syndrome of inappropriate antidiuretic hormone secretion (SIADH) and, 217
Lung compliance, worsening, high peak pressures and, 456
Lung Injury, acute, mechanical ventilation for, 442
Lung volumes, in cough, 88
Lungs
  examination of
  in abdominal pain, 4
  in acidosis, 15
  in anaphylaxis, 25
  in aspiration, 37
  in bradycardia, 42
  in chest pain, 61
  in cough, 88
  in dyspnea, 113–114
  in fever, 130
    in HIV-positive patient, 138
  in hyperglycemia, 181
  in hypertension, 196
  in hyponatremia, 218
  in hypophosphatemia, 221
  in hypothermia, 231
  in insomnia, 236
  in leukocytosis, 253
  in leukopenia, 258
  in oliguria/anuria, 270
  in overdose, 278
  pacemaker complications and, 285
  in polycythemia, 293
  in seizures, 311
  interstitial disease of. *See* Interstitial lung disease
  water loss via, hypernatremia and, 192
Lupron. *See* Leuprolide
Lupus anticoagulant, 349
Lupus erythematosus, systemic (SLE)
  antinuclear antibodies in, 348
  arthritis and, 246, 248
  hemoptysis and, 172
  hyperkalemia and, 188
  thrombocytopenia and, 335
Luvox. *See* Fluvoxamine
Lyme disease, arthritis in, 247
Lyme disease vaccine, 538
Lymerix. *See* Lyme disease vaccine
Lymph nodes, examination of
  in cough, 88
  in fever, 130
  in hypercalcemia, 177
  in leukocytosis, 253
  in leukopenia, 258
  in pruritus, 300
Lymphocytes, **387–388**
  atypical, **388**
  laboratory reference/normal values for, 354*t*, 369, 387, 388
  total, **369**
Lymphocytosis, 254
Lymphoma
  bowel, diarrhea and, 99
  cutaneous T-cell, pruritus and, 298
  pruritus and, 299
Lysodren. *See* Mitotane

M

Ma huang (ephedra), 591
  hypertension and, 195
  toxicity of, 591, 594
Maalox. *See* Aluminum hydroxide, with magnesium hydroxide
Maalox Plus. *See* Aluminum hydroxide, with magnesium hydroxide and simethicone
Macrobid. *See* Nitrofurantoin
Macrodantin. *See* Nitrofurantoin
Mag-Ox 400. *See* Magnesium oxide
Magaldrate, 538
Magnesium, **369**, 590
  disorders of balance of. *See also* Hypermagnesemia; Hypomagnesemia
  in alcohol withdrawal/delirium tremens, 94
  coma/acute mental status changes and, 74, 94
  hypokalemia and, 208
  metabolic alkalosis and, 22
  in hyperglycemia, 182
  in hypophosphatemia, 222
  serum, in hypomagnesemia, 211
  supplementary
  for alcohol withdrawal/delirium tremens, 96
  for hypocalcemia, 201
  for hypomagnesemia, 201, 212–213
  for tachycardia, 332
  urine, **369**
  in hypomagnesemia, 211, 212
Magnesium carbonate, with aluminum hydroxide, 475
Magnesium citrate, 85*t*, 538
Magnesium hydroxide, 85*t*, 538
  with aluminum hydroxide, 475
  with aluminum hydroxide and simethicone, 475
Magnesium oxide, 538
  for hypomagnesemia, 213
Magnesium retention test, 212
Magnesium sulfate, 539
  for alcohol withdrawal/delirium tremens, 96
  for hypomagnesemia, 212–213
  IM, 213
  IV, 212–213
Magnesium trisilicate, with aluminum hydroxide, 475
Magnetic resonance imaging (MRI)
  in fever, 131
  in headache, 148
  in oliguria/anuria, 271
  in polycythemia, 294
  in seizures, 313
Malabsorption
  diarrhea and, 100

Malabsorption, *(cont)*
 hypocalcemia and, 199
 hypomagnesemia and, 211
 hypophosphatemia and, 221
Malaise, in HIV-positive patient, fever and, 135
Male breast, examination of, in jaundice, 243
Males, bladder catheterization in, 396
Malignancy. *See* Cancer
Malignant carcinoid syndrome, diarrhea and, 99
Malignant hypertension, 196
 oliguria/anuria/acute renal failure and, 268, 269
Malignant neuroleptic syndrome
 fever and, 128, 134
 management of, 134
Mallory-Weiss tear
 hematemesis/melena and, 159, 161
 management of, 161
Malnutrition
 hypocalcemia and, 199
 hypoglycemia and, 203
 hypophosphatemia and, 221
 thrombocytopenia and, 334
Mandol. *See* Cefamandole
Mannitol, 539
 for coma/acute mental status changes in CNS tumor, 82
 hypernatremia and, 190, 191
 hyponatremia and, 214, 216
 for oliguria/anuria/acute renal failure, 272
MAOI. *See* Monoamine oxidase inhibitors
Marcaine. *See* Bupivacaine
Margination, neutrophil, 257
Marinol. *See* Dronabinol
Mast cell stabilizers, ophthalmic, 609*t*
MAST suit, 227
Mastocytosis, pruritus and, 299
Matulane. *See* Procarbazine
Mavik. *See* Trandolapril
Maxair. *See* Pirbuterol
Maxalt. *See* Rizatriptan
Maxipime. *See* Cefepime
Maxitrol. *See* Neomycin, with polymyxin B and dexamethasone, ophthalmic
Maxzide. *See* Hydrochlorothiazide, with triamterene
Mazaquin. *See* Lomefloxacin
MCH. *See* Mean cellular hemoglobin
MCV. *See* Mean cell volume
MDMA (3,4-methylenedioxymethamphetamine/ecstasy), toxicity of, 276–277
Mean cell volume (MCV), 377
 in anemia, 29–30
 laboratory reference/normal values for, 354*t*
Mean cellular hemoglobin concentration (MCHC), 377
 laboratory reference/normal values for, 354*t*
Mean cellular hemoglobin (MCH), 377
 laboratory reference/normal values for, 354*t*
Mechanical ventilation, **442–460**
 agitated patient and, **448–450**
 for aspiration, 39
 endotracheal intubation for, **407–410**, 409*f*, 444
 high peak pressures and, **456–458**
 hypercarbia in patient with, **454–455**
 hypoxemia in patient with, **450–454**
 indications for, **442–444**
 management of, **442–460**
 modes of, 445–446
 partial ventilatory assistance, 443–444
 pneumothorax and, 59
 agitation and, 448
 high peak pressures and, 457, 458
 hypoxemia and, 451, 453
 respiratory acidosis and, 18
 respiratory alkalosis and, 23
 settings for
 initial, 446
 reviewing/adjusting
  in agitated patient, 448, 450
  in hypoxemic patient, 451, 453
  routine modification of, **447–448**
 ventilator setup for, **444–447**
 weaning from, **458–460**
Mechlorethamine, 539
Meclizine, 539
 for dizziness/vertigo, 110
Median basilic vein, for central venous catheterization, 406–407
Medic Alert bracelet, for anaphylaxis patients, 27
Medications. *See* Drugs/toxins
Medihaler-ISO. *See* Isoproterenol
Mediquell. *See* Dextromethorphan
Medrol. *See* Methylprednisolone
Medroxyprogesterone, 539
Medullary thyroid carcinoma
 diarrhea and, 99
 hypocalcemia and, 200
Mefoxin. *See* Cefoxitin
Megace. *See* Megestrol acetate
Megaloblastic anemia, 29–30
 treatment of, hypokalemia and, 206
Megaloblastic syndromes, leukopenia and, 256
Megestrol acetate, 539–540
Melatonin, 592–593
 for insomnia, 237
Melena, **158–162**
 anemia and, 28
Mellaril. *See* Thioridazine
Meloxicam, 606*t*
Melphalan, 540
MEN. *See* Multiple endocrine neoplasia
Menest. *See* Esterified estrogens
Ménière's disease, 106
 surgery for, 110
Meningitis
 bacterial, cerebrospinal fluid findings in, 419*t*
 coma/acute mental status changes and, 72, 92
 delirium and, 92
 in HIV-positive patient, 137, 140
 management of, 134, 140
 nausea and vomiting and, 263
Menorrhagia, anemia and, 28
Menstrual history, in abdominal pain, 2
Mental status. *See also* Neurologic examination
 acute changes in, **72–82**
 differential diagnosis/causes of, 73–77
 exogenous causes of, 74, 81
 initial evaluation of, 72–73
 laboratory findings/data in, 80–81
 management of, 81–82
 physical examination/findings in, 77–80
 time course of, 72
 alcohol withdrawal/delirium tremens and, 90
 alkalosis and, 19

anaphylaxis and, 26
body temperature alteration and, 76
bradycardia and, 42
dizziness/vertigo and, 108
drugs/toxins and, 72, 74, 81
endocrine status and, 75
fluid/electrolyte status and, 74–75
hypernatremia and, 74, 75, 190
hypoglycemia and, 75, 92, 94, 202, 204
hypomagnesemia and, 212
hyponatremia and, 74, 94, 218
hypotension and, 224
infections and, 76, 82
insomnia and, 234
intracranial hemorrhage and, 77, 82
metabolic status and, 74–76, 81
nausea and vomiting and, 264
organ failure and, 75
psychiatric disorders and, 76–77
seizures and, 311
shock and, 224
trauma patient and, 73, 73–74
tumors and, 76, 82
vitamin deficiency states and, 75–76

Meperidine, 290, 540
Meprobamate, 540
Mepron. *See* Atovaquone
Mercaptopurine (6-MP), 540
Meridia. *See* Sibutramine
Meropenem, 540
Merrem. *See* Meropenem
Mesalamine, 540–541
Mesenteric ischemia/infarction, leukocytosis and, 252
Mesna, 541
Mesnex. *See* Mesna
Mesoridazine, 541
Metabolic acidosis. *See also* Acidosis
characteristics of, 9–11, 350*t*
chloride-responsive, 21
chloride-unresponsive, 22
compensation in, 11, 350*t*
differential diagnosis/causes of, 12–15
gap, 13–15
laboratory findings/data in, 16
initial evaluation of, 9–11
management of, 17–18, 228
nausea and vomiting and, 263
nongap, 12–13
laboratory findings/data in, 16
in shock, 228
Metabolic alkalosis. *See also* Alkalosis
characteristics of, 18–20, 350*t*
compensation in, 20, 350*t*
differential diagnosis/causes of, 21–22
hypokalemia and, 206
in hypophosphatemia, 222
initial evaluation of, 18–20
laboratory findings/data in, 23
management of, 23–24
Metabolic disorders
arthritis and, 247
coma/acute mental status changes and, 74–76, 81
constipation and, 83
delirium and, 92
falls and, 124–125
hypothermia and, 230
pre-syncope and, 107
pruritus and, 299
seizures and, 310
Metabolic encephalopathy, falls and, 125
Metabolism, increased, hypercarbia in ventilator patient caused by, 454
Metamucil. *See* Psyllium
Metanephrines, urine, **369**
Metaprel. *See* Metaproterenol
Metaproterenol, 541
Metaxalone, 541
Metformin, 183, 541
diarrhea caused by, 100
Methadone, 541
Methanol
metabolic acidosis caused by, 13, 16, 18
overdose/toxicity of, antidote for, 282
Methenamine, 541–542
Methergine. *See* Methylergonovine
Methimazole, 542
Methocarbamol, 542
Methotrexate, 542
Methyldopa, 542
3,4-Methylenedioxymethamphetamine (MDMA/ecstasy), toxicity of, 276–277
Methylergonovine, 542
N-Methyl-histamine, in anaphylaxis, 26
Methylprednisolone, 597*t*
for anaphylaxis, 27
for bronchospasm, 334
for dyspnea in asthma, 116
for stridor, 344
Methylprogesterone, with conjugated estrogens, 512–513
4-Methylpyrazole. *See* Fomepizole
Methyltestosterone
with conjugated estrogens, 513
with esterified estrogens, 512
Metipranolol, 607*t*
Metoclopramide, 543
for nausea and vomiting, 266
Metolazone, 543
for oliguria/anuria/acute renal failure, 272
Metopirone. *See* Metyrapone
Metoprolol, 601*t*
for tachycardia, 331
Metrogel. *See* Metronidazole
Metronidazole, 543
for *Clostridium difficile* diarrhea, 103
Metyrapone, 543–544
Mevacor. *See* Lovastatin
Mexiletine, 544
Mexitil. *See* Mexiletine
Mezlin. *See* Mezlocillin
Mezlocillin, 600*t*
Miacalcin. *See* Calcitonin
Micardis. *See* Telmisartan
Miconazole, 544
Micro-K. *See* Potassium, supplementary
Microalbuminuria, 346
Microcytic anemia, 29, 29*t*
Micronase. *See* Glyburide
Micturition syncope, 317
management of, 323
Midamor. *See* Amiloride
Midazolam, 544
for seizures, 314, 315
Midepigastric pain, 1
Midrin. *See* Isometheptene/dichloralphenazone/acetaminophen
Miglitol, 544
Migraine headache, 144
abdominal pain and, 4
with aura (classic migraine), 145
without aura (common migraine), 145
complicated, 145
management of, 149–150
nausea and vomiting and, 263
prophylactic therapy for, 150
syncope and, 318
Milk, phosphate content of, 223, 223*t*

Milk-alkali syndrome
hypercalcemia and, 176
metabolic alkalosis and, 22
Milk of Magnesia. *See* Magnesium hydroxide
Milrinone, 544
Miltown. *See* Meprobamate
Milwaukee shoulder syndrome, 249
Mineral oil, 85*t*, 545
Mineralocorticoids
excess, hypokalemia and, 207
hypernatremia and, 192
Minerals, 469*t*, **589–590**. *See also specific type*
Minipress. *See* Prazosin
Minoxidil, 545
Minute ventilation ($\dot{V}_e$)
high, high peak pressures and, 456
inadequate, in hypercarbic ventilator patient, 454
ventilator setup and, 444
ventilator weaning guidelines for, 458
Miotics, for glaucoma, 607*t*
Mirapex. *See* Pramipexole
Mirtazapine, 545
Misoprostol, 545
Mithracin. *See* Plicamycin
Mithramycin. *See* Plicamycin
Mitomycin C, 545
Mitotane, 545
Mitoxantrone, 546
Mitral regurgitation, heart murmur in, 154
congestive failure and, 152
myocardial infarction and, 152
Mitral stenosis
heart murmur in, 153, 155
hemoptysis and, 171, 172
Mitral valve prolapse, heart murmur in, 152, 154–155
Mixed connective tissue disease. *See also* Connective tissue/collagen-vascular disorders
arthritis and, 248
Mixed venous blood gases, 350*t*
Mixed venous oxygen saturation (SvO_2)
pulmonary artery catheter measurement of, 428*t*
in hypoxemic ventilator patient, 452
in shock, 423*t*
Moban. *See* Molindone
Mobic. *See* Meloxicam
Mobitz type I second-degree atrioventricular block (Wenckebach), 41, 239–240
ECG/rhythm strip in, 42
Mobitz type II second-degree atrioventricular block, 41, 239–240
ECG/rhythm strip in, 42
management of, 241
Modafinil, 546
Moduretic. *See* Hydrochlorothiazide, with amiloride
Moexipril, 598*t*
Molindone, 546
Monistat. *See* Miconazole
Monitoring
arterial line, **390–391**
problems with, **34–36**
central venous catheter, **399–407**, 403*f*
problems with, **53–57**
pulmonary artery catheter, **421–429**, 423*t*, 424*f*, 427*f*, 428*t*, 429*t*
problems with, **303–307**
Monitors, for pulmonary artery catheter, problems related to, 304
Monoamine oxidase inhibitors (MAOI), interactions of, hypertensive crisis and, 194
Monocid. *See* Cefonicid
Monoclate. *See* Antihemophilic factor
Monocytes, **388**
laboratory reference/normal values for, 354*t*, 388
Monopril. *See* Fosinopril
Monosodium urate crystals, in gout, 249
Monospot test, **369**
Montelukast, 546
Monurol. *See* Fosfomycin
Morphine, 290, 546
for aortic dissection, 65
for congestive heart failure, 116
for myocardial infarction, 64, 157
for pain management, 290
for pulmonary edema, 344
Moschowitz's syndrome (thrombotic thrombocytopenia purpura/TTP), 67, 335
management of, 337
Motor examination, in seizures, 312
Motrin. *See* Ibuprofen
Mouth, examination of
in arthritis, 248
in cough, 88
in headache, 147
in hypernatremia, 193
Moxifloxacin, 546
6-MP. *See* Mercaptopurine
MS Contin. *See* Morphine
Mucolytic agents, 465–466*t*. *See also specific agent*
Mucomyst. *See* Acetylcysteine
Mucosa/mucous membranes, examination of
in leukocytosis, 253
in thrombocytopenia, 336
in transfusion reaction, 340
Mucosil. *See* Acetylcysteine
Mucous membranes. *See* Mucosa
Mucous plugging, wheezing and, 342
Mucus, in urine, microscopic appearance of, 385
Multifocal atrial tachycardia, 326
Multiple endocrine neoplasia (MEN), hyperparathyroidism/hypercalcemia and, 175
Multiple myeloma
protein electrophoresis in, 374*f*
pruritus and, 299
Multiple sclerosis, dizziness/vertigo and, 106
Multisensory deficit disorder, disequilibrium and, 107
Mupirocin, 546–547
Murmurs. *See* Heart murmurs
Muromonab-CD3, 547
Murphy's sign
in fever, 130
in jaundice, 243
Muscle relaxants, 468*t*. *See also specific agent*
Muscle strain/spasm, chest pain and, 60
Musculoskeletal system
disorders of
chest pain associated with, 60
falls and, 124
examination of
in arthritis, 248
in diarrhea, 101
in hypercalcemia, 177
in hypercarbic ventilator patient, 455
in hypophosphatemia, 221
in overdose, 278
Muse. *See* Alprostadil, urethral suppository

Mustargen. *See* Mechlorethamine
Mutamycin. *See* Mitomycin C
Myambutol. *See* Ethambutol
Mycelex. *See* Clotrimazole
Mycetoma, hemoptysis and, 171
Mycobacterial infection, leukocytosis and, 252
Mycobacterium tuberculosis infection. *See also* Tuberculosis
  in HIV-positive patient, 136
  management of, 140
Mycobutin. *See* Rifabutin
Mycophenolate mofetil, 547
Mycostatin. *See* Nystatin
Myelodysplasia (preleukemic syndrome)
  leukopenia and, 256
  thrombocytopenia and, 334
Myeloma
  protein electrophoresis in, 374*f*
  pruritus and, 299
Myelosuppression, chemotherapy/radiation causing, 256
Mylanta/Mylanta II. *See* Aluminum hydroxide, with magnesium hydroxide and simethicone
Myleran. *See* Busulfan
Mylicon. *See* Simethicone
Mylotarg. *See* Gemtuzumab ozagamicin
Myocardial edema, at pacemaker catheter tip, failure to capture and, 284
Myocardial infarction. *See also* Chest pain
  cardiopulmonary arrest and, 45
  chest pain and, 57, 58, 64–65
  dyspnea and, 112
  falls and, 124
  heart murmur and, 152, 157
  hyperglycemia and, 181
  hypertension and, 196
  hypomagnesemia and, management of, 213
  leukocytosis and, 252
  management of, 64–65, 157
  Mobitz type I (Wenckebach) second-degree AV block and, 41
  Mobitz type II second-degree AV block and, 41
  nausea and vomiting and, 263
  pacemaker failure to capture and, 284
  pericarditis and, 58
  premature ventricular contractions after, 241
  sinus bradycardia and, 40
  syncope and, 318
Myocardial ischemia. *See also* Myocardial infarction
  dyspnea and, 112, 116
  heart murmur and, 152, 157
  hyperglycemia and, 181
  management of, 64–65, 116
Myocardial perforation, pacemaker complications and, 285
Myoglobin, urine, **369–370**. *See also* Myoglobinuria
  in overdose, 278
Myoglobinuria, oliguria/anuria/acute renal failure and, 268
Myxedema, hypothermia and, 230
Myxoma, atrial
  heart murmur in, 153, 155
  syncope and, 318

N

N-acetylprocainamide (NAPA), therapeutic/toxic levels of, 613*t*
N-methyl-histamine, in anaphylaxis, 26
Nabumetone, 605*t*
Nadolol, 601*t*
Nafcil. *See* Nafcillin
Nafcillin, 600*t*
Naftifine, 547
Naftin. *See* Naftifine
Nalbuphine, 547
Nalfon. *See* Fenoprofen
Nalidixic acid, 547
Nallpen. *See* Nafcillin
Naloxone, 547–548
  for coma/acute mental status changes, 81
  for overdose, 275, 281
Naltrexone, 548
NAPA (*N*-acetylprocainamide), therapeutic/toxic levels of, 613*t*
Naphazoline
  with antazoline, 609*t*
  with pheniramine acetate, 609*t*
Naphcon A. *See* Naphazoline, with pheniramine acetate
Naprosyn. *See* Naproxen
Naproxen, 606*t*
Naproxen sodium, 606*t*
Naratriptan, 548
Narcan. *See* Naloxone
Narcotics
  overdose/toxicity of, 275
  management of, 275, 281, 547–548
  in pain management, 290
Nardil. *See* Phenelzine
Nasal inhalants, 468*t*. *See also specific agent and* Bronchodilators
Nasalcrom. *See* Cromolyn sodium
Nasalide. *See* Flunisolide
Nasogastric intubation
  in hematemesis/melena, 160
  in hematochezia, 164
  in hypotension/shock, 227
  ventilator setup and, 446
Nasogastric tubes, 410, 411
  alkalosis and, 19, 21
  aspiration prevention and, 38
  potassium loss through, hypokalemia and, 206
  water and sodium loss through, hypernatremia and, 191
Nasopharynx
  disorders of, cough and, 87
  examination of. *See also* HEENT examination
  in coma/acute mental status changes, 79
Nasotracheal intubation, 444. *See also* Endotracheal tube; Mechanical ventilation
Natural products, 469–470*t*, **590–594**. *See also specific type*
Nausea and vomiting, **261–266**
  abdominal pain and, 2, 262
  alkalosis and, 19, 21
  characteristics/timing of, 261
  coma/acute mental status changes and, 73, 78
  differential diagnosis/causes of, 262–263
  dizziness and, 105
  hypernatremia and, 191
  hypokalemia and, 206, 207
  hyponatremia and, 214
  hypophosphatemia and, 221
  imaging/clinical studies in, 265
  initial evaluation of, 261–262
  intra-abdominal/thoracic causes of, 262–263
  intracranial causes of, 263
  laboratory findings/data in, 264–265

Nausea and vomiting, *(cont)*
management of, 265–266
metabolic causes of, 263
physical examination/findings in, 263–264
Navane. *See* Thiothixene
Navelbine. *See* Vinorelbine
Nebcin. *See* Tobramycin
NebuPent. *See* Pentamidine
Necator americanus, pruritus caused by, 297, 298, 299
Neck/neck veins
examination of. *See also* HEENT examination; Jugular venous distention
in alcohol withdrawal/delirium tremens, 93
in aspiration, 37
in bradycardia, 41–42
in cardiopulmonary arrest, 46
in chest pain, 61
in coma/acute mental status changes, 79
in cough, 88
in dizziness/vertigo, 108
in fever, 130
in HIV-positive patient, 138
in headache, 147
in heart murmur, 154
in hypotension/shock, 225
in hypoxemic ventilator patient, 452
in oliguria/anuria, 270
pain management and, 288
in tachycardia, 328
pain in, in nausea and vomiting, 264
surgery on, hypocalcemia and, 199
Neck massage, for chronic tension-type headache, 149
Nedocromil, 548
ophthalmic, 609*t*
Nefazodone, 548
Neggram. *See* Nalidixic acid
Neisseria gonorrhoeae. See also under Gonococcal
pruritus caused by, 297
urethritis caused by, dysuria in men and, 118
urine test for (ligase chain reaction), 120, **368**
Nelfinavir, 548
Nembutal. *See* Pentobarbital
Neo-Synephrine. *See* Phenylephrine
Neodecadron Ophthalmic. *See* Neomycin, with dexamethasone, ophthalmic
Neomycin
with bacitracin and polymyxin B
ophthalmic, 484
topical, 483
with bacitracin and polymyxin B and hydrocortisone
ophthalmic, 484, 608*t*
topical, 483
with bacitracin and polymyxin B and lidocaine, topical, 483
with colistin and hydrocortisone, otic, 548–549
with colistin and hydrocortisone and thonzonium, otic, 548–549
with dexamethasone, ophthalmic, 609*t*
with polymyxin B
for bladder irrigation, 549
topical, 549
with polymyxin B and dexamethasone, ophthalmic, 609*t*
with polymyxin B and hydrocortisone
ophthalmic, 549, 609*t*
otic, 548–549, 549
with polymyxin B and prednisolone, ophthalmic, 609*t*
Neomycin sulfate, 549
Neoplasia. *See specific type and* Cancer; Tumors
Neoral. *See* Cyclosporine
Neosar. *See* Cyclophosphamide
Neosporin. *See* Bacitracin, with polymyxin B and neomycin; Neomycin, with polymyxin B
Nephritis, interstitial, oliguria/anuria/acute renal failure and, 268
Nephrogenic diabetes insipidus
hypernatremia and, 191, 192, 193, 194
management of, 194
water deprivation/vasopressin test in diagnosis of, 193
Nephrolithiasis
Foley catheter problems and, 142
hematuria and, 168
nausea and vomiting and, 262
Nephrotic syndrome
hyponatremia and, 214, 217, 220
management of, 220
oliguria/anuria/acute renal failure and, 268
protein electrophoresis in, 374*f*
Nephrotoxic drugs, oliguria/anuria and, 267
Nerve infiltration/compression, in cancer, pain caused by, 288
Neumega. *See* Oprelvekin
Neupogen. *See* Filgrastim
Neuralgia, glossopharyngeal, syncope and, 317
Neurodegenerative disorders, seizures and, 310
Neurogenic shock, 225. *See also* Shock
management of, 228
Neuroimaging
in dizziness/vertigo, 109
in fever, in HIV-positive patient, 139–140
Neurologic deficits
dizziness and, 105
headache and, 146
in heart murmur, 155
nausea and vomiting and, 264
Neurologic disorders
constipation and, 83–84
falls and, 124
in HIV-positive patient, 137–138
hyponatremia and, 215
pruritus and, 300
seizures and, 310
syncope and, 317–318
syndrome of inappropriate antidiuretic hormone secretion (SIADH) and, 217
Neurologic examination. *See also* Mental status
in alcohol withdrawal/delirium tremens, 93–94
in alkalosis, 22
in anemia, 31
in aspiration, 37
in chest pain, 62
in coagulopathy, 69
in coma/acute mental status changes, 79–80
in constipation, 84
in dizziness/vertigo, 108
in dyspnea, 114
in falls, 125
in fever, in HIV-positive patient, 138
in headache, 147–148
in heart murmur, 155
in hypercalcemia, 177
in hyperglycemia, 181
in hypernatremia, 193
in hypertension, 196–197

in hypoglycemia, 204
in hypokalemia, 208
in hypomagnesemia, 212
in hyponatremia, 218
in hypophosphatemia, 221
in hypotension, 226
in hypothermia, 231
in insomnia, 236
in leukocytosis, 253
in nausea and vomiting, 264
in overdose, 278
pacemaker complications and, 285
pain management and, 289
in polycythemia, 293
in pruritus, 300
in seizures, 311–312
in shock, 226
in syncope, 319
in thrombocytopenia, 336
Neuromas, acoustic, dizziness/vertigo and, 106
Neuromuscular disease
dyspnea and, 113
hypoxemia in ventilator patient caused by, 451
respiratory failure in, mechanical ventilation for, 442–443
Neuromuscular examination
in acidosis, 15
in hyperkalemia, 189
in hypocalcemia, 200
Neuromuscular irritability, hypernatremia and, 190
Neuronitis, vestibular, 106
Neurontin. *See* Gabapentin
Neuropathy
autonomic, constipation and, 84
peripheral, falls and, 124
Neurotic excoriations, 298
Neutra-Phos, 223
for alcohol withdrawal/delirium tremens, 96
Neutrexin. *See* Trimetrexate
Neutropenia, 255–261. *See also* Leukopenia
cyclic, 256, 257
definition of, 255
fever and, 133–134
management of, 259–260
racial/familial, 256, 257
Neutrophil count, absolute, 255
Neutrophils, **387**
accelerated removal/consumption of, 257, 260
banded (stab), laboratory reference/normal values for, 354*t*, 387
inadequate production of, 256–257
redistribution of, 257, 260
segmented, laboratory reference/normal values for, 354*t*, 387
Nevirapine, 549
Nexium. *See* Esomeprazole
Niacin (vitamin B_3), 549–550
deficiency of, coma/acute mental status changes and, 75–76
Niaspan. *See* Niacin
Nicardipine, 550
Nicloar. *See* Niacin
Nicoderm. *See* Nicotine, transdermal
Nicorette/Nicorette DS. *See* Nicotine gum
Nicotine, transdermal, 550
Nicotine gum, 550
Nicotine nasal spray, 550
Nicotrol. *See* Nicotine, transdermal
Nicotrol NS. *See* Nicotine nasal spray
Nifedipine, 550
Nilandron. *See* Nilutamide
Nilstat. *See* Nystatin
Nilutamide, 550–551
Nimodipine, 551
Nimotop. *See* Nimodipine
Nipride. *See* Nitroprusside
Nisoldipine, 551
Nitrates, for myocardial infarction, 64
Nitrite, urine, 385
Nitro-Bid IV. *See* Nitroglycerin
Nitro-Bid Ointment. *See* Nitroglycerin
Nitrodisc. *See* Nitroglycerin
Nitrofurantoin, 551
Nitroglycerin, 551
for chest pain, 63, 64
for myocardial infarction, 64, 116, 157
for pulmonary edema, 344
Nitrolingual. *See* Nitroglycerin
Nitropress. *See* Nitroprusside
Nitroprusside, 551–552
for hypertensive emergency, 197–198
for pulmonary edema, 344
Nitrostat. *See* Nitroglycerin
Nix. *See* Permethrin
Nizatidine, 552
for gastritis/esophagitis, 66
Nizoral. *See* Ketoconazole
Noise, insomnia and, 236
Nolvadex. *See* Tamoxifen
Nonepileptic psychogenic seizures, 310
Nongap acidosis, 12–13
Nongonococcal urethritis, dysuria in men and, 118
Nonsteroidal anti-inflammatory drugs (NSAIDs), 289–290, 605–606*t*
anemia and, 28
for arthritis, 250
for chronic tension-type headache, 149
for episodic tension-type headache, 148
for migraine headache, 149
nausea and vomiting and, 262
ophthalmic, 608*t*
in pain management, 289–290
platelet function affected by, 68
Non–tonic-clonic seizures, coma/acute mental status changes and, 73, 77
Norcuron. *See* Vecuronium
Norepinephrine
serum/urine levels of, laboratory reference/normal values for, 354*t*
therapeutic, 552
Norethindrone acetate/ethinyl estradiol, 552
Norflex. *See* Orphenadrine
Norfloxacin, 552
Norgestrel, 552
Normal saline, composition of, 435*t*
Normiflo. *See* Ardeparin
Normodyne. *See* Labetalol
Noroxin. *See* Norfloxacin
Norpace. *See* Disopyramide
Norplant. *See* Levonorgestrel implant
Norpramin. *See* Desipramine
Nortriptyline, 552–553
Norvasc. *See* Amlodipine
Norvir. *See* Ritonavir
Norwalk virus, diarrhea caused by, 98
Nose, examination of, in alcohol withdrawal/delirium tremens, 93
Nosocomial infection, fever and, 127
Novafed. *See* Pseudoephedrine
Novantrone. *See* Mitoxantrone
Novolin, 597*t*
Novolog. *See* Aspart
NPH Iletin II, 597*t*

NSAIDs. *See* Nonsteroidal anti-inflammatory drugs
Nubain. *See* Nalbuphine
Nuclear scans
in hypotension/shock, 227
in jaundice, 244
in oliguria/anuria, 271
Nuclear venogram, in central venous line problems, 55
Nucleated red blood cells, 378
Nucleolar RNA, antibodies to, 348
5N-Nucleotidase, **370**
Numorphan. *See* Oxymorphone
Nupercainal. *See* Dibucaine
Nutrition
for oliguria/anuria/acute renal failure, 274
reviewing/adjusting, in hypercarbic ventilator patient, 455
thrombocytopenia and, 334
Nylen-Barany (Hallpike-Dix) maneuver, in dizziness/vertigo, 108
Nystagmus
in alcohol withdrawal/delirium tremens, 93
in coma/acute mental status changes, 79, 93
in dizziness/vertigo, 108
testing for, 108
Nystatin, 553

O

O_2. *See* Oxygen
Obesity
respiratory acidosis and, 12
type 2 diabetes and, 180
Obstipation
abdominal distension and, 82
abdominal pain and, 2
Obstructive cardiomyopathy, hypertrophic, heart murmur in, 153, 155
Obstructive extracardiac shock. *See also* Shock
pulmonary artery catheter monitoring in, 423*t*
Obturator sign, abdominal pain and, 5
Occult blood, in stool, testing for, **379**
in anemia, 30
in constipation, 84
in diarrhea, 102
Occupational exposures, coma/acute mental status changes and, 73, 74
Octamide. *See* Metoclopramide
Octreotide, 553
for esophageal varices, 161
Ocufen. *See* Flurbiprofen
Ocuflox ophthalmic. *See* Ofloxacin
Ocular decontamination, 281
Ocular disease
headache and, 145
in HIV infection/AIDS, 136
Ocular fundus
in coma/acute mental status changes, 78–79
in dizziness/vertigo, 108
in heart murmur, 155
in hyperglycemia, 181
Ocular movements, in coma/acute mental status changes, 79
Oculocephalic reflex, assessment of, in coma/acute mental status changes, 80
Ocupress. *See* Carteolol, ophthalmic
Ofloxacin, 553
Oil retention enema, 85, 85*t*
Olanzapine, 553
Oligemic shock. *See also* Shock
pulmonary artery catheter monitoring in, 423*t*
Oliguria, **266–274**
definition of, 266
diagnostic/therapeutic maneuvers in, 271–273
differential diagnosis/causes of, 267–269, 386*t*
imaging/clinical studies in, 271
initial evaluation of, 266–267
laboratory findings/data in, 270
management of specific causes of, 273–274
physical examination/findings in, 269–270
urinary indices in, 386*t*
Olsalazine, 553
Omeprazole, 611*t*
for gastritis/esophagitis, 66
Omnicef. *See* Cefdinir
Omnipen. *See* Ampicillin
Oncaspar. *See* L-Asparaginase
Oncovin. *See* Vincristine
Ondansetron, 553–554
for nausea and vomiting, 265–266
Ophthalmic agents, 468*t*, 607–609*t*
Opiates
epidural, 291
overdose/toxicity of, 275
management of, 275, 281, 547–548
in pain management, 290
Opioid withdrawal, 91
Oprelvekin, 554
for thrombocytopenia prophylaxis, 338
Opticrom. *See* Cromolyn sodium
Optipranolol. *See* Metipranolol
Optivar. *See* Azelastine
Oral contraceptives, 554
Oral disease, in HIV-positive patient, 136
Oral examination. *See* Mouth, examination of
Oral hypoglycemic agents, 183
overdose/toxicity of, 276
hypoglycemia and, 203
Oral temperature, 129
Organ failure, coma/acute mental status changes and, 75
Organophosphate toxicity, antidote for, 282
Orgaron. *See* Danaparoid
Orinase. *See* Tolbutamide
Orlistat, 554–555
Oropharynx
bacteria in, aspiration of, 37
disorders of, cough and, 87
examination of, in anemia, 30
Orotracheal intubation, 408–409, 409*f*, 444. *See also* Endotracheal tube; Mechanical ventilation
Orphenadrine, 555
Orthoclone OKT3. *See* Muromonab-CD3
Orthopnea, 111
Orthostatic hypotension, 105. *See also* Hypotension
in anemia, 30
in coagulopathy, 68–69
in dizziness, 104
falls and, 124, 125
in hematemesis/melena, 158, 159
in hematochezia, 162, 163
in hyperglycemia, 181
in hypernatremia, 192–193
in hyponatremia, 217
in nausea and vomiting, 263–264
in oliguria/anuria, 269
pre-syncope and, 106
syncope and, 316, 317, 322

Orudis. *See* Ketoprofen
Oruvail. *See* Ketoprofen
Osborn wave, in hypothermia, 232
Oseltamivir, 555
Osler nodes, 155
Osler-Weber-Rendu disease, hematochezia and, 163, 164
Osmolal gap, in coma/acute mental status changes, 80
Osmolality
 disturbances in, coma/acute mental status changes and, 75
 serum, **370**
 in hyponatremia, 218
 urine, **370**
 in acute renal failure/oliguria, 386*t*
 in hypernatremia, 193
 in hyponatremia, 218
Osmolarity, serum, in overdose, 279
Osmostat, serum sodium levels and, 216
Osmotic diuresis
 hypernatremia and, 191
 hyponatremia and, 216
Osteoarthritis, 247
 falls and, 124
Osteoblastic metastases, hypocalcemia and, 200
Otic agents, 468*t*. *See also specific agent*
Otobiotic Otic. *See* Polymyxin B, with hydrocortisone
Ototoxic medications, dizziness and, 106
Ova and parasites, in stool, testing for
 in diarrhea, 102
 in HIV-positive patient, 139
 in pruritus, 301
Ovarian carcinoma, polycythemia and, 293
Overdoses, **274–282**
 antidotes for, 281–282
 decontamination and, 280–281
 differential diagnosis/causes of, 275–277
 enhanced elimination and, 282
 identification of causative agent and, 275
 imaging/clinical studies in, 279
 initial evaluation of, 274–275
 laboratory findings/data in, 278–279
 management of, 279–282
 physical examination/findings in, 277–278
Ovrette. *See* Norgestrel
Oxacillin, 600*t*
Oxaprozin, 606*t*
Oxazepam, 555
 for alcohol withdrawal, 95
Oxcarbazepine, 555
Oxicams, 605*t*
Oxiconazole, 555
Oxistat. *See* Oxiconazole
Oxybutynin, 555
Oxycodone, 555–556
 with acetaminophen, 290, 556
 with aspirin, 290, 556
Oxycontin. *See* Oxycodone
Oxygen. *See also* PaO_2/pO_2
 inspired fraction of (FiO_2)
 adjusting, for ventilator patient, 447
  high peak pressures and, 458
  hypoxemia and, 453
 ratio of to PaO_2 (P/F ratio), in respiratory failure, mechanical ventilation and, 442
 ventilator set up and, 445
Oxygen affinity of hemoglobin, polycythemia and, 292, 294
Oxygen consumption, reducing, for hypoxemic ventilator patient, 453
Oxygen saturation
 laboratory reference/normal values for, 350*t*
 mixed venous (SvO_2), pulmonary artery catheter measurement of, 428*t*
 in hypoxemic ventilator patient, 452
 in shock, 423*t*
 in polycythemia vera, 292
 pulmonary artery catheter problems and, 306
Oxygen therapy
 for anaphylaxis, 26
 for aspiration, 39
 for chest pain, 63
 for cluster headache, 150
 for dyspnea, 115
 for hypotension/shock, 227
 for pneumothorax, 66
 for pulmonary edema, 344
 for pulmonary embolism, 65
Oxyir. *See* Oxycodone
Oxymorphone, 556
Oxytocin, 556

P

^{32}P, for polycythemia vera, 295
P-ANCA. *See* Perinuclear-staining ANCA
P/F ratio (PaO_2/FiO_2 ratio), in respiratory failure, mechanical ventilation and, 442
P wave–QRS complex relationship, in supraventricular tachyarrhythmias, 324
P waves
 in bradycardia, 42
 in irregular pulse, 240–241
 pacemaker oversensing of, 285
 in supraventricular tachyarrhythmias, 324
p50. *See* Oxygen affinity of hemoglobin
PAC. *See* Premature atrial contractions; Pulmonary artery (Swan-Ganz) catheter
Pacemaker
 adjusting settings of, 286–287
 for asystole, 51
 for bradycardia, 43
 failure to capture and, 283–284, 284*f*, 286
 failure to sense and, 284–285, 284*f*, 287
 troubleshooting, **283–287**, 284*f*
Pacemaker spikes
 in bradycardia, 42
 without capture, 283, 284*f*
 failure to sense and, 284–285, 284*f*
Pacemaker syncope, 318
Pacerone. *See* Amiodarone
Pacing threshold, 286
Pacing wire, pacemaker complications and, 286
Pacis. *See* Bacillus Calmette-Guérin
Packed red blood cells (RBCs), transfusion of, 437
Paclitaxel, 556–557
$PaCO_2/pCO_2$, **353**
 in acidosis, 9, 10–11, 350*t*
 adjusting, for ventilator patient, 447–448
 in alkalosis, 19, 350*t*
 laboratory reference/normal values for, 350*t*
 in ventilatory failure, mechanical ventilation and, 442
Paget's disease, hypercalcemia and, 177

Pain
insomnia and, 234, 235
respiratory alkalosis and, 21
Pain management, **287–291**
for abdominal pain, 7
analgesics in, 289–291, 462*t*
for myocardial infarction, 64, 157
Painful rib syndrome, abdominal pain and, 4
Pamelor. *See* Nortriptyline
Pamidronate, 557
for hypercalcemia, 179
Pancreas, disorders of
abdominal pain and, 3, 3*t*
coma/acute mental status changes and, 75
in HIV-positive patient, fever and, 137
hyperglycemia and, 181
Pancrease. *See* Pancreatin/pancrelipase
Pancreatic islet cell tumor, hypoglycemia and, 203
Pancreatic juice, composition/daily production of, 436*t*
Pancreatin/pancrelipase, 557
Pancreatitis
abdominal pain and, 3, 3*t*, 6
chest pain and, 60
diarrhea and100
in HIV-positive patient, 137
hyperglycemia and, 181
hypocalcemia and, 199, 200
hypomagnesemia and, 211
nausea and vomiting and, 262
Pancuronium, 557
Pancytopenia, 29
Panorex, in leukopenia, 259
Pantoprazole, 611*t*
PaO_2/pO_2, **370**
adjusting, for ventilator patient, 447
laboratory reference/normal values for, 350*t*, **370**
in respiratory failure, mechanical ventilation and, 442
ventilator weaning guidelines for, 458
PaO_2/FiO_2 ratio (P/F ratio), in respiratory failure, mechanical ventilation and, 442
PAP. *See* Pulmonary artery pressure
Papillary muscle dysfunction/rupture, heart murmur and, 152
Papilledema
in coma/acute mental status changes, 78–79
in dizziness/vertigo, 108
in hypertension, 196
Papulosquamous diseases, pruritus in, 298
Paracentesis, **418–421**
in abdominal pain, 7
urgent surgery and, 8*t*
in hypotension/shock, 227
Paraflex. *See* Chlorzoxazone
Parafon Forte DSC. *See* Chlorzoxazone
Paraldehyde, metabolic acidosis caused by, 16
Paralysis, Todd's, in seizures, 312
Paralytic ileus
abdominal pain and, 5*t*
nausea and vomiting and, 262
Paraneoplastic syndromes
cancer pain and, 288
coma/acute mental status changes and, 76
Paraplatin. *See* Carboplatin
Parasites
diarrhea caused by infection with, 98
in HIV infection/AIDS, 98, 100, 137
pruritus caused by, 297, 298, 299
pulmonary infection caused by, in HIV-positive patient, 137
in stool, testing for
in diarrhea, 102
in HIV-positive patient, 139
in pruritus, 301
in urine, microscopic appearance of, 384
Parasympathetic nervous system, bradycardia caused by changes in, 40
Parathyroid gland disorders
coma/acute mental status changes and, 75
hypocalcemia and, 199
Parathyroid hormone (PTH), **371**
in hypocalcemia, 199, 200
management of deficiency and, 201
Parathyroid hormone–related peptide, coma/acute mental status changes and, 76
Paregoric, 103, 557
Parkinson's disease
disequilibrium and, 107
falls and, 123, 124
Parlodel. *See* Bromocriptine
Paroxetine, 557
Paroxysmal atrial tachycardia
with block, 325
syncope and, 318
Paroxysmal nocturnal hemoglobinuria
leukopenia and, 256, 257
thrombocytopenia and, 334
Partial thromboplastin time (PTT), **371**
in central venous line problems, 55
in coagulopathy, 69, 69*t*
in diarrhea, 101
in headache, 148
in hematemesis/melena, 160
in hematochezia, 164
in hemoptysis, 173
in hypotension/shock, 226
in hypothermia, 231
in thrombocytopenia, 336
in transfusion reaction, 340
Particulate aspiration, 36
PASG. *See* Pneumatic antishock garment
Pathologic fracture, in cancer, pain caused by, 288
Patient-controlled analgesia (PCA), 291
Patient positioning
aspiration and, 36, 38
for CPR, 44
for hypoxemic ventilator patient, 454
for lumbar puncture, 414–415, 416*f*
syncope and, 315
Pausinystalia yohimbe (yohimbine), 593
toxicity of, 594
Pavulon. *See* Pancuronium
Paxil. *See* Paroxetine
PCA. *See* Patient-controlled analgesia
pCO_2. *See* $PaCO_2/pCO_2$
PCP. *See Pneumocystis carinii* pneumonia
PCWP. *See* Pulmonary capillary wedge pressure
PE. *See* Pulmonary embolism
PEA. *See* Pulseless electrical activity
Peak pressures, ventilator, high, **456–458**
Pediculosis, pruritus in, 296, 297, 298
Pediculus capitis, pruritus caused by, 296, 298

Pediculus corporis, pruritus caused by, 296, 298
PEEP (positive end-expiratory pressure)
 adjusting PaO_2 for ventilator patient and, 447
 hypoxemia and, 453
 auto-PEEP
 agitation in ventilator patient and, 448
 high peak pressures and, 456, 457
 high peak pressures and, 456, 458
Peg (polyethylene glycol)–electrolyte solution, 562
Pellagra, coma/acute mental status changes and, 75–76
Pelvic computed tomography, in polycythemia, 294
Pelvic exam. *See* Gynecologic examination
Pelvic inflammatory disease, nausea and vomiting and, 262
Pelvic trauma, constipation and, 83
Pelvis, examination of, in hematuria, 168
Pemirolast, ophthalmic, 609*t*
Pemphigoid, bullous, pruritus in, 298
Pemphigus, pruritus in, 298
Pen-Vee K. *See* Penicillin V
Penbutolol, 601*t*
Penciclovir, 557–558
Penicillin
 antistaphylococcal, 600*t*
 extended-spectrum, 600*t*
Penicillin G
 aqueous (potassium or sodium), 558
 benzathine, 558
 procaine, 558
Penicillin V, 558
Pentam 300. *See* Pentamidine
Pentamidine, 558
Pentasa. *See* Mesalamine
Pentazocine, 558–559
Pentids. *See* Penicillin G, aqueous
Pentobarbital, 559
 for seizures, 314–315
Pentosan polysulfate sodium, 559
Pentoxifylline, 559
Pepcid. *See* Famotidine
Peptic ulcer disease
 chest pain and, 60
 hematemesis/melena and, 158, 159, 161
 management of, 161
 nausea and vomiting and, 262
Pepto-Bismol. *See* Bismuth subsalicylate
Percocet. *See* Oxycodone, with acetaminophen
Percodab-Demi. *See* Oxycodone, with aspirin
Percodan. *See* Oxycodone, with aspirin
Percutaneous transhepatic cholangiogram (PTC), in jaundice, 244
Perforated viscus
 abdominal pain and, 2–3, 5*t*
 nausea and vomiting and, 262
Pergolide, 559
Periactin. *See* Cyproheptadine
Pericardial friction rub, in chest pain, 61
Pericardial/cardiac tamponade
 cardiopulmonary arrest and, 45
 dyspnea and, 112
 pulseless electrical activity and, 51
 syncope and, 318
Pericardiocentesis, in hypotension/shock, 227
Pericarditis
 chest pain and, 57, 58–59, 61, 66
 dyspnea and, 112
 management of, 66
Perindopril, 598*t*
Perinuclear-staining ANCA (P-ANCA), 348
Periodic breathing (Cheyne-Stokes respiration), in coma/acute mental status changes, 78
Periodic limb movements, insomnia and, 235
Periodic paralysis
 familial, hypokalemia and, 206
 hyperkalemic, 187
Peripheral blood smear
 in anemia, 29–30, 31
 in coagulopathy, 69
 in hypertension, 197
 in hypophosphatemia, 222
 in leukocytosis, 253–254
 in leukopenia, 258
 in thrombocytopenia, 336
 in transfusion reaction, 340
Peripheral neuropathy, falls and, 124
Peripheral vascular system
 disorders of, with ischemia, leukocytosis and, 252
 examination of, in hyperglycemia, 181
Peritoneal dialysis. *See also* Dialysis
 for hyperkalemia, 190
 for oliguria/anuria/acute renal failure, 274
Peritoneal disorders, abdominal pain and, 1, 3*t*, 5*t*
Peritonitis
 abdominal pain and, 1, 3*t*, 5*t*
 ascitic fluid findings in, 421*t*
Periumbilical pain, 1
Periureteritis, hematuria and, 168
Permanent pacemaker. *See also* Pacemaker
 for bradycardia, 43
Permax. *See* Pergolide
Permethrin, 559
Permitil. *See* Fluphenazine
Pernicious anemia
 treatment of, hypokalemia and, 206
 vitamin B_{12} deficiency and, 28, 32–33
Perphenazine, 559
Persantine. *See* Dipyridamole
Peutz-Jeghers syndrome, hematochezia and, 163
Pfizerpen. *See* Penicillin G, aqueous
pH, **371**, **383**
 in acidosis, 10–11, 350*t*
 in alkalosis, 350*t*
 arterial, **371**
 in hypophosphatemia, 222
 laboratory reference/normal values for, 350*t*, 371, 383
 pleural fluid, 433*t*
 urine, **383**
 dysuria in women and, 118
Phenazopyridine, 559–560
Phencyclidine, hypertension and, 195
Phenelzine, 560
Phenergan. *See* Promethazine
Pheniramine acetate with naphazoline, 609*t*
Phenobarbital, 560
 for alcohol withdrawal/delirium tremens, 96
 with hyoscyamine/atropine/scopolamine, 527
 hypocalcemia and, 199
 therapeutic/toxic levels of, 613*t*

Phenothiazines
for dizziness/vertigo, 110
for nausea and vomiting, 265
Phenylephrine, 560
with hydrocodone/chlorpheniramine/acetaminophen/caffeine, 526
Phenytoin, 560–561
hypocalcemia and, 199
for seizures, 314
therapeutic/toxic levels of, 613*t*
Pheochromocytoma
hypertension and, 195, 198
management of, 198
polycythemia and, 293
Phlebotomy, therapeutic, for polycythemia, 295, 296
Phos-Ex. *See* Calcium acetate
Phoslo. *See* Calcium acetate
Phospholine iodide. *See* Echothiophate iodide
Phosphorus/phosphate
disorders of balance of. *See also* Hyperphosphatemia; Hypophosphatemia
in alcohol withdrawal/delirium tremens, 94
in hypercalcemia, 177
in hyperglycemia, 182
in hypocalcemia, 200
in hypomagnesemia, 212
intestinal loss of, 221
intracellular shift of, 221
in milk, 223, 223*t*
renal loss of, 221
supplementary, 222–223
for alcohol withdrawal/delirium tremens, 96
intravenous, 223
for hypercalcemia, 179
oral replacement, 223
Phthirus pubis, pruritus caused by, 297, 298
Physical therapy
for dizziness/vertigo, 110
after fall, 126
Physostigmine, 561
for anticholinergic overdose/toxicity, 281
ophthalmic, 607*t*
Phytonadione, 561. *See also* Vitamin K
Pickwickian syndrome, respiratory acidosis and, 12
PID. *See* Pelvic inflammatory disease
Pilocar. *See* Pilocarpine
Pilocarpine, 607*t*
Pilopine HS gel. *See* Pilocarpine
Pindolol, 601*t*
Pinworms *(Enterobius vermicularis),* pruritus caused by, 297, 299
Pioglitazone, 183, 561
Piper methysticum (kava kava/kava kava root extract), 592
Piperacillin, 600*t*
Piperacillin-tazobactam, 600*t*
Pipracil. *See* Piperacillin
Pirbuterol, 561
Piroxicam, 605*t*
Pitocin. *See* Oxytocin
Pitressin. *See* Vasopressin
Pituitary gland, disorders of, coma/acute mental status changes and, 75
Pityriasis rosea, pruritus in, 296, 298
Plantar reflex, in coma/acute mental status changes, 80
Plasma component therapy, **439–440**
for disseminated intravascular coagulation (DIC), 71
for vitamin K deficiency/liver disease, 72
for von Willebrand's disease, 71
Plasma protein fraction, 561
Plasma volume, increased, pseudoanemia and, 28
Plasma volume expanders, 468*t*. *See also specific agent*
Plasmanate. *See* Plasma protein fraction
Plasmapheresis, for thrombotic thrombocytopenia purpura (TTP), 337
Plasminogen, **371–372**
Platelet antibodies, in thrombocytopenia, 337
Platelet clumping, platelet count errors and, 333, 333–334
Platelet count. *See also* Thrombocytopenia
in anemia, 32
central venous line problems and, 55
in coagulopathy, 69, 69*t*
in coma/acute mental status changes, 80
in headache, 148
in hematemesis/melena, 160
in hematochezia, 164
in hemoptysis, 173
in hyperkalemia, 189
in hypophosphatemia, 222
in hypothermia, 231
laboratory reference/normal values for, 354*t*
in polycythemia vera, 292, 294
Platelet glycoprotein IIb/IIIa inhibitors
for myocardial infarction, 65
platelet function affected by, 68
Platelet transfusions, 70–71, **438–439**
for disseminated intravascular coagulation (DIC), 71
for thrombocytopenia, 70–71, 338
Platelets, **372**
disorders of function/number of, 67–68. *See also* Thrombocytopenia
decreased production and, 334
peripheral destruction and, 334–335
sequestration in spleen and, 335
tests of, in headache, 148
Platinol AQ. *See* Cisplatin
Platypnea, 111
Plavix. *See* Clopidogrel
Plendil. *See* Felodipine
Pletal. *See* Cilostazol
Plethora, in polycythemia, 293
Plethysmography, impedance, in central venous line problems, 55
Pleural effusion
diagnosis/evaluation of (thoracentesis), **431–434**, 432*f*, 433*t*
dyspnea and, 112, 116
management of, 116
respiratory acidosis and, 12
Pleural fluid
differential diagnosis of, 433, 433*t*
removal of (thoracentesis), **431–434**, 432*f*, 433*t*
Pleural friction rub, in chest pain, 61
Pleuritic pain, hemoptysis and, 171
Pleuritis, chest pain and, 60
Pleurodynia, chest pain and, 60
Plicamycin, 561–562
for hypercalcemia, 179
PM-1 antibodies, 348
PMI. *See* Point of maximal impulse

Pneumatic antishock garment, 227
Pneumococcal vaccine, polyvalent, 562
Pneumocystis carinii pneumonia (PCP), in HIV-positive patient, 137
management of, 140
Pneumonia
aspiration and, 37
chest pain and, 60
community-acquired, 89
cough and, 87, 89
dyspnea and, 112, 116
hemoptysis and, 171
in HIV-positive patient
acid-fast organisms causing, 136–137
bacterial, 136
parasitic infections and, 137
Pneumocystis carinii, 137, 140
hypoxemia in ventilator patient caused by, 451, 453
management of, 89, 116, 132–133
respiratory acidosis and, 12
respiratory alkalosis and, 21
Pneumothorax, 59–60
cardiopulmonary arrest and, 45
causes of, 59–60
chest pain and, 59–60, 66
dyspnea and, 112
management of, 66
pulseless electrical activity and, 51
respiratory acidosis and, 12
respiratory alkalosis and, 21
spontaneous, 59
in ventilator patient, 59
agitation and, 448
high peak pressures and, 457, 458
hypoxemia and, 451, 453
Pneumovax-23. *See* Pneumococcal vaccine, polyvalent
pO_2. *See* PaO_2/pO_2
Podocon-25. *See* Podophyllin
Podophyllin, 562
Poikilocytosis, 377
Point of maximal impulse, assessment of
in chest pain, 61
in cough, 88
in dyspnea, 114
Pokeweed, toxicity of, 594
Polychondritis, arthritis and, 248
Polychromasia, 378
Polycitra-K. *See* Potassium citrate, with citric acid
Polyclonal gammopathy, protein electrophoresis in, 374*f*
Polycythemia, **291–296**
differential diagnosis/causes of, 291–293
imaging/clinical studies in, 294
initial evaluation of, 291
laboratory findings/data in, 293–294
management of, 294–296
physical examination/findings in, 293
relative, 292, 294
secondary, 292–293, 294–295
vera, 292, 295–296
pruritus and, 299
Polydipsia, hypernatremia and, 191
psychogenic, 217
Polyethylene glycol (Peg)–electrolyte solution, 562
Polymox. *See* Amoxicillin
Polymyxin B
with bacitracin
ophthalmic, 484
topical, 483
with bacitracin and neomycin
ophthalmic, 484
topical, 483
with bacitracin and neomycin and hydrocortisone
ophthalmic, 484
topical, 483
with bacitracin and neomycin and lidocaine, topical, 483
with hydrocortisone, 562
with neomycin
for bladder irrigation, 549
topical, 549
with neomycin and dexamethasone, ophthalmic, 609*t*
with neomycin and hydrocortisone, ophthalmic, 549, 608*t*, 609*t*
with neomycin and prednisolone, ophthalmic, 609*t*
Poly-Pred. *See* Neomycin, with polymyxin B and prednisolone, ophthalmic
Polyps, gastrointestinal, hematochezia and, 163
Polysporin. *See* Bacitracin, with polymyxin B
Polyuria, hypernatremia and, 191
Porphyria, hepatic, coma/acute mental status changes and, 76
Positional vertigo, benign, 105, 105–106
Positive end-expiratory pressure (PEEP)
adjusting PaO_2 for ventilator patient and, 447
hypoxemia and, 453
auto-PEEP
agitation in ventilator patient and, 448
high peak pressures and, 456, 457
high peak pressures and, 456
Positive pressure breathing. *See also* Mechanical ventilation
for aspiration, 39
Posterior iliac crest, bone marrow aspiration and biopsy from, 397–399
Postictal confusion, 77
Post-lumbar puncture headache, 418
Postnasal drip, cough and, 87
Postobstructive diuresis, 273
hypernatremia and, 191
Postprandial orthostasis, syncope and, 317
Postural hypotension. *See* Orthostatic hypotension
Potassium
in body fluids, 436*t*
daily maintenance requirements for, 435
for diabetic ketoacidosis, 185
disorders of balance of. *See also* Hyperkalemia; Hypokalemia
in alcohol withdrawal/delirium tremens, 94
cardiopulmonary arrest and, 45
coma/acute mental status changes and, 74, 94
metabolic alkalosis and, 22
exogenous, hyperkalemia and, 186, 188
in hyperglycemia, 182
for hyperosmolar/hyperglycemia nonketotic syndrome, 184
in hypophosphatemia, 222
serum, **372**
in acidosis, 15–16
in hyperkalemia, 189

Potassium, *(cont)*
supplementary, 563
for alcohol withdrawal/delirium tremens, 95–96
hyperkalemia and, 186, 188
for hypokalemia, 209–210
for hyponatremia, 219
urine, **372**, 386
in hypokalemia, 209
Potassium-binding resins, for hyperkalemia, 190
Potassium citrate, 562
with citric acid, 562
Potassium hydroxide (KOH) prep, **368**
in pruritus, 301
Potassium iodide (Lugol's solution/SSKI), 563
Potassium phosphate, 223
Potassium-sparing diuretics, hyperkalemia and, 186, 188
Potomania, beer, hyponatremia and, 217
Pounds/kilograms weight conversion chart, 619*t*
PPD (purified protein derivative) skin test
in cough, 88
in hemoptysis, 173
Pralidoxime, for organophosphate and carbamate toxicity, 282
Pramipexole, 563
Pramoxine, 563
with hydrocortisone, 563
Prandin. *See* Repaglinide
Pravachol. *See* Pravastatin
Pravastatin, 612*t*
Prazosin, 563–564
Precose. *See* Acarbose
Pred Forte. *See* Prednisolone, ophthalmic
Pred-G Ophthalmic. *See* Gentamicin, ophthalmic, with prednisolone
Prednisolone, 597*t*
ophthalmic, 609*t*
with gentamicin, 609*t*
with neomycin and polymyxin B, 609*t*
with sulfacetamide, 575, 609*t*
Prednisone, 597*t*
for idiopathic thrombocytopenic purpura (ITP), 337
for thrombotic thrombocytopenia purpura (TTP), 337
Pregnancy
cholestasis of, pruritus in, 299, 302
diabetes and, 180
hepatitis B screening tests in, 364*t*
hypertension and, 196
jaundice and, 243
nausea and vomiting and, 263
respiratory alkalosis and, 21
syncope and, 318
Pregnancy test
in abdominal pain, 6
HCG beta subunit, **366**
in hypotension/shock, 226
in nausea and vomiting, 265
Preleukemic syndrome (myelodysplasia)
leukopenia and, 256
thrombocytopenia and, 334
Premarin. *See* Estrogens, conjugated
Premarin with methylprogesterone. *See* Estrogens, conjugated, with methylprogesterone
Premarin with methyltestosterone. *See* Estrogens, conjugated, with methyltestosterone
Premature atrial contractions (PACs), 238–239
Premature ventricular contractions (PVCs), 239
management of, 241
pulmonary artery catheterization and, 428
Prerenal azotemia, urinary indices in, 386*t*
Pressure control ventilation, 445
for high peak pressures in ventilator patient, 458
Pressure support (PS) ventilation, 445
for weaning, 459–460
Pre-syncope, 106–107
Prevacid. *See* Lansoprazole
Priftin. *See* Rifapentine
Prilocaine, with lidocaine, 536
Prilosec. *See* Omeprazole
Primacor. *See* Milrinone
Primaxin. *See* Imipenem-cilastin
Prinivil. *See* Lisinopril
Priscoline. *See* Tolazoline
Pro-Banthine. *See* Propantheline
Probenecid, 564
Procainamide, 564
for tachycardia, 332
therapeutic/toxic levels of, 613*t*
for ventricular fibrillation, 47
for ventricular tachycardia, 47–49
Procan. *See* Procainamide
Procarbazine, 564
Procardia/Procardia XL. *See* Nifedipine
Prochlorperazine, 564
for dizziness/vertigo, 110
for migraine headache, 150
for nausea and vomiting, 265
Procrit. *See* Epoetin alfa
Proctocort. *See* Hydrocortisone, rectal
Proctofoam-HC. *See* Pramoxine, with hydrocortisone
Proctofoam-NS. *See* Pramoxine
Proctosigmoidoscopy
in constipation, 84
in diarrhea, 102
Progesterone, respiratory alkalosis and, 20, 21
Proglycem. *See* Diazoxide
Prograf. *See* Tacrolimus
ProHIBiT. *See* *Haemophilus B* conjugate vaccine
Prokine. *See* Sargramostim
Prolactin, **372**
Prolastin. *See* Alpha$_1$ protease inhibitor
Proleukin. *See* Aldesleukin
Prolixin. *See* Fluphenazine
Proloprim. *See* Trimethoprim
Promethazine, 564–565
for dizziness/vertigo, 110
for nausea and vomiting, 265
Prone positioning, for hypoxemic ventilator patient, 454
Pronestyl. *See* Procainamide
Propafenone, 565
Propantheline, 565
Propecia. *See* Finasteride
Propine. *See* Dipivefrin
Propionic acid derivatives, as nonsteroidal anti-inflammatory drugs, 606*t*
Propofol, 565
for seizures, 315
Propoxyphene, 565
with acetaminophen, 565
with aspirin, 565
Propranolol, 565–566, 602*t*
cessation of, rebound hypertension and, 194
for tachycardia, 331
Propylthiouracil (PTU), 566
Proscar. *See* Finasteride
Prosom. *See* Estazolam

Prostaglandin agonists, for glaucoma, 608*t*
Prostate, examination of, in dysuria, 119
Prostate-specific antigen (PSA), **373**
Prostatic hypertrophy, oliguria/anuria and, 267
Prostatitis
 dysuria in men and, 117, 118, 119
 hematuria and, 168
 management of, 122
ProStep. *See* Nicotine, transdermal
Prosthetic heart valves
 dysfunction of, heart murmur in, 153
 fever and, 128
Protamine sulfate, 566
Protein
 ascitic fluid, 421*t*
 cerebrospinal fluid, 419*t*
 pleural fluid, 433*t*
 serum, **373**
 sodium levels affected by, 215
 total, in hypercalcemia, 178
 urine, **373–376**
 in oliguria/anuria, 270
Protein C, plasma, **376**
Protein calorie malnutrition (kwashiorkor), hypoglycemia and, 203
Protein electrophoresis, **373**, 374*f*, 375*t*
Protein (pleural fluid-to-serum) ratio, 433*t*
Protein S, plasma, **376**
Protein-to-albumin ratio, in hypercalcemia, 178
Proteinuria, 373–376
 Bence-Jones, **350**, 373, 374*f*
 in oliguria/anuria, 270
Prothrombin time (PT), **376**
 central venous line problems and, 55
 in coagulopathy, 69, 69*t*
 in diarrhea, 101
 in headache, 148
 in hematemesis/melena, 160
 in hematochezia, 164
 in hemoptysis, 173
 in hypotension, 226
 in hypothermia, 231
 in jaundice, 244
 in shock, 226
 in thrombocytopenia, 336
 in transfusion reaction, 340
Proton pump inhibitors, 611*t*
 for gastritis/esophagitis, 66
Protonix. *See* Pantoprazole
Proventil. *See* Albuterol
Provera. *See* Medroxyprogesterone
Provigil. *See* Modafinil
Proximal renal tubular acidosis, 13, 16
Prozac. *See* Fluoxetine
Pruritus, **296–303**
 differential diagnosis/causes of, 297–300
 generalized versus localized, 296–297
 imaging/clinical studies in, 301–302
 initial evaluation of, 296–297
 laboratory findings/data in, 300–301
 management of, 302–303
 physical examination/findings in, 300
 systemic, 298–300
PS. *See* Pressure support (PS) ventilation
PSA. *See* Prostate-specific antigen
Pseudo-Pelger-Huet anomaly, in leukopenia, 258
Pseudoanemia, 28
Pseudocoma (psychogenic coma), 76
Pseudoephedrine, 566
 with hydrocodone, 526
 hypertension and, 195
Pseudohyperkalemia, 187
Pseudohyponatremia, 215
Pseudohypoparathyroidism, hypocalcemia and, 199
Pseudomembranous colitis, 99
Pseudo-obstruction, nausea and vomiting and, 262
Pseudorespiratory alkalosis, 12, 21
Pseudothrombocytopenia, 333–334
Psoas sign, abdominal pain and, 5
Psoriasis, pruritus in, 296, 297, 298
Psoriatic arthritis, 247
Psychiatric disorders
 coma/acute mental status changes and, 73, 76–77, 92
 delirium and, 92
 dizziness and, 107
 insomnia and, 236
 leukopenia and, 256
 pruritus and, 300
 syncope and, 317
Psychogenic breathlessness, 113
Psychogenic coma (pseudocoma), 76
Psychogenic polydipsia, hyponatremia and, 217
Psychogenic seizures, 310
Psychosis
 ICU, 77, 92
 agitation in ventilator patient caused by, 449, 450
 Korsakoff's, coma/acute mental status changes and, 75
Psychotherapy, for chronic tension-type headache, 149
Psyllium, 85, 85*t*, 566
PT. *See* Prothrombin time
Pteroylglutamic acid. *See* Folate/folic acid
PTH. *See* Parathyroid hormone
PTT. *See* Partial thromboplastin time
PTU. *See* Propylthiouracil
Pubic louse, pruritus caused by, 297, 298
PUD. *See* Peptic ulcer disease
Pulmicort. *See* Budesonide
Pulmonary angiography
 in dyspnea, 115
 in hemoptysis, 174
Pulmonary artery (Swan-Ganz) catheter (PAC), 424–425, 424*f*. *See also* Pulmonary artery (Swan-Ganz) catheterization
 balloon malfunction/rupture and, 304, 305, 306
 infection/sepsis and, 305
 kinked, 303, 305
 migration of, 305
 obstruction of, 303, 305
 positioning of, 425–426, 427*f*
 problems with, **303–307**
 inside patient, 305
 outside patient, 304
 thrombosis of, 303, 305
 unable to wedge, 306
 wedged (permanent), 303–304, 306
 withdrawal of, for permanent wedge, 306
Pulmonary artery (Swan-Ganz) catheterization, **421–429**, 423*t*, 424*f*, 427*f*, 428*t*, 429*t*
 for cardiac output measurement, 426, 428*t*
 inaccurate/poorly reproducible results and, 306–307
 complications of, 428–429

Pulmonary artery, *(cont)*
contraindications for, 422–423
differential diagnosis of readings and, 426–428, 429*t*
in heart murmur, 156, 157
in hypotension, 227
in hypoxemic ventilator patient, 452, 453
indications for, 422
materials for, 424–425, 424*f*
in oliguria/anuria/acute renal failure, 271
pressure waveforms of, 303, 427*f*
procedure for, 425–428
in shock, 227, 422, 423*t*
Pulmonary artery pressure (PAP), pulmonary artery catheter measurement of, 428*t*
abnormalities and, 429*t*
in shock, 423*t*
Pulmonary artery rupture/erosion, pulmonary artery catheterization and, 307, 428–429
Pulmonary artery waveform, 303, 427*f*
Pulmonary capillary wedge pressure. *See also* Pulmonary wedge pressure
pulmonary artery catheter measurement of, 428*t*
Pulmonary consolidation, in cough, 88
Pulmonary contusion
hemoptysis and, 172
hypoxemia in ventilator patient caused by, 451
Pulmonary diffusing capacity, decreased, pO_2 in, 370
Pulmonary disorders
dyspnea and, 111–112
hemoptysis and, 171–172
in HIV-positive patient, fever and, 136–137
hyponatremia and, 215
insomnia and, 235
respiratory alkalosis and, 21
syndrome of inappropriate antidiuretic hormone secretion (SIADH) and, 217
Pulmonary edema
cardiogenic
hemoptysis and, 172
in ventilator patient
high peak pressures and, 456
hypoxemia and, 451, 453
wheezing and, 342
cardiopulmonary arrest and, 45
hypertension and, 196
management of, 344
respiratory acidosis and, 11
respiratory alkalosis and, 21
Pulmonary embolism, 59
aspiration and, 37
cardiopulmonary arrest and, 45
chest pain and, 59, 62, 65–66
dyspnea and, 111–112
hemoptysis and, 171, 174
leukocytosis and, 252
management of, 65–66, 174
respiratory alkalosis and, 21
syncope and, 318
in ventilator patient
agitation and, 449
hypercarbia and, 454
hypoxemia and, 451
wheezing and, 342
Pulmonary function tests
in cough, 88–89
in dyspnea, 115
in polycythemia, 294
Pulmonary hypertension, primary
chest pain and, 59
syncope and, 318
Pulmonary infarction
chest pain and, 59
hemoptysis and, 171
leukocytosis and, 252
pulmonary artery catheterization and, 428–429
Pulmonary-renal syndrome
hemoptysis and, 173, 175
management of, 175
Pulmonary wedge pressure (PWP), pulmonary artery catheter measurement of
abnormalities and, 429*t*
in shock, 423*t*
Pulmozyme. *See* Dornase alfa
Pulse
assessment of
arterial line problems and, 35
in cardiopulmonary arrest, 44
in fever, 129–130
in heart murmur, 153, 155
in hematochezia, 163
in hemoptysis, 172
in hyperglycemia, 181
irregular, **238–241**. *See also* Arrhythmias; Bradycardia; Tachycardia
Pulse-temperature dissociation, 129–130
Pulseless electrical activity (PEA), management of, 51–53, 52–53*f*
Pulseless ventricular tachycardia, management of, 47, 48–49*f*
Pulsus paradoxus
in dyspnea, 113
in heart murmur, 153
in oliguria/anuria, 269
tachycardia and, 323
Pulsus parvus et tardus, in aortic stenosis, 154
Punch biopsy, 430–431
Pupils
in coma/acute mental status changes, 78
in dizziness/vertigo, 108
in seizures, 311
Purified protein derivative (PPD) skin test
in cough, 88
in hemoptysis, 173
Purinethol. *See* Mercaptopurine
Purple top tubes, 622*t*
Purpura
idiopathic thrombocytopenic, 67, 334
management of, 71, 337
thrombotic thrombocytopenic, 67, 335
management of, 337
PVC. *See* Premature ventricular contractions
PWP. *See* Pulmonary wedge pressure
Pyelography
intravenous
in dysuria, 120
in hematuria, 169
in oliguria/anuria, 271
retrograde, in oliguria/anuria, 271
Pyelonephritis, 117. *See also* Urinary tract infection
dysuria and, 117, 120–121
in men, 118
in women, 117
hematuria and, 167
management of, 120–121
nausea and vomiting and, 262
urologic evaluation in, 120
Pyrazinamide, 566
Pyridium. *See* Phenazopyridine
Pyridoxine (vitamin B_6), 566–567, 595
for ethylene glycol toxicity, 282
Pyuria, 119
in HIV-positive patient, 139

Q

QRS complexes
 in bradycardia, 42
 in supraventricular tachyarrhythmias, 324
Quazepam, 567
Quelicin. *See* Succinylcholine
Questran. *See* Cholestyramine
Quetiapine, 567
Quinaglute. *See* Quinidine
Quinapril, 598*t*
Quincke's sign, 156
Quinidex. *See* Quinidine
Quinidine, 567
 diarrhea caused by, 99
 therapeutic/toxic levels of, 613*t*
Quinupristin/dalfopristin, 500, 567
QVAR. *See* Beclomethasone, oral metered-dose inhaler

R

RA latex test (rheumatoid factor), **378**
Rabeprazole, 611*t*
Racemic epinephrine, for stridor, 344
Racial/familial neutropenia, 256, 257
Radial artery
 arterial line placement and, 390–391
 arterial puncture and, 391
Radiation
 leukopenia and, 256, 257
 thrombocytopenia and, 334
Radiation therapy, emergent, for coma/acute mental status changes in CNS tumor, 82
Radionuclide scans. *See* Nuclear scans
Raloxifene, 567
Ramipril, 598*t*
Ranitidine, 567–568
 for gastritis/esophagitis, 66
RAP. *See* Right artery pressure
Rapamune. *See* Sirolimus
Rapid-acting insulins, 597*t*. *See also* Insulin
Rapid plasma reagin (RPR) test, **387**
 in dizziness/vertigo, 109
Rapid shallow breathing index, ventilator weaning guidelines and, 458
Rapidly progressive glomerulonephritis,
 oliguria/anuria/acute renal failure and, 268
Rash, pruritus and, 296
 medications causing, 299
RBBB. *See* Right bundle branch block
RBC (red blood cell) casts, in urine
 in hematuria, 167, 168
 microscopic appearance of, 385
RBC (red blood cell) count. *See also* Hematocrit
 laboratory reference/normal values for, 354*t*
RBC (red blood cell) indices, 354*t*, **377**
 in anemia, 29–30, 31
RBC (red blood cell) morphology, **377–378**
RBC (red blood cell) transfusions, **437**
RDW (red cell distribution width), 377
 laboratory reference/normal values for, 354*t*
Reactive arthritis, 246
Reactive hypoglycemia, 203
Rebetron. *See* Interferon alfa-2B and ribavirin combination
Rebound insomnia, 234
Recombivax HB. *See* Hepatitis B vaccine
Recreational water activities, diarrhea and, 98
Rectal bleeding
 constipation and, 83
 hematuria and, 168
Rectal examination
 in abdominal pain, 5
 in anemia, 30
 in constipation, 84
 in diarrhea, 101
 Foley catheter problems and, 142
 in hematemesis/melena, 159
 in hematochezia, 164
 in hematuria, 168
 in hypotension, 226
 in jaundice, 243
 in nausea and vomiting, 264
 in pruritus, 300
 in seizures, 311
 in shock, 226
Rectal temperature, 129
Red and black (hot pink) tubes, 622*t*
Red blood cell (RBC) casts, in urine
 in hematuria, 167, 168
 microscopic appearance of, 385
Red blood cell (RBC) count. *See also* Hematocrit
 laboratory reference/normal values for, 354*t*
Red blood cell (RBC) indices, 354*t*, **377**
 in anemia, 29–30, 31
Red blood cell (RBC) mass
 in polycythemia vera, 292, 294
 in pruritus, 302
Red blood cell (RBC) transfusions, **437**
Red blood cells (RBCs)
 morphology of, **377–378**
 in urine, microscopic appearance of, 384
Red cell distribution width (RDW), 377
 laboratory reference/normal values for, 354*t*
Red top tubes, 622*t*
Reducing substance, urine, 385
Reentrant supraventricular tachycardia, 326
Refeeding
 hypophosphatemia and, 221
 metabolic alkalosis and, 22
Referred pain, abdominal, 1
Reflexes, assessment of
 in alcohol withdrawal/delirium tremens, 93
 in coma/acute mental status changes, 79–80, 93
 in hyponatremia, 218
 in pruritus, 300
Refludan. *See* Lepirudin
Reglan. *See* Metoclopramide
Regranex Gel. *See* Becaplermin
Regular Iletin II, 597*t*
Relafen. *See* Nabumetone
Relative polycythemia, 292
 management of, 294
Relaxation therapy, for chronic tension-type headache, 149
Relenza. *See* Zanamivir
Remeron. *See* Mirtazapine
Remicade. *See* Infliximab
Renagel. *See* Sevelamer
Renal artery occlusion, oliguria/anuria/acute renal failure and, 268
Renal biopsy, in oliguria/anuria/acute renal

Renal biopsy, *(cont)*
failure, 271
Renal cancer
hematuria and, 167, 168, 170
polycythemia and, 293
Renal cysts, polycythemia and, 293
Renal disease
hematuria and, 167, 167–168
hypernatremia and, 191
hypertension and, 195
hypocalcemia and, 199
hypoglycemia and, 203
hyponatremia and, 214, 216, 217
polycythemia and, 292
Renal duplex Doppler, in oliguria/anuria/acute renal failure, 271
Renal failure
acidosis and, 13, 17
coma/acute mental status changes and, 75
differential diagnosis/causes of, 267–269
hyperkalemia and, 188
hyponatremia and, 217, 220
management of, 220, 273–274
oliguria/anuria and, 267–269
recovery from, hypercalcemia and, 176
urinary indices in, 386*t*
Renal failure index, 386*t*
Renal function tests
in coagulopathy, 69
in dyspnea, 114
in heart murmur, 156
in seizures, 312
Renal scans, in oliguria/anuria, 271
Renal transplant
hyperkalemia and, 188
polycythemia and, 293
Renal tubular acidosis, 13, 16
hypokalemia and, 208
type I (distal), 208
type II (proximal), 208
Renal tubular disease. *See also* Acute tubular necrosis
hypomagnesemia and, 211
hypophosphatemia and, 221
Renal ultrasound, in oliguria/anuria, 271
Renovascular hypertension, 195
Reopro. *See* Abciximab
Repaglinide, 568
Requip. *See* Ropinirole
Rescriptor. *See* Delavirdine
Rescue breathing, in cardiopulmonary resuscitation, 44
Respiratory acidosis. *See also* Acidosis
characteristics of, 9, 350*t*
compensation in, 11, 350*t*
differential diagnosis/causes of, 11–12
laboratory findings/data in, 16
management of, 18
Respiratory alkalosis. *See also* Alkalosis
characteristics of, 18–20, 350*t*
compensation in, 20, 350*t*
differential diagnosis/causes of, 20–21
hypokalemia and, 206
in hypophosphatemia, 222
imaging/clinical studies in, 23
initial evaluation of, 18–20
laboratory findings/data in, 22
management of, 23
Respiratory disorders. *See* Pulmonary disorders
Respiratory distress, aspiration causing, **36–39**. *See also* Aspiration
Respiratory examination. *See* Lungs, examination of
Respiratory failure
cardiopulmonary arrest and, 45
coma/acute mental status changes and, 75
hypoxemic, mechanical ventilation for, 442
mixed, mechanical ventilation for, 442
in neuromuscular disease, mechanical ventilation for, 442–443
Respiratory inhalants, 468*t*. *See also specific agent and* Bronchodilators
Respiratory rate/pattern. *See also* Tachypnea
in coma/acute mental status changes, 78
in dyspnea, 113
in hemoptysis, 172
in hypophosphatemia, 221
in polycythemia, 293
wheezing and, 341
Restless leg syndrome, insomnia and, 235
Restoril. *See* Temazepam
Restraints, for alcohol withdrawal/delirium tremens, 96
Restrictive pattern, in cough, 88
Retavase. *See* Reteplase
Reteplase, 568
Reticulocyte, definition of, 30
Reticulocyte count, **378**
in anemia, 30, 31, 33
Reticulocytosis, anemia and, 30, 31, 33
Retin-A. *See* Tretinoin (retinoic acid), topical
Retinitis, in HIV-positive patient, 136
management of, 140
13-*cis* Retinoic acid (Isotretinoin), 531, 532
Retinoic acid (tretinoin), topical, 582
Retinopathy, in hyperglycemia, 181
Retrograde pyelogram, in oliguria/anuria, 271
Retrograde urethrogram/cystogram, in hematuria, 169
Retroperitoneal disorders, abdominal pain and, 3*t*
Retrovir. *See* Zidovudine
Reversible obstructive defect, in cough, 88
Revia. *See* Naltrexone
Rewarming, after hypothermia
cardiopulmonary arrest and, 45
techniques for, 233
Reye's encephalopathy, coma/acute mental status changes and, 76
Rhabdomyolysis, phosphate release in, hypocalcemia and, 200
Rheomacrodex. *See* Dextran 40
Rheumatic disease. *See also* Collagen-vascular/connective tissue diseases
pruritus and, 300
workup for, in arthritis, 246, 249–250
Rheumatic fever, arthritis and, 247
Rheumatoid arthritis, 248
juvenile, 248
leukopenia and (Felty's syndrome), 256, 257, 258
Rheumatoid factor
in arthritis, 249
in leukopenia, 258
test for (RA latex test), **378**
Rheumatrex. *See* Methotrexate
Rhinitis

cough and, 87, 89
management of, 89
Rhinocort. *See* Budesonide
Rhinophyma, in alcohol withdrawal/delirium tremens, 93
Rhonchi, in cough, 88
Rhythm strip. *See* Electrocardiogram (ECG)/rhythm strip
Rib fractures, 60
Ribavirin, 568
with interferon-2B, 530
Rifabutin, 568
Rifadin. *See* Rifampin
Rifampin, 568
Rifapentine, 568
Right artery pressure (RAP), pulmonary artery catheter measurement of, 428*t*
Right bundle branch block (RBBB), pulmonary artery catheterization and, 428
Right internal jugular vein, for central venous catheterization, 400–402
Right-to-left shunts
pO_2 in, 370
polycythemia and, 292
Rimantadine, 568–569
Rimexolone, 609*t*
RIMSO 50. *See* Dimethyl sulfoxide
Ringer's solution, lactated, composition of, 435*t*
Rinne test, in dizziness/vertigo, 107
Riopan. *See* Magaldrate
Risedronate, 569
Risperdal. *See* Risperidone
Risperidone, 569
Ritonavir, 569
with lopinavir, 537
Rivastigmine, 569
Rizatriptan, 569
RNA
HCV (hepatitis C virus), 364*t*, 365
nucleolar, antibodies to, 348
RNP antibodies, 348
Robaxin. *See* Methocarbamol
Robitussin. *See* Guaifenesin
Robitussin AC. *See* Guaifenesin, with codeine
Rocaltrol. *See* Calcitriol
Rocephin. *See* Ceftriaxone
Rocuronium, 569–570
Rofecoxib, 606*t*
for arthritis, 250
Roferon-A. *See* Interferon alfa
Rogaine. *See* Minoxidil
Rolaids. *See* Dihydroxyaluminum sodium carbonate
Romazicon. *See* Flumazenil
Romberg test, in dizziness/vertigo, 109
Ropinirole, 570
Rosiglitazone, 183, 570
Rotavirus, diarrhea caused by, 98
Roth spots, 155
Roundworms, pruritus caused by, 299
Roving eye movements, in coma/acute mental status changes, 79
Rowasa. *See* Mesalamine
Roxanol. *See* Morphine
Roxicodone. *See* Oxycodone
RPG. *See* Retrograde pyelogram
RPR (rapid plasma reagin) test, **387**
in dizziness/vertigo, 109
Rubex. *See* Doxorubicin
Rufen. *See* Ibuprofen
Rythmol. *See* Propafenone

S

S_3. *See* Heart sounds
S_4 *See* Heart sounds
Sacroiliac joint, arthritis affecting, 247
SAH. *See* Subarachnoid hemorrhage
Salem sump, 410, 411
Salicylates, 605*t*
metabolic acidosis caused by, 13, 16, 17–18
overdose/toxicity of, 276
respiratory alkalosis caused by, 20, 22, 23
Reye's encephalopathy and, 76
therapeutic/toxic levels of, 613*t*
Saline
composition of, 435*t*
for hypercalcemia, 178
for hyperosmolar/hyperglycemia nonketotic syndrome, 184
hypertonic
hypernatremia and, 192
for hyponatremia, 219
for hyponatremia, 219
Saline enemas, hypertonic, hypernatremia and, 192
Saliva, composition/daily production of, 436*t*
Salmeterol, 570
Salmonella, diarrhea caused by, 98
in HIV infection/AIDS, 100, 137
management of, 103
Salt wasting, cerebral, hyponatremia and, 216
Sandimmune. *See* Cyclosporine
Sandoglobulin. *See* Immune globulin, intravenous
Sandostatin. *See* Octreotide
Saquinavir, 570
Sarafem. *See* Fluoxetine
Sarcoidosis
arthritis and, 248
hypercalcemia and, 176
Sarcoptes scabiei, pruritus caused by, 296, 297, 298
Sargramostim (GM-CSF), 570
leukocytosis and, 251
for leukopenia, 260
Sassafras, toxicity of, 594
Saw palmetto *(Serenoa repens),* 593
Scabies, pruritus in, 296, 298
Scalp
examination of, in headache, 147
pruritus affecting, 296
Schilling's test, in vitamin B_{12} deficiency, 32–33
Schistocytes (helmet cells), 378
Scleroderma
antinuclear antibodies in, 348
arthritis and, 248
chest affected in, respiratory acidosis and, 12
Sclerosing cholangitis-like syndrome, in HIV-positive patient, 137
Scopolamine
for dizziness/vertigo, 110
with hyoscyamine/atropine/phenobarbital, 527
transdermal, 570
Sea water ingestion, hypernatremia and, 192
Secobarbital, 570
Seconal. *See* Secobarbital
Second-degree atrioventricular block, 239–240
Mobitz type I (Wenckebach), 41, 239–240
ECG/rhythm strip in, 42
Mobitz type II, 41, 239–240
ECG/rhythm strip in, 42

Second-degree atrioventricular block, *(cont)*
management of, 241
syncope and, 318
Sectral. *See* Acebutolol
Sedatives, 468*t*. *See also specific agent and* Hypnotic medications
hypercarbia in ventilator patient caused by, 454, 455
hypoxemia in ventilator patient caused by, 451
overdose/toxicity of, 275
Sedimentation test (ESR), **378–379**
in arthritis, 249
in constipation, 84
in diarrhea, 101
in headache, 148
Segmented neutrophils, **387**
laboratory reference/normal values for, 354*t*, 387
Seizures, **308–315**
alcohol withdrawal, 91, 309, 314
differential diagnosis/causes of, 309–310
disorders simulating, 308
emergency management of, 313
falls and, 124
focal, 308, 308*t*
generalized, 308, 308*t*
idiopathic, 308
imaging/clinical studies in, 313
initial evaluation of, 308–309
laboratory findings/data in, 312
management of, 313–315
neurologic examination in, 311–312
non–tonic-clonic, coma/acute mental status changes and, 73, 77
partial, 308, 308*t*
physical examination/findings in, 310–312
psychogenic, 310
symptomatic, 308
syncope and, 316
types of, 308, 308*t*
Selegiline, 570–571
Selenium, 590
Selenium sulfide, 571
Self-induced (factitious) fever, 129
Self-limiting febrile transfusion reaction, 339–340
management of, 341
Selsun Shampoo/Selsun Blue Shampoo. *See* Selenium sulfide
Sengstaken-Blakemore tube, 410
Senna, 85*t*
Senokot. *See* Senna
Sensing failure (pacemaker), 284–285, 284*f*
management of, 287
Sensory examination, in seizures, 312
Sepsis. *See also* Infection
acute renal failure and, 268
central line, 54
coma/acute mental status changes and, 76, 93
delirium and, 93
heart murmur and, 152
hypoglycemia and, 203
hypothermia and, 229–230, 230
jaundice and, 243
metabolic acidosis caused by, 17
oliguria/anuria and, 268
pacemaker complications and, 285
pyelonephritis and, 120
in ventilator patient
agitation and, 449
hypercarbia and, 455
Septic arthritis, 246, 249
management of, 250
Septic shock. *See also* Shock
management of, 228
pulmonary artery catheter monitoring in, 423*t*
Septra. *See* Trimethoprim-sulfamethoxazole
Serax. *See* Oxazepam
Serenoa repens (saw palmetto), 593
Serentil. *See* Mesoridazine
Serevent/Serevent Diskus. *See* Salmeterol
Seroquel. *See* Quetiapine
Serotonin agents, overdose/toxicity of, 276
Sertraline, 571
Serum chemistry. *See* Blood/serum chemistry
Serum gamma-glutamyltransferase (SGGT). *See* Gamma-glutamyltransferase/transpeptidase
Serum glutamic-oxaloacetic transferase (SGOT). *See* AST
Serum glutamic-pyruvic transferase (SGPT). *See* ALT
Serum osmolarity, in overdose, 279
Serum protein electrophoresis (SPEP), **373**, 374*f*, 375*t*
Serum sickness, anaphylaxis and, 25
Serum toxicology screening. *See* Toxicology screening
Serums, 469*t*. *See also specific type*
Serutan. *See* Psyllium
Serzone. *See* Nefazodone
Sevelamer, 571
Sexual protection/contraception, dysuria and, 117
SGGT (serum gamma-glutamyltransferase). *See* Gamma-glutamyltransferase/transpeptidase
SGOT (serum glutamic-oxaloacetic transferase). *See* AST
SGPT (serum glutamic-pyruvic transferase). *See* ALT
Shigella (shigellosis), diarrhea and, 98
management of, 103
Shock, **224–229**
acute renal failure and, 268
anaphylactic, 24, 228–229
in aspiration, 36
cardiogenic, 225, 229
differential diagnosis/causes of, 224–225
hemorrhagic, 224–225
hypovolemic, 224–225, 228
imaging/clinical studies in, 227
initial evaluation of, 224
laboratory findings/data in, 226–227
management of, 227–229
metabolic acidosis and, 17
neurogenic, 225, 228
oliguria/anuria and, 268
physical examination/findings in, 225–226
pulmonary artery catheter monitoring in, 422, 423*t*
septic, 228
vasogenic, 225, 228–229
Short gut syndrome, hypocalcemia and, 199
Shortness of breath. *See* Dyspnea
Shunts, hypoxemia in ventilator patient caused by, 451
Shy-Drager syndrome, syncope and, 317

SIADH. *See* Syndrome of inappropriate antidiuretic hormone secretion
Sibutramine, 571
Sick sinus syndrome, 40
Sickle cell disease
hematuria and, 167, 169
hyperkalemia and, 188
Sickle cell screen, in hematuria, 169
Sickling, red blood cell, 377
Sideroblastic anemia, 29, 29*t*
Sigmoidoscopy, in hematochezia, 164
Signal-averaged electrocardiogram, in syncope, 321
Sildenafil, 571
Silvadene. *See* Silver sulfadiazine
Silver nitrate, 571
Silver sulfadiazine, 572
Simethicone, 572
with aluminum hydroxide and magnesium hydroxide, 475
Simulect. *See* Basiliximab
SIMV (synchronized intermittent mandatory ventilation), 445
for ventilator weaning, 459
Simvastatin, 612*t*
Sinemet. *See* Carbidopa/-levodopa
Sinequan. *See* Doxepin
Single-donor plasma, transfusion of, 439
Singulair. *See* Montelukast
Sinoatrial exit block, 239
Sinoatrial node dysfunction, 40
syncope and, 318
Sinus arrhythmia, 239
Sinus bradycardia, 40. *See also* Bradycardia
dyspnea and, 113
syncope and, 318
Sinus computed tomography
in fever, 131
in headache, 148
Sinus films
in fever, 131
in headache, 148
in leukopenia, 259
Sinus node dysfunction. *See* Sinoatrial node dysfunction
Sinus tachycardia, 324. *See also* Tachycardia
in chest pain, 61
Sinuses, examination of
in cough, 88
in headache, 147
Sinusitis
cough and, 87, 89
headache and, 145
in HIV-positive patient, 136
management of, 89
Sirolimus, 572
Sjögren's syndrome, antinuclear antibodies in, 348
Skelaxin. *See* Metaxalone
Skeletal survey, in hypercalcemia, 178
Skeletal x-rays, in falls, 126
Skin
biopsy of, **430–431**
disorders of
in HIV-positive patient, 137
pruritus and, 296, 297–298
dry (xerosis), pruritus and, 298, 302
examination of
in acidosis, 15
in agitated ventilator patient, 449
in alcohol withdrawal/delirium tremens, 93
in alkalosis, 22
in anaphylaxis, 26
in anemia, 30
in arthritis, 248
in aspiration, 37
in bradycardia, 42
central venous line problems and, 55
in coagulopathy, 69
in coma/acute mental status changes, 79
in diarrhea, 101
in fever, 130
in HIV-positive patient, 138
in heart murmur, 155
in hematemesis/melena, 159
in hematochezia, 163–164
in hematuria, 168
in hemoptysis, 173
high peak pressures in ventilator patient and, 457
in hypercalcemia, 177
in hypernatremia, 193
in hypocalcemia, 200
in hypoglycemia, 204
in hyponatremia, 218
in hypotension, 225
in hypothermia, 231
in hypoxemic ventilator patient, 452
in jaundice, 243
in leukocytosis, 253
in leukopenia, 257–258
in nausea and vomiting, 264
in oliguria/anuria, 269
in overdose, 277
pain management and, 288
in pruritus, 300
in seizures, 311
in shock, 225
in thrombocytopenia, 336
in transfusion reaction, 340
in wheezing, 343
water loss through
hypernatremia and, 191, 192
hyponatremia and, 216
Skin biopsy, in pruritus, 301
Skin test, PPD (purified protein derivative/tuberculin)
in cough, 88
in hemoptysis, 173
Skull films, in hypercalcemia, 178
SLE. *See* Systemic lupus erythematosus
Sleep apnea, polycythemia and, 292
Sleep disorders, insomnia, **234–238**
Sleep latency, prolonged, 235
Sleep pattern, customary, insomnia and, 234–235
Slow-K. *See* Potassium, supplementary
Sm antibodies, 348
Small bowel obstruction. *See also* Intestinal obstruction
nausea and vomiting and, 262
Smoking
cough and, 87
hematemesis/melena and, 158
hemoptysis and, 171
insomnia and, 234, 235
Snake bite, thrombocytopenia and, 335
Sodium
administration of. *See also* Saline
hypernatremia and, 192
in body fluids, 436*t*
daily maintenance requirements for, 435
disorders of balance of. *See also* Hypernatremia; Hyponatremia
coma/acute mental status changes and, 74, 94
delirium and, 94
fractional excreted, in oliguria/anuria/acute renal failure, 270, 386*t*
in hyperglycemia, 182
in hypernatremia

Sodium, *(cont)*
without change in body water, 192, 194
management of, 194
with water loss, 191–192, 194
management of, 194
serum, **379**
in hypernatremia, 193
urine, **379**, 386
in hypokalemia, 209
in oliguria/anuria/acute renal failure, 270, 386*t*
spot, in hypernatremia, 193
Sodium bicarbonate. *See* Bicarbonate therapy
Sodium chloride tablets, hypernatremia and, 192
Sodium citrate, 572
Sodium phosphate, 223, 572
Sodium polystyrene (Kayexalate), 572–573
for hyperkalemia, 190
Sodium Sulfamyd. *See* Sulfacetamide
Solu-Medrol. *See* Methylprednisolone
Soma. *See* Carisoprodol
Somophyllin. *See* Theophylline
Sonata. *See* Zaleplon
Sorbitol, 573
for hyperkalemia, 190
Sorbitrate. *See* Isosorbide dinitrate
Soriatane. *See* Acetretin
Sotalol, 573, 602*t*
for ventricular tachycardia, 49
Sparfloxacin, 573
Specific gravity
pleural fluid, 433*t*
urine, **383**
in oliguria/anuria, 270
Specimen tubes, for venipuncture, 622*t*
Spectazole. *See* Econazole
SPEP. *See* Serum protein electrophoresis
Spermatozoa, in urine, microscopic appearance of, 384
Spermicides, dysuria associated with use of, 117
Spherocytes, 378
Spinal analgesia, 291
Spinal cord transection, hypothermia and, 230
Spinal tap. *See* Lumbar puncture
Spinal trauma, constipation and, 83
Spine, arthritis affecting, 247
Spiral computed tomography, in chest pain, 63
Spironolactone, 573
with hydrochlorothiazide, 525
Spleen
disorders of, abdominal pain and, 3, 3*t*
platelet sequestration in, 335, 336
Spleen scan
in pruritus, 302
in thrombocytopenia, 337
Splenectomy
for idiopathic thrombocytopenic purpura (ITP), 337
leukocytosis and, 252
Splenomegaly
in anemia, 30
platelet sequestration and, 335, 336
in polycythemia vera, 292
Spondyloarthropathies, 247–248
Spontaneous pneumothorax, 59
Sporanox. *See* Itraconazole
Spot urine sodium, in hypernatremia, 193
Sprue
celiac/tropical, diarrhea and, 100
hypocalcemia and, 199
Sputum
analysis of
in aspiration, 38
in cough, 86, 88
in dyspnea, 114
in fever, 131
in hemoptysis, 173
in HIV-positive patient, 139
in hypoxemic ventilator patient, 452
production of
abdominal pain and, 2
cough and, 86
Sputum culture, in dyspnea, 114
SS-A antibodies, 348
SSKI (potassium iodide/Lugol's solution), 563
St. John's wort *(Hypericum perforatum),* 593
St. Joseph Aspirin. *See* Aspirin
Stab (banded) neutrophils, **387**
laboratory reference/normal values for, 354*t*, 387
Stadol. *See* Butorphanol
Staphylococcus, diarrhea caused by, 98
Starvation
hypomagnesemia and, 211
ketoacidosis/ketosis and, 13, 17
leukopenia and, 256, 257
refeeding after
hypophosphatemia and, 221
metabolic alkalosis and, 22
Status asthmaticus, high peak pressures and, 456
Status epilepticus, 314–315
Stavudine, 573
Stelazine. *See* Trifluoperazine
Steroids. *See also* Corticosteroids; Glucocorticoids
17-ketogenic (17-KGS), **367**
17-ketosteroids (17-KS), **367**
exogenous, hypernatremia and, 192
for idiopathic thrombocytopenic purpura (ITP), 337
metabolic alkalosis and, 22
therapeutic
comparison of, 597*t*
ophthalmic, 609*t*
systemic, 573–574
Still's disease, 248
Stimate. *See* Desmopressin
Stimulant use/abuse, insomnia and, 235
Stokes-Adams attacks, syncope caused by, 315
Stool
fat in, testing for in diarrhea, 101
leukocytes/white blood cells in, testing for, **379**
in diarrhea, 102
in HIV-positive patient, 139
occult blood in, testing for, **379**
in anemia, 30
in constipation, 84
in diarrhea, 102
ova and parasites in, testing for
in diarrhea, 102
in HIV-positive patient, 139
in pruritus, 301
volume of in diarrhea, 98
Stool culture, in diarrhea, 102
in HIV-positive patient, 139
Streptase. *See* Streptokinase
Streptokinase, 574
Streptomycin, 574–575
Streptozocin, 575
Stress
acute, hyperglycemia and, 181
leukocytosis and, 251, 252
syndrome of inappropriate antidiuretic hormone secre-

tion (SIADH) and, 217
Stridor, 342. *See also* Wheezing
  anaphylaxis and, 25
  in cough, 88
  management of, 344
  in pruritus, 300
  upper airway obstruction in aspiration and, 37
Stroke. *See* Cerebrovascular accident
Strongyloides stercoralis, pruritus caused by, 299
Subarachnoid hemorrhage
  bloody cerebrospinal fluid and, 418
  headache and, 146
  hypertension and, 196
  syncope and, 318
Subclavian steal syndrome
  dizziness/vertigo and, 106
  syncope and, 318
Subclavian vein, left/right
  for central venous catheterization, 402–405, 403*f*
  kinking of catheter and, 54
  misdirected placement and, 54, 55–56
Subdural hematoma, coma/acute mental status changes and, 73
Subhyaloid hemorrhage, in coma/acute mental status changes, 79
Sublimaze. *See* Fentanyl
Substance abuse. *See also specific drug*
  coma/acute mental status changes and, 74
  jaundice and, 242
  overdose/toxicity and, 276–277
  withdrawal seizures and, 309
Succimer, 575
Succinylcholine, 575
  hyperkalemia and, 187
Sucostrin. *See* Succinylcholine
Sucralfate, 575
Sucrose water test, in leukopenia, 258
Suctioning (airway)
  for agitated ventilator patient, 450, 452
  for high peak pressures, 458
  for hypoxemic ventilator patient, 452
Sudafed. *See* Pseudoephedrine
Sudan stain, positive, pleural fluid, 433*t*
Sufak (docusate calcium). *See* Docusate calcium/potassium/sodium
Sular. *See* Nisoldipine
Sulfacetamide, 608*t*
  with prednisolone, 575, 609*t*
Sulfadiazine (silver sulfadiazine), 572
Sulfasalazine, 576
Sulfinpyrazone, 576
Sulfonylureas, 183, 610*t*
Sulindac, 605*t*
Sumatriptan, 576
  for cluster headache, 150
  for migraine headache, 149–150
Sump tubes (Salem sump), 410, 411
Sumycin. *See* Tetracycline
"Sundowning," 92
Superchar. *See* Charcoal, activated
Supplements, 468–469*t*. *See also specific agent and* Minerals; Natural products; Vitamins
Suppositories, for constipation, 85
Suprapubic pain, oliguria/anuria and, 267
Supraventricular tachyarrhythmia/tachycardia, 324–326
  automatic, 325–326
  dyspnea and, 113
  reentrant, 326
Suprax. *See* Cefixime
Sus-Phrine. *See* Epinephrine
Sustiva. *See* Efavirenz
SvO_2. *See* Mixed venous oxygen saturation
SVR. *See* Systemic vascular resistance
SVT. *See* Supraventricular tachyarrhythmia/tachycardia
Swallow syncope, 317
Swallowing, impaired, aspiration and, 37
Swan-Ganz catheter. *See* Pulmonary artery (Swan-Ganz) catheter
Sweat
  composition/daily production of, 436*t*
  magnesium loss through, hypomagnesemia and, 211
  potassium loss through, hypokalemia and, 206, 207
  sodium loss through
  hypernatremia and, 191
  hyponatremia and, 216
  water loss through
  hypernatremia and, 191
  hyponatremia and, 216
Symmetrel. *See* Amantadine
Sympathomimetic agents
  hypertension and, 195
  overdose/toxicity of, 275
Synchronized intermittent mandatory ventilation (SIMV), 445
  for ventilator weaning, 459
Syncope, **315–323**. *See also* Pre-syncope
  cardiac, 82, 316, 318, 321, 322
  coma/acute mental status changes and, 77, 82
  convulsive, 316
  cough, 317
  definition of, 315
  differential diagnosis/causes of, 317–318
  exertional, 315
  initial evaluation of, 315–317
  laboratory findings/data in, 319–322, 320–321*f*
  management of, 322–323
  micturition, 317, 323
  neural-mediated reflexes and, 317
  pacemaker, 318
  physical examination/findings in, 319
  swallow, 317
  unexplained
  in elderly, 321
  with heart disease/abnormal ECG, 321
  with no coronary artery disease, 321–322
  vasovagal, 315, 316, 317, 322
Syndrome of inappropriate antidiuretic hormone secretion (SIADH)
  coma/acute mental status changes and, 76
  hyponatremia and, 215, 217
  management of, 219–220
Synercid. *See* Dalfopristin/quinupristin
Synovial fluid analysis. *See also* Arthrocentesis
  in arthritis, 248–249
Synthroid. *See* Levothyroxine
Syntocinon. *See* Oxytocin
Syphilis tests
  in dizziness/vertigo, 109
  FTA-ABS test, 361
  RPR test, 387

Syphilis tests, *(cont)*
VDRL test, 387
Syrup of ipecac, 530
Systemic lupus erythematosus (SLE)
antinuclear antibodies in, 348
arthritis and, 246, 248
hemoptysis and, 172
hyperkalemia and, 188
thrombocytopenia and, 335
Systemic vascular resistance (SVR), pulmonary artery catheter measurement of, 428*t*
in shock, 423*t*
Systolic pressure, pulmonary artery catheter measurement of, 428*t*

T

T_3 (triiodothyronine) radioimmunoassay, **380**
T_3 (triiodothyronine) resin uptake, **380**
T_4 (thyroxine)
in coma/acute mental status changes, 80, 94
in delirium, 94
in hypothermia, 231
overproduction of, leukocytosis and, 253
total, **380**
t-PA (alteplase, recombinant), 474
T-piece/T-tube bypass, for ventilator weaning, 458–459
T waves, pacemaker oversensing of, 285
Tabloid. *See* 6-Thioguanine
Tachyarrhythmias. *See also specific type and* Tachycardia
dyspnea and, 113
falls and, 124
supraventricular, 324–326
Tachycardia, **323–333**. *See also specific type and* Supraventricular tachyarrhythmia/tachycardia; Ventricular tachycardia
in abdominal pain, 1
in alcohol withdrawal/delirium tremens, 93
in anaphylaxis, 24
in aspiration, 36
in cardiopulmonary arrest, 47–49, 48–49*f*, 50–51*f*
in chest pain, 61
in coma/acute mental status changes, 78
in diarrhea, 100–101
differential diagnosis/causes of, 324–328
dyspnea and, 113
electrocardiogram/rhythm strip in, 329
falls and, 123, 124, 125
in heart murmur, 153
in hematemesis/melena, 158
in hematochezia, 162
in hyperglycemia, 180
in hypoglycemia, 204
in hypotension, 224
in hypothermia, 232
initial evaluation of, 323
in jaundice, 242
laboratory findings/data in, 328–329
in leukocytosis, 253
management of, 329–332
carotid sinus massage in, 330
electrical cardioversion in, 329–330
medications in, 330–332
pain management and, 288
physical examination/findings in, 328
in shock, 224
sinus, 324
supraventricular, 324–326
syncope and, 316, 318
ventricular, 327
Tachypnea
in acidosis, 9
in alkalosis, 22
in aspiration, 36
in coma/acute mental status changes, 78
in cough, 86, 87
in diarrhea, 100–101
in dizziness, 104
in dyspnea, 113
in falls, 123, 125
in heart murmur, 154
in hyperglycemia, 180
in hyponatremia, 217
in hypotension, 224
in shock, 224
tachycardia and, 323
Tacrine, 576
Tacrolimus (FK 506), 576
therapeutic levels of, 613*t*
Tactile fremitus, in cough, 88
Tagamet. *See* Cimetidine
Talwin. *See* Pentazocine
Tambocor. *See* Flecainide
Tamiflu. *See* Oseltamivir
Tamoxifen, 576–577
Tamponade
cardiopulmonary arrest and, 45
dyspnea and, 112
pulseless electrical activity and, 51
syncope and, 318
Tamsulosin, 577
Tanacetum parthenium (feverfew), 591
Tapazole. *See* Methimazole
Target cells, 378
Targretin. *See* Bexarotene
Tasmar. *See* Tolcapone
Tavist. *See* Clemastine fumarate
Taxol. *See* Paclitaxel
Taxotere. *See* Docetaxel
Tazarotene, 577
Tazicef. *See* Ceftazidime
Tazidime. *See* Ceftazidime
Tazobactam-piperacillin, 600*t*
Tazorac. *See* Tazarotene
TB. *See* Tuberculosis
TBG. *See* Thyroid-binding globulin
TCP. *See* Transcutaneous cardiac pacing
TdT. *See* Terminal dexoynucleotidal transferase
Tears Naturale. *See* Artificial tears
Technetium-labeled bleeding scan
in hematemesis/melena, 160
in hematochezia, 165
Teeth
disease involving, headache and, 146
examination of, in headache, 147
Tegopen. *See* Cloxacillin
Tegretol. *See* Carbamazepine
Telemetry, in dizziness/vertigo, 109
Telmisartan, 599*t*
Temazepam, 577
for insomnia, 237
Temperature. *See* Body temperature
Temperature conversion chart, 618*t*
Temporal arteries, evaluation of, in headache, 147
Temporal arteritis, headache and, 145
Temporary pacemakers. *See also* Pacemaker
for bradycardia, 43
failure to capture and, 283–284, 284*f*, 286

failure to sense and, 284–285, 284*f*, 287
Temporomandibular joint disease, headache and, 146
Tenecteplase (TNKase), 577
Tenex. *See* Guanfacine
Teniposide, 577
Tenormin. *See* Atenolol
Tensilon. *See* Edrophonium
Tension pneumothorax, 59–60. *See also* Pneumothorax
cardiopulmonary arrest and, 45
causes of, 59–60
chest pain and, 59–60, 66
high peak pressures and, 457
management of, 66
pulseless electrical activity and, 51
Tension-type headache, 144
management of, 148–149
Tequin. *See* Gatifloxacin
Terazol 7. *See* Terconazole
Terazosin, 577
Terbinafine, 578
Terbutaline, 578
Terconazole, 578
Terminal dexoynucleotidal transferase, in leukocytosis, 254
Tessalon Perles. *See* Benzonatate
Tetanus immune globulin, 578
Tetanus toxoid, 578
Tetany, of hypocalcemia, 201
specific tests of, 200
Tetracycline, 578
Teveten. *See* Eprosartan
6-TG. *See* 6-Thioguanine
Thalassemia, 29, 29*t*, 31
Thalidomide, 578–579
Thalomid. *See* Thalidomide
THAM (*N* tromethamine), for metabolic acidosis, 17
Theo-Dur. *See* Theophylline
Theolair. *See* Theophylline
Theophylline, 579
therapeutic/toxic levels of, 613*t*
Theracys. *See* Bacillus Calmette-Guérin
Therapeutic drug monitoring, 613*t*
in tachycardia, 329
Thermodilution technique, for cardiac output, 307
Thermoregulatory disorders, fever and, 128
Thiamine (vitamin B_1), 579, 594
for alcohol withdrawal/delirium tremens, 96
for coma/acute mental status changes, 81
deficiency of, Wernicke's encephalopathy caused by, 75, 92
for ethylene glycol toxicity, 282
for seizures, 314
for unconscious patient, 274
Thiazide diuretics
hypercalcemia and, 176
for oliguria/anuria/acute renal failure, 272
Thiazolidinediones, 183
Thiethylperazine, 579
6-Thioguanine (6-TG), 579
Thioplex. *See* Thio-tepa
Thioridazine, 579
Thio-tepa, 579–580
Thiothixene, 580
Third-degree atrioventricular block, 41
cardiopulmonary arrest and, 45
dyspnea and, 113
ECG/rhythm strip in, 42
syncope and, 318
Third heart sound. *See* Heart sounds
Third-space fluid loss
hyponatremia and, 216
hypovolemic shock and, 225
oliguria/anuria/acute renal failure and, 268
Thonzonium, with neomycin and colistin and hydrocortisone, otic, 548–549
Thoracentesis, **431–434**, 432*f*, 433*t*
for dyspnea in pleural effusion, 116
in fever, 131
in hypotension/shock, 227
Thoracic aneurysm, cough and, 87
Thorazine. *See* Chlorpromazine
Thrombasthenia, Glanzmann's, 68
Thrombin time (TT), **380**
in coagulopathy, 70
in thrombocytopenia, 336
in transfusion reaction, 340
Thrombocytopenia, 67, **333–338**
artifactual (pseudothrombocytopenia), 333–334
bleeding time in, 70
chemotherapy-related, management of, 338
differential diagnosis/causes of, 333–335
in hematemesis/melena, 160
hemoptysis and, 172
imaging/clinical studies in, 337
initial evaluation of, 333
laboratory findings/data in, 336–337
management of, 70–71, 337–338
physical examination/findings in, 335–336
Thrombocytopenic purpura
idiopathic (ITP), 67, 334
management of, 71, 337
thrombotic (TTP), 67, 335
management of, 337
Thrombolytic therapy, 463*t*. *See also specific agent*
for myocardial infarction, 65, 157
for pulmonary embolism, 66
Thromboplastin time, partial (PTT). *See* Partial thromboplastin time
Thrombosis
central venous line problems and, 54, 55, 56
hematuria and, 167
oliguria/anuria/acute renal failure and, 268
renal, hematuria and, 167
Thrombotic thrombocytopenia purpura (TTP), 67, 335
management of, 337
Thunderclap headaches, subarachnoid hemorrhage and, 146
Thyro-Block. *See* Potassium iodide
Thyroglobulin, **380–381**
Thyroid/antithyroid agents, 469*t*. *See also specific agent*
Thyroid-binding globulin (TBG), **381**
Thyroid carcinoma, medullary
diarrhea and, 99
hypocalcemia and, 200
Thyroid function tests. *See also specific type*
in bradycardia, 42
in constipation, 84
in delirium, 94
in dizziness/vertigo, 109
in dyspnea, 114
in heart murmur, 156

Thyroid function tests, *(cont)*
in hyponatremia, 218
in insomnia, 236
in pruritus, 301
in respiratory alkalosis, 22
in tachycardia, 329
Thyroid gland disorders. *See also* Hyperthyroidism; Hypothyroidism
coma/acute mental status changes and, 75
Thyroid-stimulating hormone (TSH), **381**
in coma/acute mental status changes, 80, 94
in delirium, 94
in hypothermia, 231
Thyroid storm
fever and, 128, 134
management of, 134
nausea and vomiting and, 263
Thyrotoxicosis. *See also* Hyperthyroidism
coma/acute mental status changes and, 75
Thyroxine (T_4)
in coma/acute mental status changes, 80, 94
in delirium, 94
in hypothermia, 231
overproduction of, leukocytosis and, 253
total, **380**
TIA. *See* Transient ischemic attack
Tiagabine, 580
Tiazac. *See* Diltiazem
TIBC. *See* Total iron binding capacity
Ticar. *See* Ticarcillin
Ticarcillin, 600*t*
Ticarcillin-clavulanate, 600*t*
Tice Bcg. *See* Bacillus Calmette-Guérin
Ticlid. *See* Ticlopidine
Ticlopidine, 580
Tidal breathing, pulsus paradoxus and, 113
Tidal volume, for ventilator patient
adjusting, 447
high peak pressures and, 456, 457
hypercarbia and, 454
setup and, 444
weaning guidelines for, 458
Tigan. *See* Trimethobenzamide
Tikosyn. *See* Dofetilide
Tilade. *See* Nedocromil
Tilt table, head-up, in syncope, 322
Timentin. *See* Ticarcillin-clavulanate
Timolol, 602*t*
ophthalmic, 607*t*
with dorzolamide, 608*t*
Timoptic. *See* Timolol, ophthalmic
Tinactin. *See* Tolnaftate
Tinea, pruritus in, 296, 297, 298
Tinnitus, dizziness and, 105
Tinzaparin, 580
Tioconazole, 580
Tirofiban, 580
for myocardial infarction, 65
Tissue breakdown, hyperkalemia and, 187
TMP-SMX. *See* Trimethoprim-sulfamethoxazole
TNKase. *See* Tenecteplase
Tobacco use
cough and, 87
hematemesis/melena and, 158
hemoptysis and, 171
insomnia and, 234, 235
Tobramycin, 581
dosing guidelines for, 614*t*, 616–617*t*
ophthalmic, 608*t*
therapeutic levels of, 613*t*
Tobrex. *See* Tobramycin, ophthalmic
Todd's paralysis, in seizures, 312
Tofranil. *See* Imipramine
Tolazamide, 610*t*
Tolazoline, 581
Tolbutamide, 610*t*
Tolcapone, 581
Tolectin. *See* Tolmetin
Tolinase. *See* Tolazamide
Tolmetin, 605*t*
Tolnaftate, 581
Tolterodine, 581
Toluene, metabolic acidosis caused by, 13
Tonic-clonic seizures, 308*t*, 309
syncope and, 316
Tonic-clonic status epilepticus, 314–315
Tooth. *See* Teeth
Topamax. *See* Topiramate
Topical decontamination, 281
Topiramate, 581
Topotecan, 582
Toprol XL. *See* Metoprolol
Toradol. *See* Ketorolac
Torecan. *See* Thiethylperazine
Tornalate. *See* Bitolterol
Torsades de pointes, 328
cardiopulmonary arrest and, 44, 49
syncope and, 318
Torsemide, 582
for oliguria/anuria/acute renal failure, 272
Total body water, excess, pseudoanemia and, 28
Total iron binding capacity (TIBC), **367**
in anemia, 29*t*, 31
Total parenteral nutrition (TPN)
abrupt discontinuation of, hypoglycemia and, 203
hypomagnesemia and, 211
jaundice and, 243
Total protein, in hypercalcemia, 178
Total protein-to-albumin ratio, in hypercalcemia, 178
Toxic granulation, white blood cell, 389
Toxicology screening
in coma/acute mental status changes, 80
in dizziness/vertigo, 109
in hypoglycemia, 204
in hypothermia, 232
in overdose, 278
in seizures, 312
Toxins. *See* Drugs/toxins
Toxoids, 469*t*. *See also specific type*
Toxoplasma gondii infection, in HIV-positive patient, management of, 140
t-PA (alteplase, recombinant), 474
T-piece/T-tube bypass, for ventilator weaning, 458–459
TPN. *See* Total parenteral nutrition
Tracheal deviation
in cardiopulmonary arrest, 46
in dyspnea, 113
in hypotension/shock, 225
Tracheal intubation, 444. *See also* Endotracheal tube; Mechanical ventilation
Tracheal tumor, stridor and, 201
Tracheobronchial tree, disorders of, cough and, 87
Tracheostomy, 444
for stridor, 344
Tracrium. *See* Atracurium

Tramadol, 582
Trandate. *See* Labetalol
Trandolapril, 598*t*
Transaminases. *See also* ALT; AST
  in abdominal pain, 6
  pain management and, 289
Transcutaneous cardiac pacing, for bradycardia, 43
Transderm-Nitro. *See* Nitroglycerin
Transderm-Scop. *See* Scopolamine, transdermal
Transducer error, pulmonary artery catheter problems related to, 304
Transferrin, **381**
  serum levels of, in anemia, 31
Transfusion reaction, **338–341**
  contaminated blood and, 340, 341
  hemolytic, 339, 341
  delayed, 340
  oliguria/anuria/acute renal failure and, 268
  self-limiting febrile, 339–340, 341
Transfusions, blood/blood components, **437–441**. *See also specific type and* Transfusion reaction
  alkalosis and, 21
  for anemia, 32, **437–438**
  for coagulopathy, 70
  contaminated, 340, 341
  for disseminated intravascular coagulation (DIC), 71
  fever and, 128
  hypokalemia and, 206
  plasma, **439–440**
  platelet, **438–439**
  red blood cell, **437**
  for von Willebrand's disease, 71
Transient ischemic attack (TIA), syncope and, 317–318
Transudate, pleural, 433*t*
Transvenous pacemakers. *See also* Pacemaker
  complications of, 283–285, 284*f*
Tranxene. *See* Clorazepate
Trastuzumab, 582
Trasylol. *See* Aprotinin
Trauma
  arthritis and, 246
  coma/acute mental status changes and, 73, 73–74
  head. *See* Head trauma
  hematuria and, 167
  rectal examination and, 168
  hemoptysis and, 172
  joint swelling and, 246
  leukocytosis and, 252
  pneumothorax and, 60
  respiratory alkalosis and, 21
  spinal/pelvic, constipation and, 83
Travel history, fever and, 128
Trazodone, 582
  for insomnia, 237
Tremulousness, in alcohol withdrawal/delirium tremens, 93
Trendelenburg position, in hypotension/shock, 227
Trental. *See* Pentoxifylline
Trepopnea, 111
Tretinoin (retinoic acid), topical, 582
Triamcinolone, 597*t*
  inhalation, 582
  with nystatin, topical, 583
Triamterene, 583
  with hydrochlorothiazide, 525
Triazolam, 583
  for insomnia, 237
Trichinella, pruritus caused by, 299
Trichomoniasis (trichomonal vaginitis)
  dysuria and, 118
  management of, 121
Trichuris trichiura, pruritus caused by, 297, 299
Tricor. *See* Fenofibrate
Tricuspid valve dysfunction, pacemaker complications and, 285
Tricyclic antidepressants, overdose/toxicity of, antidote for, 281
Triethanolamine, 583
Trifluoperazine, 583
Trifluridine, 583
Trigeminal neuralgia, headache and, 145
Triglycerides, **381**
  pleural fluid, 433*t*
  sodium levels affected by, 215
Trihexyphenidyl, 583
Triiodothyronine (T_3) radioimmunoassay, **380**
Triiodothyronine (T_3) resin uptake, **380**
Trilafon. *See* Perphenazine
Trileptal. *See* Oxcarbazepine
Trimethobenzamide, 583
Trimethoprim, 584
Trimethoprim-sulfamethoxazole, 584
  hyperkalemia and, 188
Trimetrexate, 584
Trimpex. *See* Trimethoprim
N Tromethamine (THAM), for metabolic acidosis, 17
Tropical sprue, diarrhea and, 100
Troponin I, **382**
  in chest pain evaluation, 62
  in hypotension/shock, 226
Troponin T, **382**
  in hypotension/shock, 226
Trousseau's sign, 200
  delirium and, 93
  in hypocalcemia, 200
  in hypomagnesemia, 212
Trovafloxacin, 584
Trovan. *See* Trovafloxacin
Trunk, pruritus affecting, 296
Trusopt. *See* Dorzolamide
Tryptase, **382**
  serum levels of, in anaphylaxis, 26
TSH. *See* Thyroid-stimulating hormone
TT. *See* Thrombin time
TTP. *See* Thrombotic thrombocytopenia purpura
T-tube/T-piece bypass, for ventilator weaning, 458–459
Tube feedings, aspiration prevention and, 38
Tuberculin skin test (PPD skin test)
  in cough, 88
  in hemoptysis, 173
Tuberculosis
  hematuria and, 167, 170
  hemoptysis and, 171
  in HIV-positive patient, 136, 140
  management of, 140, 170
Tuberculous meningitis, cerebrospinal fluid findings in, 419*t*
Tubular necrosis, acute
  dopamine for, 273
  hypernatremia and, 191
  oliguria/anuria/acute renal failure and, 268, 273
  urinary indices in, 386*t*
Tumor lysis
  oliguria/anuria/acute renal failure and, 268
  phosphate release by, hypocalcemia and, 200
Tumor markers, in leukocytosis, 254

Tumor plop, 155
Tumors. *See also specific type and* Cancer
arthritis and, 247
coma/acute mental status changes and, 73, 76, 82
constipation and, 83
diarrhea and, 99
dizziness/vertigo and, 106
fever and, 128
hematuria and, 170
hemoptysis and, 171
hypoglycemia and, 204
joint swelling and, 247
leukocytosis and, 252
nausea and vomiting and, 263
pain caused by, 288
respiratory alkalosis and, 21
stridor and, 201
wheezing and, 342
Tums. *See* Calcium carbonate
Tylenol. *See* Acetaminophen
Tylenol Nos. 1-4. *See* Acetaminophen, with codeine
Tylox. *See* Oxycodone, with acetaminophen
Tympanic membrane, examination of, in dizziness/vertigo, 107
Type and cross-match
for coagulopathy, 70
in hematemesis/melena, 160
in hematochezia, 164
for hypotension, 226
for shock, 226

U

UC. *See* Ulcerative colitis
Ulcerative colitis
diarrhea and, 99
hematochezia and, 163
Ulcers. *See* Peptic ulcer disease
Ultracef. *See* Cefadroxil
Ultralente insulin, 597*t*. *See also* Insulin
Ultram. *See* Tramadol
Ultrase. *See* Pancreatin/pancrelipase
Ultrasound
in abdominal pain, 7
central venous line problems and, 55
in fever, 131
Foley catheter problems and, 143
in jaundice, 244
in nausea and vomiting, 265
oliguria/anuria and, 271
Unasyn. *See* Ampicillin-sulbactam
Unipen. *See* Nafcillin
Univasc. *See* Moexipril
Unsafe herbs, 470*t*
UPEP. *See* Urine protein electrophoresis
Upper airway obstruction. *See also* Airway obstruction
anaphylaxis and, 25
aspiration and, 37
respiratory acidosis and, 12
Upper GI endoscopy
in hematemesis/melena, 160
in hematochezia, 164
Upper GI series, with small bowel follow-through, in diarrhea, 102
Upper respiratory procedures, endocarditis prophylaxis for, 621*t*
Urate crystals, in gout, 249
Urea, hypernatremia and, 191
Urea nitrogen. *See* Blood urea nitrogen
Urecholine. *See* Bethanechol
Uremia
hemoptysis and, 172
hypothermia and, 230
nausea and vomiting and, 263
pericarditis and, 58
platelet function affected by, 68
pruritus and, 299, 302
Ureteral obstruction
management of, 273
oliguria/anuria/acute renal failure and, 269, 273
Ureterosigmoidostomy, hypokalemia and, 208
Urethral discharge, gram-stain/culture of, in dysuria, 119–120
Urethral meatus, examination of, in hematuria, 168
Urethral obstruction, oliguria/anuria/acute renal failure and, 269
Urethral syndrome
dysuria in women and, 118, 122
management of, 122
Urethritis, 117, 118
dysuria and, 117, 121–122
in men, 118
in women, 118
hematuria and, 168
management of, 121–122
Urethrogram, retrograde, in hematuria, 169
Urex. *See* Methenamine
Uric acid, **382**
in hypophosphatemia, 222
oliguria/anuria/acute renal failure and, 268
in pruritus, 301
Urinalysis, **382–385**
in abdominal pain, 6
in arthritis, 249
in dysuria, 119
in falls, 126
in fever, 131
in HIV-positive patient, 139
in hematuria, 168
in hemoptysis, 173
in hypercalcemia, 178
in hypertension, 197
in hypoglycemia, 204
in nausea and vomiting, 264
in oliguria/anuria, 270
routine, **382–385**
Urinary casts
in hematuria, 167, 168
microscopic appearance of, 385
Urinary (bladder) catheterization, **394–397**. *See also* Foley catheter
dysuria after catheter removal and, 117
hematuria and, 166
in oliguria/anuria, 271–272
problems with catheter and, **141–143**
Urinary cyclic AMP, in hypocalcemia, 200
Urinary cytology, in hematuria, 169
Urinary indices, **386**, 386*t*
Urinary stones
Foley catheter problems and, 142
hematuria and, 168, 169–170
management of, 169–170
Urinary tract, disorders of, abdominal pain and, 3, 3*t*
Urinary tract agents, 469*t*. *See also specific agent*
Urinary tract infection
dysuria and, 117, 121
in men, 118
in women, 117–118
hematuria and, 166, 168, 169
management of, 121, 169
Urine
alkalinization of
in overdose management, 282
for salicylate intoxication, 17–18

bloody, **383**. *See also* Hematuria
Foley catheter problems and, 141, 141–142
for drug screen. *See* Toxicology screening
examination of. *See* Urinalysis
ketones in, in hyperglycemia, 182
specific gravity of, **383**
in oliguria/anuria, 270
tea-colored, leukopenia and, 256
Urine culture
in arthritis, 249
in coma/acute mental status changes, 80
in dysuria, 119
in fever, 131
in hematuria, 169
in leukopenia, 258
Urine microscopy, **384–385**
Urine osmolality, **370**
in acute renal failure/oliguria, 386*t*
in hypernatremia, 193
Urine output
changes in, hematuria and, 166
Foley catheter problems and, 141
in hyperkalemia, 186
in oliguria/anuria, 266. *See also* Oliguria
monitoring, 273
Urine protein electrophoresis (UPEP), **373**, 374*f*
Urine sediment, Foley catheter problems and, 142
Urine sodium, spot, in hypernatremia, 193
Urine toxicology screening. *See* Toxicology screening
Urispas. *See* Flavoxate
Urobilinogen, 385
Urocit-K. *See* Potassium citrate
Urokinase, 584
Urolithiasis
Foley catheter problems and, 142
hematuria and, 168, 169–170
management of, 169–170
Urologic disorders
dysuria and, 117
hematuria and, 167
Urticaria
anaphylaxis and, 25
pruritus in, 296, 298
in wheezing, 343
US. *See* Ultrasound
Uterine leiomyomas, polycythemia and, 292
UTI. *See* Urinary tract infection

V

$\dot{V}/\dot{Q}$ scan. *See* Ventilation-perfusion ($\dot{V}/\dot{Q}$) scan
Vaccines, 469*t*. *See also specific type*
Vagal response disorders, falls and, 124
Vaginal bleeding, hematuria and, 168
Vaginal discharge, in dysuria, 120
Vaginitis
dysuria in women and, 117, 118, 121
management of, 121
Vagistat. *See* Tioconazole
Valacyclovir, 584
Valerian *(Valeriana officinalis)*, 593
Valium. *See* Diazepam
Valproic acid, 585
for seizures, 314
therapeutic/toxic levels of, 613*t*
Valrubicin, 585
Valsalva maneuver, syncope and, 317
Valsartan, 599*t*
with hydrochlorothiazide, 599*t*
Valstar. *See* Valrubicin
Valtrex. *See* Valacyclovir
Valvular heart disease
dyspnea and, 113
fever and, 128
murmur in, 151, 152–153
Vancenase nasal inhaler. *See* Beclomethasone, nasal inhaler
Vanceril inhaler. *See* Beclomethasone, oral metered-dose inhaler
Vancocin. *See* Vancomycin
Vancoled. *See* Vancomycin
Vancomycin, 585
for *Clostridium difficile* diarrhea, 103
for endocarditis prophylaxis, 621*t*
therapeutic levels of, 613*t*
Vanillylmandelic acid (VMA), urine, **386–387**
Vantin. *See* Cefpodoxime
Vaqta. *See* Hepatitis A vaccine
Varicella virus vaccine, 585
Varices, esophageal
hematemesis/melena and, 158, 159, 161
management of, 161
Sengstaken-Blakemore tube for, 410
Varivax. *See* Varicella virus vaccine
Vascor. *See* Bepridil
Vascular disorders, abdominal pain and, 3, 3*t*
Vasculitis, arthritis and, 248
Vasodilation, syncope and, 317
Vasogenic shock, 225. *See also* Shock
management of, 228–229
Vasopressin, 585. *See also* Antidiuretic hormone
deamino-8-D-arginine (DDAVP), for von Willebrand's disease, 71
in hypernatremia, 193
for ventricular fibrillation, 47
Vasopressors
for anaphylaxis, 27
for hypovolemic shock, 228
Vasotec. *See* Enalapril
Vasovagal reaction, pre-syncope and, 106
Vasovagal syncope, 315, 316, 317
management of, 322
symptoms prior to, 316
VDRL (Venereal Disease Research Laboratory) test, **387**
in dizziness/vertigo, 109
$\dot{V}_e$. *See* Minute ventilation
Vecuronium, 585–586
Veetids. *See* Penicillin V
Velban. *See* Vinblastine
Velbe. *See* Vinblastine
Velosef. *See* Cephradine
Venipuncture, specimen tubes for, 622*t*
Venlafaxine, 586
Veno-caval filter, for pulmonary embolism, 65
Venofer. *See* Iron sucrose
Venogram, nuclear, in central venous line problems, 55
Venography, in central venous line problems, 55
Venous access, cannulation/catheterization for, 411–412, 413*f*, 414*f*
in hypotension/shock, 227
Venous blood gases, 350*t*, **351**
Venous line, central. *See* Central venous catheterization
Venous oxygen saturation, mixed (SvO_2), pulmonary

Venous oxygen saturation, *(cont)*
artery catheter measurement of, 428*t*
in hypoxemic ventilator patient, 452
in shock, 423*t*
Venous thrombosis
central line problems and, 54, 55, 56
pacemaker complications and, 285
Ventilation, inadequate. *See* Hypoventilation
Ventilation-perfusion abnormalities
hypoxemia in ventilator patient caused by, 451, 452
pO_2 in, 370
Ventilation/perfusion ($\dot{V}/\dot{Q}$) scan
in chest pain, 63
in cough, 88
in dyspnea, 115
in hemoptysis, 173
in hypotension/shock, 227
Ventilator management, **442–460**. *See also* Mechanical ventilation
high peak pressures and, **456–458**
hypercarbia and, **454–455**
hypoxemia and, **450–454**
indications/setup and, **442–447**
routine modification of settings and, **447–448**
troubleshooting agitation and, **448–450**
weaning and, **458–460**
Ventilator settings
initial, 446
reviewing/adjusting
in agitated patient, 448, 450
high peak pressures and, 456
in hypercarbic patient, 455
in hypoxemic patient, 451, 453
routine, **447–448**
Ventilatory failure, mechanical ventilation for, 442
Ventolin. *See* Albuterol
Ventricular arrhythmias, 327–328. *See also specific type*
cardiopulmonary arrest and, 45
in hyperkalemia, 186, 189
Ventricular ectopy, pacemaker complications and, 285
Ventricular fibrillation, 327–328
in hypothermia, 232
management of, 46–47, 48–49*f*
Ventricular pressure, abnormalities of, pulmonary artery catheter measurements in, 429*t*
Ventricular septal defect (VSD)
heart murmur in, 152, 153, 155
hypoxemia in ventilator patient caused by, 451
Ventricular tachycardia, 327. *See also* Tachycardia
in chest pain, 61
dyspnea and, 113
with pulse, management of, 47–49
stable monomorphic with decreased ejection fraction, 47
stable monomorphic with normal ejection fraction, 47–49
stable polymorphic, 49
unstable, 49
pulseless, management of, 47, 48–49*f*
syncope and, 318
Ventricular wall rupture, heart murmur and, 152
VePesid. *See* Etoposide
Verapamil, 586
for tachycardia, 332
Versed. *See* Midazolam
Vertebral artery dissection, headache and, 147
Vertigo, 105–106
benign positional, 105, 105–106
management of, 109–110
onset and duration of, 105
Vestibular disorders
central, 106, 109
falls and, 124
peripheral, 105–106, 109–110
Vestibular neuronitis, 106
Vestibular rehabilitation, for dizziness/vertigo, 110
Vexol. *See* Rimexolone
VF. *See* Ventricular fibrillation
Viagra. *See* Sildenafil
Vibramycin. *See* Doxycycline
Vibrio, diarrhea caused by, 98
Vicodin. *See* Hydrocodone, with acetaminophen
Vicoprofen. *See* Hydrocodone, with ibuprofen
Videx. *See* Didanosine
Villous adenoma, diarrhea and, 99
Vinblastine, 586
Vincasar PFS. *See* Vincristine
Vincristine, 586
Vinorelbine, 586–587
Vioxx. *See* Rofecoxib
Viracept. *See* Nelfinavir
Viral infection. *See also* Infection
diarrhea and, 98
leukopenia and, 255
meningitis, cerebrospinal fluid findings in, 419*t*
thrombocytopenia and, 333, 334, 335
Viramine. *See* Nevirapine
Virazole. *See* Ribavirin
Viroptic. *See* Trifluridine
Visceral pain, 1
Viscus
cancer pain and, 288
perforation of
abdominal pain and, 2–3, 5*t*
nausea and vomiting and, 262
Visicol. *See* Sodium phosphate
Visken. *See* Pindolol
Vistaril. *See* Hydroxyzine
Vistide. *See* Cidofovir
Visual field defects, seizures and, 312
Visual input, altered, disequilibrium and, 107
Vital capacity, ventilator weaning guidelines for, 458
Vital signs
in abdominal pain, 1, 4
in acidosis, 9, 15
in agitated ventilator patient, 449
in alcohol withdrawal/delirium tremens, 90, 93
in alkalosis, 19, 22
in anaphylaxis, 24, 25
in anemia, 28, 30
in aspiration, 36
in bradycardia, 39, 41
central venous line malfunction and, 54
in chest pain, 61
in coagulopathy, 68–69
in coma, 72, 77–78
in constipation, 84
in cough, 87
in diarrhea, 97, 100–101
in dizziness, 104
in dyspnea, 113
in dysuria, 119
in falls, 123, 125
in fever, 129–130

in HIV-positive patient, 138
Foley catheter problems and, 142
in headache, 144
in heart murmur, 153–154
in hematemesis, 158, 159
in hematochezia, 162, 163
in hemoptysis, 172
high peak pressures in ventilator patient and, 457
in hypercalcemia, 177
in hypercarbic ventilator patient, 455
in hyperglycemia, 180, 181
in hyperkalemia, 186
in hypernatremia, 192–193
in hypertension, 196
in hypoglycemia, 202, 204
in hypokalemia, 206
in hypomagnesemia, 210, 211–212
in hyponatremia, 217
in hypophosphatemia, 221
in hypotension, 224, 225
in hypothermia, 231
in hypoxemic ventilator patient, 452
irregular pulse and, 238, 240
in jaundice, 242, 243
in leukocytosis, 253
in leukopenia, 257
in melena, 158, 159
in mental status changes, 72, 77–78
in nausea and vomiting, 261, 263–264
in oliguria/anuria, 269
in overdose, 274–275, 277
pacemaker complications and, 283, 285
pain management and, 288
in polycythemia, 293
pulmonary artery catheter problems and, 305
in seizures, 310–311
in shock, 224, 225
in syncope, 316, 319
in tachycardia, 323, 328
in thrombocytopenia, 336
in transfusion reaction, 338–339, 340
in wheezing, 341, 343
Vitamin A, 594
Vitamin A intoxication, hypercalcemia and, 176
Vitamin B_1 (thiamine), 579, 594
for alcohol withdrawal/delirium tremens, 96
for coma/acute mental status changes, 81
deficiency of, Wernicke's encephalopathy caused by, 75, 92
for ethylene glycol toxicity, 282
for seizures, 314
for unconscious patient, 274
Vitamin B_3 (niacin), 549–550
deficiency of, coma/acute mental status changes and, 75–76
Vitamin B_6 (pyridoxine), 566–567, 595
for ethylene glycol toxicity, 282
Vitamin B_{12}, **349**, 595
deficiency of, 29–30, 31, 32–33, 349
coma/acute mental status changes and, 75
in leukocytosis, 254
in leukopenia, 258
in polycythemia vera, 292, 294
supplementary, 498, 595
Vitamin C (ascorbic acid), 595
Vitamin D, 595
in hypocalcemia, 199, 200
management of deficiency and, 201
hypophosphatemia and, 221
supplementary, hypomagnesemia and, 211
Vitamin D intoxication, hypercalcemia and, 176
Vitamin D_2 (ergocalciferol), for hypocalcemia, 201
Vitamin D_2 analogue (dihydrotachysterol), for hypocalcemia, 201
Vitamin D_3 (cholecalciferol), 493
Vitamin E, 595–596
Vitamin K, 596
deficiency of
bleeding and, 68
management of, 72
supplementary, 561
for vitamin K deficiency/liver disease, 72
Vitamin K-dependent factor concentrates, transfusion of, 72, 440
Vitamins, 470*t*, **594–596**. *See also specific type*
deficiency of, coma/acute mental status changes and, 75–76
supplementary, for alcohol withdrawal/delirium tremens, 96
Vitrasert. *See* Ganciclovir
Vitravene. *See* Fomivirsen
Vivonex tube, 410
VM-26. *See* Teniposide
VMA. *See* Vanillylmandelic acid
vO_2. *See* Mixed venous oxygen saturation
$\dot{V}O_2$. *See* Oxygen consumption
Vocal cord dysfunction, stridor and, 342
Voltaren. *See* Diclofenac
Volume challenge, in oliguria/anuria, 272
Volume resuscitation. *See also* Fluid management
in hematemesis/melena, 161
in hematochezia, 165
Volume status
constipation and, 83
falls and, 124
in hyperglycemia, 181
in hyponatremia, 214
management of. *See also* Fluid management
in hypoxemic ventilator patient, 453
Vomiting, 261–266. *See also* Nausea and vomiting
blood. *See* Hematemesis
Vomitus, appearance/volume of, 261–262
von Willebrand's disease, 67, 71
bleeding time in, 70
management of, 71
VP-16. *See* Etoposide
$\dot{V}/\dot{Q}$ scan. *See* Ventilation-perfusion ($\dot{V}/\dot{Q}$) scan
VSD. *See* Ventricular septal defect
VT. *See* Ventricular tachycardia
Vumon. *See* Teniposide
vWD. *See* von Willebrand's disease

W

Wandering spleen syndrome, abdominal pain and, 4
Warfarin, 587
Warning headache, before subarachnoid bleed, 146
Washed red blood cells (RBCs), transfusion of, 438
Water deprivation/vasopressin test, in hypernatremia, 193
Water-hammer pulse, 154

Water intoxication, hyponatremia and (hypotonic hyponatremia), 216
Water loss, in hypernatremia
with sodium loss, 191–192, 194
management of, 194
without sodium loss, 192, 194
management of, 194
Waxy casts, in urine, microscopic appearance of, 385
WBC (white blood cell) count. *See also* Leukocytosis; Leukopenia
high peak pressures in ventilator patient and, 457
in hypercarbic ventilator patient, 455
in hyperkalemia, 189
in hypophosphatemia, 222
laboratory reference/normal values for, 354*t*
pleural fluid, 433*t*
in polycythemia, 294
WBC (white blood cell) differential. *See* Differential count
WBC (white blood cell) morphology, **389**
Weaning, ventilator, **458–460**
Weber test, in dizziness/vertigo, 107
Wedge pressure, pulmonary (PWP), pulmonary artery catheter measurement of
abnormalities and, 429*t*
in shock, 423*t*
Wegener's granulomatosis, hemoptysis and, 172
Weight conversion chart (pounds/kilograms), 619*t*
Weight loss
in HIV-positive patient, fever and, 135
hyponatremia and, 215
for type 2 diabetes, 180
Welchol. *See* Colesevelam
Wellbutrin. *See* Bupropion
Wellcovorin. *See* Leucovorin
Wenckebach second-degree AV block (Mobitz type I), 41, 239–240
ECG/rhythm strip in, 42
Wernicke's encephalopathy, 92
coma/acute mental status changes and, 75, 92
hypothermia and, 230–231
Westergren scale, for sedimentation test, 378
in arthritis, 249
Westerman needle, for bone marrow aspiration and biopsy, 397
Western blot assay, for HIV antibody, 366
Wheezing, **341–344**. *See also* Bronchospasm; Stridor
anaphylaxis and, 25
in chest pain, 61
in cough, 88
diffuse, 342
localized, 342
in pruritus, 300
Whipple's disease, diarrhea and, 100
Whipworm *(Trichuris trichiura)*, pruritus caused by, 299
White blood cell (WBC) count. *See also* Leukocytosis; Leukopenia
high peak pressures in ventilator patient and, 457
in hypercarbic ventilator patient, 455
in hyperkalemia, 189
in hypophosphatemia, 222
laboratory reference/normal values for, 354*t*
pleural fluid, 433*t*
in polycythemia, 294
White blood cell (WBC) differential. *See* Differential count
White blood cells (WBCs)
morphology of, **389**
in stool, **379**
in diarrhea, 102
in HIV-positive patient, 139
in urine
hematuria and, 168
microscopic appearance of, 384
Whole blood, transfusion of, 437
Wintrobe scale, for sedimentation test, 378
Withdrawal syndromes. *See also specific type*
alcohol
major, **90–97**
minor, 91
barbiturate, 91
opioid, 91
seizures and, 91, 309, 314
Wolff-Parkinson-White syndrome (atrioventricular reciprocating tachycardia), 326
management of, 332
syncope and, 318
Wood's ultraviolet light, in pruritus, 301
WPW syndrome. *See* Wolff-Parkinson-White syndrome
Wrist, arthrocentesis of, 393–394, 395*f*
Wycillin. *See* Penicillin G, procaine

X

Xalatan. *See* Latanoprost
Xanax. *See* Alprazolam
Xeloda. *See* Capecitabine
Xenical. *See* Orlistat
Xerosis (dry skin), pruritus and, 298, 302
Xopenex. *See* Levalbuterol
Xylocaine. *See* Lidocaine
D-Xylose test, in diarrhea, 102

Y

Yeasts, in urine, microscopic appearance of, 384
Yellow top tubes, 622*t*
Yersinia, diarrhea caused by, 98
Yohimbine *(Pausinystalia yohimbe)*, 593
toxicity of, 594

Z

Zaditor. *See* Ketotifen
Zafirlukast, 587
Zagam. *See* Sparfloxacin
Zalcitabine, 587
fever caused by, 136
Zaleplon, 587–588
for insomnia, 237
Zanamivir, 588
Zanosar. *See* Streptozocin
Zantac. *See* Ranitidine
Zarontin. *See* Ethosuximide
Zaroxolyn. *See* Metolazone
Zebeta. *See* Bisoprolol
Zefazone. *See* Cefmetazole
Zemuron. *See* Rocuronium
Zenapax. *See* Daclizumab
Zerit. *See* Stavudine
Zestril. *See* Lisinopril
ZETA scale, for sedimentation test, 378
Ziagen. *See* Abacavir
Ziditor. *See* Ketotifen
Zidovudine (AZT), 588
fever caused by, 136
with lamivudine, 588
Zileuton, 588
Zinacef. *See* Cefuroxime

Zinc, **389**, 590
Zinecard. *See* Dexrazoxane
Zingiber officinale (ginger), 591–592
Zithromax. *See* Azithromycin
Zocor. *See* Simvastatin
Zofran. *See* Ondansetron
Zoladex. *See* Goserelin
Zolmitriptan, 588
for migraine headache, 150
Zoloft. *See* Sertraline
Zolpidem, 588
for insomnia, 237
Zomig. *See* Zolmitriptan
Zonalon. *See* Doxepin, topical
Zonegran. *See* Zonisamide
Zonisamide, 588
Zostrix. *See* Capsaicin
Zosyn. *See* Piperacillin-tazobactam
Zovirax. *See* Acyclovir
Zyban. *See* Bupropion
Zyflo. *See* Zileuton
Zyloprim. *See* Allopurinol
Zyprexa. *See* Olanzapine
Zyrtec. *See* Cetirizine
Zyvox. *See* Linezolid